THE
ULTIMATE MEDICAL
ENCYCLOPEDIA

THE
ULTIMATE MEDICAL
ENCYCLOPEDIA

Understanding, Preventing, and Treating Medical Conditions

FIREFLY BOOKS

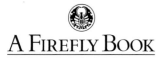

A FIREFLY BOOK

Published by Firefly Books Ltd. 2010

First printing

Publisher Cataloging-in-Publication Data (U.S.)

The ultimate medical encyclopedia : understanding, preventing, and treating medical conditions / collective work of some 300 physicians, medical specialists and university professors.
[602] p. : col. ill., col. photos. ; cm.
Includes index.
Summary: Illustrations and explanations addressing general family health and well-being, with topics such as: pregnancy, child growth, nutrition, physical exercise and aging.
ISBN-13: 978-1-55407-731-1
ISBN-10: 1-55407-731-1
1. Medicine, Popular—Encyclopedias. I. Title.
616/.02 dc22   RC81.A2.F3 2010

Published in the United States by
Firefly Books (U.S.) Inc.
P.O. Box 1338, Ellicott Station
Buffalo, New York 14205

Printed and bound in Singapore

10 9 8 7 6 5 4 3 2 1   14 13 12 11 10
432, Version 1.0

The publisher gratefully acknowledges the financial support for our publishing program by the Government of Canada through the Canada Book Fund as administered by the Department of Canadian Heritage.

The Ultimate Medical Encyclopedia was created and designed by
QA International
329, rue de la Commune Ouest, 3ʳᵈ floor
Montreal (Quebec) H2Y 2E1 Canada
T: 514.499.3000 F: 514.499.3010
www.qa-international.com

EDITORIAL DIRECTOR
Martine Podesto

EDITORS-IN-CHIEF
Marie-Anne Legault
Stéphane Batigne

EDITORIAL STAFF
Mathieu Burgard
Myriam Caron Belzile
Julie Cailliau
Ophélie Delaunay
Claire de Guillebon
Christine Leroy
Jean-François Noulin
Aurélie Olivier
Olivier Peyronnet
Rose-Hélène Philippot

PRINT DESIGN
Mélanie Giguère-Gilbert

GRAPHIC DESIGN
Johanne Plante

LAYOUT
Julien Brisebois
Émilie Corriveau
Pascal Goyette
Caroline Grégoire
François Hénault
Cécile Lalonde
Karine Lévesque
Danielle Quinty
Shadia Toumani

ILLUSTRATION
Danielle Bader
Manuela Bertoni
Jocelyn Gardner
Mélanie Giguère-Gilbert
Alain Lemire
Raymond Martin
Émilie McMahon
Anouk Noël
Under the direction of
Sylvain Bélanger, medical illustration specialist

PHOTOGRAPHIC RESEARCH
Olivier Delorme
Gilles Vézina

IT MANAGER
Martin Lemieux

PROGRAMMING
Éric Gagnon
Gabriel Trudeau-St-Hilaire

PROJECT MANAGEMENT
Nathalie Fréchette
Véronique Loranger

TRANSLATION
TransPerfect

COPYEDITING
Veronica Schami Editorial Services

INDEX
François Trahan

PRINT MANAGEMENT
Salvatore Parisi

ACKNOWLEDGMENTS

This work is the work of a team of experienced and passionate medical illustrators, graphic artists and editors. It was developed based on the needs of the general public from an initial work validated by almost 300 professionals in the field of health, specialists in cardiology, oncology, genetics, obstetrics, pediatrics, immunology, neurology, surgery, urology, nutrition, psychology, rheumatology, toxicology, pneumology, hepatology, orthopedics, traumatology, gastroenterology, opthalmology and other life sciences. We would like to thank these doctors, professors and researchers affiliated with North American and European institutions.

Very special recognition is given to Dr. Éric Philippe, professor at the University of Laval Medical School, who reviewed *The Ultimate Medical Encyclopedia* and who made sure that we had presented with rigor and clarity the different systems and parts of the human body, as well as the diseases which may affect it and the treatments that they require. His assistance as well as that of the other technical reviewers were essential in order to make this book a basic reference for the whole family.

CONTRIBUTORS

QA International thanks the following people for their contribution to this work:

Émilie Bellemare, Dr. Vincent Bernier, Pascal Bilodeau, Sonia Charette, Mathieu Douville, François Fortin, Véronique Gosselin, Dr. Claude Lamarche, Pascal Laniel, Samuel Larochelle, Benoit Nantais, Josée Noiseux, Odile Perpillou, Serge Robert, Anne Rouleau, Sylvain Simard, Kien Tang and Anne Tremblay.

SCIENTIFIC REVIEW OF THIS EDITION

Principal Reviewer: Dr. Éric Philippe, PhD

St. John Ambulance (*First Aid*)
Extenso - Nutrition Reference Center of the University of Montréal, www.extenso.org (*The Digestive System — The Health of the Digestive System; Childhood and Adolescence — Diet diversification; Prevention — Nutrition*)
Dr. Isabelle Arsenault (*The Reproductive System — Sexually Transmitted Infections*)
Christina Blais, M.Sc., professional dietitian (*The Senses — Smell, Taste*)
Dr. Pierre Blondeau (*The Senses — Eye Diseases*)
Dr. Olivier Deguine (*The Senses — Balance Disturbances*)
Dr. Louis-Gilles Durand (*The Cardiovascular System*)
Dr. Daniel Grenier (*The Digestive System— Oral Diseases, Cavities*)
Dr. Sylvain Ladouceur (*Directory of Symptoms*)
Dr. Bernard Lambert (*The Reproductive System — Diseases Affecting Women*)
Dr. Robert Patenaude (*Directory of Symptoms*)
Dr. Claude Poirier (*The Respiratory System*)
Dr. Claude Rouillard (*The Nervous System — Drug Addiction*)
Dr. Julio Soto (*The Immune System — p.292 to 301, 380, 381*)
Dr. Julie Thibault (*Directory of Symptoms*)
Dr. Catherine Vincent (*The Digestive System — Hepatitis*)

LANGUAGE REVIEW

Claude Frappier

DISCLAIMER

HOW TO USE THIS BOOK

The *Ultimate Medical Encyclopedia* is divided into 20 themes which most often correspond to a mechanism or system in the human body. The themes are divided into sub-themes, then into subjects that describe the anatomy, functioning and diseases associated with a group of organs. The contents of the encyclopedia can be accessed in several ways:

- from the table of contents, which presents the detailed outline of the work;
- from the index, which lists the work's keywords and makes it possible to quickly find the information required on a particular subject;
- from the directory of symptoms, which makes it possible to find, based on a symptom, diseases that can be connected with it, and the corresponding pages in the book.

Subjects
The subjects covering diseases are identifiable by the colored outline.

Introduction
The text of the introduction states the basis of the subject and is completed by articles.

Article

Footnote
The footnote directs the reader to a page of the encyclopedia which contains additional information.

Sub-theme

Theme
Each theme is marked by a distinct color.

Glossary term
The shaded terms are defined in the glossary.

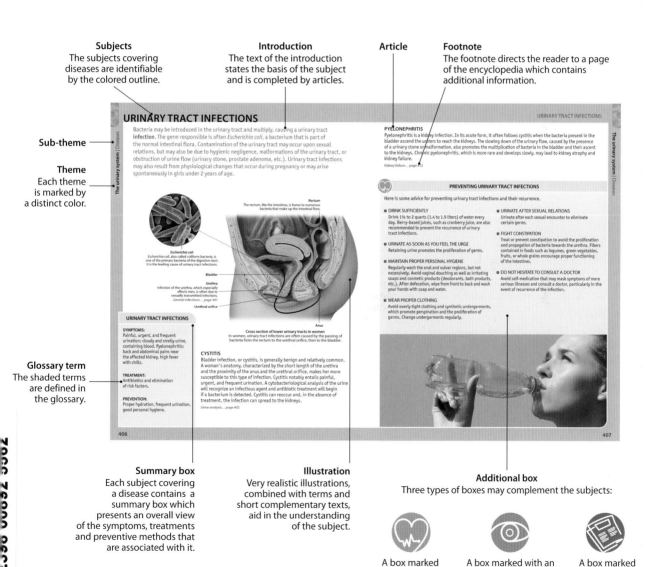

Summary box
Each subject covering a disease contains a summary box which presents an overall view of the symptoms, treatments and preventive methods that are associated with it.

Illustration
Very realistic illustrations, combined with terms and short complementary texts, aid in the understanding of the subject.

Additional box
Three types of boxes may complement the subjects:

A box marked with a heart indicates lifestyle habits to adopt in order to prevent or treat a disease.

A box marked with an eye offers surprising information connected with a subject.

A box marked with a press clipping provides information on current affairs debated in the media.

TABLE OF CONTENTS

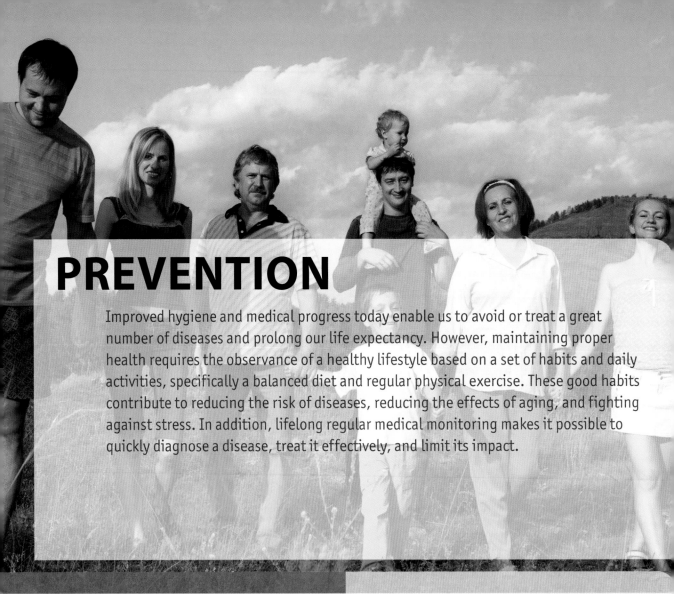

PREVENTION

Improved hygiene and medical progress today enable us to avoid or treat a great number of diseases and prolong our life expectancy. However, maintaining proper health requires the observance of a healthy lifestyle based on a set of habits and daily activities, specifically a balanced diet and regular physical exercise. These good habits contribute to reducing the risk of diseases, reducing the effects of aging, and fighting against stress. In addition, lifelong regular medical monitoring makes it possible to quickly diagnose a disease, treat it effectively, and limit its impact.

NUTRITION

Nutrition is the set of mechanisms responsible for the transformation of food into nutrients, substances assimilated by the body and vital for its functioning. Carbohydrates, proteins, fats, minerals, vitamins, and water are nutrients. Each of them must be obtained from regular meals, in proportions corresponding to the body's needs. Once ingested, they are absorbed by the digestive system (digestion), then converted to produce energy, among other things. Excess nutrients are stored in the fatty tissues, the muscles, and the liver. A diversified and balanced diet is indispensable for maintaining good health.

A **BALANCED DIET**

A balanced diet provides all of the nutrients and energy the body needs, on a daily basis, without deficiency or excess. The daily recommended energy needed for an average adult is approximately 2,000 to 2,500 calories for a man and 1,800 to 2,000 calories for a woman. However, needs vary according to age, height, weight, profession, physical activity, and certain circumstances (pregnancy, nursing, disease). The diet must be adapted in the cases of high blood pressure, diabetes, dietary intolerances, or other specific conditions.

CALORIES

The calorie (cal) is a unit of measurement of energy that is absorbed in the form of food or used by the body. In nutrition, we primarily use its multiple, the kilocalorie (kcal) or Calorie (Cal), equal to 1,000 calories. Food labels sometimes use another unit, the joule (J), with the equivalence: 1 kcal = 4.1855 kJ.

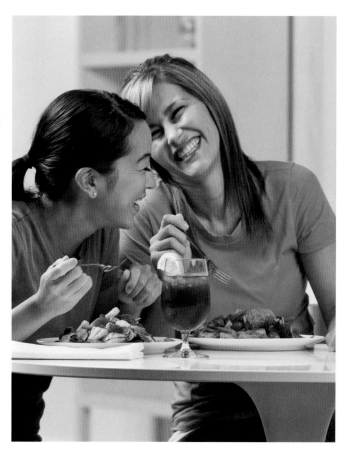

WATER

Water, which represents approximately 60% of the body mass (blood, lymph, etc.), is the most abundant chemical substance in the human body. Its properties make it an essential nutrient for transporting chemical components in the body: hormones, nutrients, metabolic waste, respiratory gases, etc. Water has other important functions, including temperature regulation and protecting the organs against shock. Its daily supply, provided by beverages and foods, must be approximately 2.5 quarts (2.4 liters), of which at least 1.5 quarts (1.4 liters) is water. Needs may increase under certain conditions (high heat, physical activity). A water deficiency rapidly results in dehydration, then death, after only two or three days of deprivation.

THE **FOOD GUIDE**

The various nutrients (carbohydrates, proteins, fats, minerals, vitamins) are distributed in four major food groups: grain products, vegetables and fruit, milk and milk alternatives, and meat and meat alternatives. The Food Guide specifies the daily recommended portions for each of these groups. The guidelines vary slightly from one country to another (e.g. with regard to recommended portions), but the order of importance of each group remains the same. Thus, eating large quantities of grain products, vegetables and fruit is recommended. Dairy products and meats are to be consumed more moderately. Finally, the recommended servings vary according to age, height, sex, weight, and level of physical activity.

DAILY RECOMMENDED SERVINGS ACCORDING TO CANADA'S FOOD GUIDE

	Children			Adolescents		Adults			
Age (years)	2-3	4-8	9-13	14-18		19-50		51+	
Sex	Girls and boys			Girls	Boys	Women	Men	Women	Men
Vegetables and fruit	4	5	6	7	8	7-8	8-10	7	7
Grain products	3	4	6	6	7	6-7	8	6	7
Milk and alternatives	2	2	3-4	3-4	3-4	2	2	3	3
Meats and alternatives	1	1	1-2	2	3	2	3	2	3

Source: Based on Canada's Food Guide, http://www.hc-sc.gc.ca/fn-an/food-guide-aliment/index-eng.php

Milk and milk alternatives
1 serving equals 1 cup (250 mL) of milk or enriched soy beverage; 1.76 oz. (50 g) of cheese; ¾ cup (175 g) of yogurt.

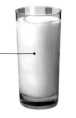

Vegetables and fruit
1 serving equals 1 fruit of average size; ½ cup of vegetables or fruit, fresh, frozen, or canned; ½ cup of juice; 1 cup of salad (raw leafy vegetables).

Meats and meat alternatives
1 serving equals 2.65 oz (125 mL) of meat, poultry, fish, or shellfish; ¾ cup (175 mL) of cooked legumes; 2 eggs; ¾ cup (175 mL) of tofu; ¼ cup (60 mL) of nuts or shelled seeds; or 2 tablespoons (30 mL) of peanut butter or nut butter.

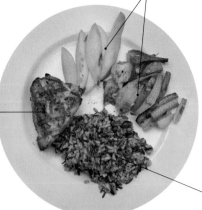
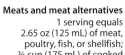

Grain products
1 serving equals one slice of bread (1.23 oz., or 35 g); 1.06 oz. (30 g) of cold cereal; ¾ cup (175 mL) of hot cereal; ½ cup (125 mL) of rice, couscous, or pasta.

THE PREGNANT OR NURSING WOMAN

The energy needs of a pregnant or nursing woman are much greater. In Canada, for example, the Food Guide recommends having two to three additional servings from any of the food groups daily. In order to prevent fetal anomalies and anemia, it is also recommended they take a daily vitamin supplement containing folic acid and iron.

CARBOHYDRATES

Carbohydrates constitute the body's main source of energy. They alone should constitute more than half of the daily recommended calorie requirement. Carbohydrates are primarily present in foods of plant origin such as grain products, legumes, vegetables, and fruit. A distinction is made between simple carbohydrates, complex carbohydrates and dietary fiber. Complex carbohydrates and dietary fiber are particularly beneficial for the body and should therefore be favored in a balanced diet.

SIMPLE CARBOHYDRATES

Simple carbohydrates are assimilated by the body in very little time because they are digested quickly. They therefore constitute an immediately usable source of energy and are particularly effective in the context of an intense effort. However, certain simple carbohydrates, such as sucrose (or saccharose) should be consumed in moderation because excesses promote obesity and type 2 diabetes. The principal simple carbohydrates are glucose, fructose, sucrose, lactose, and galactose. They are present in milk, corn, honey, and fruit, but particularly (and often in excessive quantity) in baked goods, candy, fruit juices, and carbonated beverages, in the form of white sugar, light and dark brown sugar, corn syrup, or molasses.

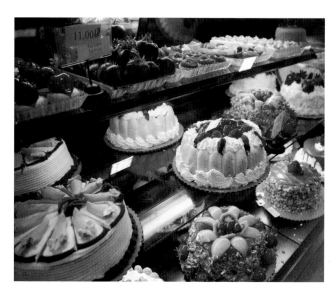

COMPLEX CARBOHYDRATES

Complex carbohydrates, also called polysaccharides, are formed by a grouping of simple carbohydrates. They are assimilated more slowly by the body and have less harmful effects on the health than simple carbohydrates. The principal complex carbohydrates are starch and glycogen. Starch, of plant origin, comes from starchy foods such as grains, bread, pasta, rice, corn, legumes, and potatoes. Glycogen, of animal origin, is present in trace form in red meat.

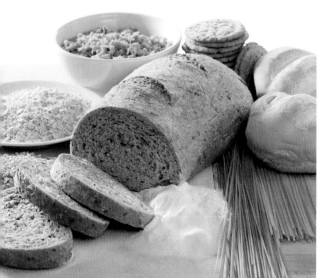

DIETARY FIBER

Dietary fiber consists of complex carbohydrates of plant origin that cannot be absorbed, that is, cannot be digested. Cellulose, hemicellulose, pectin, and mucilage are the main dietary fibers. They come from whole grains, legumes, vegetables, and fruit. Dietary fiber is particularly beneficial for health because it forms a system that retains water. The fibers limit the absorption of certain substances such as cholesterol and produce a feeling of fullness, thus contributing in fighting against obesity and certain cardiovascular diseases. They also increase the volume of fecal matter and soften it, which facilitates its transit and reduces the risks of hemorrhoids, anal fissures, diverticulosis, and colorectal cancer.

FATS

Fats are particularly represented by fatty acids and cholesterol. The former are present in numerous foods such as oils, butter, margarine, meat, fish, eggs, dairy products, nuts, and seeds, while cholesterol is present only in products of animal origin. Lipids are stored in the fatty tissue, where they provide energy storage and thermal insulation. Certain dietary lipids increase the risk of developing cardiovascular disease or cancer; others play a protective role.

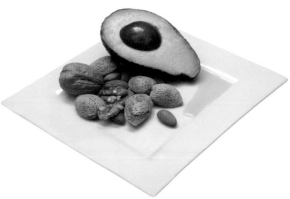

Unsaturated fatty acids
Unsaturated fatty acids are present in plant oils (olive, canola, corn, sunflower, walnut, soy oils, etc.), avocados, fatty fish (salmon, mackerel, smelt, herring, and trout) as well as in seeds and nuts (flax, sunflower, walnut, cashews, pecans, almonds, peanuts, etc.).

FATTY ACID

A distinction is made between saturated and unsaturated fatty acids. Unsaturated fatty acids come primarily from plant fats. If excesses are avoided, they generally have a beneficial effect on the health by reducing the blood cholesterol level. As for saturated fatty acids, they come primarily from animal fats (butter, eggs, meat, processed meat products, fish, milk, cheese). Some plant oils contain them too, such as palm and coconut oil. Consumed in excess, saturated fatty acids increase the blood cholesterol level and the risk of cardiovascular diseases, as do trans-fatty acids, a category of unsaturated fatty acids present primarily in industrial foods (pastries, fried goods).

CHOLESTEROL

Cholesterol is a lipid naturally produced by the body, specifically by the liver. It enters into the composition of cellular membranes and several hormones. It is transported from the liver to the cells by blood proteins. Cholesterol that comes from food may, in certain cases, be added to that which is produced by the body and contribute to the increase in the blood cholesterol level. Excess cholesterol tends to deposit on the artery walls, thus increasing the risk of cardiovascular disease.

Heart disease... page 256
Good and bad cholesterol... page 258

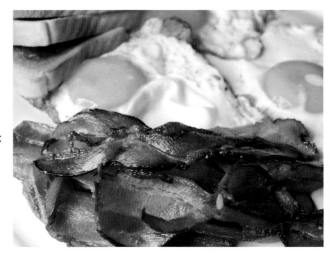

OMEGA 3s

Omega 3s are unsaturated essential fatty acids that have a protective effect against cardiovascular diseases and inflammatory diseases such as arthritis. They also play a role in the proper functioning of the nervous system, specifically the brain. Omega 3s are present in certain oils (canola, wheat germ, soy) and in nuts and seeds (flax, hemp, pumpkin). They are also present in algae and fatty fish (salmon, herring, sardines, mackerel, anchovies) and their consumption is particularly beneficial. Due to our dietary habits, the minimum recommended daily requirements are rarely achieved.

VITAMINS

Vitamins, 13 in number, are present in very small quantities in the body, but they are indispensable for its functioning. They play a role in numerous functions: metabolism, cellular division, growth, coagulation, etc. With the exceptions of Vitamins B_3 and D, which can be synthesized by the body under certain conditions, vitamins must be obtained from food. Any deficiency will result in health problems, which can sometimes be severe.

THE 13 VITAMINS

	Other name	Role	Source	Deficiency
A	Retinol	Vision, growth, immunity, protection of tissues, antioxidant	Eggs; dairy products; yellow, orange, and dark green vegetables and fruit; liver	Decreased night vision, xerophthalmia, blindness, sensitivity to infections
B_1	Thiamine	Metabolism, functioning of nervous system	Meat (pork), fish, eggs, legumes, whole grains, nuts and seeds, wheat germ	Beriberi (cardiac insufficiency and neurological problems)
B_2	Riboflavin	Metabolism, muscle tissue repair	Dairy products, eggs, meats, fish, whole grains, legumes, nuts and seeds	Delayed growth, dermatosis
B_3	Nicotinamide, vitamin PP	Metabolism, functioning of nervous system, hormone synthesis, transporting oxygen in the blood	Meats (poultry, rabbit), fish, legumes, nuts and seeds	Pellagra, tingling in the hands and feet, fatigue, headaches, dizziness
B_5	Pantothenic acid	Metabolism, regeneration of the skin and mucous membranes	Meats, fish, eggs, whole grains, legumes, mushrooms	Fatigue and depression, insomnia, leg cramps
B_6	Pyridoxin	Metabolism, formation of red blood cells, immunity, regulation of glycemia	Enriched grains, legumes, vegetables and fruit, meats	Dermatosis, anemia, irritability
B_8	Biotin	Metabolism	Meats (poultry), raw vegetables, legumes, eggs, whole grains	Neurological problems, hair loss
B_9	Folic acid, folate	DNA and RNA synthesis, formation of red blood cells	Green vegetables, legumes, liver, enriched grains	Anemia, loss of appetite, irritability, spina bifida (fetus)
B_{12}	Cobalamin	DNA and RNA synthesis, formation of red blood cells, nervous system	Fish, meat, dairy products, eggs, enriched soy beverages	Anemia, fatigue, weakness
C	Ascorbic acid	Antioxidant, collagen synthesis, iron absorption, immunity	Vegetables and fruit (including red pepper, kiwi, orange, broccoli, strawberry)	Scurvy, intense fatigue, joint pains
D	Calciferol	Absorption of calcium, mineralization of bones, growth	Fatty fish, egg yolk, enriched dairy products	Rickets, weakening of muscles and bones, osteoporosis
E	Tocopherol	Antioxidant, protection of tissues	Vegetable oils, nuts and seeds, green and orange vegetables	Weakness of red blood cells, nervous system development problems (child)
K	Phylloquinone, menaquinone	Blood clotting, bone formation	Green vegetables, vegetable oils, tofu, margarine	Hemorrhages (newborn)

MINERALS

Minerals are inorganic chemical elements that are indispensable for the body. Based on the quantity normally present in the body, a distinction is made between macroelements and oligoelements.

MACROELEMENTS

A macroelement is a mineral present in a relatively large quantity in the body (more than 5 g for a 154 pounds [70 kg] man). There are seven of them: phosphorus, potassium, calcium, magnesium, sodium, chlorine, and sulfur. Macroelements enter into the composition of certain tissues (bones, teeth) and fluids (blood, saliva, tears, sweat, urine). They are fundamental to the conduction of nerve impulses and muscular contraction, and participate in numerous metabolic reactions.

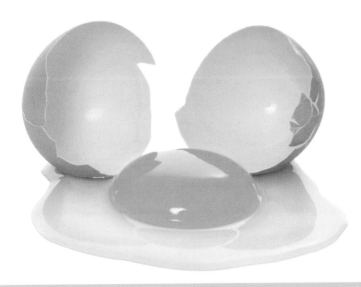

Macroelement	Role	Source	Deficiency
MINERALS (MACROELEMENTS)			
Phosphorus	Composition of bones and teeth, maintenance of normal blood acidity	Meats, fish, milk, grains, eggs, nuts, seeds, legumes	Bone demineralization, problems with sensitivity (tingling, stinging), cardiac, respiratory, and neurological problems
Potassium	Metabolism, blood pressure regulation, nerve conduction, muscular contraction	Vegetables, fruit, dairy products, legumes	Neuromuscular and cardiac problems, confusion
Calcium	Composition of bones, muscular contraction, nerve conduction, blood clotting	Dairy products, canned fish, leafy vegetables	Tetanus, neurological problems, osteoporosis
Magnesium	Metabolism, muscular contraction, blood clotting, health of bones and teeth	Whole grains, legumes, nuts, artichokes	Depression, confusion, cramps, numbness, cardiac problems, loss of appetite, tetanus
Sodium	Composition of fluids (plasma, tears, sweat), nerve conduction	Table salt, soy sauce	Digestive and neurological problems, muscle cramps
Chlorine	Composition of gastric juice	Table salt	Digestive problems, muscle cramps, apathy
Sulfur	Metabolism, immune system, composition of bones and teeth	Grains, milk, eggs, legumes	Metabolism problems, vulnerability to infections

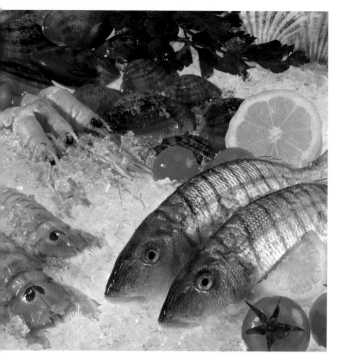

OLIGOELEMENTS

An oligoelement is a mineral present in the body in a very small quantity yet indispensable to its functioning. The most important oligoelements are iron, iodine, fluorine, cobalt, chromium, selenium, zinc, copper, and manganese.

ANTIOXIDANTS

Antioxidants are substances capable of neutralizing the excess of free radicals produced by the metabolism. These free radicals contribute to the acceleration of aging and diseases such as cancer, certain cardiovascular problems, senile dementia, and other diseases related to aging. The main antioxidants are the phenolic compounds (substances produced by plants); Vitamins A, C, and E; selenium; and zinc.

MINERALS (OLIGOELEMENTS)

Oligoelement	Role	Source	Deficiency
Iron	Composition of hemoglobin, metabolism	Red meats, liver, shellfish, egg yolk, green vegetables, enriched grains, lentils	Anemia
Iodine	Synthesis of steroidal hormones	Sea salt and iodized table salt, fish, shellfish, algae	Thyroid insufficiency, mental retardation (newborn)
Fluorine	Composition of teeth and bones	Fluoridated water, supplements	Increase in susceptibility to dental cavities
Cobalt	Maturation of red blood cells	Meats, fish, milk, legumes, whole grains	Anemia
Chromium	Regulation of blood glucose and cholesterol	Whole grains, liver, green vegetables	Increase in blood cholesterol level and risk of diabetes
Selenium	Antioxidant	Meats, shellfish, fish, whole grains, eggs	Muscle pain, increase in susceptibility to infections
Zinc	Metabolism, antioxidant	Shellfish, fish, whole grains, nuts	Fatigue, gout and smell problems, delayed growth, lowered immunity
Copper	Metabolism, immunity, bone and cartilage health	Shellfish, whole grains, legumes, liver, nuts	Anemia, osteoporosis
Manganese	Metabolism	Whole grains, nuts, legumes, green vegetables, fruit	Increase in cholesterol level, glucose intolerance

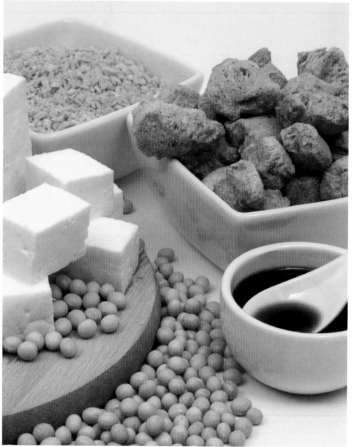

PROTEINS

Proteins are complex substances made of amino acids arranged in chains. They are very diversified in their composition, form, and role. Some are involved in the structure of the body, such as collagen. Others participate in its functioning while contributing to, for example, muscle contraction, nervous conduction, and immunity. Proteins of the body are manufactured using amino acids resulting mostly from the digestion of proteins contained in food. Meat, fish, eggs, and dairy products constitute the main sources of animal protein. Cereal products (bread, rice, cereals, etc.), nuts, grains and legumes (including soy) are sources of vegetable protein. An insufficient level of protein can cause growth problems in children, general weakening, muscle atrophy, and a greater susceptibility to infections. A surplus of proteins, particularly of animal origin, can constitute a risk factor for obesity and increase the risk of cardiovascular disease and cancer.

COFFEE AND TEA

Coffee and tea are noncaloric drinks, as long as they do not contain sugar, milk, or cream. These two drinks contain caffeine, a stimulating substance that temporarily increases vigilance, arterial pressure, and heartbeat frequency. The effects, variable depending on the sensitivity of the individual, increase with the quantity absorbed. The recommended limit for an adult in good health is 400 mg per day, that is, 3–4 cups of filtered coffee or 9–12 cups of tea, or 300 mg per day for a pregnant or nursing woman. People suffering from high blood pressure, cardiovascular diseases, or sleeping disorders should also decrease their consumption. Too much caffeine can cause irritability, anxiety, tremors, palpitations, and heartburn. Recent studies attribute beneficial effects to green tea in cancer prevention due to the antioxidants it contains.

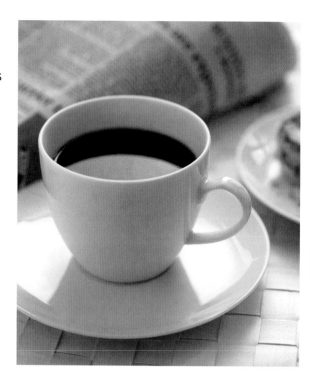

RULES FOR A HEALTHY DIET

Even though many foods present a detailed nutritional label, it is useless to attempt to perfectly control the quantities of various nutrients absorbed daily. Observing the recommendations of the dietary guide for the four main food groups and following a few golden rules is sufficient.

- Have three main meals a day and complement them with one or two snacks.

- Eat fruit, vegetables, and whole grain cereal products with each meal. They are an excellent source of vitamins, minerals, fiber, and antioxidants.

- Nuts and grains are excellent. They are sources of protein, good lipids (unsaturated fats), and antioxidants.

- Limit fats, particularly those that are used for cooking and seasonings and those that are hidden in baked goods, crusts, etc.

- Steam vegetables and cook meat and fish on a grill, in an oven, on the stove, etc., adding little or no oil. Avoid frying.

- Use olive oil and canola oil. They contain good lipids.

- Limit sugars, baked goods, carbonated soft drinks, etc.

- Drink plenty of water, at least 6–8 cups (1.5–2 liters) per day, and reduce your alcohol consumption, if necessary.
  Alcohol consumption, a few guidelines... page 26

- Limit your meat consumption and substitute it regularly with fish, legumes, or soybean-based products. Choose lean meats, notably poultry and pork.

- Reduce your salt consumption. Season your food with spices and fines herbes and limit your consumption of commercially processed foods.

- Control your diet by reducing the number of meals eaten in restaurants and the purchase of prepared meals (which often contain too much sugar, salt, or fat).

- Take the time to savor food and enjoy meal hours. Eat a wide range of foods in moderation.

FOOD LABELING

The labeling on packaged foods provides information on the nutritional value of their contents. The first line of a label indicates the serving size of the nutritional data. To compare two different brands, you must compare identical servings. The quantity of calories and content of various nutrients in this serving are then listed. The quantities are generally given in milligrams (mg) or grams (g), and in a percentage of a daily recommended value. When the percentage of a nutritious element is below 5%, its dietary contribution is considered to be low. Above 20%, it is high. Choose products that are low in sugar, sodium (salt), and saturated and trans fats.

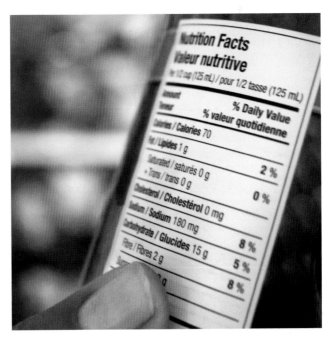

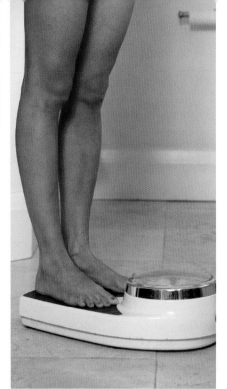

HEALTHY WEIGHT

Healthy weight, or ideal weight, is an interval within which weight variations have no repercussions on the state of health. It is personalized to each individual and depends, among other things, on height, age, and gender. When weight strays from its ideal value, the risk of developing certain diseases increases. The greater the deviation, the more the danger increases. Excess weight increases the risk of high blood pressure, coronary diseases, cerebrovascular accident, type 2 diabetes, sleep apnea, arthrosis, and colorectal cancer. On the other hand, excessive weight loss can lead to nutritional deficiencies and stop menstruations in women. It also promotes osteoporosis after menopause.

BODY MASS INDEX

The body mass index (BMI) is a measure of body fat and is used to estimate the risk of diseases that are associated with it. The BMI of an individual is obtained by dividing their weight (in kilograms) by the square of their height (in meters). Thus, the BMI of an individual who weighs 165 pounds (75 kg) and measures 5 feet 9 inches (1.75 m) is equal to 75/(1.75 x 1.75), which is 24.5. A body mass index between 18.5 and 25 corresponds to a healthy weight. BMI categories apply to adults between the ages of 18 and 65 and are not valid for children, pregnant or nursing women, high-level athletes, and older or seriously ill individuals. Furthermore, the quantity of adipose tissue may be overestimated in stocky or athletic people and underestimated in individuals who have a lower bone density.

CALCULATING YOUR HEALTHY WEIGHT

Weight and body mass index (BMI) are related. The weight of a person (in kilograms) is equal to the BMI multiplied by the height (in meters) squared. Knowing that healthy weight corresponds to a body mass index between 18.5 and 25, it is easy to calculate the interval corresponding to ideal weight. For example, the healthy weight of a woman who is 5 feet 6 inches (1.70 m) tall is between 118 pounds (53.5 kg) (18.5 x 1.70 x 1.70) and 158 pounds (72 kg) (25 x 1.70 x 1.70).

Obesity... page 355

BMI AND HEALTH RISKS		
Category	**BMI in kg/m²**	**Risk**
Underweight	Below 18.5	+
Healthy weight	From 18.5–24.9	–
Overweight	From 25–29.9	+
Class I obesity	From 30–34.9	++
Class II obesity	From 35–39.9	+++
Class III obesity (morbid obesity)	40+	++++

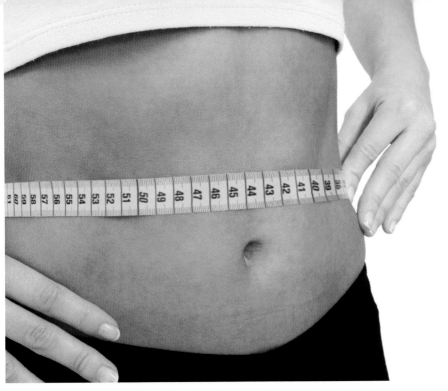

WAIST SIZE

Waist size is an additional risk indicator of diseases associated with excess weight. It must be measured halfway between the lowest rib and the highest point of the hip bone. Values greater than or equal to 40 inches (102 cm) in men and 35 inches (88 cm) in women expose the person to a higher risk of disease (notably high blood pressure, coronary diseases, and type 2 diabetes).

WAIST SIZE, BMI, AND HEALTH RISKS

Waist size \ BMI	Normal	Overweight	Obesity
Less than 40 in (102 cm) (men) Less than 35 in (88 cm) (women)	Low risk	Heightened risk	Elevated risk
Greater than or equal to 40 in (102 cm) (men) Greater than or equal to 35 in (88 cm) (women)	Heightened risk	Elevated risk	Very elevated risk

MAINTAINING A HEALTHY WEIGHT

In healthy adults, weight fluctuations are mainly due to a gain or loss of adipose tissue mass. As these variations are directly influenced by diet and physical activity, it is possible for you to exert control over your weight by having a balanced diet and practicing regular physical activity. Your diet must be low in animal fats, particularly found in red meat. It must not contain too much sugar, particularly simple sugars, which are contained in sweets, baked goods, carbonated soft drinks, etc. Alcohol is also a caloric substance and its consumption must be limited. Physical activity must be daily, progressive, and adapted to each person. Half an hour of activity per day is enough to have a beneficial effect on health.

WEIGHT LOSS

To be lasting, weight loss must be progressive, at about 1 pound (0.5 kg) per week. Weight loss that is too fast is harmful for the body. It generally results in regain, even exceeding the initial weight, caused by the reflex storage of calories by the body to compensate for the deprivation. This is the yo-yo effect induced by rapid weight loss diets, based on the sudden decrease in caloric intake, without any profound change in lifestyle habits.

EXERCISE

Regular and adapted physical exercise is beneficial for health. It decreases the effects of aging and the risk of certain diseases. People who exercise regularly, even moderately, have a higher life expectancy compared to sedentary people in the same age group. A complete exercise program includes limbering, muscle-building, and endurance exercises. The intensity and duration of these exercises must be adjusted to each individual to avoid injury.

LIMBERING EXERCISES

Limbering exercises, also called "stretching," stretch and relax the muscles to increase the amplitude of movements. All physical exercise sessions should begin and end with a series of stretches (flexion, extension) to prevent muscle soreness or limit its intensity. Limbering exercises facilitate daily gestures, maintain the elasticity of the body, eliminate tension in the muscles and tendons accumulated during the day (overexertion, work in front of the computer, etc.), and extend the autonomy of older individuals. Activities such as tai chi, yoga, and dancing are excellent limbering exercises.

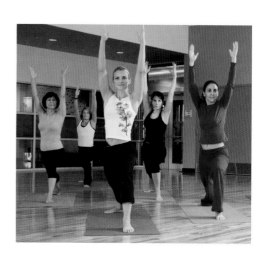

MUSCLE-BUILDING EXERCISES

Muscle building consists in building resistance to movement commanded by a group of muscles. This resistance, adapted to each person, can be obtained by lifting weight, using muscle-building machines, or simply using one's own weight (push-ups, sit-ups, etc.). During the exercise, a series of a dozen identical movements are repeated two to four times, with a pause between each series to let the muscles rest and avoid muscular contractions and tears. Contrary to endurance exercises, the demanded effort is intense, but of a short duration.

BENEFICAL EFFECTS OF MUSCLE BUILDING

Muscle-building exercises, when they are practiced in a regular manner, lead to the formation of new muscle fibers, which increase the strength and volume of muscles. Blood capillaries develop to carry out better oxygenation of muscle mass. The increase in muscle force, which is exerted on the bones by the tendons, also stimulates the formation of bone tissues. It therefore slows down osteoporosis and also reduces the risk of fracture in older individuals. Muscle building also helps control weight by reducing the mass of adipose tissue. It decreases the risks of type 2 diabetes and hypercholesterolemia. It also improves movement coordination and contributes to reducing back pain symptoms.

ENDURANCE EXERCISES

Physical endurance is the ability of the body to maintain an effort for several minutes without experiencing signs of fatigue (decrease in strength, cramps, shortness of breath). It can be reinforced by appropriate physical activities practiced in a regular manner: walking, swimming, cycling, jogging, etc. The benefits of endurance exercises are significant and varied: strengthening of skeletal and heart muscles, improvement in respiration, oxygenation of organs, and blood circulation. By promoting the use of lipid reserves by the muscles, endurance exercises help control weight problems. They also improve the sensation of well-being and contribute to fighting stress and anxiety.

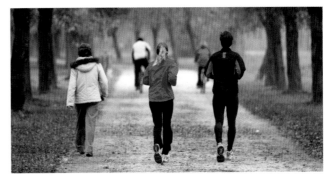

Walking and jogging
Walking can be practiced anywhere, without equipment. It burns approximately 300 calories per hour and is a good exercise for leg muscles. Walking must be relatively rapid and last at least 30 minutes per day. Jogging is more intense than walking. One hour of jogging at the rate of 7.5 miles per hour (12 km/h) burns approximately 900 calories. It must be practiced with the appropriate shoes to reduce the risk of joint trauma in the knees and ankles.

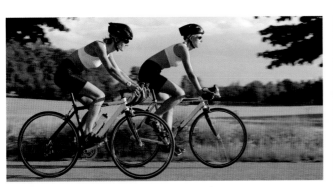

Cycling
In addition to being an ecological method of transportation, cycling is an excellent endurance and muscle-building exercise for the legs and back. A distance of approximately 12½ miles (20 km) per hour can be equivalent to burning 500 calories.

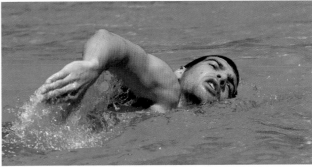

Swimming
Swimming is a cardiovascular activity, but also a complete muscle-building exercise, particularly recommended for people who suffer from back pain. One hour of swimming is equal to burning 600 calories.

WARMING UP

All physical exercise must begin with a 10-minute warm-up. Warming up consists of gentle and progressive exercises that allow the body to adapt to effort. While warming up, the body temperature slightly rises, which increases the effectiveness of the metabolism to produce energy. Cardiac rhythm progressively accelerates to adapt to the transportation of oxygen as needed. The elasticity of the muscles, tendons, and ligaments increases and joint lubrication is stimulated. Warming up includes stretching (flexion, extension), joint rotations, muscle exercises (sit-ups, push-ups, etc.), and cardiovascular exercises (running in place, rapid walking, etc.). In the absence of warming up, the sudden passage from the resting state to effort can cause cardiac arrhythmia and joint traumas.

PHYSICAL BENEFITS OF EXERCISE

Physical exercise has a number of beneficial effects on the body. One of the main benefits is reducing the risk of cardiovascular diseases thanks to the strengthening of muscles of the cardiovascular system, a better oxygenation of tissues, a decrease in arterial pressure, and the reduction of "bad cholesterol" responsible for atherosclerosis. With a balanced diet, physical exercise stimulates the metabolism and eliminates excess calories, which allows for better weight control and reduces the risk of obesity and type 2 diabetes. It also decreases the risk of colorectal cancer and breast cancer, possibly also the risk of prostate cancer and endometrial (uterine) cancer. Physical activity stimulates the immune system and protects against infections, particularly those of the respiratory system (cold, flu, etc.). In older individuals and women who have experienced menopause, physical exercise slows down the loss of muscle mass, maintains joint flexibility, and fights against osteoporosis. It also contributes to reducing falls and the risk of fractures.

PSYCHOLOGICAL BENEFITS

By stimulating the liberation of natural morphines (endorphins) by the brain, physical exercise helps to reduce stress, mental fatigue, and anxiety. It provides a sense of pleasure and helps fight against depression. Physical activity also helps reduce the symptoms of premenstrual syndrome. It improves sleep and increases energy.

MUSCLE SORENESS

Muscle soreness is the painful manifestation of microtears in the muscle fibers, most often caused by an intense or irregular muscular effort. These microscopic tears lead to a localized and temporary inflammation. Generally, muscle soreness disappears on its own after a few days.

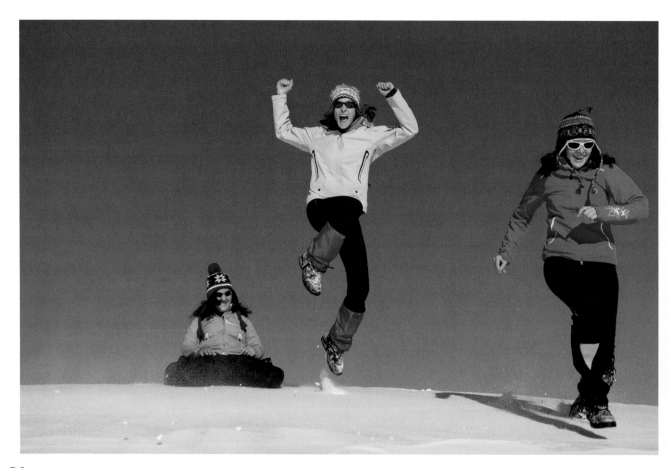

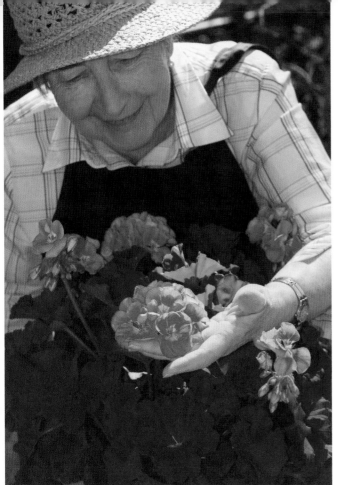

CHANGING LIFESTYLE HABITS

Daily life is filled with opportunities to exercise. Moreover, such exercise provides the added advantage of being affordable and beneficial to the environment. Thus, using public transportation instead of a car increases the time dedicated to walking, a natural exercise that should be practiced at least 30 minutes per day. Bicycling is another means of transportation for short trips. At work or in public buildings, taking the stairs more often than elevators or escalators is excellent for endurance and building leg muscles. At home, a manual lawn mower is a better choice than a motorized lawn mower for building arm muscles. In general, gardening provides an opportunity for limbering and relaxation. Come wintertime, shoveling provides more effective cardiovascular exercise and muscle building than pushing a snowblower, assuming you warm up and respect your limits.

A WEEKLY SCHEDULE

A complete exercise program includes regular sessions of limbering, muscle-building, and endurance exercises. Each exercise session must start with a warm-up period (stretching, joint rotation, running in place, etc.) and end with stretching exercises, particularly after an intense workout (muscle building, endurance), to avoid injuries and muscle soreness.

Example:

- **Day 1:** 30–60 minutes of endurance, progressively increasing the intensity of the effort.
- **Day 2:** 15–30 minutes of muscle building (push-ups, sit-ups, weights, or machines).
- **Day 3:** 30 minutes of limbering (yoga, tai chi, etc.).
- **Day 4:** 30–60 minutes of endurance by progressively increasing the intensity of the effort.
- **Day 5:** 15–30 minutes of muscle building (push-ups, sit-ups, weights, or machines).
- **Day 6:** 30 minutes of limbering (yoga, tai chi, etc.).
- **Day 7:** 30–60 minutes of endurance, progressively increasing the intensity of the effort.

TOBACCO, ALCOHOL, AND DRUGS

Certain substances used over the long term, whether they are legal (tobacco, alcohol, sedatives, etc.) or illegal (marijuana, heroin, cocaine, etc.), lead to an addiction that results in abusive consumption that is harmful to the health.

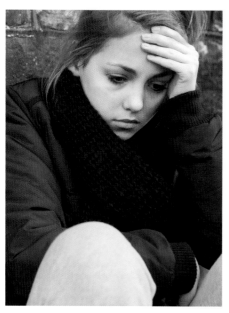

FROM OCCASIONAL USE TO ADDICTION

It is easier to diagnose a state of addiction than it is to define the limits of consumption that induce it. These depend on numerous factors: the chemical composition of the drug, its effects on the body, its method of absorption, its dose, the frequency of use, as well as the sensitivity of the user (genetic predisposition; exposure to substances during fetal life; personal and family history; social, personal, and psychological situation).

SIGNS OF ADDICTION

Addiction can be recognized in several signs: pressing desire to consume, difficulty controlling the consumed quantity, physical or psychic symptoms after a period of abstinence (palpitations, transpiration, nervousness, irritability, etc.), necessity to increase the dose to obtain an effect, loss of interest in other pleasures, interference with daily activities, continuation of consumption in spite of its harmful effects, etc.

ALCOHOL CONSUMPTION, A FEW GUIDELINES

According to the World Health Organization (WHO), regular use consisting of less than three standard glasses per day for men or two glasses per day for women presents only minimum risks and is individually and socially acceptable. These thresholds must be lowered depending on the circumstances (pregnancy, driving a vehicle, a situation requiring attention, following a treatment or specific state of health). The WHO also recommends, in the case of regular use, to respect a day of abstinence per week. Finally, it is preferable to consume alcohol while eating. A standard drink of alcohol defined by the WHO corresponds to 10 g of pure alcohol, as follows:

- One glass or 3½ oz. (100 mL) of wine or champagne (alcohol content: 11%-13%)

- One glass 8¾ oz. (250 mL) of beer (alcohol content: 5%)

- 2½–3 oz. (70–85 mL) of an aperitif (alcohol content: 18%-20%)

- 1 oz. (30 mL) of liqueur (alcohol content: 40%-45%)

- 8¾ oz. (250 mL) of cider (alcohol content: 6%)

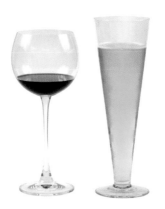

THE DANGERS OF DRUGS

Smoking kills millions of people worldwide each year and constitutes, easily, the first cause of lung cancer. Alcoholism is often responsible for cancers of the esophagus and liver, cirrhosis of the liver, epilepsy, homicides, and car accidents. Alcoholism and drug addiction have significant social and economic repercussions: law violations, acts of violence, accidental traumas, professional absenteeism, deterioration of social and family life. Finally, drug consumption during pregnancy can cause miscarriage or premature birth. It also has consequences on the development of the fetus and the child: low birth weight, growth delay, intellectual retardation, malformations, death.

PREVENTING ADDICTION

Awareness and information campaigns contribute to preventing drug addiction in the general public and groups at risk, such as adolescents. Nevertheless, family and friends remain best suited to intervene if they detect high-risk consumption behavior in those around them.

- Stay informed on the dangers of consumption of a substance likely to create addiction.
- Ask your family and friends what they think of your consumption. Analyze the circumstances surrounding the abusive consumption and avoid situations that might contribute to abuse. Change your habits and hobbies if needed. Do not isolate yourself; on the contrary, maintain or renew contact with your family and friends.
- If you think that a loved one's consumption presents a risk, remain nonjudgmental and keep the lines of communication open. Suggest that the person seek help (specialized center, telephone hotline, psychologist, etc.) and offer to accompany him or her in their efforts.

WITHDRAWAL FROM TOBACCO AND ITS BENEFITS

Time elapsed since the last cigarette	Effects on the body
20 minutes	Return to normal of blood pressure, pulse, and temperature of hands and feet.
8 hours	Return to normal of cell oxygenation. Level of carbon monoxide in the blood decreased by half.
1 day	Complete elimination of carbon monoxide. Lungs begin to reject combustion residue. Risk of infarction begins to decrease.
2 days	Complete elimination of nicotine. Taste and smell begin to improve.
3 days	Dilation of bronchial tubes. Pulmonary capacity begins to improve. Alleviation of fatigue and regain of energy.
2 weeks to 3 months	Improvement of blood circulation. More facility in exerting physical effort. Decrease in cough caused by smoking. Return to normal of taste and smell. Improvement in quality of sleep.
1 to 9 months	Clarification of voice. Decrease in shortness of breath during effort and in nasal congestion. Beginning of regeneration of cilia present in bronchial tubes. Less sensitivity to infections of the respiratory tract.
1 year	Risk of cardiovascular diseases decreased by half. Return to normal of the risk of cervical cancer.
5 years	Risk of cancer of the mouth, throat, esophagus, and lungs decreases by half. Risks of mortality due to tobacco decreases by half.
10 years	Return to normal of risk of cerebral vascular accident. Return to normal of mortality rate by lung cancer. Significant decrease in risk of cancer of the mouth, throat, esophagus, bladder, and pancreas.
15 years	Return to normal of risk of coronary disease.

STRESS CONTROL

Stress is an increasingly widespread disease, due in most part to our lifestyle. Underestimated for a long time, its repercussions on the body are now known and the methods of fighting it are becoming increasingly popular.

Stress... page 224

RECOGNIZING STRESS

Stress is a psychological response of the body to what we perceive, consciously or not, as aggression. It is accompanied by physical and psychological symptoms of varying intensity, depending on the individual, but are aggravated when stress becomes chronic. Recognizing the signs of stress, even if delayed, is the first step in controlling it.

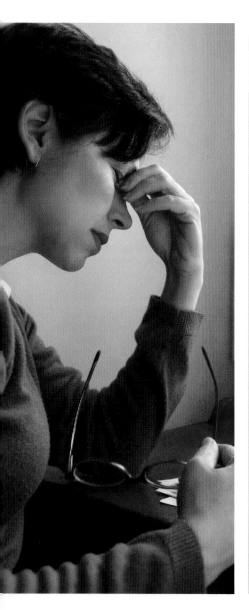

SIGNS OF STRESS	
Physical signs	**Psychological signs**
• Muscle tension: often clenched fists and jaw, shoulder and neck contraction, difficulty relaxing muscles	• Weariness
• Headaches	• Irregular or frequent mood changes: agitation, nervousness, irritability, sadness, melancholy
• Fatigue	• Indecision
• Change in appetite	• Anxiety, panic attacks
• Digestive problems: stomach pains, ulcers, nausea, vomiting, constipation, diarrhea	• Loss of desire
• Cardiovascular problems: heart palpitations, increase in heart rhythm, arterial hypertension	• Low self-esteem
• Superficial breathing	• Loss of memory, difficulty concentrating
• Sensitivity to infectious diseases: colds, flu, reactivation of herpes, herpes zoster	• Phobias
• Sleeping disorders	• Depression
• Erectile dysfunction	• Increase in tobacco, alcohol, or mood-enhancing foods, such as chocolate, consumption
• Irregularity or stopping of periods	
• Vertigo	

STRESS MANAGEMENT

To manage stress, its causes must be recognized first: family obligations, daily management, overburdened schedule, academic success of children, conflicting family or professional relations, performance desire, deadlines, traffic, lack of privacy in public transportation, etc. Subsequently, several approaches may be followed to attempt to ease its effects.

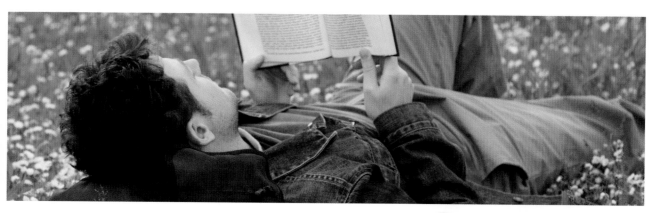

REMOVE ITS CAUSES

Certain sources of stress may be eliminated by changing habits: modifying one's work hours, method of transportation, or commute to work; transferring from one departement to another; improving the distribution of chores at home; hiring domestic help, etc. When stress is caused by poor personal relations, communicating with others or seeking mediator can often help to resolve the problem. Vacations can also be a good way to break the daily routine and provide distance from a situation.

FIGHT ITS EFFECT

Another approach to stress management consists in releasing nervous tension or fighting its effects. There are several specific relaxation techniques (yoga, meditation, tai chi, massage, etc.), but any leisure activities contribute to relieving stress: reading, shows, nature walks, gardening, meetings and social activities. Practicing a sport is also an excellent means of alleviating stress.

Exercise... page 22

CHANGE OF ATTITUDE

Certain people will foresee a problematic situation like a challenge to overcome; others, like a mountain to move. This perception of events and the reaction that it creates are personal components of stress. A variety of techniques can be learned to approach problems more positively, through stress management, personal growth or development, visualization, sophrology, etc. When stress becomes invasive and disturbs daily life, it may be necessary to seek help from a specialist (psychologist, psychoanalyst, psychiatrist, etc.), who may recommend appropriate therapy.

ANTISTRESS TIPS

- Have a balanced diet.
- Reduce your consumption of coffee, especially in the afternoon.
- Exercise regularly.
- Get enough sleep by going to bed earlier.
- Take breaks during the day, even if they are short.
- Know how to turn down work or delegate.
- Let go and accept the opinion of others on occasion.
- Do not get angry.
- Isolate yourself and breathe deeply for three to five minutes while focusing your attention on your breathing.
- Talk about your problems with your loved ones.

HYGIENE AND THE
PREVENTION OF INFECTIONS

Certain changes in lifestyle—such as increase in international exposure, the development of public transportation services, and day care centers, as well as the increased use of **antibiotics**—facilitate and accelerate the dissemination of **infectious** agents. Given the increased risk of infection, basic hygiene measures remain the most effective way to prevent infections.

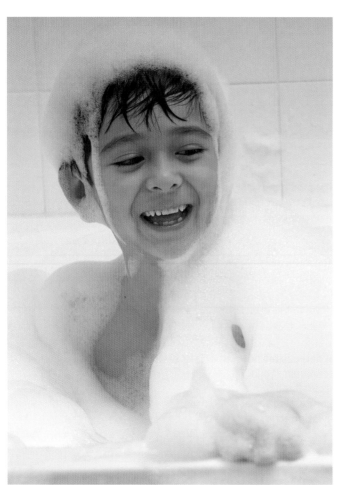

PHYSICAL HYGIENE

By avoiding the proliferation of pathogenic agents (bacteria, viruses, fungi, parasites) on the surface of the skin and mucous membranes, physical hygiene contributes to keeping us free of infection. Good hygiene consists in simple gestures such as:

• Washing your hands after having touched an animal or dirty object, after having used the bathroom, before touching food, before eating, and before touching a person at risk of infection (newborns, the elderly, or immunodeficient individuals).

• Wash daily (particularly between the fingers and toes, the navel, the underarms, and private parts).

• Wash your hair once a week (or more, if needed).

• Brush your teeth after meals or at least twice a day, and use dental floss at least once a day.

• Change your underwear daily.

THE FIGHT AGAINST THE SPREAD OF INFECTIONS

A person who is afflicted with an infectious disease of the respiratory tract, such as a cold, can avoid spreading the infection by coughing or sneezing into a handkerchief or into the crease of the elbow. Blowing the nose and washing the hands as often as possible, as well as postponing visits to weak individuals (e.g. newborns, the elderly, immunodeficient individuals) can also help to minimize the spread of infection. In children, it is best to avoid sharing clothing such as hats and scarves, which are conducive to the transmission of lice and the spread of respiratory infections.

Respiratory infections... page 318
The flu... page 320

DOMESTIC HYGIENE

At home, the places where food is handled and stored, as well as humid places, are conducive to the proliferation of bacteria and fungi. Therefore, the kitchen, bathrooms, and toilets require particular cleaning and ventilation. Showers, toilets, plumbing, and doorknobs must be disinfected regularly, as do the sink, refrigerator, countertops, and kitchen trash can. Napkins, linens, and dishcloths must be dried rapidly and cleaned frequently. Bedding and floors must also be washed periodically. The vaccination schedule for domestic animals must be respected. Also, animals must be forbidden access, as much as possible, to bedding, kitchen tables, and countertops, and to food that is not their own. Objects or areas that they come into contact with must be cleaned regularly.

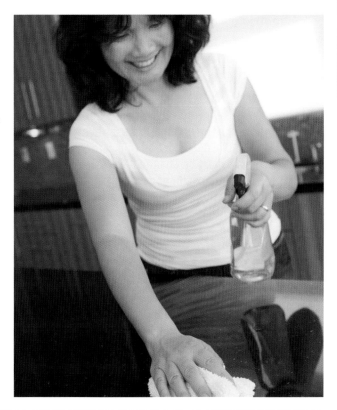

PREVENTING GASTROENTERITIS AND FOOD POISONING

In Canada, close to half of the cases of gastroenteritis and food poisoning happen at home. They are caused when food is insufficiently cooked, by contamination through handling or during production (poor hygiene, washing with contaminated water, etc.), or by the poor storage of food, either stored too long or at an inadequate temperature. Contamination, most often by salmonella and *Escherichia coli*, more rarely by the bacterium *Listeria*, primarily affects poultry and meats, and, secondly, fish and seafood. To avoid poisoning by contaminated food, certain rules must be followed:

• Be sure, at the moment of purchase, of the origin of food and check the expiration date.

• When you are buying groceries, buy refrigerated or frozen foods last. Put them away immediately when you return home. Transport them in insulated bags, particularly if it is hot or if the trip is long.

• Wash your hands before handling food and wash fruit and vegetables before consuming them.

• Wash utensils and countertops with soap and water if they have been in contact with raw meat before using them for other foods.

• Place foods that must be kept cold in the correct location in the refrigerator. Separate raw and cooked foods. To let air circulate, do not overfill the refrigerator. Keep the temperature of the refrigerator between 32°F and 39°F (0°C and 4°C).

• Do not refreeze food that has been defrosted.

CONTROL OF THE ENVIRONMENT

A good knowledge of the risks present in our environment—at home, at work, or while enjoying leisure activities—helps to prevent accidents.

A SAFE HOME

The home must be arranged in a safe manner for each occupant, from newborns to the elderly. It must have a fire extinguisher and at least one smoke detector and one carbon monoxide detector, whose batteries must be changed every year. Also, it is important to learn about the toxicity of certain construction materials (plumbing, insulation, etc.). The home must also be correctly and regularly ventilated to avoid the formation of moisture or the accumulation of pollutants and thus minimize the risk of respiratory diseases.

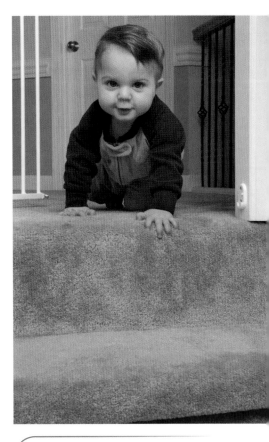

CHILD SAFETY

Dangers that affect children vary depending on their degree of autonomy. A child under 10 years of age should never be left home alone. For children under the age of 1, the main risks are asphyxiation and falling. To minimize these risks:

- Keep the temperature in a newborn's room around 65°F (19°C). Do not allow the child to become overheated with excessive bedding.

- Verify the stability of the crib or bed. The bars should be spaced 1¾–2½ inches (45–65 mm) apart.

- Avoid curtains with cords and jewelry around the neck of the baby.

- Avoid letting a newborn sleep with stuffed animals or pets.

From the age of 1, the child becomes more autonomous and dangers multiply. Be sure to:

- Equip windows with hooks or guards and balconies with protection. Access to stairs should be blocked.

- Place nonslip adhesive mats in the bathtub and shower.

- Block electrical sockets.

- Turn the handles of saucepans towards the back of the stove and keep electrical cords out of reach.

- Place sharp objects, plastic bags, matches, lighters, domestic products, medications, alcoholic beverages, and toxic plants out of reach of children.

SAFETY FOR THE ELDERLY

The reduced mobility of an elderly person increases the risk of falls and traumas. To avoid accidents:

- Eliminate obstacles (low furniture, plants, electrical cords, etc.) in passageways.

- Cover slippery surfaces with nonslip materials.

- Increase points of support: stair ramps; support bars around toilets, in the bath, and in the shower.

- Raise toilet seats and adjust the height of the bed.

- Keep a cordless telephone nearby.

WORRY-FREE LEISURE ACTIVITIES

In order for leisure activities to remain a source of pleasure and satisfaction, they should be practiced using caution. You must:

- Check weather conditions before practicing an activity outdoors.
- Protect yourself from the sun (lotion, sunglasses, hat) and plan for clothes to protect against the cold and rain.
- Bring plenty of water, food, and a first aid kit when going on a long hike.
- Protect yourself again insect bites.
- Avoid feeding or getting close to wild animals, even if they seem harmless, and make noise so as not to surprise them (if you happen to come face to face, distance yourself without looking the animal in the eye and without running or turning your back).
- Verify the state of outdoor equipment before using it.
- Wear a helmet to play sports when there is an elevated risk of shock to the head (bicycling, skiing, etc.).
- Wear a life jacket for water activities.
- Supervise children at all times when near water.
- Forbid access to pools to children in the absence of an adult (all pools must be enclosed by a fence).
- Progressively enter water when it is hot outside to avoid immersion hypothermia (thermal shock).
- Warm up before practicing any physical activity.
- Avoid leaving alone, without notifying anyone.

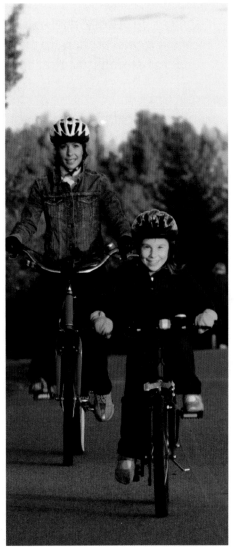

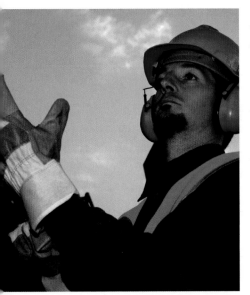

SAFETY AT WORK

Work should not be a source of health problems. A poor position, inadequate movements, and a work space that is poorly organized or ill-adapted to a person's physiognomy can create painful joint and muscle problems over the long term. These may be prevented by calling on **ergonomic** specialists. Reducing accidents and diseases inherent to the practice of a profession is a collective responsibility. Employers must not only apply safety norms and rules, they must also promote them among their employees and consider any improvements that they suggest. Employees must know and apply safety measures, promote them among their colleagues, and suggest improvements. When the situation requires it, it is particularly important to wear protective equipment. It is also necessary to know evacuation plans in the event of fire.

MEDICAL EXAMINATIONS

Our family history, age, and lifestyle predispose us to certain diseases that, in most cases, can be treated if they are diagnosed and treated early. It is thus often recommended to undergo periodic medical examinations.

MEDICAL CHECKUP DURING PREGNANCY

Monitoring pregnancy consists of a series of medical visits, with regular blood tests, urine analyses, and screening tests to ensure the health of the mother and fetus during the entire pregnancy. The first appointment is generally between the 8th and 12th weeks following the last period. During the first exam, the doctor normally establishes the health report of the mother using a questionnaire, a complete physical exam, and a gynecological exam. Generally a cervical cancer test (PAP smear) is completed and a blood analysis is prescribed to determine blood type, verify if the patient is anemic, control her glycemia, and screen certain infectious diseases (gonorrhea, chlamydia, syphilis, AIDS, hepatitis B, rubella, toxoplasmosis). A urine analysis also indicates whether she is suffering from a urinary infection. Other visits will follow, normally once a month until the 32nd week, then once a week during the last month, in order to monitor the weight of the mother, her arterial tension, height and position of her uterus, and the heart rhythm of the fetus. These exams are completed by ultrasounds, normally performed around the 12th, 22nd and 32nd weeks of amenorrhea. These help to determine the date of fertilization, the gender of the fetus, and the position of the placenta, as well as detect potential anomalies.

Other tests may be proposed during pregnancy, particularly:

• The sampling and analysis of amniotic fluid (amniocentesis), between the 14th and 18th weeks of pregnancy, when a chromosomal problem, hereditary or infectious disease, or even a malformation of the fetus is suspected

• The screening for gestational diabetes between the 24th and 28th weeks of pregnancy

• The screening for group B streptococcus, between the 34th and 37th weeks of pregnancy

Prenatal examinations… page 468

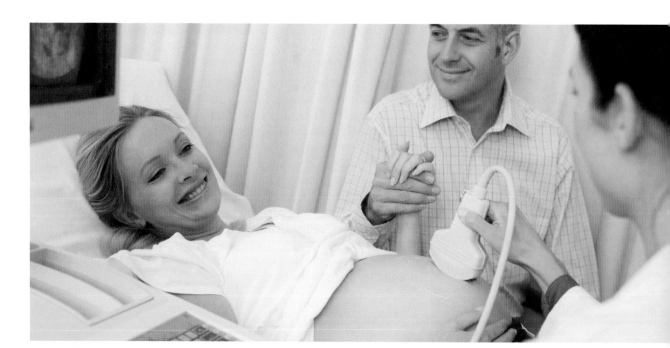

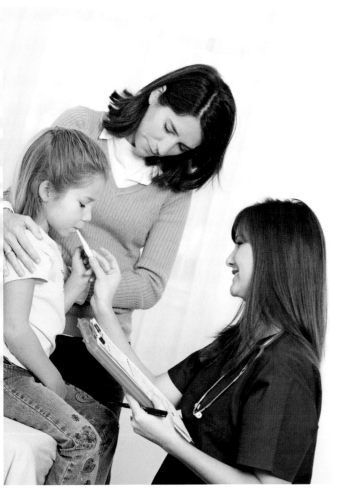

MEDICAL CHECKUPS FOR CHILDREN

At birth, a newborn is subjected to a blood analysis to screen for certain hereditary metabolic diseases. This screening can be completed by a urine analysis that can detect other anomalies, if the parents request it. Periodic medical examinations are therefore advised for the medical follow-up of children.

Be sure to:

• Follow the vaccination schedule.

• Be attentive to the weight, height, and stages of psychomotor development in children: speech, mobility, attention, behavior, etc.

• Have their teeth examined regularly. A first visit to the dentist is advised in the months following the eruption of the first tooth.

• Have your children's eyes examined by an optometrist or ophthalmologist at 3 months, 1 year, and between 3 and 5 years of age. Later, it is recommended to have an eye exam every two years until 10 years old and every 3 years up to 18 years of age.

MEDICAL CHECKUPS FOR ADULTS

Every adult in good health should have a medical exam every year. Preferably, it should be completed by a family doctor who is familiar with the patient's medical file, family history, and lifestyle habits. This exam allows the doctor to follow the development of the patient's state of health and to screen for potential diseases.

To be monitored:

• Dental exam, every year.

• Lipid screening, every 5 years, as of 40 years of age for men and 50 for women.

• Body mass index, every year.

• Screening for high blood pressure, every year, by measuring arterial pressure.

• Colorectal cancer, as of 50 years of age, every 1 to 2 years by screening for blood in the stools (blood culture test) or every 5 years by having a sigmoidoscopy or colonoscopy.

• Breast cancer, by having an annual clinical exam as of 25 years of age and a mammography every 2 years for women over 50 years of age (or as of 40 years of age if there is a family history of breast cancer).

• Cervical cancer, by having an annual gynecological cytology (PAP smear) up to 30 years of age, repeated every 3 years afterward.

• Prostate cancer, every year as of 50 years of age.

HEALTH WHILE TRAVELING

Climate and lifestyle, but also the organization of treatment and the type of health problems (particularly **infectious** diseases), can be very different from one area of the globe to another. In planning for a trip, the health risks that a sudden, sometimes radical, change in environment can cause must be considered.

BEFORE LEAVING

Four to eight weeks before leaving, it is important to consult a doctor or travel health clinic to learn about preventive treatments (antimalarials), **vaccinations**, and the precautions to take depending on the destination. Certain countries require an international vaccination record and an updated vaccination against yellow fever. Here are other precautions to take before leaving:

• Obtain good travel insurance and bring a list of people to contact in the event of emergency, including your doctor.

• Put together a medical kit that could contain, depending on needs, **antipyretic** medications (fever reduction), **anti-inflammatories**, **antalgics** (pain reducers), **antihistamines** (allergy treatment), antidiarrhea medications, a product for disinfecting water, sunscreen with an elevated sun protection factor, repellent, and contraceptives.

• People suffering from a **chronic** disease must bring enough medication and syringes for their needs during the stay as well as a medical certificate justifying their use. Prescription renewal must indicate the name of the active ingredient rather than the brand name.

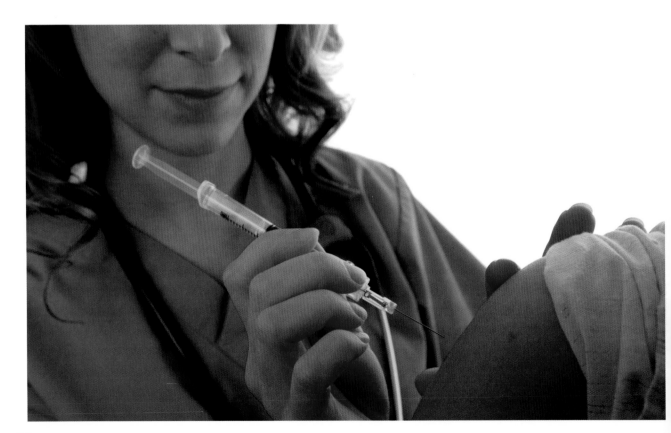

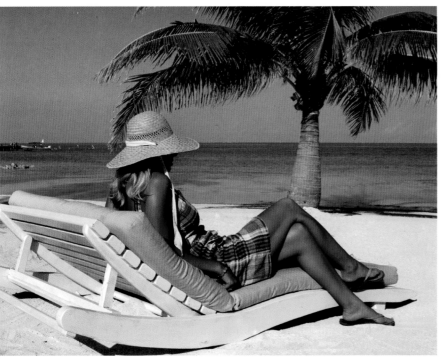

AT THE **DESTINATION**

In warm countries, the sun represents one of the main dangers. Avoid activities during the strongest hours of sun (between 10 a.m. and 3 p.m.), wear protective sunglasses, a hat, and long-sleeved clothes (dark and thick clothes provide better protection from UV rays), stay hydrated by drinking regularly and not waiting until you're thirsty. Showering or sponging also helps to fight against heat.

Here are other precautions that will help you avoid injuries and contaminations, particularly in tropical countries:

- Drink only purified water (i.e. water that has been adequately filtered, boiled, or treated with a disinfectant, or water that is sold in a sealed container).

- Wash your hands before eating (but avoid wiping your hands on a public towel).

- Only consume properly and recently prepared dishes and preferably eat pasteurized dairy products.

- Peel vegetables and fruit.

- Do not consume tap water (not even to brush your teeth), ice, reheated food, or raw food such as salads, vegetables, seafood, or fish.

- Avoid walking barefoot to avoid injuries or bites by venomous animals or even an infection by parasites that can travel through the skin.

- Avoid all direct skin contact with the ground (use lounge chairs to tan).

- Avoid bathing in freshwater or walking in mud and puddles of water.

UPON RETURN

Upon returning from a country that is at risk for malaria, the prescribed treatment must be followed until it is finished. It is not necessary to consult a physician unless the person who returns from a trip suffers from chronic illness, consulted a doctor while traveling, stay or presents specific symptoms that appeared during the trip and that persist upon return: fever, headache, neck pains, persistent diarrhea, skin problems, urinary or genital problems, cough, or thoracic pains.

THE **SYSTEMS**

Each **system** of the human body is composed of a group of organs that share a common function. The organs of the digestive system (stomach, liver, intestine, etc.), for example, are mainly responsible for making it possible for the body to assimilate food. Although each system is responsible for a specific function, each interacts closely with the others to ensure the general proper functioning of the human body.

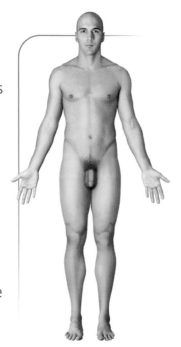

Integumentary system
The integumentary system includes the skin, hair, body hair, nails, sebaceous glands, and sweat glands. It is involved in the protection of the body against the aggressions of the surrounding environment.
The skin… page 62

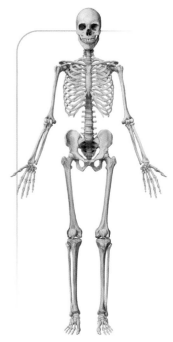

Skeleton
The skeleton is made up of all the bones. It supports the body, protects the vital organs, and participates in the movement of the body.
The bones, joints, and muscles… page 92

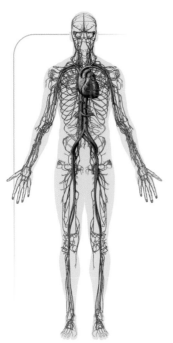

Cardiovascular system
The cardiovascular system, made up of the heart and blood vessels, ensures the blood irrigation of the body and the oxygenation of the blood in the lungs.
The cardiovascular system… page 246

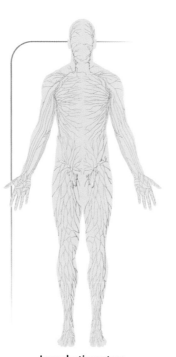

Lymphatic system
The lymphatic system includes all the lymph nodes and lymphatic vessels that ensure the drainage of lymph to the blood circulation and participates in the immune protection of the body.
The immune system… page 276

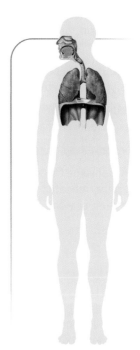

Respiratory system
The structures that make up the respiratory system (nasal cavity, larynx, pharynx, lungs, etc.) provide the oxygen necessary to the body while eliminating the carbon gas that it produces.
The respiratory system… page 308

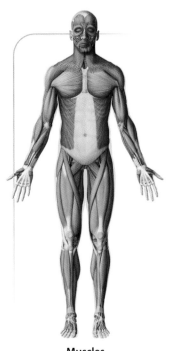

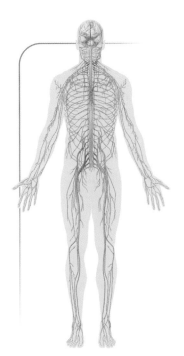

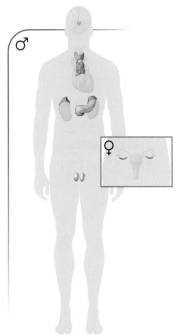

Muscles
The muscles ensure the involuntary contractions of blood vessels and hollow organs, as well as voluntary movement.
The bones, joints, and muscles... page 92

Nervous system
The nervous system, made up of the brain, spinal cord, and nerves, allows the body to perceive sensations, think and carry out all movement.
The nervous system... page 132

Endocrine system
The endocrine system includes all the cells and endocrine glands that regulate certain functions of the body releasing hormones in the blood.
The endocrine system... page 218

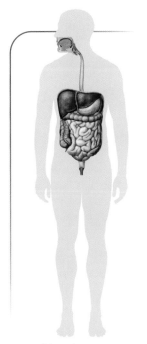

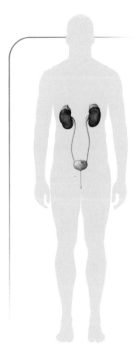

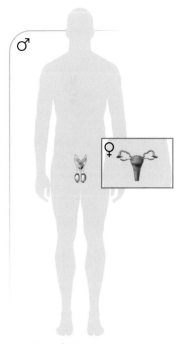

Digestive system
e digestive system, formed of the mouth, digestive tract, and accessory glands, transforms the food into elements assimilable by the body.
The digestive system... page 340

Urinary system
The urinary system is made up of the kidneys, ureters, bladder, and urethra. It creates, transports, stores, and eliminates urine from the body.
The urinary system... page 398

Reproductive system
The reproductive system ensures the reproductive functions with a set of organs (sex glands, genital tracts, external organs, etc.).
The reproductive system... page 414

GENERAL ANATOMY
OF THE **HUMAN BODY**

Anatomy is the science that studies the form and structure of organs and the relationships between them. It is very closely related to physiology, which studies the functioning of the organs. Anatomical vocabulary names each body part and places it in relation to the whole. The human body is divided into four large anatomical areas: head, trunk, upper limbs and lower limbs. These areas are further divided into subregions. They are all connected by complex joints that allow them to move in an independent manner.

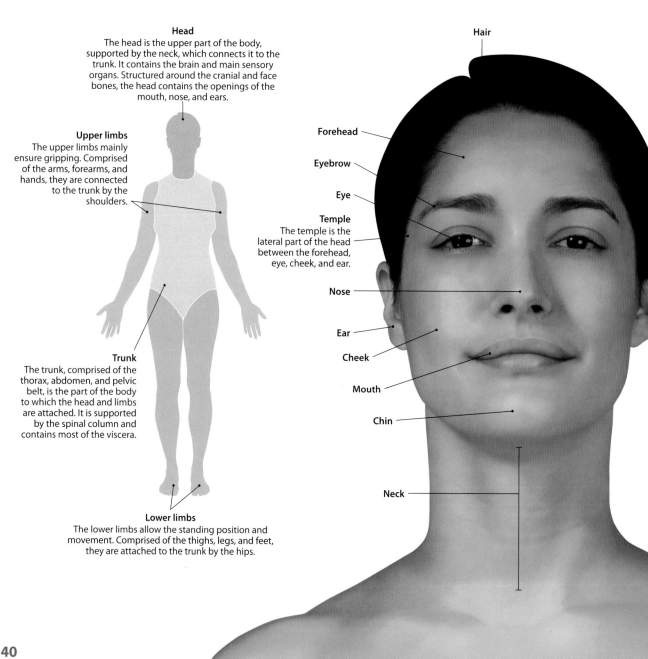

Head
The head is the upper part of the body, supported by the neck, which connects it to the trunk. It contains the brain and main sensory organs. Structured around the cranial and face bones, the head contains the openings of the mouth, nose, and ears.

Upper limbs
The upper limbs mainly ensure gripping. Comprised of the arms, forearms, and hands, they are connected to the trunk by the shoulders.

Trunk
The trunk, comprised of the thorax, abdomen, and pelvic belt, is the part of the body to which the head and limbs are attached. It is supported by the spinal column and contains most of the viscera.

Lower limbs
The lower limbs allow the standing position and movement. Comprised of the thighs, legs, and feet, they are attached to the trunk by the hips.

Hair

Forehead

Eyebrow

Eye

Temple
The temple is the lateral part of the head between the forehead, eye, cheek, and ear.

Nose

Ear

Cheek

Mouth

Chin

Neck

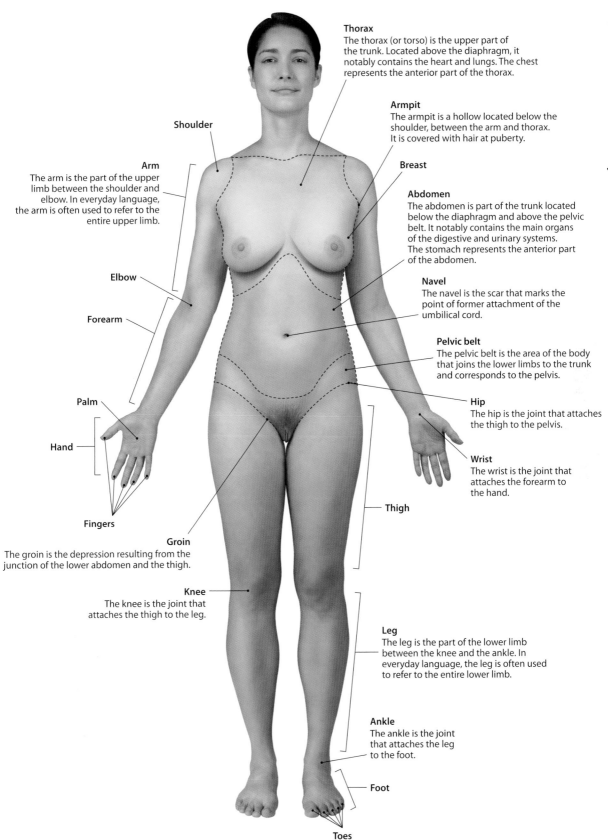

Thorax
The thorax (or torso) is the upper part of the trunk. Located above the diaphragm, it notably contains the heart and lungs. The chest represents the anterior part of the thorax.

Armpit
The armpit is a hollow located below the shoulder, between the arm and thorax. It is covered with hair at puberty.

Breast

Abdomen
The abdomen is part of the trunk located below the diaphragm and above the pelvic belt. It notably contains the main organs of the digestive and urinary systems. The stomach represents the anterior part of the abdomen.

Navel
The navel is the scar that marks the point of former attachment of the umbilical cord.

Pelvic belt
The pelvic belt is the area of the body that joins the lower limbs to the trunk and corresponds to the pelvis.

Hip
The hip is the joint that attaches the thigh to the pelvis.

Wrist
The wrist is the joint that attaches the forearm to the hand.

Thigh

Shoulder

Arm
The arm is the part of the upper limb between the shoulder and elbow. In everyday language, the arm is often used to refer to the entire upper limb.

Elbow

Forearm

Palm

Hand

Fingers

Groin
The groin is the depression resulting from the junction of the lower abdomen and the thigh.

Knee
The knee is the joint that attaches the thigh to the leg.

Leg
The leg is the part of the lower limb between the knee and the ankle. In everyday language, the leg is often used to refer to the entire lower limb.

Ankle
The ankle is the joint that attaches the leg to the foot.

Foot

Toes

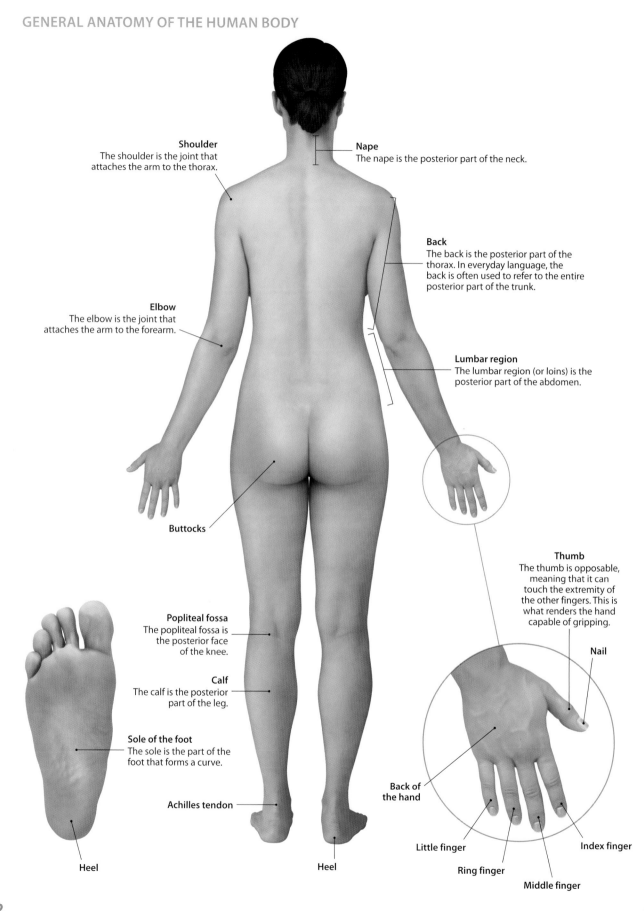

Shoulder
The shoulder is the joint that attaches the arm to the thorax.

Nape
The nape is the posterior part of the neck.

Back
The back is the posterior part of the thorax. In everyday language, the back is often used to refer to the entire posterior part of the trunk.

Elbow
The elbow is the joint that attaches the arm to the forearm.

Lumbar region
The lumbar region (or loins) is the posterior part of the abdomen.

Buttocks

Thumb
The thumb is opposable, meaning that it can touch the extremity of the other fingers. This is what renders the hand capable of gripping.

Nail

Popliteal fossa
The popliteal fossa is the posterior face of the knee.

Calf
The calf is the posterior part of the leg.

Sole of the foot
The sole is the part of the foot that forms a curve.

Back of the hand

Achilles tendon

Heel

Heel

Little finger

Ring finger

Middle finger

Index finger

FROM THE **SYSTEM** TO THE **CELL**

The human body is made up of billions of small base units: cells. Invisible to the naked eye, they group together to form different tissues, which themselves make up organs. The organs in turn form the systems that ensure all the functions of the body.

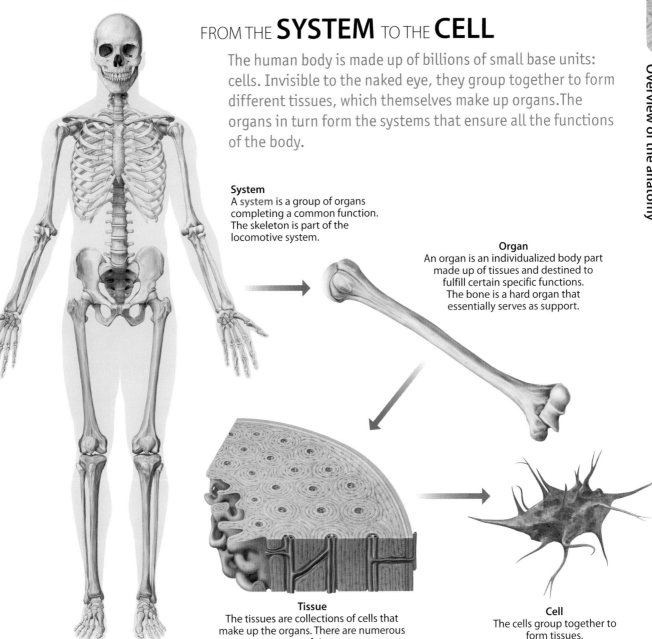

System
A **system** is a group of organs completing a common function. The skeleton is part of the locomotive system.

Organ
An organ is an individualized body part made up of tissues and destined to fulfill certain specific functions. The bone is a hard organ that essentially serves as support.

Tissue
The tissues are collections of cells that make up the organs. There are numerous types of tissues.

Cell
The cells group together to form tissues.

TISSUES

A tissue is a collection of cells that possess a similar structure and fulfill a common function. Thus, muscle cells, which form muscle tissue, have the capacity to contract, generating different movements of the body. Four types of primary tissue make up the entire body: epithelial tissue, conjunctive tissue, muscular tissue, and nervous tissue. Epithelial tissue, which includes the superficial layer of the skin, provides a covering and secretion. It covers and protects the exterior of the body and its internal cavities, in addition to constituting glands. The conjunctive tissue supports and connects the various tissues and organs of the body. It is subdivided into several varieties, including bone tissue, cartilage, blood, adipose tissue (fat), and fibrous tissue (which forms the deep layer of skin, tendons, and ligaments).

Bone tissue... page 95
Muscular tissue... page 99

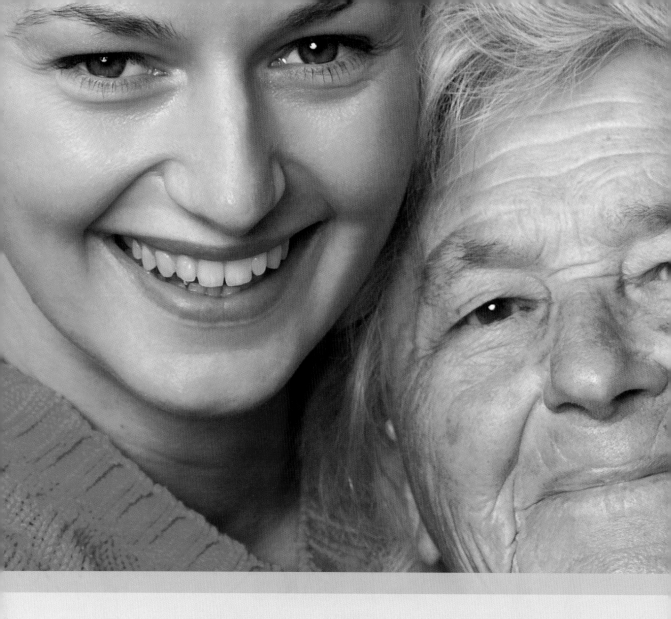

CELLS

Our body is made up of billions of cells. These cells form tissues that make up organs. Despite their diversity, all of the cells in our body are made from the division of one cell that was formed by the union of an ovum and a sperm cell. Most cells renew themselves through cell division. Among other functions, they have the ability to create proteins that allow our body to function properly. Within their nucleus, they also hold **genetic** material that is unique to each one of us.

Some diseases are the result of cell malfunctioning or the malfunctioning of the tissues that they make up. When a tissue is not properly nourished by blood circulation, it dies from **necrosis** (or gangrene). If a tissue retains an excessive quantity of fluid, an **edema** forms. Also, sometimes cells can multiply in an abnormal manner, leading to the development of a cyst or tumor. A malignant tumor, or cancer, is made up of abnormal cells that invade a tissue and then migrate to different places within the body. Certain cell malfunctions that are present at the beginning of embryo formation can cause incurable genetic or chromosomal diseases, like trisomy.

THE **HUMAN CELL**

The cell is the basic unit that makes up tissues in the human body. The human body is made up of 60,000 billion cells. In general, their diameter does not exceed a few hundredths of a millimeter, which makes them invisible to the naked eye. Despite their small size, cells are living and organized elements that are born, nourished, multiply, and die. The human body has about 200 types of cells. Even though they have distinctive features and are very different, depending on the functions that they perform in the body, almost all cells have the same general structure.

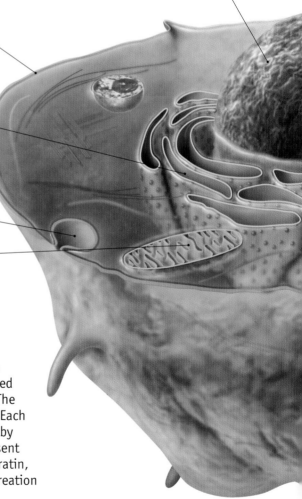

Cell nucleus
The cell nucleus contains genetic material and controls the creation of proteins.

Cell membrane
The cell membrane forms the exterior boundary of the cell. It controls what enters and exits the cell.

Endoplasmic reticulum
The endoplasmic reticulum participates in the creation of proteins.

Vacuole
Vacuoles are small cavities in the cell that contain substances intended to be stored or evacuated. The number of vacuoles is variable.

Mitochondrion
Mitochondria, present in a variable number, ensure the production and storage of the energy that is necessary for the functioning of the cell.

PROTEINS

Proteins are in the makeup of all living beings. Those that are present in food are broken down during digestion and absorbed by the cells that then use them to create their own proteins. The cells of the human body create millions of different proteins. Each one participates in the structure and functioning of the body by performing a specific task. For example, the hemoglobin present in red blood cells transports oxygen throughout the body. Keratin, another protein, is produced by skin cells and is used in the creation of nails and hair.

CELL LONGEVITY

Some cells, such as white blood cells, can die only hours after their birth. Others live for months and even years. Neurons, which are incapable of reproducing, hold the record for longevity: their life span can be equal to that of the body, that's more than 100 years!

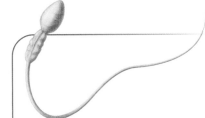

Sperm cells
Sperm cells are the only cells that have a flagellum, allowing them to propel themselves.

Cytoplasm
The cytoplasm is a gelatinous substance in which the organelles (microscopic organs of the cell) are submerged.

Golgi apparatus
The Golgi apparatus participates in the maturing and transport of proteins in the cell.

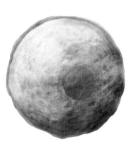

Ovum
The ovum is the largest cell of the body.

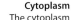

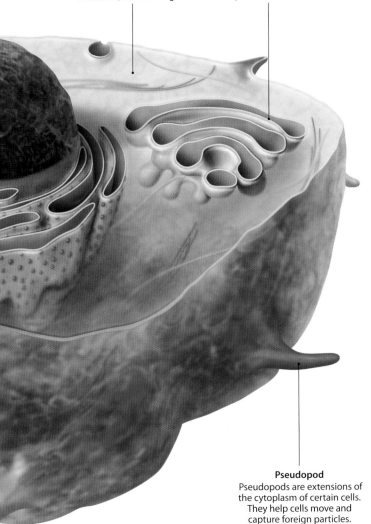

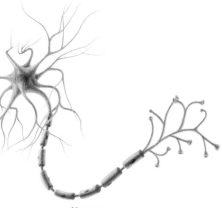

Neurons
Neurons are nerve cells that can reach a length of as long as one meter.

Pseudopod
Pseudopods are extensions of the cytoplasm of certain cells. They help cells move and capture foreign particles.

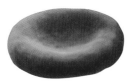

Red blood cells
Red blood cells are cells that can change shape to pass through the narrowest blood vessels.

DNA AND GENES

It is at the heart of cells that **genetic** information is inscribed, which determines the unique nature of each person. This information is carried by genes, united in one large molecule: deoxyribonucleic acid, or DNA. DNA is present in the nucleus of cells in the form of long chromatin entangled filaments. During the process of cell division, the chromatin condenses to form 46 small X-shaped rods, the chromosomes. Whether in the form of chromatin or chromosomes, DNA is made up of about 25,000 genes that constitute the human genetic material.

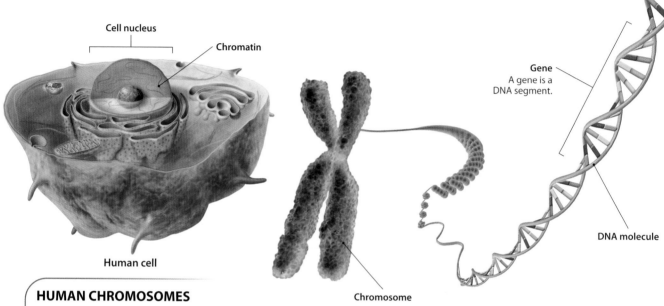

Cell nucleus

Chromatin

Gene
A gene is a
DNA segment.

DNA molecule

Human cell

Chromosome

HUMAN CHROMOSOMES

The human cell contains 23 pairs of chromosomes. The chromosomes of just one pair are inherited from each parent at the time of fertilization. There are 22 pairs of autosomes and one pair of sex chromosomes. Autosomes are the chromosomes that carry hereditary characteristics that are not related to sex. The sex chromosomes are responsible for determining sex. They are identical for women (two Xs) and different for men (one X and one Y, which is smaller).

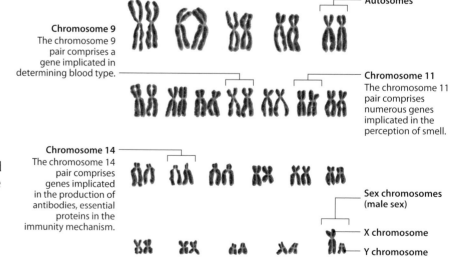

Autosomes

Chromosome 9
The chromosome 9 pair comprises a gene implicated in determining blood type.

Chromosome 11
The chromosome 11 pair comprises numerous genes implicated in the perception of smell.

Chromosome 14
The chromosome 14 pair comprises genes implicated in the production of antibodies, essential proteins in the immunity mechanism.

Sex chromosomes (male sex)

X chromosome

Y chromosome

The 23 pairs of human chromosomes

CELL DIVISION

Every day, cells renew themselves by dividing at a continuous rate. Billions die that are then replaced by just as many new cells. Cell division is the formation of two identical daughter cells from one mother cell. During this process, the **genetic** material, or DNA, is identically reproduced. The daughter cells in turn divide, and so on and so forth. Cell division allows for the healing and regeneration of tissues. It also allows for the development and growth of the body, from an embryo to adulthood.

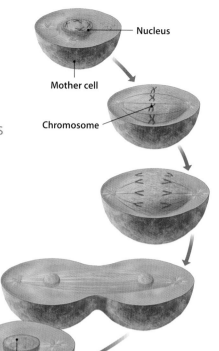

Nucleus

Mother cell

Chromosome

Daughter cells

New nucleus

STEM CELLS

A stem cell is a cell that is capable, through cell division, of creating different, specialized types of cells. Bone marrow stem cells, for example, are at the origin of all blood cells. Even more remarkable are the stem cells that make up a human embryo that is only a few days old. In a short period of time, these cells can create practically all of the tissues and organs of the body.

In medicine, stem cells can be introduced to a sick organ to regenerate tissues. For several decades now, stem cells taken from bone marrow have been used to treat blood pathologies, such as leukemia. Experiments with stem cells originating from human embryos began in 1998, raising controversy for ethical reasons. Defenders of this research emphasize that it could allow for the treatment of a multitude of afflictions: cancer, Parkinson's disease, Alzheimer's, paralysis, myocardial infarction, etc. Opponents maintain that these experiments promote the destruction of human embryos.

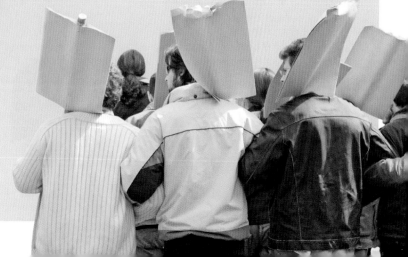

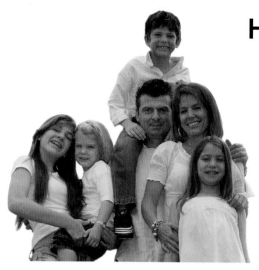

HEREDITY

Hair color, eye color, skin color, the shape of the nose, or predisposition to certain diseases are some hereditary characteristics, meaning that they are transmitted from one generation to another, from one individual to their descendants. During fertilization, the genes from two parents combine in a random manner to form the **genetic** material of the child.

DOMINANT AND RECESSIVE GENES

A hereditary characteristic, hair color, for example, is the expression of a gene. Each individual possesses two samples of each gene, one coming from the father, and the other coming from the mother. These samples are situated at the same level on each of the chromosomes of a pair. The genes are said to be dominant or recessive, depending on their mode of expression. A dominant gene is a hereditary characteristic that expresses itself in being present on only one of the chromosomes of a pair. Dark hair, for example, is coded by a dominant gene. A recessive gene is a hereditary characteristic that must be present on both chromosomes of a pair to be expressed. Blond hair is coded by a recessive gene. At the time of fertilization, there are four genetic combination possibilities for each hereditary characteristic, depending on the ovum and the sperm cell that are present.

CHROMOSOMAL AND GENETIC DISEASES

A chromosomal disease is caused by a defect in chromosome structure (a break, for example) or in the number of chromosomes: presence of an additional chromosome (trisomy) or absence of a chromosome (monosomy) in one of the pairs. A genetic disease is a disease caused by an abnormal gene. When it is transmitted to descendants, this disease is said to be hereditary.

DNA and genes... page 48

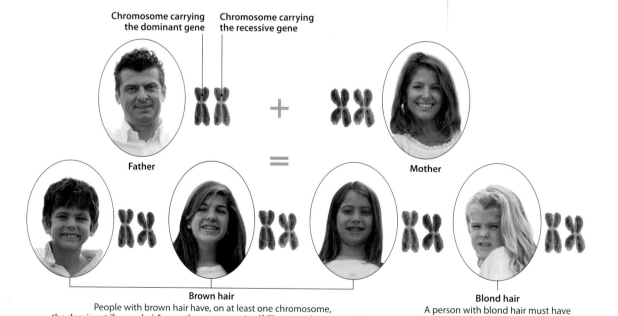

Chromosome carrying the dominant gene   Chromosome carrying the recessive gene

Father   +   =   Mother

Brown hair
People with brown hair have, on at least one chromosome, the dominant "brown hair" gene that expresses itself. They can also possess the recessive "blond hair" gene that is not expressed, but can be passed to descendants.

Blond hair
A person with blond hair must have received the "blond hair" gene from both parents.

TRISOMIES

Trisomies are chromosomal diseases that are characterized by the presence of an extra chromosome in the cells of the body. Most trisomies lead to spontaneous abortion or the death of an infant within a few days. Otherwise, trisomic people demonstrate symptoms and, more or less, significant complications that reduce their life expectancy. Trisomies are often indicated by the number of the abnormal chromosome pair. Trisomy 21 is the most frequent: it affects, on average, 1 in 700 children, without distinction of sex.

TRISOMY 21

Trisomy 21, or Down Syndrome, is characterized by the presence of an extra chromosome in the 21st pair. In addition to mental and psychomotor retardation, children with trisomy 21 demonstrate several typical morphological characteristics, immune deficiency, anatomical malformations, and metabolic disorders that reduce their life expectancy to 50 years old. The incidence of the disease increases with the age of the mother, because the chromosomal defect generally occurs during the formation of ova. In certain countries, a prenatal screening (amniocentesis) test is recommended for pregnant women over 35 years old.

Prenatal exams... page 468

TRISOMIES 13 AND 18

More rare than trisomy 21, trisomy 13 and trisomy 18 lead to severe mental retardation, in addition to multiple malformations that seriously reduce the life expectancy of the child. In the case of trisomy 18, diagnosed in 1 out of 10,000 newborns, the survival rate in the first year is less than 10%.

TRISOMIES

SYMPTOMS:
Trisomy 21: distinctive morphological characteristics, mental and psychomotor retardation, cardiac malformations, metabolic disorders.

TREATMENTS:
Trisomies are incurable diseases. Trisomy 21: surgery allows for the correction of certain cardiac malformations.

PREVENTION:
Prenatal screening (amniocentesis, first-trimester diagnostic ultrasound).

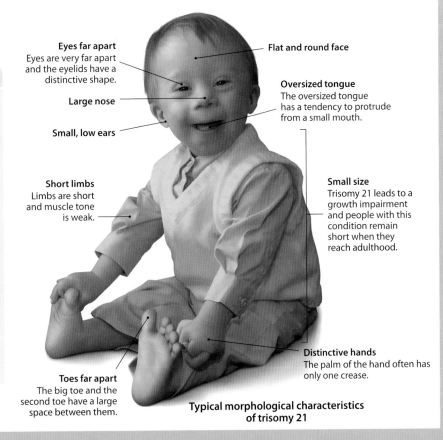

Eyes far apart
Eyes are very far apart and the eyelids have a distinctive shape.

Large nose

Small, low ears

Flat and round face

Oversized tongue
The oversized tongue has a tendency to protrude from a small mouth.

Short limbs
Limbs are short and muscle tone is weak.

Small size
Trisomy 21 leads to a growth impairment and people with this condition remain short when they reach adulthood.

Distinctive hands
The palm of the hand often has only one crease.

Toes far apart
The big toe and the second toe have a large space between them.

Typical morphological characteristics of trisomy 21

GANGRENE

Gangrene is the death of a tissue, generally caused by a local interruption of blood circulation. This interruption can be generated by a disease, such as diabetes. It can also be of external origin (frostbite, prolonged compression). The cells of the affected region are not sufficiently oxygenated and die, which causes the destruction of tissues. A bacterial **infection** can develop on the gangrenous tissues and spread to neighboring tissues, increasing the severity of the affliction.

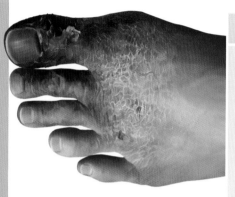

Gangrenous tissues
Tissues that are not supplied blood first become painful and purplish. When they die, they become hard and blacken. In the case of infection, the tissues redden, swell, and ooze.

GANGRENE

SYMPTOMS:
Progressive blackening of tissues with blisters and oozing in the case of infection. Insensitivity of gangrenous tissues.

TREATMENT:
Reestablishment of blood circulation and ablation of affected tissues. Antibiotics in the case of infection. Amputation when an entire limb is affected, or to stop the spread of an infection. Hyperbaric oxygen therapy.

PREVENTION:
Avoid long exposure to cold and prolonged compression. Treat diseases that can cause an interruption in blood circulation. Clean and disinfect wounds.

CYSTS

A cyst is an abnormal cavity filled with a liquid, semi-liquid, or gaseous substance that forms in a tissue or organ and is defined by one of its walls. Cysts can appear on any part of the body. Their size varies and most are not serious. Sebaceous cysts are painless accumulations of sebum under the skin. They are susceptible to infection and can then become red and painful. Synovial cysts develop in the joints, particularly in the knees and wrists. Some cysts, like ovarian or renal cysts, can disrupt the proper functioning of the affected organ.

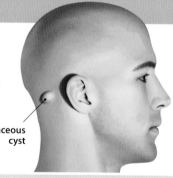

Sebaceous cyst

CYSTS

SYMPTOMS:
More or less voluminous growth, sensation of compression, pain, functional discomfort. Some cysts show no symptoms.

TREATMENT:
Puncturing of cyst or surgical ablation. Hormonal treatment can repair some cysts (breasts, ovaries). Sometimes cysts can disappear spontaneously.

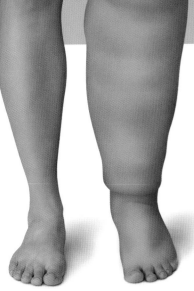

EDEMA

Edema is an accumulation of serous fluid in tissues. It results in swelling, sometimes very localized (insect bite), sometimes it spreads to an organ, limb, or the entire body. Edema is often caused by poor blood or lymph circulation. It can also be caused by a blood imbalance due to liver or kidney disease, by an **inflammatory** reaction (prick, allergy), or by taking certain medications. When it affects vital organs, like the lungs, respiratory tract, or the brain, an edema can be fatal.

Lymphatic system... page 281

Edema affecting only one leg

EDEMA IN THE LOWER LIMBS

The most frequent types of edema affect the lower limbs. When edema only affects one leg, its main cause is a restriction of vein circulation from phlebitis or varicose veins. When it affects both legs, it may be caused by cardiac or renal insufficiency, or by cirrhosis of the liver.

EDEMA

SYMPTOMS:
More or less significant swelling, weight gain, pain, difficulty moving, sensation of heat, and compression.

TREATMENT:
Treatments stimulating blood circulation (cardioactive, vasodilators, phlebotonic, anticoagulants) or the elimination of organic waste (diuretics, lymphatic drainage). Wearing of compression stockings, surgery, low-salt diet.

PREVENTION:
Treat diseases that can cause edema.

EDEMA DURING PREGNANCY

Swelling, notably in the feet and ankles, is common in pregnant women, in which pregancy hormones can cause water retention. This type of edema is common and, for the most part, is not dangerous.
To relieve edema:

- Raise your legs when you are seated or lying down.
- Wear compression stockings and slip them on before getting up.
- Avoid standing for prolonged periods.
- Wash feet in cold water.

   Warning! Swelling accompanied with an increased weight gain, headaches, vision troubles, and ringing in the ears are signs of preeclampsia and require immediate medical attention.

BENIGN TUMORS

A tumor is a localized growth in the volume of a tissue. It is caused by the proliferation of new cells that resemble the cells of the affected tissue. A tumor can be benign or malignant (cancer). A benign tumor develops slowly, without invading neighboring tissues. The cells that it is made up of do not have a morphological anomaly. Generally speaking, this type of tumor does not endanger a person's life. A benign tumor can nevertheless prevent the affected organ from functioning correctly and some can degenerate into cancer. There are several types of benign tumors, depending on the tissue where they develop.

ADENOMAS

Adenomas are tumors that essentially develop on the glands. The main glands affected are the prostate, hypophysis, thyroid, parathyroid, and adrenal glands. Adenomas can also affect certain types of mucous membranes, like those of the colon or the uterus.

FIBROMAS

Fibromas are more rare tumors that form in fibrous tissues, particularly in that of the skin, bones, kidneys, ovaries, blood vessels, and mouth. Uterine fibromas are actually myomas because they affect the muscular tissue of the uterus.

LIPOMAS

Lipomas are tumors that appear in the fatty tissues of the body, specifically under the skin, where they form painless, flabby, and mobile masses.

MYOMAS

Myomas are tumors that affect muscular tissue, like that of the uterus, and specifically affect adults 25 to 40 years of age.

POLYPS

Polyps are tumors that develop on a mucous membrane, notably the mucous membranes of the uterus, digestive tube (stomach, colon, rectum), and upper respiratory tract (nasal cavities, vocal cords), where they can affect breathing or hearing, or even result in voice changes. They are often pedicles, meaning that a foot (pedicle) connects the mucous membrane and the polyp. Some polyps present a strong risk of becoming cancerous, particularly polyps in the colon. They must be removed and analyzed.

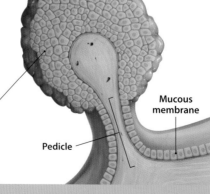

Polyp head
The polyp head, with a rounded or oval shape, is made of cells that have multiplied.

Pedicle

Mucous membrane

BENIGN TUMORS

SYMPTOMS:
Palpable mass or visible on an X-ray, leading to various problems. Some tumors are asymptomatic.

TREATMENT:
Surgical or cryotherapy ablation, if the tumor affects the functioning of the concerned organ or presents a risk of becoming cancerous.

PREVENTION:
Avoid tobacco and prolonged exposure to the sun without protection. A balanced diet rich in fiber reduces the formation of polyps in the colon.

CANCER

Each year, more than 10 million new cases of cancer are reported in the world. Cancer is one of the main causes of death in Western countries, where it is responsible for approximately one in four deaths. Cancer (malignant tumors) is characterized by the spreading of abnormal cells. These cells invade neighboring tissues and, in the absence of diagnosis and early treatment, can spread throughout the entire body. Cancer can affect any body tissue. However, cells that reproduce infrequently, such as muscle fibers and neurons, are very rarely affected by the disease. Some types of cancer, like breast or colon cancer, are encouraged by hereditary predispositions. However, it is estimated that 90% of cancer cases are due to external factors, of which 80% could be linked to an individual's lifestyle. Tobacco, poor dietary habits, viruses, chemical substances, and radiation are among the main causes of cancer.

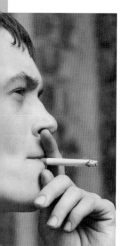

TOBACCO

Between 80% and 90% of lung cancer cases are caused by tobacco, which releases toxic substances during consumption. Tobacco is also responsible for mouth and larynx cancer and it promotes numerous other cancers (bladder, esophagus, etc.). The carcinogenic effect of tobacco is multiplied when it is combined with alcohol.

POOR DIETARY HABITS

There are correlations between certain dietary habits and certain cancers, particularly the overconsumption of fat and a lack of fiber (colon cancer) or vitamins. Alcohol is a risk factor for cancer of the liver, mouth, pharynx, and esophagus.

CHEMICAL SUBSTANCES

Several chemical substances have been recognized as carcinogenic, meaning susceptible to causing cancer: tar, asbestos, heavy metals, paint solvents, pesticides, etc.

VIRUSES

Certain viruses can promote genetic modifications of the cells that they infect. Also, the hepatitis B virus can cause liver cancer. Certain types of papillomavirus, which are sexually transmitted, can cause cervical cancer. In addition, a virus leads to the weakening of the immune system, which can prevent the body from efficiently fighting the appearance of abnormal cells.

RADIATION

An individual can be exposed to radiation that is natural (from the sun) or artificial (radiological exams, nuclear tests, tanning lamps, etc.). Their carcinogenic effects are observed above a certain dose that can vary depending on the individual.

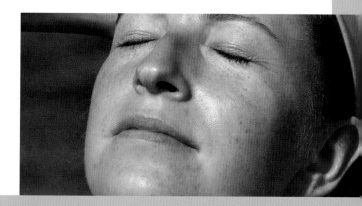

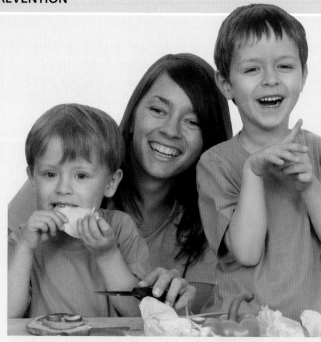

CANCER PREVENTION

Some cancers are caused by factors that are beyond our control, but for the majority of them, their occurrence can be prevented by modifying our lifestyle habits. Here are a few precautions to take to lower the risks of developing cancer, or to quickly stop its progression.

■ PAY ATTENTION TO WARNING SIGNS

Cancer does not always manifest itself with specific signs, but certain perpetuated or intensified symptoms require particular attention, specifically if you are an at-risk individual (smoker, alcoholic, person with a family history of cancer). Consult a doctor if you experience any of the following symptoms:

- Abnormal, lasting, and growing fatigue
- Loss of appetite or significant weight loss
- Resistant fever
- Specific points of pain that may intensify
- Abnormal bleeding
- Repeated infections
- Nodule or hardening, painful or not, of the skin, muscle, breast, or testicle
- Lesion that does not heal and spreads
- Wart or beauty mark that changes: thickening, color change, bleeding

■ HAVE REGULAR SCREENING TESTS

Early cancer screenings thanks to different exams allow for more rapid and less intensive treatment, which noticeably increases the chances of recovery. You should regularly have these exams, if possible, specifically if you are an at-risk individual: mammograms starting at 40 years of age for breast cancer, cervical smears for cervical cancer, a colonoscopy for cancer of the colon and rectum, a rectal exam for prostate cancer, self-checks for skin cancer, testicular cancer, breast cancer, etc.

■ ADOPT A HEALTHY AND BALANCED DIET

A varied and balanced diet is the key to good health and preventing cancer. It is important to limit your consumption of food that is rich in salt, in calories, or in fatty animal materials, like red meat, deli meat, fast foods, or soft drinks. The consumption of 5 to 10 servings of fruit and vegetables per day is also recommended. Eat foods that are rich in fiber, vitamins, and antioxidants like whole grains, nuts, vegetable oils, red fruit, green vegetables, tomatoes, cauliflower, and fish.

Nutrition... page 11

■ MAINTAIN A HEALTHY WEIGHT

Being overweight is an aggravating factor for some cancers, like lung cancer, uterine cancer, and colon cancer. To maintain a healthy weight, adopt a balanced diet and exercise regularly.

Healthy weight... page 20

■ CONSUME ALCOHOL IN MODERATION

The excessive consumption of alcohol promotes damage that can cause cancer of the liver, esophagus, mouth, and throat. The risk increases if you combine alcohol consumption with cigarettes.

CANCER PREVENTION

■ **DON'T SMOKE**

Smoking is the number one cause of lung cancer, but it can also cause other cancers (mouth, larynx, liver, esophagus, etc.). Second-hand smoke is also a non-negligible risk factor.

■ **EXERCISE REGULARLY**

Physical activity decreases the risks of cancer by stimulating the immune system. You should regularly do endurance, flexibility, and muscle strengthening exercises.

Exercising... page 22

■ **PROTECT YOURSELF AGAINST SEXUALLY TRANSMITTED INFECTIONS**

Short of having a stable relationship with your partner, use a condom during every sexual encounter. Certain sexually transmitted viruses, such as human papillomavirus, can lead to cancer (cervical cancer).

■ **PROTECT YOUR SKIN FROM THE SUN**

Intensive exposure to rays from the sun can lead to skin cancer, even several years after exposure. Protect yourself from the sun and avoid using tanning beds or lamps.

■ **TAKE CARE OF AND PREVENT DISEASES THAT MAY LEAD TO CANCER**

Certain diseases, like hepatitis B, can lead to cancer. It is important to treat them or to protect yourself against them through vaccination.

■ **HANDLE HAZARDOUS PRODUCTS CAREFULLY**

Certain substances or chemical products, like asbestos, pesticides, or paint, contain hazardous elements that may cause cancer. To protect yourself, avoid them, or use them with caution: work in a well-ventilated place, wear protective clothing, a mask, etc.

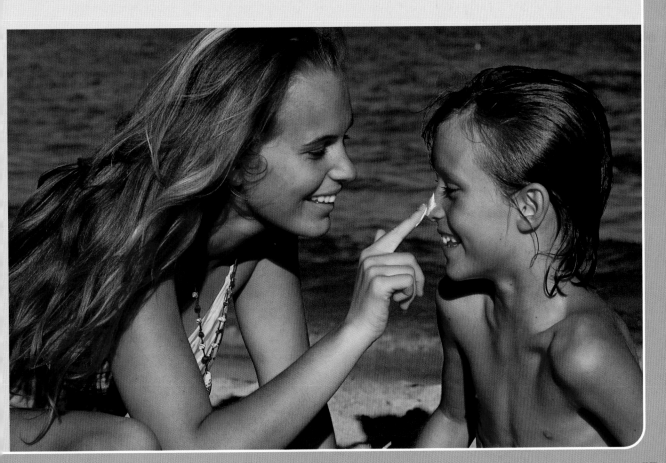

FORMATION AND EVOLUTION OF CANCER

Cancer develops in various stages. The process begins with **genetic** mutations in a cell, often under the effect of an exterior carcinogenic factor (tobacco, diet, radiation, virus, etc.). This cell multiplies in transmitting the genetic anomaly to its descendants, which then undergo new alterations, making the cancer more aggressive. The cancerous cells spread and form a malignant tumor in the tissue where they are implanted. When the extent of a tumor is limited to its original tissue, the cancer is said to be "in situ." Treated in this initial stage, the disease has a high chance for recovery. When the tumor has spread to neighboring tissues, the cancer is considered to be invasive and becomes more difficult to treat. Certain cancerous cells detach themselves and move using lymphatic and blood vessels. Generally, they first attach to lymph nodes, sometimes causing their swelling. They then migrate to other organs where they form tumors called metastases. The appearance of metastases characterizes cancers at the most advanced stage (spread cancer).

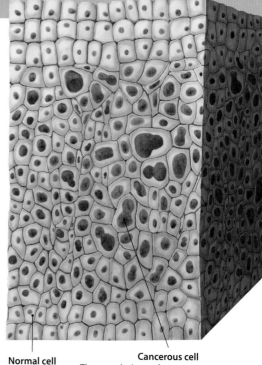

Normal cell

Cancerous cell
The morphology of cancerous cells is more or less abnormal depending on the degree of aggressiveness of the cancer: various sizes and shapes, voluminous nuclei often containing an abnormal number of chromosomes.

THE GRADE AND STAGE OF CANCER

A malignant tumor spreads and becomes increasingly aggressive. This double evolution is expressed using two scales: the grade (which reflects its degree of aggressiveness) and the stage (indicator of the extent of the tumor). Generally, the grade of a cancer ranges from 1 to 4: with grade 1 corresponding to not very abnormal cells that closely resemble the cells from their original tissue, while grade 4 corresponds to very abnormal cells. TNM classification (Tumor Node Metastasis) is the most frequently used system to describe the stage of cancer.

TNM CLASSIFICATION OF CANCER STAGES					
T (size and propagation in neighboring tissues)		**N** (propagation in lymph nodes)		**M** (metastasis)	
T1	In situ of small size	**N0**	Absence	**M0**	Absence
T2	In situ of average size	**N1**	Cancer present in some lymph nodes close to the tumor	**M1**	Presence
T3	In situ of large size	**N2**	Average lymph node invasion	–	–
T4	Invasive cancer	**N3**	Cancer present in numerous lymph nodes or in distant lymph nodes	–	–

METASTASES

Metastases are secondary sources of cancer. They can develop in most organs, but the most frequently affected are the liver, lungs, bones, and brain. Cancerous cells that make up a metastasis conserve the characteristics of their original tissue, which allows them to recognize and localize the initial cancer. The treatment of metastases is difficult and reoccurrences are frequent.

TYPES OF CANCER

The incidence of different types of cancer in a population varies depending on the level of development, lifestyle, and genetic factors. Lung cancer is one of the most common and biggest killers in the world, essentially due to the widespread use of tobacco. Cancer caused by viral or bacterial infections is more widespread in poor countries in Asia, Africa, and Latin America. They especially affect the liver (hepatitis B virus), cervix (human papillomavirus), and stomach (*Heliobacter pylori* bacterium). Prostate, breast, and colon cancer are the most frequent in wealthy countries. They are in part attributed to being overweight, physical inactivity, and a diet rich in fat and low in fresh fruit and vegetables.

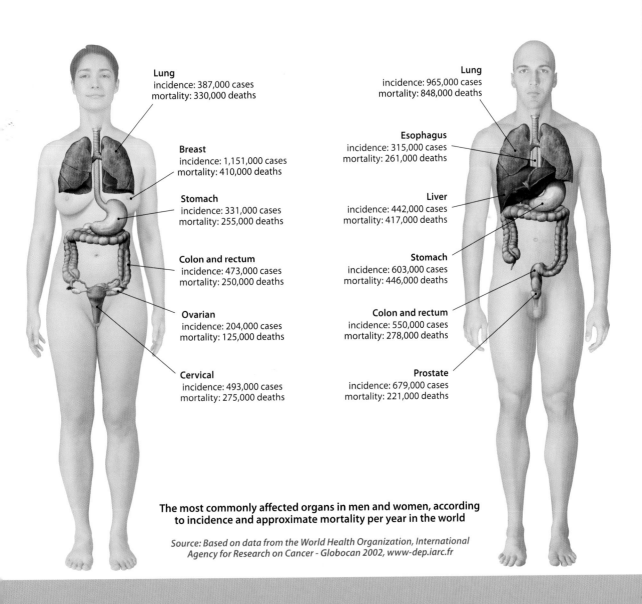

Lung
incidence: 387,000 cases
mortality: 330,000 deaths

Breast
incidence: 1,151,000 cases
mortality: 410,000 deaths

Stomach
incidence: 331,000 cases
mortality: 255,000 deaths

Colon and rectum
incidence: 473,000 cases
mortality: 250,000 deaths

Ovarian
incidence: 204,000 cases
mortality: 125,000 deaths

Cervical
incidence: 493,000 cases
mortality: 275,000 deaths

Lung
incidence: 965,000 cases
mortality: 848,000 deaths

Esophagus
incidence: 315,000 cases
mortality: 261,000 deaths

Liver
incidence: 442,000 cases
mortality: 417,000 deaths

Stomach
incidence: 603,000 cases
mortality: 446,000 deaths

Colon and rectum
incidence: 550,000 cases
mortality: 278,000 deaths

Prostate
incidence: 679,000 cases
mortality: 221,000 deaths

The most commonly affected organs in men and women, according to incidence and approximate mortality per year in the world

Source: Based on data from the World Health Organization, International Agency for Research on Cancer - Globocan 2002, www-dep.iarc.fr

CANCER TREATMENTS

The efficiency of cancer treatments essentially depends on the swiftness of the diagnosis and the stage of the disease. The more advanced the cancer (invasive), the more complicated it is to treat. Ablation of the tumor through surgery is the main treatment, but this is often combined with **chemotherapy, radiation therapy,** or **hormone therapy** sessions. Recovery comes often after several years of remission because metastases can develop after a preliminary treatment. If the disease is incurable, **palliative treatment** is implemented.

SURGICAL TREATMENT OF CANCER

Surgery aims for the ablation of a tumor, or of the entire affected organ. The ablation of lymph nodes close to the initial tumor is often done as a preventative measure. It eliminates secondary cancerous foci and diminishes the risk of the disease reappearing. Metastases are also removed when their placement and size allow it.

ANTICANCER CHEMOTHERAPY

Anticancer chemotherapy aims to destroy cancerous cells or prevent them from developing, with the assistance of medications. These medications are administered to the patients, often intravenously, at a rate that depends on the condition of the patients and their disease. Very exhausting, chemotherapy treatments are followed by periods of rest. Since it acts without distinction on all of the cells that develop quickly (notably blood cells, digestive cells, and epithelial cells), chemotherapy has numerous side effects: nausea, canker sores, diarrhea, constipation, temporary hair loss (partial or total), increased sensitivity to infections, anemia, bleeding (nose, gums), etc.

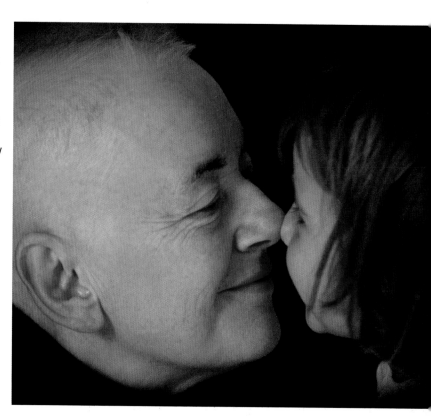

ANTICANCER HORMONE THERAPY

Anticancer hormone therapy halts the growth of certain hormone-dependent tumors, whose appearance and development are promoted by sex hormones (breast, prostate, and endometrium cancer). It calls for various techniques aiming to suppress the effects of hormones on the tumor. Surgical castration consists in the ablation of a gland producing the hormones (testicles or ovaries). It is a permanent operation. On the contrary, chemical castration is reversible: it consists in administering medication that blocks the production of hormones by the glands. Another hormone therapy technique aims to administer molecules that block the action of hormones on the hormonal receptors of cancerous cells.

CANCER

SYMPTOMS:
Intense fatigue, significant weight loss, various pains, bleeding, palpable mass increasing in volume, repeated infections, malfunction of the affected organ. Certain cancers are asymptomatic for a long period of time.

TREATMENT:
Surgery (ablation of the tumor or affected organ), radiation therapy, chemotherapy, immunotherapy, hormone therapy.

PREVENTION:
Avoid unprotected exposure to the sun, do not smoke, adopt a healthy diet, protect yourself against sexually transmitted diseases. Screening (mammogram, rectal exam, colonoscopy, etc.), particularly for at-risk individuals. Anti-papmoma virus vaccination.

RADIATION THERAPY
Radiation therapy consists of administering specific rays, called ionizing rays. These rays cause DNA damage that leads to the death of cells. It is carried out in daily sessions, each lasting several minutes, for several weeks. The objective of radiation therapy is to destroy cancerous cells. Damage, reversible or not, can nevertheless appear in the surrounding healthy tissues. When possible, curietherapy prevents some of these side effects. This radiation therapy technique consists in introducing a radioactive substance in a cancerous tumor or in an organ affected by cancer. It allows for the concentration of radioactive emissions on the tumor to destroy it, while reducing side effects on the neighboring tissues.

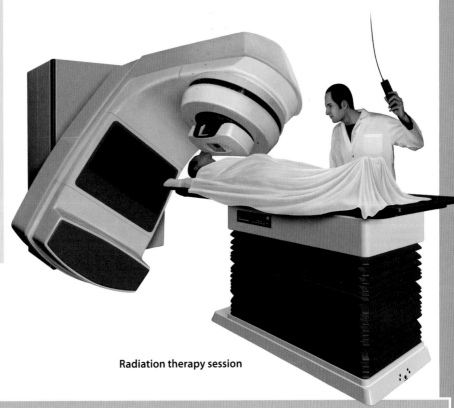

Radiation therapy session

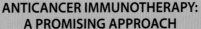

ANTICANCER IMMUNOTHERAPY: A PROMISING APPROACH

Immunotherapy consists of stimulating the body's immune system so that it can correctly decelerate cancerous cells and destroy them. This stimulation is currently obtained by administering artificial antigens or cytokines. The antigens allow the formation of antibodies that destroy the cancerous cells, while cytokine, a substance that is naturally present in the body, plays a major role in defense reactions. Still in the experimental stage, these processes have opened the door to optimistic prospects for the treatment and cure of cancer, notably because immunotherapy destroys cancerous cells without harming healthy cells. It could even lead to the creation of a vaccine against cancer.

The immune system... page 278

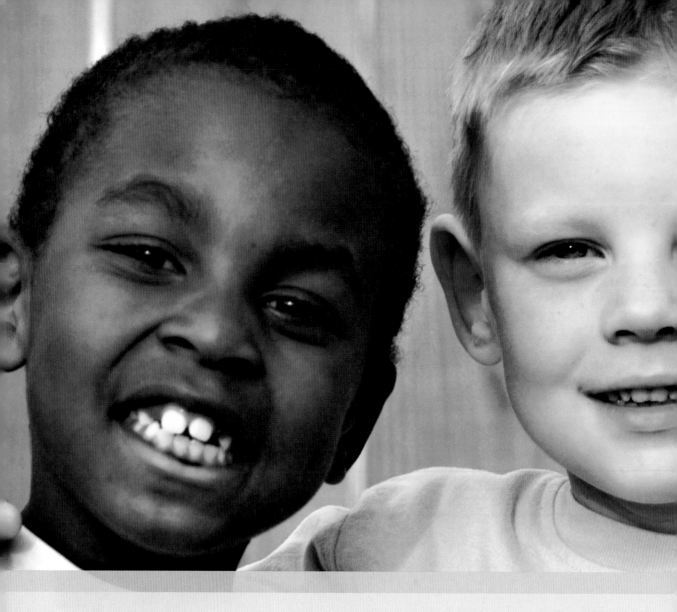

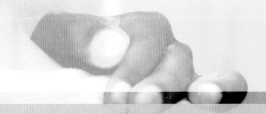

THE **SKIN**

The skin is an organ that covers our entire body, accounting for approximately 7% of our body mass. Along with the nails and hair, it forms the integumentary system. Supple, elastic, and of varying color, skin is also highly resistant. It provides real protective armor against harmful external elements such as ultraviolet rays and **infections.** Our skin contains cells, fibers, and specialized structures that, in addition to protecting the body, also contribute to the regulation of our body temperature and our perception of the world through touch.

Despite its great resistance, the skin can suffer a variety of lesions, caused by **trauma** (cuts, burns, etc.) or diseases (**inflammations** or bacterial, viral, or fungal infections). It can also be affected by tumors and parasites such as lice. However, its great capacity for regeneration often allows it to repair itself, particularly by means of the healing process.

STRUCTURE OF THE SKIN

The skin is a supple, resistant organ that covers the entire body and plays a protective role against physical, chemical, and biological attacks from the surrounding environment. Its total thickness varies from ³/₅₀–⁴/₂₅ inches (1.5–4 mm), depending on the part of the body and the individual. The skin comprises three superimposed layers: the epidermis, the dermis, and the hypodermis.

SLIP INTO A NEW SKIN

Every year, 6½–9 pounds (3–4 kg) of old skin detaches from the surface of the body. The epidermis renews itself completely every 35–45 days.

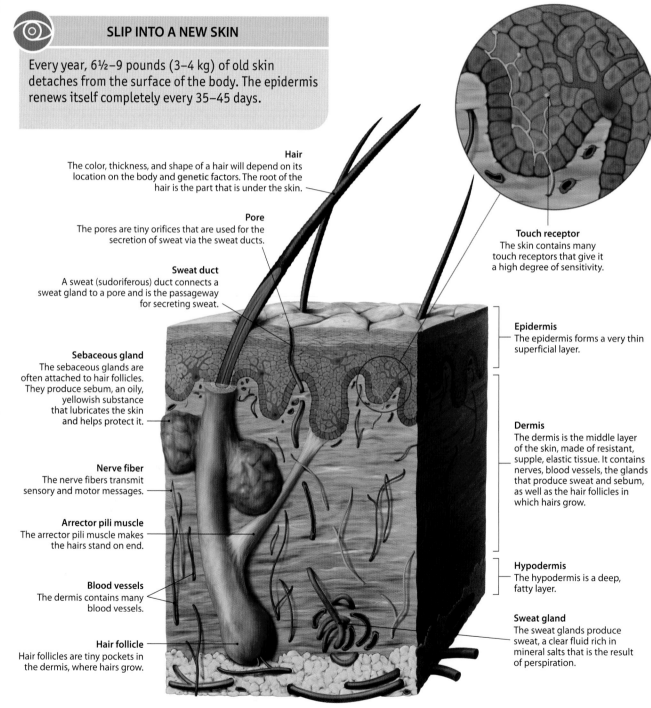

Hair
The color, thickness, and shape of a hair will depend on its location on the body and **genetic** factors. The root of the hair is the part that is under the skin.

Pore
The pores are tiny orifices that are used for the secretion of sweat via the sweat ducts.

Sweat duct
A sweat (sudoriferous) duct connects a sweat gland to a pore and is the passageway for secreting sweat.

Sebaceous gland
The sebaceous glands are often attached to hair follicles. They produce sebum, an oily, yellowish substance that lubricates the skin and helps protect it.

Nerve fiber
The nerve fibers transmit sensory and motor messages.

Arrector pili muscle
The arrector pili muscle makes the hairs stand on end.

Blood vessels
The dermis contains many blood vessels.

Hair follicle
Hair follicles are tiny pockets in the dermis, where hairs grow.

Touch receptor
The skin contains many touch receptors that give it a high degree of sensitivity.

Epidermis
The epidermis forms a very thin superficial layer.

Dermis
The dermis is the middle layer of the skin, made of resistant, supple, elastic tissue. It contains nerves, blood vessels, the glands that produce sweat and sebum, as well as the hair follicles in which hairs grow.

Hypodermis
The hypodermis is a deep, fatty layer.

Sweat gland
The sweat glands produce sweat, a clear fluid rich in mineral salts that is the result of perspiration.

Cross section of skin

THE **EPIDERMIS**

The epidermis is usually less than 1/32 inches (1 mm) thick. It is composed of several layers of live cells and a layer of dead cells called the stratum corneum (horned layer). The epidermis chiefly contains two types of cells: melanocytes and keratinocytes. The melanocytes produce melanin pigments, which are responsible for skin color. The keratinocytes enable the continuous renewal of the epidermis by constantly moving the deeper layers up towards the surface of the skin. These cells also produce and gather keratin, a protein that is abundant in the stratum corneum, the nails, and the hair. Keratin limits the dehydration of the skin and forms a protective barrier against external infectious agents.

THE BIGGEST ORGAN

Covering an area of approximately 21½ sq. ft. (2 m²), with a weight of around 11 pounds (5 kg), the skin is the largest and heaviest organ of the body.

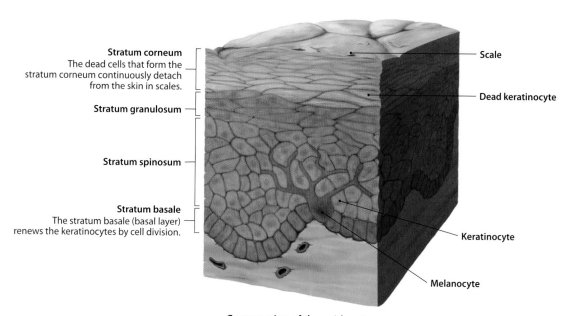

Stratum corneum
The dead cells that form the stratum corneum continuously detach from the skin in scales.

Stratum granulosum

Stratum spinosum

Stratum basale
The stratum basale (basal layer) renews the keratinocytes by cell division.

Scale

Dead keratinocyte

Keratinocyte

Melanocyte

Cross section of the epidermis

PERSPIRATION

Perspiration is the secretion of sweat through the pores of the skin. In particular, this helps to regulate body temperature: when it evaporates, the sweat releases heat, cooling the body. Perspiration can be stimulated by high ambient temperatures, an increase in the body's internal temperature (physical activity or fever), or by other factors such as emotions or stress. Abnormally heavy perspiration over the whole body can be a symptom of a disease, such as hyperthyroidism or diabetes.

WRINKLES

With age, the elasticity of the dermis decreases and furrows appear in the skin. These are wrinkles. They are mainly present on the face, where they are shaped by our facial expressions. Prolonged exposure to the sun, dryness, smoking, and certain hormonal factors can contribute to the appearance of wrinkles. The application of creams and certain cosmetic surgery techniques can be used to smooth them.

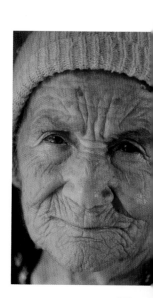

The skin | The body

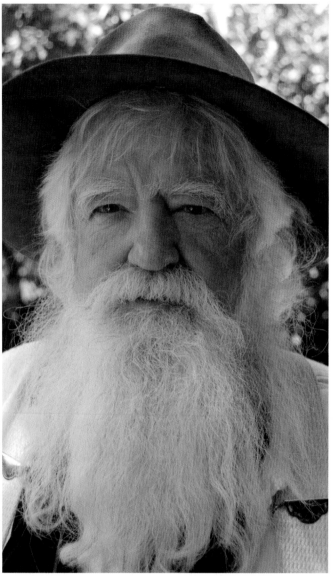

HAIR

Hair is an ancillary structure of the skin. It is fine, flexible, resistant, and rich in keratin. It is present nearly everywhere on the surface of our bodies, especially on the head (head of hair, beard, mustache, eyebrows) and at the groin (pubic hair). Hair color is determined by the melanin pigments that it contains. Hair production, which increases at puberty, is linked to hormonal, metabolic, and hereditary factors. The cause of total or partial hair loss (head and body) may be mechanical, physiological (baldness), pathological (thyroid gland disorders, psychological shock, tinea capitis), or medicinal (cancer chemotherapy).

GOOSE BUMPS

The phenomenon of our hair standing on end, called goose bumps, is the body's automatic response to cold or fear. The muscles at the base of the hairs contract, causing small bumps in the skin to appear. In furry and feathered animals, this mechanism normally traps a layer of insulating air close to the skin, to protect them from the cold. It also increases the animal's apparent size, so that it looks more impressive in the eyes of predators. This reflex has become outdated in humans, as we now have less body hair than our ancestors.

BALDNESS

Gradual, permanent hair loss, called baldness, affects men more commonly and more intensely than women. Linked to the production of hormones (androgens), baldness is also influenced by hereditary factors. It starts between the ages of 20 and 50 and can lead to total hair loss. Certain lotions can slow hair loss and sometimes even encourage its regrowth. Baldness can also be treated surgically, using a variety of transplant techniques.

 HAIR: KEY FIGURES

A typical human head of hair has 100,000 to 150,000 individual hairs. These hairs grow at a rate of roughly ½ inch (1 cm–1.5 cm) per month and remain attached to the scalp for three to six years. Between 50 and 100 hairs fall out each day, but these are normally replaced by new growth. This means that a total of 3 million hairs can grow on our heads over a lifetime.

THE **NAILS**

Each of the 10 fingers and 10 toes has a nail, which is a dense, transparent, flexible strip very rich in keratin. The nails are the product of a change in the superficial layers of the epidermis. In addition to protecting the tips of our fingers and toes, they also allow us to take hold of small objects and to scratch. The nails are subject to various diseases, especially mycosis (fungal infection).

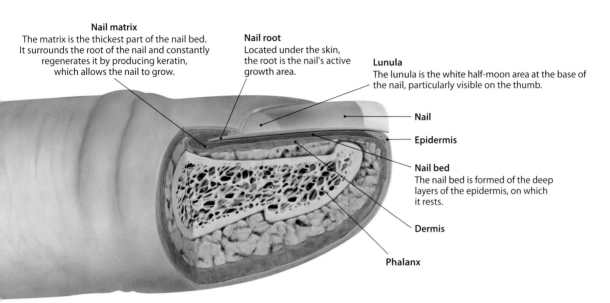

Nail matrix
The matrix is the thickest part of the nail bed. It surrounds the root of the nail and constantly regenerates it by producing keratin, which allows the nail to grow.

Nail root
Located under the skin, the root is the nail's active growth area.

Lunula
The lunula is the white half-moon area at the base of the nail, particularly visible on the thumb.

Nail

Epidermis

Nail bed
The nail bed is formed of the deep layers of the epidermis, on which it rests.

Dermis

Phalanx

Cross section of the thumb

THE NAILS: A REFLECTION OF HEALTH

Our nails' appearance can sometimes indicate a health problem. For example, purplish nails can be the result of insufficient blood oxygen levels (respiratory failure). Pale nails or fingers can sometimes be a sign of anemia or poor circulation (Raynaud's disease), while bulging nails may be caused by a chronic disease affecting the lungs or the heart. Infection of the nails by a microscopic fungus (onychomycosis) can cause them to turn yellow and thicken and, in some cases, trigger the appearance of white spots.

Skin mycosis… page 84

NONSTOP GROWTH

The nails grow continuously over a lifetime, at an average of $^3/_{32}$–$^4/_{32}$ inch (3–4 mm) per month.

FINGERPRINTS

Fingerprints are furrows that create patterns in the skin of our fingers. They are thought to provide a better grip, a bit like the grooves in tires and the tread of shoes. Each individual's fingerprints are unique, so much so that, at the scene of a crime, they can be used to identify the guilty parties.

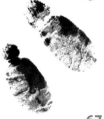

SKIN COLOR

Skin color is genetically determined and is primarily due to the presence of a pigment called melanin. Melanin is produced by specialized cells (melanocytes) in the epidermis and plays a crucial role in protecting the skin from the sun's ultraviolet rays. White skin, which contains less melanin, is more vulnerable to sunburn and skin cancer. Melanin is also responsible for the color of our hair and of the irises in our eyes.

PHOTOTYPES

A phototype is a type of natural skin, hair, and eye pigmentation, characterized by the skin's level of responsiveness to the sun. There are six different phototypes, determined by melanin quantity and color (yellow, red, brown, or black). Sun protection should be adapted to suit the individual's phototype.

MELANIN PIGMENTS

Produced by the melanocytes, melanin pigments are present in the skin in the form of granules. They are yellow or red in lighter skin and brown or black in darker skin.

Structure of the skin... page 64

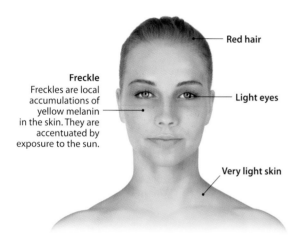

Red hair

Freckle
Freckles are local accumulations of yellow melanin in the skin. They are accentuated by exposure to the sun.

Light eyes

Very light skin

Phototype 1
Phototype 1 is characterized by very light skin, which never tans, with many freckles. This phototype is the most vulnerable to sunburns.

Black hair

Dark brown eyes

Very dark skin

Phototype 6
Phototype 6 can be distinguished by very dark skin that is highly resistant to sunburns. This phototype produces large quantities of black-colored melanin.

TANNING

Under the effect of ultraviolet rays, the melanocytes multiply in the epidermis and increase their production of melanin. This process, called tanning, results in a brown coloration of the skin, of variable duration, which improves the skin's resistance to sunburns. However, frequent, excessive exposure to the sun is a major factor of skin cancer.

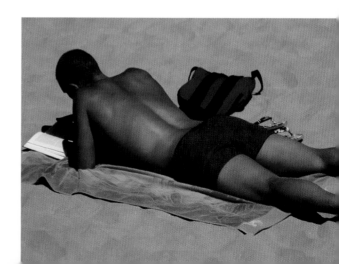

HEALING

Healing is a physiological process through which injury to a tissue, especially the skin, is repaired. It generally ends with the formation of a scar. The healing process can be triggered by an injury, a burn, a surgical incision, or a lesion caused by a disease.

THE **STAGES** OF **HEALING**

Superficial wounds heal in several stages, the length of which will vary depending on the appearance and severity of the lesion.

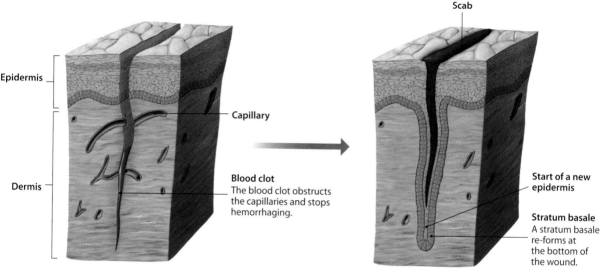

1. Stoppage of hemorrhaging (blood clot)
When an injury reaches down to the dermis, the capillaries within it burst, causing hemorrhaging. A blood clot forms at the bottom of the wound.

- Epidermis
- Dermis
- Capillary
- **Blood clot**
  The blood clot obstructs the capillaries and stops hemorrhaging.

2. Formation of a protective scab
The blood clot turns into a scab, which protects the injured tissues from **infection** and prevents their dehydration.

- Scab
- **Start of a new epidermis**
- **Stratum basale**
  A stratum basale re-forms at the bottom of the wound.

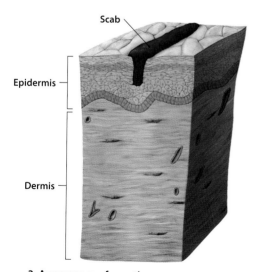

3. Appearance of new tissue
The cells in the dermis and in the capillaries multiply to form a new tissue that pushes the scab up to the surface of the epidermis. Once the healing process is complete, the scab drops off, leaving a scar in its place.

- Scab
- Epidermis
- Dermis

SUTURE

A suture is a surgical operation that consists of bringing together the edges of a wound (caused by injury or surgical incision), to accelerate or encourage the healing process. A suture is performed using adhesive strips or threads (stitches) that are removed once healing is complete. However, some threads are designed to spontaneously disintegrate after a few weeks or a few months and therefore do not need to be removed.

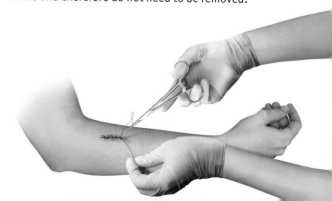

SKIN LESIONS

The skin can be injured by a **trauma**: a cut, burn, scratch, bite, rubbing, surgical incision, etc. It can also be damaged by an **infectious** disease or **inflammation**. Skin lesions vary in terms of appearance and size. Some are isolated, while others appear in bunches or patches. Lesions such as rashes, papules, blisters, pustules, maculas, and nodules are the first signs of a skin disease or trauma.

RASH

A rash is a red patch on the skin that disappears when pressed. This symptom, caused by the dilation of the capillaries, is common to many ailments, such as eczema and sunburns. Often combined with other lesions (papules, blisters), a rash can be accompanied by a burning sensation or itching.

CALLOSITIES

Pressure or repeated rubbing can cause the localized hardening and thickening of the outer layers of the skin. These callosities, or calluses, mainly affect the feet. They are called corns when on the toes, hard skin on the sole, and bunions on the big toe. These are benign lesions that can cause pain and may, in some cases, encourage infection. Callosities are treated by good foot hygiene, regular pumicing, or wearing comfortable or adapted shoes, as well as by the application of a pad to the sensitive area or by a salicylic acid treatment.

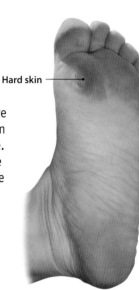

Hard skin

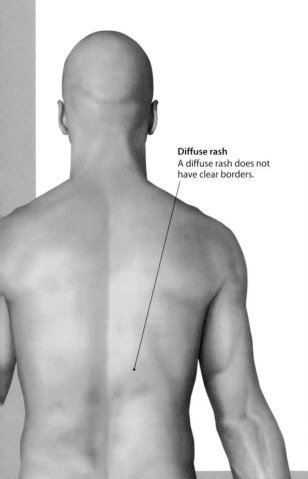

Diffuse rash
A diffuse rash does not have clear borders.

WOUNDS

Wounds are openings in a tissue caused by injury (scratches, cuts, nicks, stings, bites) or by a surgical operation. Superficial wounds affect the skin and underlying tissues. Deep wounds reach as far as the internal organs. Wounds must be carefully cleansed and treated with an antiseptic. Use of an antiseptic and sterile protection can reduce the risk of infection and help with the healing process. Deep, long, or broad wounds or wounds that bleed heavily, heal slowly, or present a risk or signs of infection require medical attention. The doctor will determine whether stitches, a tetanus vaccination, or antibiotics are necessary. Medical examination is also recommended for face, joint, and genital wounds.

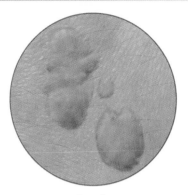

Papule
A papule is a few millimeters wide and clearly demarcated; it protrudes from the skin and is firm. Multiple papules side by side form a patch. Their appearance may be a symptom of hives or lichen planus.

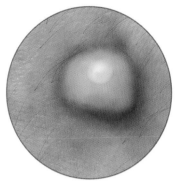

Pustule
A pustule is a clearly demarcated raised area of the epidermis, containing pus. Examples of pustules include boils and pimples.

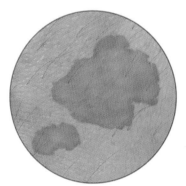

Macula
A macula is a flat spot on the skin of variable color and size. It can have different causes, such as an anomaly in the skin's pigmentation or a rash.

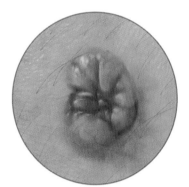

Nodule
A nodule is a round lesion on the skin or on a mucous membrane, with well-defined contours, that is fairly hard to the touch.

Vesicle
A vesicle is a blister on the skin measuring less than ½ inch (1 cm) in diameter.

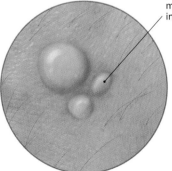

Blister
A blister is a raised portion of the epidermis that contains a clear fluid (serosity). Types of blisters include the vesicle, which is small, and the bulla, which is larger in size. Blisters are caused by burning, repeated rubbing, or skin diseases such as cold sores and eczema.

INGROWN NAILS

An ingrown nail is an inflammation of a finger or toe, especially the big toe, caused by the gradual penetration of the edges of the nail into the surrounding flesh. The flesh swells, reddens, and may become infected if the wound is not treated. Ingrown nails are more common in men than in women. They can be avoided by wearing shoes that do not compress the toes and by cutting the toenails straight and not too short. They are treated with anti-inflammatories, antiseptics, or surgery.

BURNS

Burns are deep or shallow lesions of the skin or mucous membranes, caused by heat, a corrosive substance, radiation, or an electric current. The severity of a burn will depend on the area of skin affected and on the depth of the lesion. Burns are categorized into one of three degrees. First-degree and superficial second-degree burns are usually benign, unless they involve a large portion of the body. Deep second-degree burns and third-degree burns, which are much more serious, can be life-threatening and require emergency hospitalization.

First aid: Burns and electrocution... page 557

SUNBURN

A sunburn occurs when the epidermis is burned by exposure to the sun's ultraviolet rays at a level greater than the skin's resistance. Sunburns are usually first-degree burns that cause redness, followed by peeling of the burned area a few days later. People with light skin can have second-degree sunburns, which can be identified by the rapid appearance of blisters. Repeated sunburns, especially in light-skinned people, increase the risk of skin cancer and accelerate the skin's aging process.

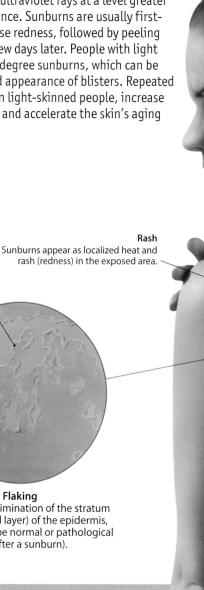

Rash
Sunburns appear as localized heat and rash (redness) in the exposed area.

Scale

Flaking
Flaking is the elimination of the stratum corneum (dead layer) of the epidermis, in scales. It can be normal or pathological (e.g. after a sunburn).

FIRST-DEGREE BURNS

First-degree burns are limited to the epidermis, the superficial layer of the skin. They appear as a red patch, or rash. This may be accompanied by slight swelling (edema) and itching. Flaking will then occur a few days later. First-degree burns are benign, though painful, lesions that heal on their own after a few days, with no aftereffects.

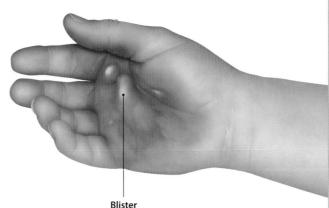

Rash
First-degree burns are characterized by the appearance of a rash.

SECOND-DEGREE BURNS

Second-degree burns involve the epidermis and some portion (greater or lesser) of the dermis, the middle layer of the skin. They result in the formation of a blister. When the lesion does not extend beyond the superficial layers of the dermis, it will heal in two to three weeks, without leaving a scar. The deeper the damage to the dermis, the longer the healing process will take and the more visible the scar will be. A second-degree burn should be examined by a doctor when the deepest layers of the dermis have been destroyed, in the case of a chemical or electrical burn, or when the burned area is larger than the palm of the hand or is located on the face, neck, genital area, or joints. A skin graft may be necessary.

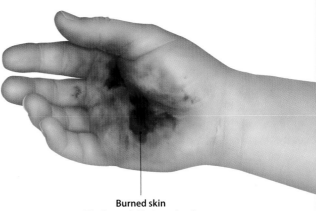

Blister
The burned tissues separate from the healthy tissues, forming a blister, a small pouch filled with a clear fluid (serosity). When the blister bursts, the dermis is exposed, and the risk of infection is high.

THIRD-DEGREE BURNS

Third-degree burns are deep burns characterized by the complete destruction of the skin and, in some cases, the underlying tissues (muscle). They are very serious lesions that do not heal on their own. When a burn covers a large area, it can be life-threatening to the victim, requiring emergency hospitalization, rehydration by IV drip, and a skin graft. Infection is very common and generalized infection (septicemia) is a threat. Skin with a third-degree burn is not sensitive to pain, because the touch receptors in the dermis have been destroyed, but the area around the burn is extremely painful.

Burned skin
The burned skin has a hard, uneven surface, with a waxy appearance that is brown or whitish in color.

SUN PROTECTION

Good sun protection can considerably reduce the harmful effects of the sun on the skin (burns, cancer, aging of the skin, etc.), especially in children and light-skinned people. Here is some advice to follow, particularly during the hottest times of the year and while on trips to the mountains or tropical countries. These precautions also apply when the sky is overcast because ultraviolet rays can cross through the cloud layer.

■ DO NOT EXPOSE YOUR SKIN IN THE MIDDLE OF THE DAY
The sun's rays are strongest when it is at its zenith (10 a.m. to 3 p.m.). The best protection against the sun is to avoid exposing your skin to it during these hours. Otherwise, it is imperative that you protect yourself as much as possible.

■ COVER UP
For effective protection of your body from the sun, wear a hat, sunglasses, and clothing that covers your legs and arms. Dark clothes block ultraviolet rays better than light-colored clothes.

■ USE SUNSCREEN
Apply sunscreen to the exposed and sensitive parts of your body (especially your face, neck, and ears). Choose a lotion with a high sun protection factor (SPF) and apply it at least 20 minutes before going into the sun. In the case of extended exposure, reapply at least every two hours, particularly after going in the water.

■ DO NOT EXPOSE NEWBORNS TO THE SUN
Babies under the age of 6 months should not be exposed to direct sunlight.

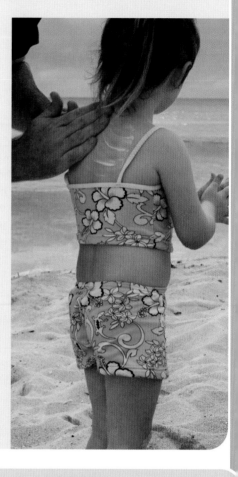

SKIN GRAFTS

A skin graft is a surgical operation in which a section of skin is transferred to an area of damaged skin. It is performed when healing is difficult or impossible, especially in the case of deep burns. To limit the risk of rejection, the grafted skin is usually taken from the patient's own body, from an area that is covered up most of the time. When the burn is over a large area, the skin may also come from a donor or be developed in a laboratory.

BURNS

SYMPTOMS:
First degree: rash, pain. Second degree: blister, pain. Third degree: destruction of the skin, leaving brown and whitish tissue in its place.

TREATMENTS:
First degree: cooling and rehydration of the skin, analgesics. Second degree: disinfection, sterile protection, rehydration as needed, sometimes antibiotics.Third degree: rehydration, removal of dead tissue, skin graft, cosmetic surgery, sometimes antibiotics, rehabilitation.

WARTS

Warts are outgrowths from the epidermis that can be more or less raised and colored. They are caused by a papillomavirus, transmitted by direct contact or by indirect contact (with a contaminated surface). Warts are common lesions that can appear on different parts of the body, either separately or in groups, and tend to multiply and spread. There are several different types, defined by their appearance and location. Verrucas and plantar warts, which are highly contagious, are the most common types. Plane warts are relatively discreet and mainly affect children, adolescents, and people with weakened immune systems. Genital warts (condyloma), likewise caused by a papillomavirus, are another type of wart. Warts disappear spontaneously, sometimes after several years, although their surgical removal can prevent them from spreading.

Genital warts… page 448

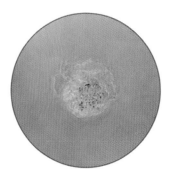

Plantar wart
Located on the soles of the feet, plantar warts are hard, dry, and sometimes black in color. They tend to grow deep inside the foot and are often painful under pressure.

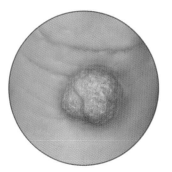

Verruca
Verrucas are raised, round, soft, lumpy, and gray, beige, or sometimes black in color. They are typically located on the hands, knees, elbows, and face.

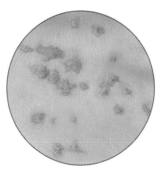

Plane wart
Plane warts are relatively flat, supple and smooth, and gray, pink, or brown in color. They generally appear on the backs of the hands, the feet, legs, face, and neck. Plane warts often spread in lines.

WART TREATMENTS

The main treatments for warts are surgical. **Cryotherapy** is based on the application of a cold source, typically liquid nitrogen. This treatment causes the **necrosis** of the wart, which detaches from the underlying tissues and falls off a few weeks later, usually leaving no visible scars. This operation may cause blistering. Electrosurgery uses the heat emitted by an electric current. It is often employed to remove warts and small tumors.

WARTS

SYMPTOMS:
Small, usually painless, smooth or rough, more or less raised, pigmented outgrowth on the skin.

TREATMENTS:
Cryotherapy, electrosurgery, application of salicylic acid or Vitamin A by-products (retinoids).

PREVENTION:
Not walking barefoot in public places (plantar warts). Not touching the warts, so as not to encourage their spread.

ULCERS

An ulcer is the localized destruction of the tissues of the skin or mucous membrane, to varying depths. These lesions do not heal easily and tend to become **chronic**. Most often, ulcers are caused by a problem with blood circulation (leg ulcer, bedsores, etc.), an **infection**, a tumor, or a **trauma**. They are frequently painful and are particularly vulnerable to infection. Their treatment is based on addressing the factors that contributed to their onset and on local, long-term care.

LEG ULCERS

Leg ulcers cause the chronic destruction of the skin, due to problems with the blood's circulation (venous or arterial insufficiency). They are typically localized in the lower third of the legs and in the protruding part of the ankles. Relatively pain-free, venous ulcers are caused by varicose veins or are an aftereffect of phlebitis. High blood pressure, diabetes, smoking, and high blood cholesterol levels can contribute to the appearance of painful arterial ulcers.

Ulcer
An ulcer should be cleaned by a health care professional and covered with appropriate bandaging.

Malleolus
In severe cases, the bone (malleolus) may appear.

BEDSORES

Bedsores, or decubitus ulcers, are skin ulcers that mainly affect bedridden individuals. They are caused by insufficient blood supply to the regions of the body subjected to prolonged pressure (e.g. the buttocks, heels, and elbows). They can form in just a few hours, especially in the case of complete immobilization (coma or paralysis). A red area appears, then the skin blackens and comes off. This necrosis leaves the underlying tissues exposed. Bedsores are painful wounds that are easily infected and often take a long time to heal. Preventive measures should be taken systematically in the case of confinement of a patient to bed.

ULCERS

SYMPTOMS:
More or less painful chronic wound on the skin.

TREATMENTS:
Treatment of the causes. Cleansing, disinfection, appropriate bandaging, sometimes a skin graft.

PREVENTION:
Leg ulcer: treatment of varicose veins, reduction of risk factors such as diabetes, hypercholesterolemia, smoking, etc. Bedsores: good personal hygiene and regular mobilization for bedridden patients.

PREVENTING BEDSORES

Bedsores mainly appear in people with reduced mobility, either bedridden or in a wheelchair. Here are some suggestions for preventing bedsores.

■ INSPECT THE SKIN AND MAINTAIN GOOD HYGIENE

Regularly inspect the skin at the tips of the fingers and watch for the appearance of red patches and pain. To avoid the moisture and infections that contribute to bedsores, maintain good hygiene by gently washing the skin with a mild soap. Hydrate the skin with creams or oils. Use absorbent surfaces to remove moisture, and change soiled or wet clothes as quickly as possible.

■ CHANGE THE PATIENT'S POSITION REGULARLY

Change the patient's position every two hours if in bed and every hour if in a chair. This will vary the points of compression, especially on the bony parts of the skin, which are very fragile. In addition, you can use an adapted anti-bedsore mattress and place pillows between the knees or the ankles, and under the calves.

■ APPROPRIATE DIET

A balanced diet and sufficient hydration can prevent the appearance of bedsores.

Nutrition... page 11

■ WHAT TO AVOID

We now know that a number of practices used in the past should actually be avoided: overly strong rubbing or massage on fragile areas (instead, give light, superficial massages), alternating hot and cold against the skin, the sidelying position (opt for the semisupine position), waterbeds, and protective films.

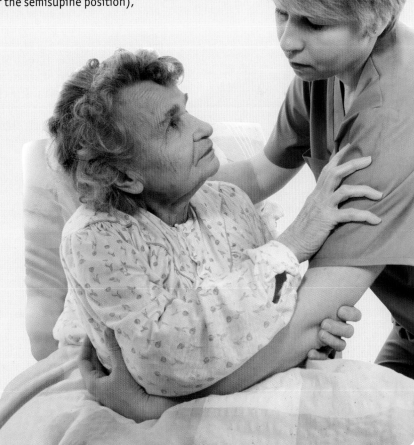

DERMATITIS

Dermatitis, or dermatite, is an **inflammation** of the skin. There are many different forms, which are differentiated by their causes and symptoms. Some forms of dermatitis have no known cause. Others are linked to the drying out of the skin, contact with an allergen or an irritant, a physical factor (water, cold, sun), or a psychological factor (stress, emotional **trauma**). Scratching or rubbing the lesions can lead to secondary infection and scarring.

ECZEMA

Eczema is an allergic form of dermatitis characterized by the presence of red patches on the skin, covered with small blisters. It causes a great deal of itching. Eczema is becoming more and more widespread, with around 20% of the populations of Western countries affected today. The most common form, atopic eczema, develops in people who are predisposed to allergies by heredity and often appears in combination with asthma or allergic rhinitis. Although it can occur at any age, this type of eczema particularly concerns infants and children and usually resolves spontaneously by the time a child reaches 10 years of age. Atopic eczema flare-ups are unpredictable and cause no aftereffects.

Allergies... page 288

CONTACT ECZEMA

Contact eczema is caused by contact with an allergen (in cosmetics, clothing, medications, plants, or metals). Lesions reappear after each contact and, over time, tend to spread beyond the point of contact. People with dry skin or white skin are more likely to develop contact eczema than those with other skin types.

CHEMICAL CONTACT DERMATITIS

Chemical contact dermatitis (or orthoergic dermatitis) is a skin irritation caused by contact of a chemical agent with the skin. Irritants can be contained in cosmetics, household detergents, and professional products. These substances cause acute or chronic lesions. The acute form appears as an outbreak of painful red patches, often covered with blisters, potentially leading to destruction of the skin. The chronic form results in dry, painful skin that may thicken or crack. Chemical contact dermatitis should not be confused with contact eczema, which is caused by an allergic reaction.

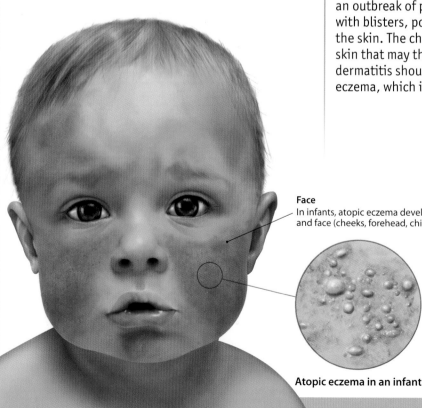

Face
In infants, atopic eczema develops on the scalp, shoulders, and face (cheeks, forehead, chin), in particular.

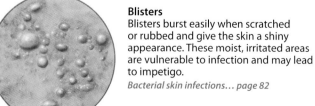

Blisters
Blisters burst easily when scratched or rubbed and give the skin a shiny appearance. These moist, irritated areas are vulnerable to infection and may lead to impetigo.
Bacterial skin infections... page 82

Atopic eczema in an infant

HIVES

Hives are characterized by the outbreak of pinkish papules or raised patches, accompanied by intense itching. There is an acute form that can last anywhere from several hours to several weeks and a chronic form that may persist over several years. Hives can be triggered by physical factors (water, sun, cold) or by allergy (insect bites, pollen, dust, medications, food). They can also be a symptom of a disease like hepatitis or mononucleosis. In many cases, the cause of hives remains unknown.

LICHEN PLANUS

Lichen planus is characterized by shiny papules that form patches criss-crossed with white lines. The papules often appear symmetrically on the body and are accompanied by intense itching. The disease can also appear as a whitish coating over the mucous membranes in the mouth. The cause of lichen planus is unknown. It typically arises between the ages of 30 and 60. The papules can remain for several weeks to several months, leaving colored marks (maculas) on the skin after their disappearance.

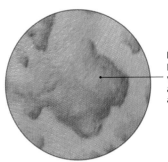

Hives papule
Hives form raised papules of varying sizes that disappear after a few hours, then reappear at other places on the body.

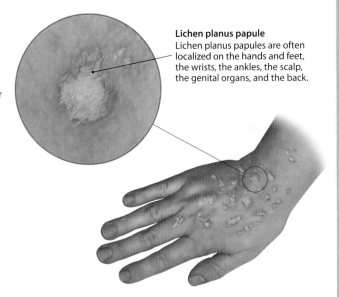

Lichen planus papule
Lichen planus papules are often localized on the hands and feet, the wrists, the ankles, the scalp, the genital organs, and the back.

ITCHING

Itching (or pruritus) is a sensation felt on the skin, triggering the desire to scratch. Itching can last for short or long periods and can affect the whole body or just a particular part. It can be caused by a skin disease (psoriasis, eczema, hives), by a disease of the liver or the gallbladder (cholelithiasis), by an endocrine disease (diabetes, hyperthyroidism), or by dried-out skin due to aging, contact with certain products, or exposure to cold. Transitory itching occurs frequently, with no apparent cause. It is not usually indicative of anything serious.

CAN YOU BE TOO CLEAN?

Excessive washing of the skin, especially using very aggressive products, removes the protective layer of the skin, contributing to its drying out and to the appearance of dermatitis, such as atopic eczema.

DERMATITIS

SYMPTOMS:
Skin lesions (red patches, blisters, papules, scabs, scales), itching, sometimes pain or a burning sensation.

TREATMENTS:
Eczema: corticosteroids, antiseptics, antibiotics in the case of infection. Hives: antihistamines. Lichen planus: corticosteroids, anxiolytics, phototherapy. Chemical contact dermatitis: oily ointments rich in Vitamin A.

PREVENTION:
Use gentle soaps and moisturizing creams, wear cotton underwear. Avoid contact with irritants and allergens.

PSORIASIS

Psoriasis is a **chronic** disease of unknown origin, characterized by the presence of scaly red spots on the skin. Psoriasis causes the **inflammation** and accelerated replacement of the epidermis, leading to significant flaking. Existing treatments can only reduce the symptoms of the disease. In some cases, psoriasis may be accompanied by joint problems that can be very debilitating.

Structure of the skin... page 64

SYMPTOMS OF PSORIASIS

Psoriasis appears as red spots that vary in size and location, covered with thick, whitish scales. These lesions, which are accompanied by itching, typically remain localized and unobtrusive. In the most severe cases, they can, however, spread, covering the whole body. Psoriasis tends to be hereditary (in one-third of cases) and is found most often in adults. It evolves in unpredictable flare-ups, sometimes caused by infection, stress, or certain medications.

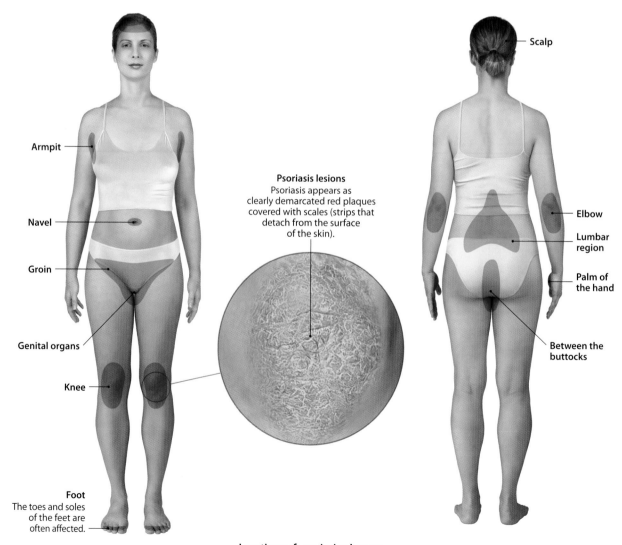

Armpit

Navel

Groin

Genital organs

Knee

Foot
The toes and soles of the feet are often affected.

Psoriasis lesions
Psoriasis appears as clearly demarcated red plaques covered with scales (strips that detach from the surface of the skin).

Scalp

Elbow

Lumbar region

Palm of the hand

Between the buttocks

Locations of psoriasis plaques

PSORIATIC ARTHRITIS

In about 10%–20% of cases, psoriasis is combined with psoriatic arthritis. This chronic inflammatory joint disease can arise before, during, or after the onset of the symptoms of psoriasis, in the form of pain, deformation, and gradual loss of mobility (ankylosis). It affects the joints in the limbs in particular and, more rarely, the spine.

PHOTOTHERAPY

Phototherapy is used to treat a variety of ailments, such as psoriasis, vitiligo, eczema, seasonal depression, and icterus of the newborn. It consists in exposing the skin to light or to a portion of its rays (ultraviolet or infrared). When treating psoriasis, ultraviolet rays block the proliferation of skin cells and reduce the inflammation of the psoriasis plaques. Despite good results, these rays do not cure the disease, and lesions may reappear after a few months, requiring a repeat of the process. In such cases, the risks of premature aging of the skin and skin cancer must be taken into consideration.

PSORIASIS

SYMPTOMS:
Clearly defined red plaques, of varying sizes, covered with whitish scales, either localized or generalized. Psoriatic arthritis: pain, stiffness, and deformation in the joints.

TREATMENTS:
Local: application of corticosteroids, salicylic acid, Vitamins A and D by-products, tar by-products, and emollient by-products. General: phototherapy, corticosteroids, immunosuppressants. Psoriatic arthritis: nonsteroidal anti-inflammatories, analgesics, immunosuppressants, physical therapy.

A COMMON AILMENT

Psoriasis is one of the most common skin ailments. It affects approximately 3% of the global population.

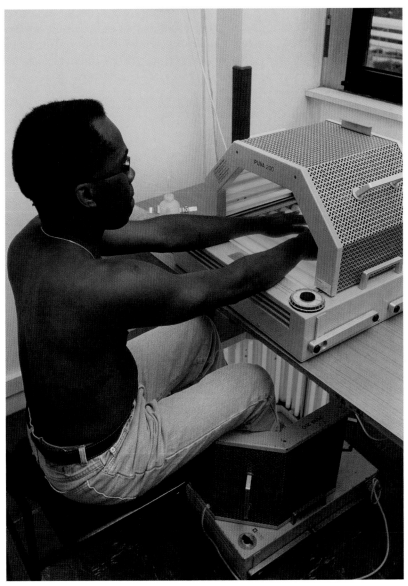

Phototherapy

BACTERIAL SKIN INFECTIONS

Bacteria can attack the skin, causing **infectious** diseases, especially when the immune system is weakened or when skin lesions provide the bacteria with a point of entry into the body. These infections, which are characterized by the presence of red patches, pustules, or scabs, are usually benign. However, if left untreated, they can lead to complications, such as the spread of the infection. The treatment of bacterial infections is primarily based on the administration of **antibiotics** and **antiseptics**.

CUTANEOUS FLORA

"Cutaneous flora" refers to all of the microorganisms (bacteria, microscopic fungi) present on the skin. Resident cutaneous flora is always present and its composition varies very little. It plays a major role in protecting the body from infection by preventing its colonization by foreign microorganisms. Transient cutaneous flora, comprised of microbes from the environment, may be pathogenic. Antiseptics have little effect on resident flora, but they do eliminate the bacteria in transient flora.

FOLLICULITIS

Folliculitis is the inflammation of a hair follicle (the base of a hair). It is often caused by a bacterial infection or, less frequently, by microscopic fungi. Superficial folliculitis is a benign ailment that appears as small pustules around hairs, particularly on the face, arms, and legs. Deep folliculitis, called a boil, is often caused by a staphylococcus aureus bacterial infection. Boils must be handled with care, due to the risk of spreading the infection. The presence of multiple boils at a single location creates a thick red, painful patch, called anthrax. Personal hygiene and the application of local antiseptics will usually cure folliculitis.

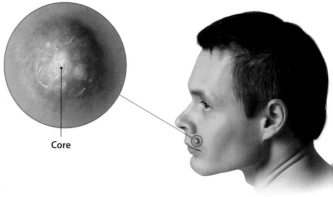

Core

Boil
Boils are usually located on the face, scalp, armpits, and buttocks. The accumulation of pus leads to the appearance of warm, thick, painful swelling, then of a white pustule (a core). Boils on the face require medical attention as soon as possible.

WHITLOW

Whitlow is an acute bacterial infection of the skin on a finger, or sometimes a toe, caused by staphylococcus aureus. This common ailment is brought about by an injury (wound, bite, torn cuticles). The infection appears as a painful inflammation, generally located at the edge of a nail. Once pus has appeared under the nail, the infected tissues will need to be surgically removed, to prevent the spread of the infection.

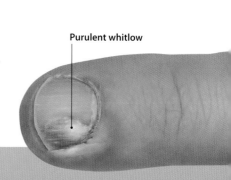

Purulent whitlow

IMPETIGO

Impetigo is a bacterial skin infection caused by staphylococcus aureus or by streptococcus. It may be due to a secondary infection of eczema. Impetigo appears as the outbreak of red patches covered with small, pus-filled blisters around the mouth, nose, or eyes. It is a common, highly contagious ailment that mainly affects children under 10 years of age.

Eczema... page 78

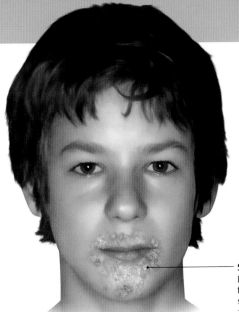

Scabs
Impetigo blisters burst easily, causing the formation of yellowish scabs. Scratching these scabs can contribute to the spread of the lesions and slow the healing process.

Impetigo

ERYSIPELAS

Erysipelas, or St. Anthony's fire, is an acute infectious skin disease, usually caused by streptococcus. It is characterized by an intense inflammation that appears as puffy red patches, often topped with blisters. These very painful lesions are typically localized on the face or the legs. They spread rapidly and are accompanied by high fever. Erysipelas requires emergency antibiotic treatment. In the vast majority of cases, it heals with no aftereffects, but it does tend to recur. The disease may lead to complications in the legs, such as edema (swelling).

BACTERIAL SKIN INFECTIONS

SYMPTOMS:
Inflammation (redness, patches, swelling), pustules that may become scabs, pain, sometimes itching or fever.

TREATMENTS:
Antiseptics, antibiotics. Surgery for whitlow.

PREVENTION:
Personal hygiene, skin and nail care treatments. Wearing protective gloves for certain types of work.

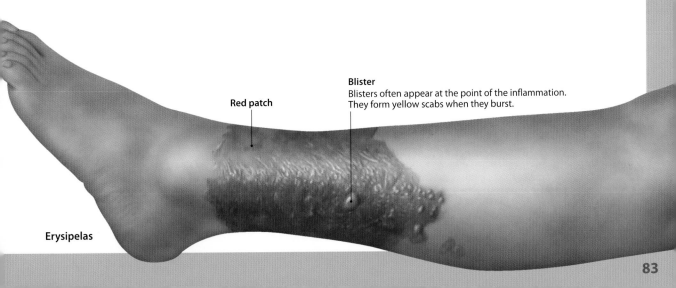

Red patch

Blister
Blisters often appear at the point of the inflammation. They form yellow scabs when they burst.

Erysipelas

SKIN MYCOSIS

Skin mycosis is an **infection** of the skin, nails, hair, or scalp by a microscopic fungus present on the skin (cutaneous flora) or in the environment. Its onset often occurs following a skin lesion, although it can also appear on apparently healthy skin, in the case of poor hygiene, a weakened immune system, or excessive heat, humidity, or perspiration. Although common and contagious, skin mycosis is usually benign. In unusual cases, it can spread to the underlying tissues, which can lead to serious complications (generalized infection). Its treatment is primarily based on the administration of **antifungals**.

TYPES OF MYCOSIS

There are multiple types of mycosis, appearing as a variety of lesions, sometimes accompanied by itching. Athlete's foot and tinea corporis (ringworm of the body) are infections caused by dermatophytes. These parasitic fungi feed on keratin, a protein that is particularly abundant in the skin, hair, and nails. Dermatophytes can be transmitted by another person, a pet, water, or contaminated objects. Other forms of skin mycosis, such as onychomycosis and intertrigo, can be caused by mold or the proliferation of a yeast from the Candida genus, a fungus that is naturally present on the skin.

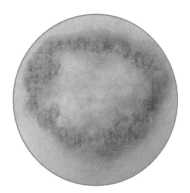

Tinea corporis
Tinea corporis appears as round, scaly red patches on the skin, edged with microblisters that scab over when they burst. These lesions spread rapidly around the edges, while the center gradually returns to a normal appearance.

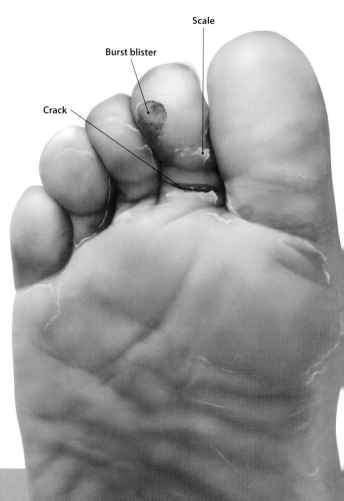

Scale

Burst blister

Crack

Athlete's foot
Athlete's foot affects the skin between the toes and appears as itching followed by painful lesions: red patches, blisters, scales, and cracks. The infection, which affects athletes in particular, is encouraged by perspiration and walking barefoot in public places. The application of antifungals can easily heal the lesions, although recurrences are common. Without treatment, the infection can spread to the rest of the foot or other parts of the body (hands, groin, scrotum).

Ringworm of the scalp

Ringworm of the scalp is an infection characterized by patches covered with pus (kerion) or scales (tinea capitis). Ringworm of the scalp mainly affects children. Its treatment is based on shaving the affected area and administering antifungals.

Tinea capitis
Dermatophytes cause the hair to break, leaving the scalp exposed.

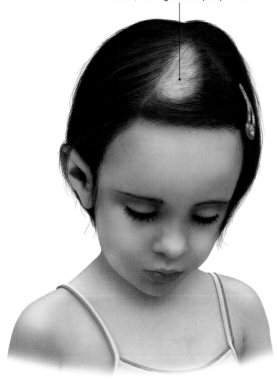

Intertrigo

Caused by a yeast from the Candida genus or a bacterium, intertrigo is characterized by an inflammation of the folds in the skin (gaps between the fingers and toes, armpits, groin, navel, between the buttocks, under the breasts). It appears as oozing red patches that cause itching. Intertrigo affects infants and obese people in particular, as they are particularly subject to perspiration. The treatment is based on good local hygiene and the application of antifungals.

Diaper rash... page 517

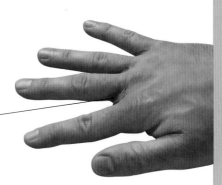

Intertrigo
When the infection is caused by a Candida fungus, the patches have a white contour.

Onychomycosis

Onychomycosis is the fungal infection of a nail, usually by a dermatophyte or sometimes a yeast (Candida) or mold. The nail thickens, yellows, and may have superficial white spots. In the advanced stages, the nail tends to detach, causing pain when pressed. Onychomycosis is treated with antifungals or by the abrasion or ablation (removal) of the infected part of the nail. After healing, the nail grows back normally.

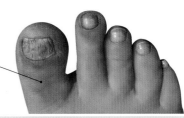

Onychomycosis
Candida infections can also cause an inflammation around the edges of the nail.

Dandruff

Dandruff is the presence of dry or oily thin scales of varying size on the scalp, which form as a response to the abnormal proliferation of a yeast present on the skin. This causes significant flaking, resulting in the spontaneous fall of dandruff, sometimes accompanied by itching. Several factors can contribute to the formation of dandruff: excess sebum, dried-out skin, irritation due to the use of cosmetics, pollution, stress, and fatigue. The application of dandruff shampoos and lotions is usually sufficient to cause it to disappear.

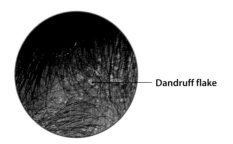

Dandruff flake

SKIN MYCOSIS

SYMPTOMS:
Inflammation (red patches, blisters), itching, burning sensation, pain, scales, deformed and discolored nails, hair alteration or breakage.

TREATMENTS:
Antifungals, antiseptics, removal of the infected part of the nail.

PREVENTION:
Personal hygiene. Not wearing tight clothes and shoes, which encourage perspiration. Not walking barefoot in public places. Disinfecting manicure and pedicure implements after use.

COLD SORES

Herpes labialis, also known as cold sores, buccal herpes, or fever blisters, is a contagious **chronic infectious** disease caused by the *Herpes simplex* virus. It appears as recurring outbreaks of characteristic blisters, typically around the mouth. The herpes labialis virus presents the same method of action as the genital herpes virus, although the two differ slightly. It remains latent in the nerve ganglions throughout the patient's life, reactivating periodically, which causes the reappearance of the symptoms at the same location. In rare cases, the virus may extend to the fingers (whitlow) or the eyes, or cause encephalitis.

Genital herpes... page 447

IS EVERYONE A CARRIER?

Contamination by the herpes labialis virus often occurs during childhood, by direct or indirect contact with herpes blisters. Approximately 9 out of 10 people carry the virus, but just 10% of the population develops the disease.

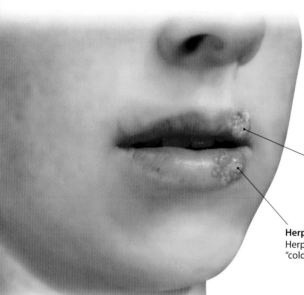

Scab
The blisters burst quickly, oozing and forming yellowish scabs when they dry. These scabs fall off in under a week, leaving no visible scarring.

Herpes blister
Herpes blisters are commonly called "fever blisters" or "cold sores."

SYMPTOMS OF COLD SORES

Initial contact with the virus is usually asymptomatic. The symptoms appear later, in unpredictable flare-ups that are more or less frequent, characterized by the outbreak of bunches of herpes blisters, usually on the lips, but sometimes elsewhere on the face or inside the mouth. A few hours before the lesions appear, the patient will experience a burning sensation, stinging, and itching, followed by redness. Herpes flare-ups can be triggered by a variety of factors: infectious diseases, stress, fatigue, emotional trauma, menstruation, pregnancy, exposure to the sun, etc.

COLD SORES

SYMPTOMS:
Burning sensation, stinging, itching, painful, oozing herpes blisters that develop into yellowish scabs.

TREATMENTS:
Antiviral (acyclovir) and local antiseptics to reduce the lesions and accelerate their disappearance.

PREVENTION:
Avoiding direct and indirect contact with the blisters of people with cold sore flare-ups. Not touching or scratching the lesions, to avoid the spread of blisters.

SKIN PARASITES

The skin can be contaminated by highly contagious parasites, such as lice, mites, ticks, and fleas. Their transmission is heightened by the crowding associated with certain places, like schools, retirement homes, and prisons. Skin parasites can be effectively eliminated by pesticides, whose instructions for use must be strictly followed, due to their harmful nature.

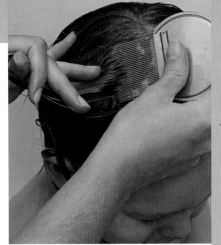

LICE

Lice are dark-colored parasitic insects that live on the skin and feed off blood. They are $\frac{1}{32}$–$\frac{3}{32}$ inches (1–3 mm) long and spread easily by direct and indirect contact (combs, clothing, bedding). They colonize the scalp and the pubis in particular. Their presence can be revealed by intense itching and the presence of red dots on the skin. Scratching can lead to secondary infection and the formation of scabs. The use of a pesticide against lice is necessary to completely eliminate the parasites and their eggs (nits).

Elimination of nits
Nits attach firmly to head and body hair. They can be dislodged by sliding fingernails or a fine comb along the entire length of the hair, starting at the root.

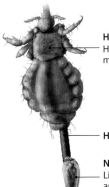

Head lice
Head lice colonize the scalp. They mainly affect school-age children.

Hair

Nit
Lice eggs, called nits, have a light color and an oblong shape, and measure less than $\frac{1}{32}$ inch (1 mm) in length.

Crabs
Crabs are lice that colonize the pubic hair. They can also affect the armpits and men's beards. Crabs are transmitted by physical contact, especially during sexual relations.

SKIN PARASITES

SYMPTOMS:
Intense itching. Red dots (lice) or small dark lines (scabies) on the skin.

TREATMENTS:
Use of a fine comb or fingernails along the entire length of the hair (lice and nits). Pesticides in the form of creams, lotions or sprays, applied to the skin, hair, bedding, and clothes. Antihistamines, corticoids in the case of persistent itching.

PREVENTION:
Avoiding contact with infected people and not sharing clothing. Use of a repellent in the case of an epidemic.

SCABIES

Scabies is a skin disease caused by a mite called *Sarcoptes scabiei*. It appears as small furrows in the skin, in which the female parasites lay their eggs. These lesions cause intense itching (especially at night) between the fingers and on the wrists, elbows, and buttocks that later becomes generalized. Scabies is highly contagious and is transmitted by direct or indirect contact (clothing, bedding).

SKIN CANCER

The two main types of skin cancer are carcinomas and melanomas. They appear mainly in adults, especially people with light skin. The frequency with which they occur has been continuously on the rise in industrialized countries. Excessive exposure to the ultraviolet rays of the sun and in tanning salons is a major risk factor for skin cancer. A **biopsy** with laboratory analysis of the skin's cells is performed to establish a diagnosis and differentiate melanoma from a benign mole.

Cancer... page 55

CARCINOMAS

Carcinomas are the most common form of skin cancer. They typically appear after the age of 40, and their incidence is directly linked to sun exposure. In the vast majority of cases, they are cured by means of early surgical ablation of the tumor. There are two main types of skin carcinomas: squamous cell carcinoma, which can form metastases, and basal cell carcinoma, which never produces metastases.

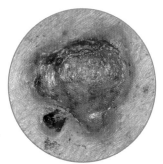

Squamous cell carcinoma
Squamous cell carcinoma develops from cells in the middle layer of the epidermis. Mainly located on the face, the oral mucous membranes, and the body's extremities, it can develop at the point of an existing lesion, like a burn scar. Squamous cell carcinoma often appears on the lips.

ACTINIC KERATOSIS

Actinic keratosis is a small, rough plaque that is clear to reddish in color, whose appearance is favored by prolonged, intense exposure to the sun over several years. Keratosis mainly develops in areas exposed to the sun (face, arms, hands). It can develop into cancer.

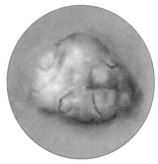

Basal cell carcinoma
Basal cell carcinoma develops from cells in the basal layer of the epidermis. It chiefly appears on the face, neck, and chest. Basal cell carcinoma does not produce metastases, but it can cause ulcers.

MELANOMAS

A melanoma is a form of skin cancer that develops from the cells responsible for the skin's pigmentation (melanocytes). Much less common than carcinomas, melanomas are also more serious, because they produce metastases. They typically appear on healthy skin, although they can also result from the transformation of an existing mole. This transformation may be spontaneous or influenced by exposure to ultraviolet rays. If treated early, the chances of recovery from a melanoma are good.

Structure of the skin... page 64

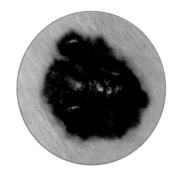

Melanoma
Melanomas may be raised and rough to varying degrees. They are characterized by poorly defined contours and uneven coloring.

MOLE

A mole, or nevus, is a small brown, more or less raised spot, resulting from the localized accumulation of pigment cells (melanocytes). Moles may be congenital or may appear anytime after birth. They vary in appearance and size, ranging from a few millimeters to an inch or more (several centimeters) in diameter, but they do not change over time. A change in the appearance of a mole, especially congenital and large ones, may be a sign of its transformation into a melanoma. In this case, medical attention should be sought immediately.

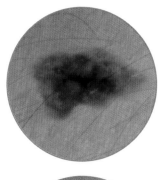

Suspicious mole
A mole that expands, bleeds spontaneously, or itches may indicate the development of a malignant melanoma.

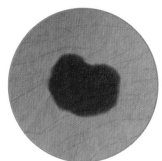

Benign mole
A benign mole has clearly defined contours and an even color.

SKIN BIOPSY

A skin biopsy involves taking a skin sample in order to diagnose the presence of cancer or a skin disease. This benign surgical operation is performed under local anesthesia, usually by means of a punch.

Punch
A punch is a surgical instrument used to gather a fragment of tissue. It is fitted with a very sharp cylindrical blade that is inserted several millimeters into the skin, down to the dermis.

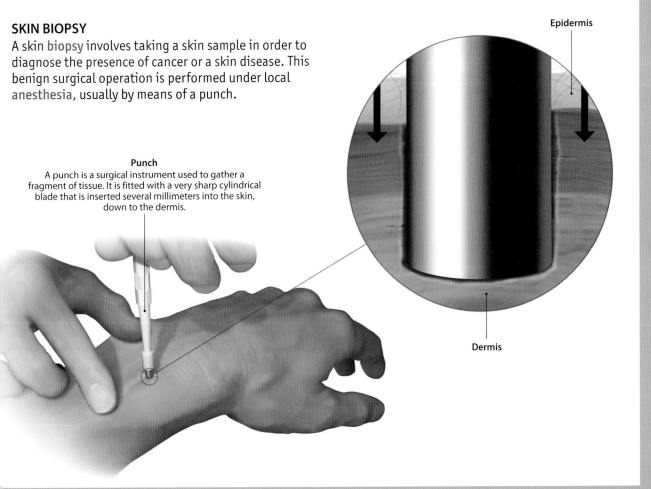

Epidermis

Dermis

PREVENTING SKIN CANCER

The prevention of skin cancer mainly involves watching the skin for any signs of change and protecting it from ultraviolet rays. The following suggestions particularly apply to people with light skin, eyes, and hair, people exposed to the sun for long periods of time, people having suffered multiple sunburns during childhood, and people with a history of skin cancer in the family.

■ PROTECT YOUR SKIN FROM THE SUN

Take all of the necessary precautions to avoid sunburns: wear a hat and long, nontransparent clothing; limit your skin's exposure to the sun (especially at high altitudes and around midday); apply sunscreen with a high sun protection factor (SPF); etc. Do not use tanning lamps or tanning products. Babies under 6 months should never be exposed to direct sunlight, and children should not stay in the sun for long periods of time.

■ EXAMINE YOUR SKIN

Perform detailed examinations of your skin on a regular basis. In particular, keep an eye on any moles, especially ones that are larger than ¼ inch (6 mm) in diameter. You should notify your doctor right away of any bleeding, itching, or changes in the shape, size, or color of your beauty marks. The same applies to any actinic keratoses that change or any wounds that do not heal. The earlier skin cancer is detected, the better the chances of recovery.

■ ASK ABOUT PHOTOSENSITIZING PRODUCTS

There are many products that make your skin more sensitive to ultraviolet rays. These include certain cosmetics (like perfumes, deodorants, and shampoos), medications (antibiotics, psychotropics, antihistamines), and natural products (phytotherapy products, essential oils). You should take extra care when combining the use of these products with exposure to the sun.

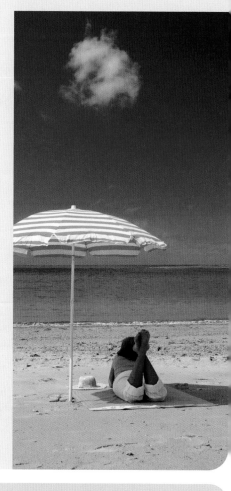

SKIN CANCER

SYMPTOMS:
Carcinoma: rounded outgrowth on the skin, wound that does not heal.
Melanoma: more or less raised spot on the skin, with blurry contours and uneven coloring.

TREATMENTS:
Ablation of the tumor. In the case of metastases: ablation of the lymph nodes, chemotherapy, and radiation therapy.

PREVENTION:
Protecting the skin against the sun's ultraviolet rays, especially for children and light-skinned people.
Melanoma: monitoring of moles, preventive removal of suspicious moles.

SKIN DISCOLORATION

The skin often undergoes temporary changes in color. Most of the time, these are physiological responses to emotion (paling or blushing), environmental factors (cold, heat, or sun), or health problems (allergy, **inflammation**, or **trauma**). The skin is also subject to permanent defects in its pigmentation. This discoloration may be localized (e.g. vitiligo) or generalized (e.g. albinism). People with such defects are more vulnerable to sunburns and skin cancer.

VITILIGO

Vitiligo is a skin disease characterized by localized depigmentation. It is caused by the loss of melanocytes, the skin cells that produce melanin pigments. Vitiligo results in white spots on the skin, that vary in size, appearance, and location, and tend to grow over time. This autoimmune disease evolves in spurts, under the influence of various factors, such as stress, anxiety, psychological shock, and rubbing. It affects about 1% of the population and can occur at any age. Existing treatments have proven ineffective in most patients. In some cases, medically supervised exposure to ultraviolet rays can cause the spots to regain their color, but it also entails the risk of skin cancer.

Structure of the skin... page 64

Vitiligo spot
Vitiligo spots are often located on the chest, hands, face, armpits, knees, and ankles. The affected areas are particularly vulnerable to sunburns and must be protected.

ALBINISM

Albinism is a recessive genetic disease characterized by the inability to produce melanin pigments. It results in the absence of pigmentation in the skin, hair, and irises. Albinism is more common in people with darker skin. It is often accompanied by vision problems and high sensitivity to light (photophobia).

Heredity... page 50

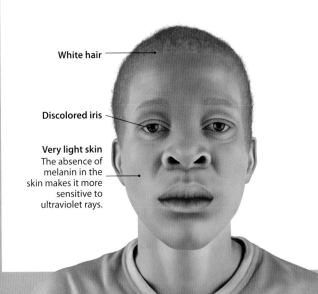

White hair

Discolored iris

Very light skin
The absence of melanin in the skin makes it more sensitive to ultraviolet rays.

SKIN DISCOLORATION

SYMPTOMS:
Vitiligo: smooth white, clearly defined spots of variable size and location, often roughly symmetrical.
Albinism: white hair, very light skin, discolored irises.

TREATMENTS:
Vitiligo: ultraviolet rays, surgery (skin autograft), local application of corticosteroids.
Albinism: no treatment.

PREVENTION:
Vitiligo: Not rubbing the spots can limit the spread of the discoloration.

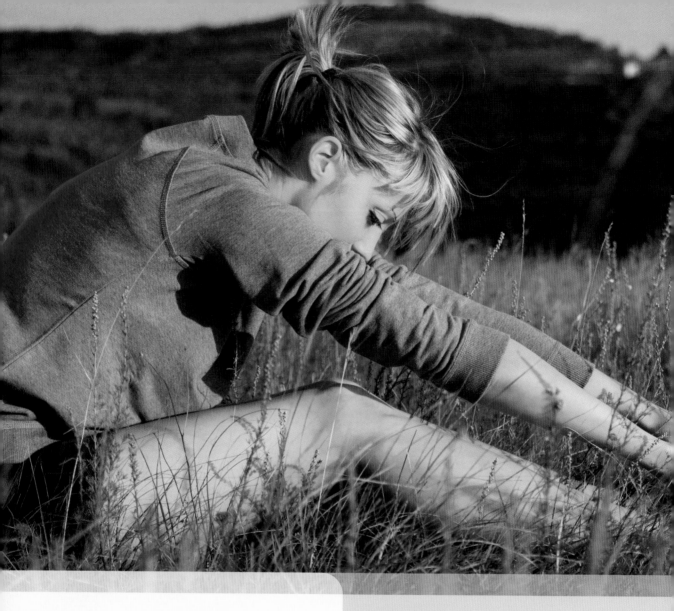

THE BONES, JOINTS, AND MUSCLES

The bones, joints, and muscles are closely interrelated. They form an inseparable trio that gives our bodies certain essential qualities: support, flexibility, and mobility. Bad habits associated with the modern lifestyle can disrupt the smooth functioning of the musculoskeletal system. A sedentary lifestyle, excess weight, stress, repetitive movements, and stationary work can lead to backache, tendinitis, and other muscle and joint pain. Excessive physical activity, whether playing sports or on the job, is another source of various problems: fractures, sprains, dislocation, lumbago, tendinitis, and torn muscles.

Some bone, joint, and muscle diseases can appear over a lifetime. A variety of them, particularly hereditary ones, appear in early childhood, such as muscular dystrophy. Others, like osteoporosis, arthrosis, and the different forms of arthritis, occur later in life and are often linked to aging.

THE **BONES**

The bones are any of the 206 rigid organs that form the skeleton, which is the framework for the human body. In addition to playing the crucial role of supporting the body, the bones also protect our vital organs, such as the brain, lungs, and heart. They actively participate in the body's movements by providing anchorage points for the muscles. The bones are also used for storing minerals and fats, while the bone marrow produces most of the body's blood cells.

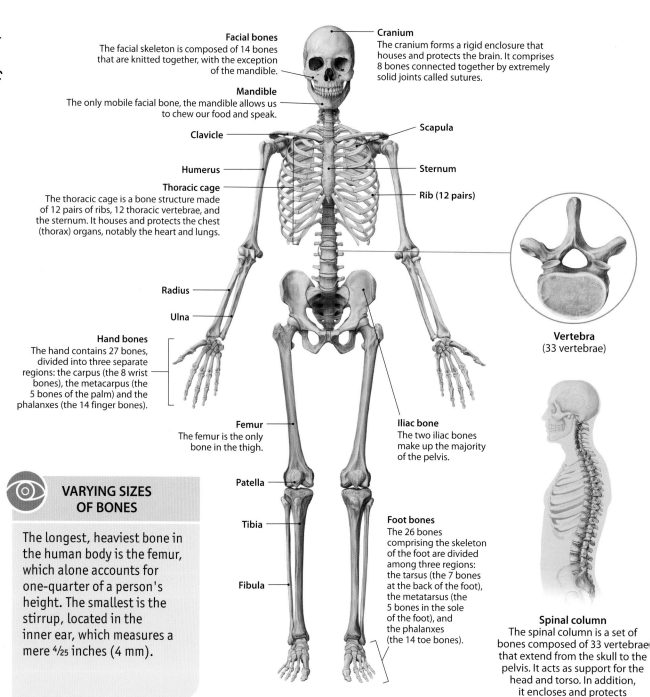

Facial bones
The facial skeleton is composed of 14 bones that are knitted together, with the exception of the mandible.

Cranium
The cranium forms a rigid enclosure that houses and protects the brain. It comprises 8 bones connected together by extremely solid joints called sutures.

Mandible
The only mobile facial bone, the mandible allows us to chew our food and speak.

Clavicle

Scapula

Humerus

Sternum

Thoracic cage
The thoracic cage is a bone structure made of 12 pairs of ribs, 12 thoracic vertebrae, and the sternum. It houses and protects the chest (thorax) organs, notably the heart and lungs.

Rib (12 pairs)

Radius

Ulna

Hand bones
The hand contains 27 bones, divided into three separate regions: the carpus (the 8 wrist bones), the metacarpus (the 5 bones of the palm) and the phalanxes (the 14 finger bones).

Vertebra
(33 vertebrae)

Femur
The femur is the only bone in the thigh.

Iliac bone
The two iliac bones make up the majority of the pelvis.

Patella

Tibia

Foot bones
The 26 bones comprising the skeleton of the foot are divided among three regions: the tarsus (the 7 bones at the back of the foot), the metatarsus (the 5 bones in the sole of the foot), and the phalanxes (the 14 toe bones).

Fibula

Spinal column
The spinal column is a set of bones composed of 33 vertebrae that extend from the skull to the pelvis. It acts as support for the head and torso. In addition, it encloses and protects the spinal cord.

VARYING SIZES OF BONES

The longest, heaviest bone in the human body is the femur, which alone accounts for one-quarter of a person's height. The smallest is the stirrup, located in the inner ear, which measures a mere 4/25 inches (4 mm).

Front view of the skeleton

BONE TISSUE

Bone is the hardest substance in the human body, after tooth enamel. The remarkable resistance of our bones comes from the nature of their tissue. Bone tissue is rich in minerals (calcium), which provide the bones with their solidity, and in collagen, a protein that gives them flexibility. Bone tissue is constantly being renewed, thanks to a balance between specialized cells, the osteoblasts (which produce it) and the osteoclasts (which destroy it). The osteoblasts are key players in the growth and maintenance of the skeleton and in bone repair after fractures.

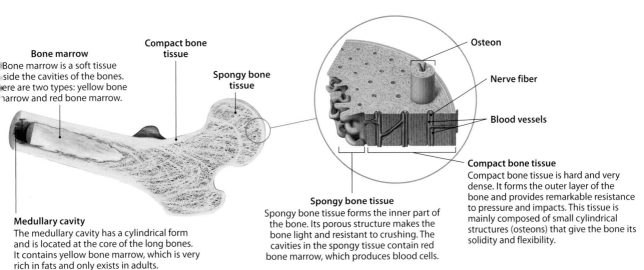

Bone marrow
Bone marrow is a soft tissue inside the cavities of the bones. There are two types: yellow bone marrow and red bone marrow.

Compact bone tissue

Spongy bone tissue

Osteon

Nerve fiber

Blood vessels

Compact bone tissue
Compact bone tissue is hard and very dense. It forms the outer layer of the bone and provides remarkable resistance to pressure and impacts. This tissue is mainly composed of small cylindrical structures (osteons) that give the bone its solidity and flexibility.

Medullary cavity
The medullary cavity has a cylindrical form and is located at the core of the long bones. It contains yellow bone marrow, which is very rich in fats and only exists in adults.

Spongy bone tissue
Spongy bone tissue forms the inner part of the bone. Its porous structure makes the bone light and resistant to crushing. The cavities in the spongy tissue contain red bone marrow, which produces blood cells.

CALCIUM

Stored in bone tissue, calcium is a mineral that gives the bones and joints resistance. You can maximize your calcium reserves by absorbing the recommended daily allowance in your food. This can help prevent or delay the onset of diseases like osteoporosis and arthrosis.

A dose of 300 mg of calcium is equivalent to approximately:

- 1 cup of milk, enriched soy beverage, or enriched orange juice
- 1.8 oz (50 g) of cheese
- ¾ cup of yogurt
- 12 sardines or 1 can of salmon
- 3 cups of broccoli or kale

If you are having a hard time reaching the recommended daily allowance, speak with a doctor to find out if dietary supplements are right for you.

Healthy bones, joints, and muscles... page 100

DAILY CALCIUM REQUIREMENTS

Age	Boys and girls
0-6 months	210 mg
6-12 months	270 mg
1-3 years	500 mg
4-8 years	800 mg
9-18 years	1300 mg
Men and women	
19-50 years	1000 mg
51 years and over	1200 mg
Pregnant and nursing women	
18 years and under	1300 mg
19-50 years	1000 mg

THE **JOINTS**

A joint is a structure that connects two or more bones. Some joints have little mobility. This is true of fibrous joints, like the cranial sutures, and cartilaginous joints, notably located between the vertebrae of the spinal column. Conversely, the synovial joints, which are more numerous, allow for a wide variety of movements. There are over 100 such joints, mainly located in the limbs.

SYNOVIAL JOINTS

The synovial joints are reinforced by ligaments and surrounded by tendons, which attach the muscles to the bones. Around the tips of the bones, these joints contain an articular capsule filled with viscous synovial fluid. Synovial fluid lubricates the articular cartilage, allowing cartilage surfaces to slide against each other.

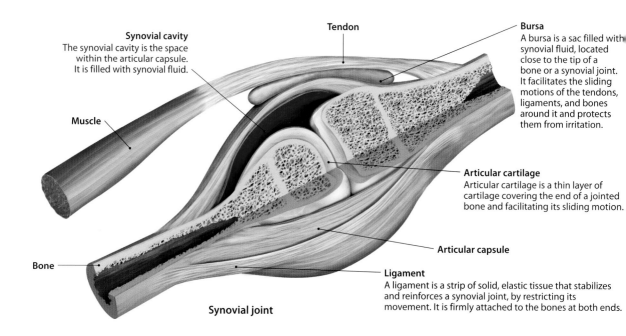

Synovial cavity
The synovial cavity is the space within the articular capsule. It is filled with synovial fluid.

Tendon

Bursa
A bursa is a sac filled with synovial fluid, located close to the tip of a bone or a synovial joint. It facilitates the sliding motions of the tendons, ligaments, and bones around it and protects them from irritation.

Muscle

Articular cartilage
Articular cartilage is a thin layer of cartilage covering the end of a jointed bone and facilitating its sliding motion.

Bone

Articular capsule

Synovial joint

Ligament
A ligament is a strip of solid, elastic tissue that stabilizes and reinforces a synovial joint, by restricting its movement. It is firmly attached to the bones at both ends.

THE KNEE

The synovial joint of the knee links the femur to the tibia, the fibula, and the patella. As a result, the knee refers to the area of the body where the thigh meets the calf. Used often, it is reinforced and stabilized by multiple ligaments and the menisci.

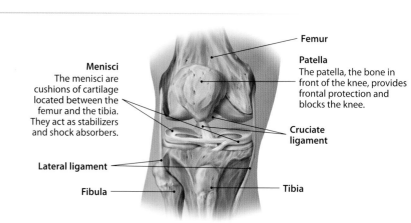

Menisci
The menisci are cushions of cartilage located between the femur and the tibia. They act as stabilizers and shock absorbers.

Femur

Patella
The patella, the bone in front of the knee, provides frontal protection and blocks the knee.

Cruciate ligament

Lateral ligament

Fibula

Tibia

Front view of the right knee

CARTILAGINOUS JOINTS

Cartilaginous joints are characterized by the presence of a cartilage plate connected to the joint surfaces of the bones. They only allow for extremely limited movements, but they are more solid and more stable than synovial joints. The cartilaginous joints include the facet joints of the spinal column.

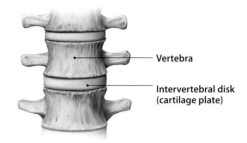

Vertebra

Intervertebral disk (cartilage plate)

Spinal column

Types of joints

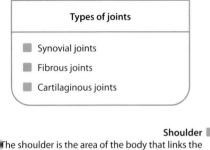

Synovial joints

Fibrous joints

Cartilaginous joints

Cranial sutures
The cranial sutures are fixed fibrous joints. However, at birth and during the first years of life, the skull bones are not completely knitted together. They retain a degree of mobility, allowing the bones in the newborn's skull to shift during childbirth, then to adapt for growth of the brain.

Shoulder
The shoulder is the area of the body that links the arm to the chest. The synovial joints in the shoulder connect the humerus, scapula, and clavicle.They allow for complete rotations of the arm.

Sternocostal joints
The sternocostal joints are the cartilaginous joints that connect the sternum and the ribs (other than the floating ribs). They give the thoracic cage its flexibility, especially for breathing movements.

Elbow
The elbow joins the upper arm to the forearm and houses a double synovial joint connecting the humerus, radius, and ulna. It allows the forearm to bend and partially rotate around its axis.

Facet joints
The facet joints are the cartilaginous joints in the spinal column. Each joint connects two adjacent vertebrae via the intermediary of a cartilage cushion, the intervertebral disk. The main function of the intervertebral disks is to absorb shocks and distribute the pressure on the spinal column, especially while walking and running.

Wrist
The wrist is the region where the forearm connects to the hand. It contains multiple synovial joints that link the radius, and the ulna to the carpal bones and that mainly provide for flexing and extending the hand.

Hip
The hip is the synovial joint that connects the femur to the iliac bone. It allows for complete rotations of the hip and is also used to transfer the body's weight to the lower limbs.

Interphalangeal joints
The interphalangeal joints are synovial joints that link the phalanxes of the fingers or the toes together. The great degree of mobility in the fingers allows them to grasp objects. The toes, which are less mobile, contribute to walking and balance when standing up. The interphalangeal joints are reinforced by a large network of tendons and ligaments.

Knee

Ankle
The ankle is the region where the leg attaches to the foot. It is home to multiple synovial joints that link the tibia and the fibula to the tarsal bones, and contains many ligaments. In particular, the ankle allows the foot to flex and extend, contributing to the ability to walk. It is a fragile area that is often subject to sprains.

The main joints

THE **MUSCLES**

A muscle is an organ that contracts when prompted by a nerve impulse. There are three types of muscles: smooth muscles, skeletal muscles, and the heart muscle. Smooth muscles are mainly located in the walls of the blood vessels and hollow organs (stomach, intestines, bladder, and uterus), where they trigger involuntary contractions. Skeletal muscles are attached to the bones by tendons. They direct the voluntary movements of the skeleton, tongue, and face. The heart muscle is one of the layers in the wall of the heart and enables its regular contraction.

The nervous system... page 132
The heart... page 250

THE **SKELETAL MUSCLES**

While the movements of the smooth muscles are always involuntary, those of the skeletal muscles are almost always the result of a conscious, voluntary command from the central nervous system. The movements of the skeletal muscles may, in some instances, be involuntary, known as reflexes. Reflexes, which are fast and automatic, are responses to external stimuli, like attacks, or reestablish the body's position and balance.

SMOOTH MUSCLES

Smooth muscles allow the involuntary movement of certain organs, prompted by the actions of the autonomic nervous system or hormones. For example, muscle contractions in the intestinal wall help to break up and eliminate the contents of the intestines.

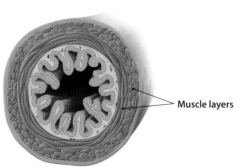

Cross section of the small intestine

Muscle layers

Frontal muscle

Orbicular muscle of eye

Zygomatics
The zygomatic muscles are used to smile.

Masseter
The masseter is a powerful muscle that connects the mandible to the upper jaw and is used in chewing.

Orbicular muscle of mouth

Sternocleidomastoid

Deltoid

Greater pectoral
The greater pectoral is the upper chest muscle. In particular, it is used to rotate the arm.

Rectus abdominis

Biceps muscle of arm

External oblique

Brachioradial

Radial flexor muscle of wrist

Quadriceps muscle of thigh
The quadriceps muscle of thigh forms the front part of the thigh. It is the most powerful muscle in the body.

Sartorius
The sartorius muscle connects the iliac bone to the tibia and allows the leg to bend and rotate.

Long fibular

Soleus

Anterior tibial muscle

Long extensor muscle of toes

Front view of the main skeletal muscles

MUSCLE TISSUE

Muscle tissue is comprised of elongated cells, the muscle fibers. These contain very fine strands called myofibrils, whose job is to contract. Their contraction is the result of a command from the nervous system, which sends a nerve impulse to the muscle fibers via the motor neurons. Even at rest, skeletal muscles never relax completely, remaining in a state of moderate contraction, called muscle tone. Muscle tone keeps the muscles ready to respond to any stimulation and continuously maintains the body's posture.

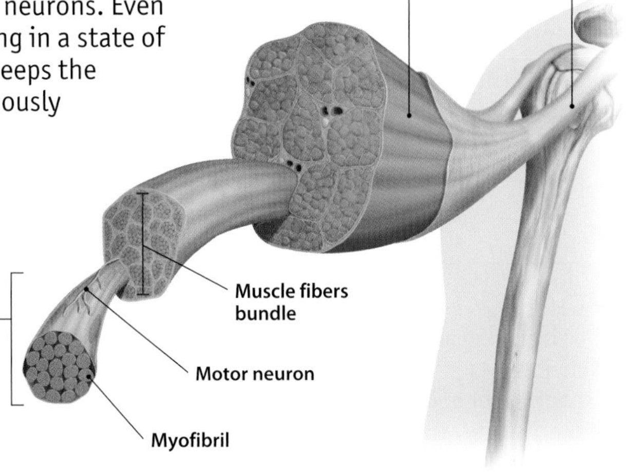

Tendon
Muscle
Muscle fibers bundle
Motor neuron
Muscle fiber
Myofibril

Structure of a skeletal muscle

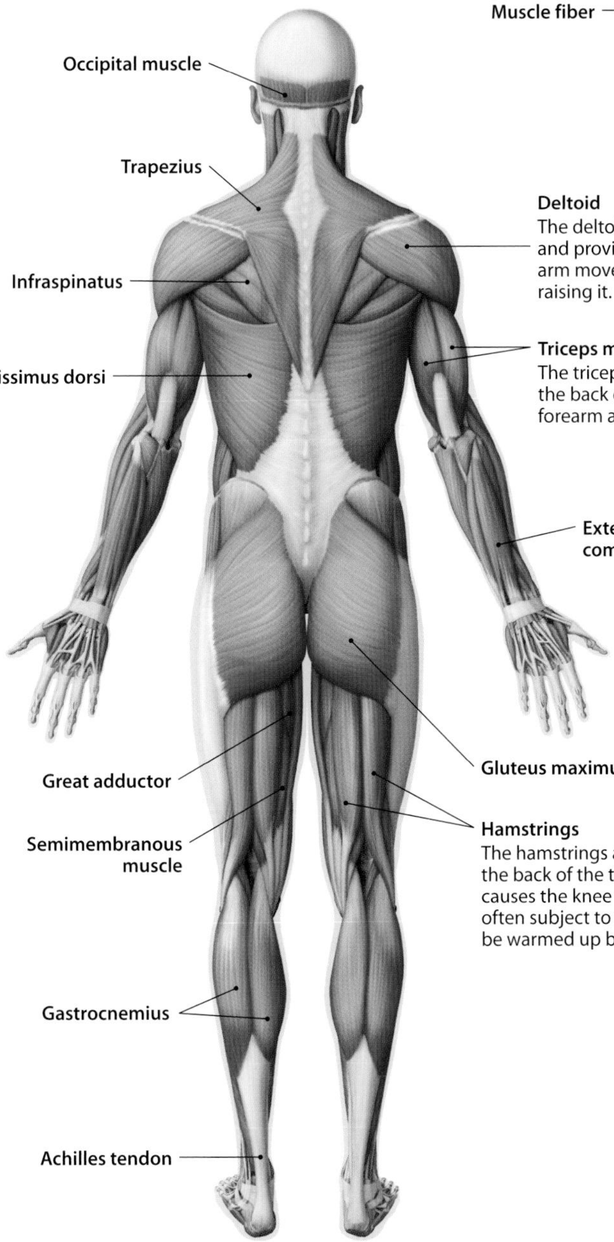

Occipital muscle
Trapezius
Infraspinatus
Latissimus dorsi

Deltoid
The deltoid covers the shoulder and provides for a number of arm movements, including raising it.

Triceps muscle of arm
The triceps muscle of arm covers the back of the arm, allowing the forearm and elbow to extend.

Extensor digitorum communis

Great adductor
Semimembranous muscle

Gluteus maximus

Hamstrings
The hamstrings are a set of muscles at the back of the thigh, whose contraction causes the knee to bend. Because they are often subject to muscle tears, they must be warmed up before physical exercise.

Gastrocnemius
Achilles tendon

Back view of the main skeletal muscles

THE TENDONS
The tendons are bands of fibrous tissue that are highly resistant, but rather inelastic. They are located at the ends of the skeletal muscles, which they anchor to the bones. The tendons may be long or short and enable transmission of the strength created by muscle contraction to the skeleton.

HEAVYWEIGHT
The 600-odd skeletal muscles in the human body generally account for approximately 40% of body mass.

HEALTHY BONES, JOINTS, AND MUSCLES

Osteoporosis, rheumatism, fractures, sprains, lumbago... a multitude of ailments can affect your bones, joints, and muscles. These common problems can be limited, or even prevented, by modifying a few of your day-to-day behaviors. This will allow you to live a full life with minimum effort and pain.

PREVENTING MUSCULOSKELETAL PROBLEMS

■ PARTICIPATE IN MODERATE PHYSICAL ACTIVITIES ON A REGULAR BASIS

Do stretching and body-building exercises or any other activity (walking, yoga, etc.) that forces your muscles to carry your body weight. These activities have many benefits. They strengthen your muscles and increase bone density, which helps to prevent muscle injury, fractures, and diseases such as osteoporosis. They also preserve the health of your joints by making them more flexible, which limits the effects of joint inflammation and degeneration (arthritis and arthrosis). In addition, these activities raise the resistance of your spinal column and of the muscles and ligaments surrounding it, which protects you against backaches. Finally, physical activity in general helps you to maintain a healthy weight, while reducing the pressure on your back and joints, particularly your knees and hips.

■ AVOID EXCESSIVE PHYSICAL ACTIVITY

Overly intense participation in a physical activity increases the pressure on your bones and muscles and is particularly hard on your joints. As a result, it increases the risk of fractures, sprains, dislocations, joint pain, and torn muscles.

■ PAY SPECIAL ATTENTION TO YOUR POSTURE

Keep your back and head in a straight position. When seated, both feet should be flat on the ground (do not cross your legs). Regular, moderate physical exercise like yoga can help correct your posture and prevent the injuries that lead to a backache.

Backache... page 114

■ WEAR COMFORTABLE SHOES

Shoes with soles that provide good cushioning, particularly at the heel, help to prevent or relieve backaches and joint pain. Avoid high heels, which, when worn regularly, deform the natural curve of the lower back and increase joint tension in the knee, in addition to causing the appearance of corns and joint pain in the feet.

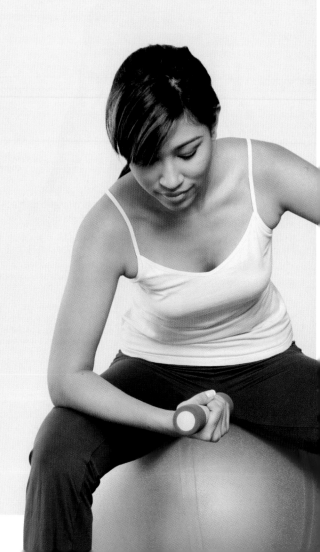

PREVENTING MUSCULOSKELETAL PROBLEMS

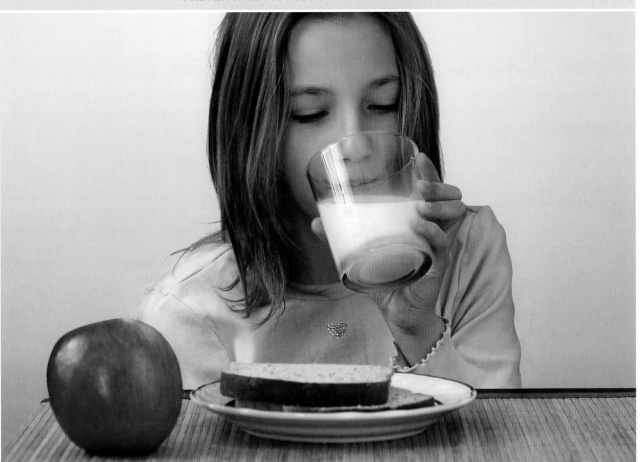

■ **FOLLOW A CALCIUM-RICH DIET**

Calcium solidifies your bones. It gives them greater density and resistance, which helps to prevent diseases like osteoporosis. Calcium also helps the muscles to contract and keeps the joints healthy by protecting them from inflammation and degeneration. Dairy products, certain fish (like sardines), and dark green vegetables are rich in calcium.

Calcium... page 95

■ **REDUCE YOUR CONSUMPTION OF CAFFEINATED DRINKS AND SOFT DRINKS**

These types of beverages inhibit the absorption of calcium by the body.

■ **TAKE VITAMIN D**

Vitamin D accelerates the body's absorption of calcium. The sun, fatty fish (like salmon), milk, and enriched drinks are excellent sources of Vitamin D. The recommended minimum dose is 5 μg (micrograms) per day up to the age of 50, 10 μg for people 51–70 years of age and 15 μg per day after the age of 70. Talk to a doctor, who can tell you whether or not taking Vitamin D in the form of dietary supplements is right for you.

■ **AVOID ALCOHOL ABUSE AND TOBACCO**

Excessive alcohol and the use of tobacco products lead to a decrease in bone mass, thereby increasing the risk of osteoporosis.

BONE FRACTURES

Despite their solidity, the bones are vulnerable to fracture. A fracture is the breakage, fragmentation, or cracking of a bone. It may be the result of an impact or prolonged, repeated effort (stress fracture). It can also occur spontaneously, when the bone has become weakened by disease, such as osteoporosis. Fractures are painful injuries, sometimes accompanied by severe hemorrhaging, an **infection**, or injury to the surrounding tissues, muscles, ligaments, tendons, and nerves. There are several types of fractures, which can be identified by X-ray.

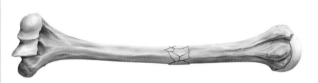

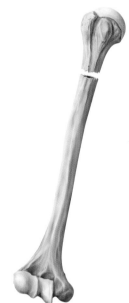

TRANSVERSE FRACTURES

A transverse fracture is a clean break in the bone of a limb. It is frequently the result of a direct impact. This is the most common type of fracture and the easiest to treat.

COMMINUTED FRACTURES

Comminuted fractures are characterized by the shattering of the bone into several pieces. This severe type of fracture is difficult to heal. Comminuted fractures primarily occur due to a violent impact, although they are also found in the elderly, whose bones are more brittle.

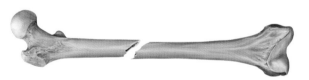

SPIRAL FRACTURES

Spiral fractures are mainly found in athletes. They occur when the bone of a limb is subjected to sudden twisting.

STRESS FRACTURES

Stress fractures are bone breaks resulting from localized weakness. They are caused by prolonged and repeated efforts. This type of fracture often occurs after intense physical activity. Rest is usually sufficient to heal stress fractures.

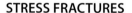

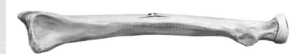

GREENSTICK FRACTURES

A greenstick fracture is an incomplete break in the bone of a limb. It is usually seen in children, whose bones are more supple than those of adults.

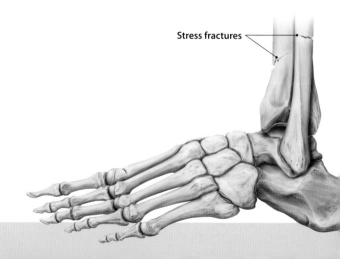

Stress fractures

FRACTURE OF THE FEMORAL NECK

The femoral neck is the narrow part of the femur, located at the hip level. The body's weight and thigh movements place a great deal of strain on this part of the skeleton. Fractures of the femoral neck are common, affecting close to 1 person in 1,000 every year in Western countries. They can be caused by a fall or an apparently insignificant impact in people whose bones have been weakened by osteoporosis. Fracture of the femoral neck leads to complete infirmity. It can be treated by the implantation of a prosthesis, which replaces the damaged end of the femur, or by metal implants attached to the bone.

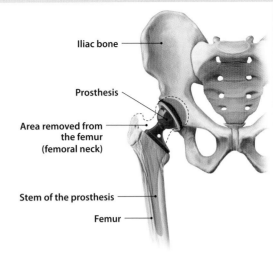

Iliac bone

Prosthesis

Area removed from the femur (femoral neck)

Stem of the prosthesis

Femur

Hip prosthesis

FRACTURES OF THE SKULL

After a head trauma, the bones of the skull may fracture and sink into the skull. Skull fractures are often accompanied by brain injuries, which may manifest as headaches, a loss of consciousness, or motor or sensory impairment.

Head trauma... page 150

COMPOUND FRACTURE OR SIMPLE FRACTURE

A fracture is simple when the fractured bone does not penetrate the skin. These fractures leave no open wounds. Conversely, a fracture is compound when the broken ends of the bones tear through the surrounding tissues and penetrate the skin. Compound fractures are less common and more serious than simple fractures. They usually cause external hemorrhaging and entail a major risk of infection of the bone tissue and neighboring tissues.

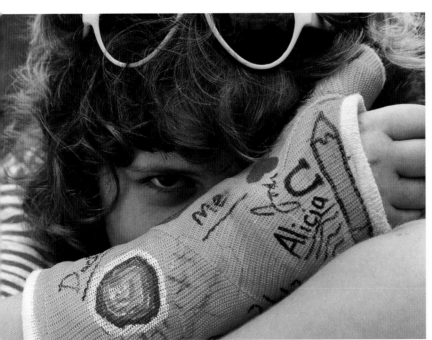

FRACTURE, SPRAIN, OR DISLOCATION?

A fracture involves the breaking of a bone: the part of the body affected by the fracture is often deformed and crippled. Sprains are the rupture or pulling of a ligament. They are characterized by the swelling of the affected joint. Dislocation is the displacement of two bones at a joint, often accompanied by full or partial infirmity and the deformation of the affected joint.

RADIOGRAPHY

There are several medical imaging techniques available for examination of a bone. Radiography (X-ray) is very commonly employed and is useful in confirming the diagnosis of a bone fracture and assessing its severity. A beam of X-rays penetrates the body, leaving its imprint on a photographic plate. The bones, which absorb a large portion of the X-rays, form white lines, while the soft tissues, which are less dense and more easily permeated by the X-rays, are displayed as different shades of gray.

Clavicle   Fracture

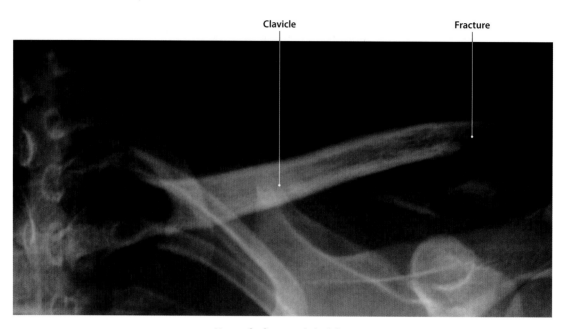

X-ray of a fractured clavicle

REPAIRING A FRACTURED BONE

When a fracture is revealed by X-ray, a number of mechanisms can be used to encourage and accelerate its consolidation. In general, a cast or other orthopedic apparatus will be used to immobilize the fractured area. If the pieces are no longer in alignment along the normal axis of the bone, it may be necessary to first perform a reduction, and in some cases, osteosynthesis.

REDUCTION OF THE FRACTURE

The reduction of a fracture is a medical or surgical intervention aiming to reposition the fragments of a fractured bone. To do this, gradual traction is performed on the fractured bone.

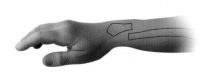

1. Fractured radius

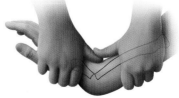

2. Gradual traction

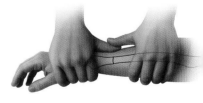

3. Repositioning the
   bone fragments

OSTEOSYNTHESIS

Osteosynthesis is a surgical technique designed to stabilize bone fractures using metal implants (plates, screws, nails, or pins) set in the bone. These implants are usually removed once bone consolidation is complete.

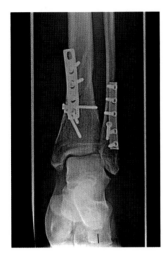

X-ray of an ankle (osteosynthesis)

CONSOLIDATION OF A FRACTURE

The consolidation of a fracture is a physiological process that ends with the knitting of the fragments of a fractured bone. When a bone is fractured, the blood vessels within it burst, causing bleeding, followed by the formation of a clot. The blood clot and the dead bone cells are gradually eliminated and replaced with a regenerative tissue, bone callus, which connects the broken parts of the bone together. With time, the callus transforms into true bone tissue. This consolidation can take several weeks to several months.
Once the bone has consolidated, only a slight bulge will remain at the site of the fracture.

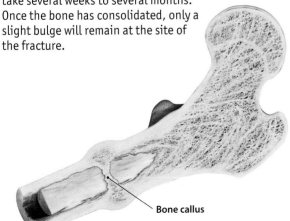

Bone callus

IMMOBILIZATION

Fractured bones are often immobilized by fitting a cast around them, possibly as a complement to osteosynthesis. The cast must be removed once the bone has consolidated. Raising the limb, especially at night, helps with the reabsorption of the swelling that accompanies fractures.

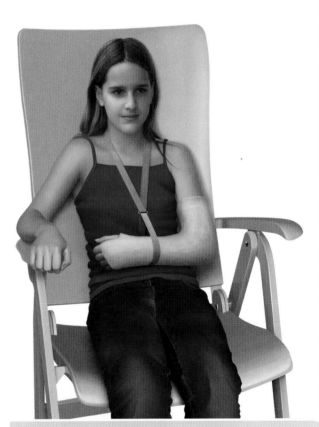

BONE FRACTURES

SYMPTOMS:
Pain, deformed limb, localized infirmity, protruding bones with external hemorrhaging (compound fracture).

TREATMENTS:
Reduction, immobilization (osteosynthesis, cast), rest (stress fractures), prosthesis if the bone is too damaged, rehabilitation.
First aid: Falls and traumas... page 552

PREVENTION:
Supervision of sports activities, osteoporosis prevention. During treatment of a fracture: raising the plastered limb to avoid the onset of edema (swelling).

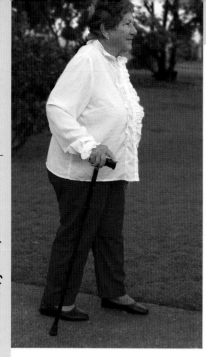

OSTEOPOROSIS

Osteoporosis is a common ailment. It is estimated that one in four women over the age of 50 is afflicted with this disease. The disease is characterized by a gradual loss of bone mass, which becomes porous and more vulnerable. Osteoporosis is responsible for bone fractures caused by minor **trauma**. It affects menopausal women in particular, but also men over the age of 70. Multiple factors lead to the development of osteoporosis, including the hormonal changes brought about by menopause, a sedentary lifestyle, calcium, Vitamin D, and protein deficiencies, as well as the consumption of alcohol and tobacco.

DEVELOPMENT OF THE SKELETON

Maintenance of bone mass in adults is the result of a balance between bone tissue production and loss. This balance depends on several factors, particularly hormonal ones. Among the sex hormones, estrogen in women and testosterone in men limit bone loss. The natural end to their production that comes with age contributes to osteoporosis, especially in menopausal women.

Bone tissue... page 95

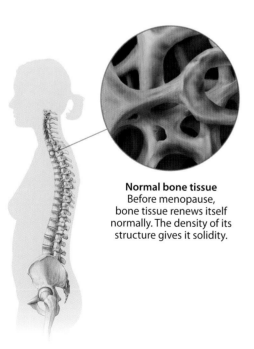

Normal bone tissue
Before menopause, bone tissue renews itself normally. The density of its structure gives it solidity.

Nonmenopausal women
Nonmenopausal women produce estrogen, which protects the bone tissue. Bone mass is stable.

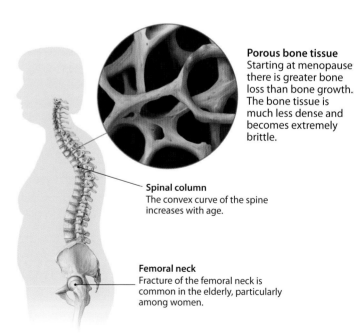

Porous bone tissue
Starting at menopause there is greater bone loss than bone growth. The bone tissue is much less dense and becomes extremely brittle.

Spinal column
The convex curve of the spine increases with age.

Femoral neck
Fracture of the femoral neck is common in the elderly, particularly among women.

Menopausal women
Menopausal women can lose up to one-third of their bone mass. The vertebrae compress, the spinal column curves, and height decreases notably. The risk of fracture (femoral neck, wrist, vertebrae, etc.) increases.

BONE MINERAL DENSITY TESTING

Bone mineral density (BMD) testing, or bone densitometry, is a medical imaging technique. It makes it possible to measure loss of bone mass, and therefore diagnose and monitor the development of osteoporosis. The amount of minerals (primarily calcium) contained in the bones is measured by a densitometer that uses X-rays. After passing through the body, the X-rays not absorbed by the calcium in the bones leave an imprint of varying strength on the detector. The more X-rays detected and the darker the outlines of the bones, the more porous the bones are.

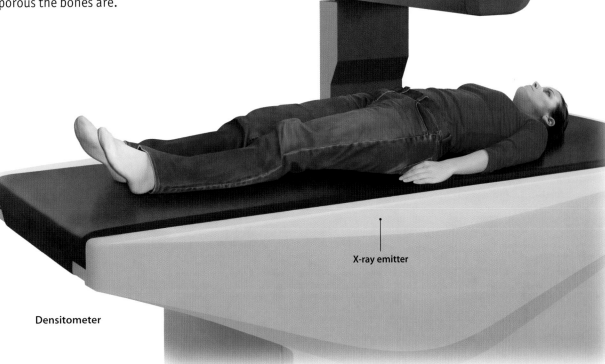

Mobile arm
The mobile arm contains an X-ray detector.

X-ray emitter

Densitometer

OSTEOPOROSIS

SYMPTOMS:
Height loss, upper and lower back pain, fractures caused by minor trauma.

TREATMENTS:
Calcium, Vitamin D, and medications that inhibit the loss of bone mass.

PREVENTION:
A diet rich in calcium and Vitamin D, moderate physical exercise, reduced consumption of alcohol, coffee and tobacco, prevention of falls for the elderly. Hormone replacement therapy (HRT) for menopausal women.

Calcium... page 95

PAGET'S DISEASE

The cause of Paget's disease is unknown. It is characterized by anomalies in the regrowth of bone tissue. These anomalies are responsible for the brittleness, deformation, and increased volume of the affected regions of bone. Paget's disease affects approximately 3% of the population, usually appearing after the age of 50. It may be revealed by spontaneous fractures, pain, or deformation of the limbs. However, Paget's disease is most often benign, presenting no symptoms.

Normal position of the tibia

Sick tibia

PAGET'S DISEASE

SYMPTOMS:
Usually asymptomatic. In some cases: bone, joint, and nerve pain; stiffness; headache; bone deformations (arched legs and arms, enlarged skull); raised skin temperature around lesions.

TREATMENTS:
Medications that inhibit the loss of bone mass, anti-inflammatories. Surgery can correct bone deformations.

Pagetic bone
The bone tissue comprises different types of cells, including osteoblasts (responsible for bone production) and osteoclasts (responsible for bone loss). In Pagetic bones, the osteoclasts rapidly destroy the bone in a disorderly manner. The osteoblasts respond by reconstructing hypertrophied bone tissue with a disorganized structure.

OSTEITIS

Osteitis is the **inflammation** of a bone, generally caused by a bacterium. When the bone marrow is affected, which is often the case, the disease is called osteomyelitis. Osteitis is caused by a direct contamination of the bone, following a **trauma** (compound fracture, infected wound), or by the circulation of blood from another point of **infection**. These infections mainly affect children, adolescents, and the elderly. Recovery is usually complete, although the treatment is long (six to eight weeks) and must be started immediately.

OSTEITIS

SYMPTOMS:
Intense pain, redness, heat and swelling in the affected bone, infirmity, fever, shivering, fatigue, nausea, malaise, refusal to walk or limping in young children.

TREATMENTS:
Prolonged antibiotic treatment (first intravenous, then oral). Rest and immobilization of the affected bone. Surgery: drainage of the infected bone, removal of the sequestra, bone transplant.

PREVENTION:
Cleansing and disinfecting wounds, especially deep wounds.

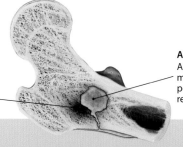

Sequestrum
A sequestrum is a fragment of **necrosed** (dead) bone that forms at the point of infection.

Abscess
An abscess (mass of pus) may appear at the point of infection, requiring drainage.

BONE CANCER

Bone cancer is, most often, caused by metastases, meaning that it develops from tumors in other organs. Primary bone tumors are rare. Bone cancer is detected via medical imaging, and diagnosis is confirmed by **biopsy**. It is treated surgically (removal of the tumor), in combination with **chemotherapy**. Bone cancer can quickly produce metastases, especially in the lungs.

PRIMARY BONE TUMORS

Of the primary bone tumors, the most common are osteosarcomas, chondrosarcomas, and Ewing's sarcomas. Osteosarcoma is a form of cancer that develops particularly in the long bones. It primarily affects male adolescents and young adults, as well as people over the age of 40 with Paget's disease. Chondrosarcoma is a form of cancer of the cartilage tissues of a bone. It chiefly affects the elderly. Finally, Ewing's sarcoma is a form of cancer that develops in the bone cavities and may spread to the marrow and other soft tissues. It especially affects male children and young adults.

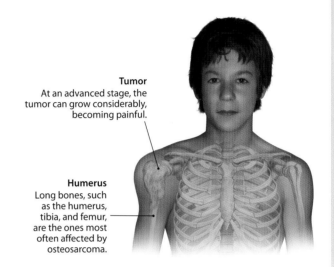

Tumor
At an advanced stage, the tumor can grow considerably, becoming painful.

Humerus
Long bones, such as the humerus, tibia, and femur, are the ones most often affected by osteosarcoma.

Osteosarcoma of the humerus

THE **GROWING PROSTHESIS**

The removal of a bone tumor may require the installation of a growing prosthesis. This internal apparatus replaces a long bone in a child and gradually lengthens as the child grows.

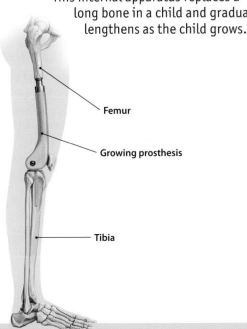

Femur

Growing prosthesis

Tibia

BONE TRANSPLANTS

A bone transplant is a surgical operation that consists of replacing a damaged bone fragment with a healthy bone fragment. The transplanted fragment, either from one of the patient's other bones or from a donor, is attached using metal implants (screws, nails, plates). A bone transplant may be performed after a trauma or after the surgical ablation of a tumor.

BONE CANCER

SYMPTOMS:
Bone pain, swelling, sometimes fever, fractures.

TREATMENTS:
Surgical ablation of the tumor, chemotherapy, sometimes radiation therapy. Surgical intervention may require installation of a prosthesis or performance of a bone transplant.

SPRAIN

A sprain is the stretching or rupture of a ligament at a joint. This common ailment, caused by torsion, stretching, or a sudden impact, results in a sharp pain and swelling of the affected region. The joints most vulnerable to sprains are those of the ankle, knee, finger, and wrist. Twisted joints are benign sprains, in which the ligaments are merely pulled. A torn, ruptured, or detached ligament is a much more serious form of a sprain. The injured ligaments heal poorly, and recovery is slow, which often leads to lasting joint fragility and instability.

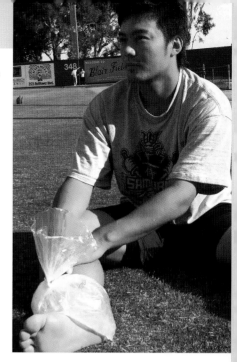

KNEE SPRAIN

The knee joint is used in many movements and is therefore particularly at risk for sprains, especially at the level of the medial collateral ligament, which is vulnerable to lateral impacts, and of the anterior cruciate ligament, which is sensitive to torsion movements. Knee sprains may be accompanied by a torn meniscus.

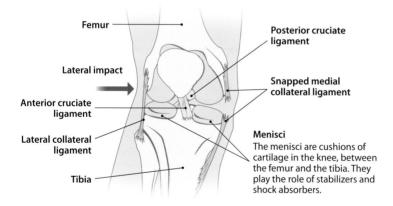

Femur

Posterior cruciate ligament

Lateral impact

Snapped medial collateral ligament

Anterior cruciate ligament

Lateral collateral ligament

Menisci
The menisci are cushions of cartilage in the knee, between the femur and the tibia. They play the role of stabilizers and shock absorbers.

Tibia

Rupture of the medial collateral ligament

TORN MENISCUS

The menisci can suffer injuries of varying severity, from fissures to complete rupture. These injuries typically arise after a forced movement of the joint, like the sudden torsion or extension of the knee. The damaged part of the meniscus may be removed or repaired by a minor surgical operation, a meniscectomy. This operation allows the patient to recover complete use of the knee after just a few weeks of rest.

SPRAIN

SYMPTOMS:
Sharp pain, swelling, sometimes hematomas. Muscle contractions. In some serious cases, the sprain may be accompanied by dislocation, bone fracture, or other injuries.

TREATMENTS:
Application of ice and pressure on the injured area for benign sprains (twisted joints). Immobilization by means of an orthosis or cast, complete rest, and sometimes surgery for severe sprains. Rehabilitation in most cases.

First aid: Falls and traumas... page 552

PREVENTION:
Wearing an orthosis can help prevent recurrences.

DISLOCATION

Dislocation is the displacement of two bones at a joint. It is often caused by an impact, fall, or forced movement. More rarely, it is **congenital**. The shoulder, elbow, fingers, and jaw are the joints most often involved in traumatic dislocations. Congenital dislocation mainly concerns the hip and may lead to limping. A dislocated joint remains fragile because the tissues pulled during injury, especially the ligaments, have difficulty recovering. Recurrences are common.

Congenital malformations... page 510

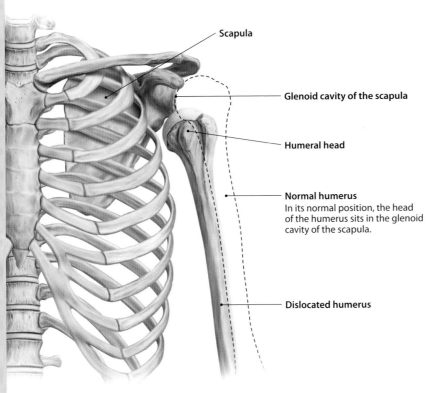

Scapula

Glenoid cavity of the scapula

Humeral head

Normal humerus
In its normal position, the head of the humerus sits in the glenoid cavity of the scapula.

Dislocated humerus

TRAUMATIC SHOULDER DISLOCATION

After an impact or fall, the head of the humerus may be displaced outside the glenoid cavity of the scapula (shoulder blade), resulting in a dislocated shoulder. Displacement of the bone is often accompanied by a sprain and sometimes by a fractured bone or by nerve or blood vessel injuries.

ORTHOSIS

An orthosis is a device used to support, protect or immobilize a joint that has been weakened by injury (sprain, dislocation, tendinitis). Orthoses are often used on a temporary or intermittent basis.

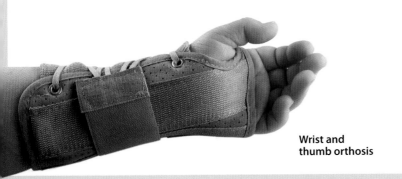

Wrist and thumb orthosis

DISLOCATION

SYMPTOMS:
Intense pain, deformed joint, limited movements or inability to move.

TREATMENTS:
Reduction of the dislocation (putting the bone back in place), usually under anesthesia, immobilization of the joint for three to four weeks, rehabilitation. Surgical operation after multiple recurrences.

First aid: Falls and traumas... page 552

PREVENTION:
Wearing an orthosis can reduce the risk of recurrences.

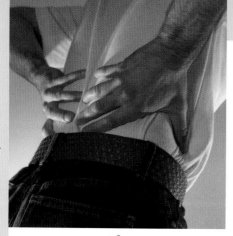

HERNIATED DISK

A herniated disk is the abnormal extrusion or crushing of an intervertebral disk. It mainly affects the lumbar region (lower back) of young adults and is often caused by an awkward movement or by lifting overly heavy loads. The main treatment is rest and **anti-inflammatories**, followed by surgery in rare cases.

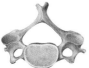

Cervical vertebra
The seven cervical vertebrae are extremely mobile bones that form the upper part of the spinal column, at the neck. They enable movement of the head.

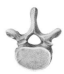

Thoracic vertebra
The 12 thoracic vertebrae are the bones in the spinal column to which the ribs are attached, at the chest.

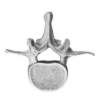

Lumbar vertebra
The five lumbar vertebrae are large vertebrae located under the thoracic vertebrae, at the abdomen.

Sacrum
The sacrum is a triangular bone resulting from the fusion of the five sacral vertebrae during childhood. It joins with the iliac bones to form the pelvis.

- Cervical vertebrae
- Thoracic vertebrae
- Lumbar vertebrae
- Sacral vertebrae
- Coccygeal vertebrae

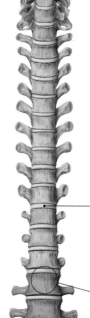

Front view of the spinal column

FACET JOINT

A facet joint (or intervertebral disk) is a cartilaginous cushion separating two adjacent vertebrae. It only allows for limited movements. The primary function of the intervertebral disks is to absorb shocks and to spread out the pressure exerted on the spinal column during effort, especially while walking and running. These solid, stable, collagen-rich disks can, however, suffer injuries in the form of herniated disks. These usually affect the lumbar region.

The joints... page 96

Intervertebral disk

Nucleus pulposus
The nucleus pulposus is a gelatinous mass that can be deformed but not compressed, located at the center of an intervertebral disk.

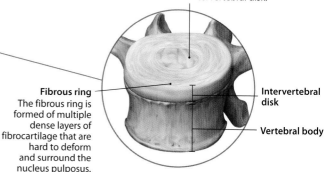

Fibrous ring
The fibrous ring is formed of multiple dense layers of fibrocartilage that are hard to deform and surround the nucleus pulposus.

Intervertebral disk

Vertebral body

Intervertebral disk (lumbar vertebra)

Coccyx
The coccyx is a small triangular bone resulting from the fusion of the four coccygeal vertebrae in early adulthood. Located below the sacrum, it is the lower tip of the spinal column.

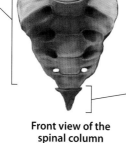

SYMPTOMS OF A HERNIATED DISK

The disks between the vertebrae of the spinal column are comprised of a nucleus pulposus surrounded by a fibrous ring. The injury of a fibrous ring leads to the protrusion of the nucleus pulposus. The herniated disk may compress the root of a spinal nerve or the spinal cord, causing very sharp pain (neuralgia) localized around the hernia and which may extend to the area innervated by the affected nerves. This pain may be accompanied by a tingling feeling, back stiffness, and muscle weakness. In unusual cases, the hernia's compression of the spinal cord can cause paralysis of the limbs.

The spinal cord... page 139

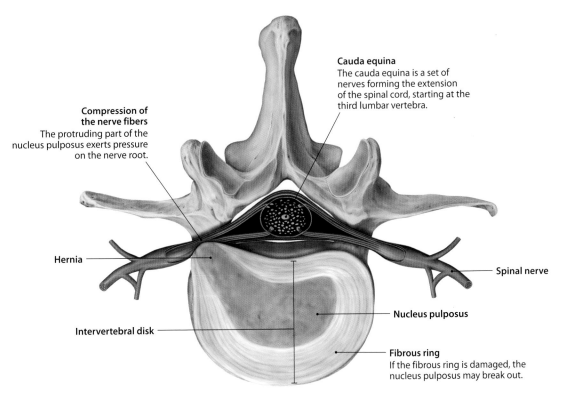

Cauda equina
The cauda equina is a set of nerves forming the extension of the spinal cord, starting at the third lumbar vertebra.

Compression of the nerve fibers
The protruding part of the nucleus pulposus exerts pressure on the nerve root.

Hernia

Spinal nerve

Nucleus pulposus

Intervertebral disk

Fibrous ring
If the fibrous ring is damaged, the nucleus pulposus may break out.

Herniated disk (lumbar vertebra)

LUMBAGO

Lumbago, also known as acute lumbar pain, is an intense pain appearing suddenly in the lower back. It may be caused by various factors, including a herniated disk or lumbar arthrosis.

HERNIATED DISK

SYMPTOMS:
Intense back pain, possibly radiating out to the limbs, tingling sensation, back stiffness.

TREATMENTS:
Rest, analgesics, anti-inflammatories, rehabilitation aiming to strengthen the muscles of the back and prevent recurrences. In the most serious cases, surgery to remove the damaged disk.

PREVENTION:
Stretching and limbering exercises when seated for long periods of time, muscle development for the back, care when lifting heavy loads.

Healthy bones, joints, and muscles... page 100
Preventing backaches... page 114

BACKACHE

Backaches are extremely common. At least one in two people will suffer from them at some point in their lives. In fact, a backache is not actually a disease: it is a symptom. It is often caused by a **trauma** or **microtrauma** affecting a disk (herniated disk), ligament (sprain), muscle (tear), or nerve (neuralgia) in the lumbar region. Many factors can trigger a backache: an awkward movement, improper handling of a heavy object, bad posture, repetitive work, fatigue, stress, weak back or abdominal muscles, being overweight, pregnancy, aging (arthrosis of the spinal column or osteoporosis), etc. Simple tricks can help to relieve or prevent backaches.

Healthy bones, joints, and muscles... page 100

PREVENTING BACKACHE

■ DO PHYSICAL EXERCISE

Participate in moderate physical activities on a regular basis. In particular, strengthen your back and abdominal muscles by means of warm-up, stretching, and body-building exercises. Here are a few simple exercises that you can do every day to prevent backaches:

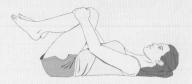

Knees to chest
Lie down on your back and bring your thighs up to your abdomen. Wrap your arms around your legs. Breathe deeply.

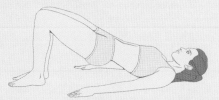

Raised pelvis
Lie down on your back and bend your knees, placing your feet close to your pelvis and slightly apart. Raise your pelvis, keeping your upper body on the ground. Hold this position for at least 30 seconds, breathing deeply.

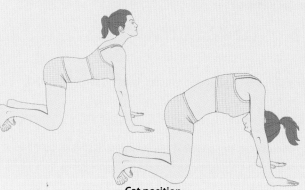

Cat position
Get on your hands and knees, with your hands aligned straight below your shoulders and your knees apart. Breathe in and slowly arch your back while raising your head. Breathe out and slowly round your back while lowering your head and stretching your arms. Repeat these movements 5–10 times.

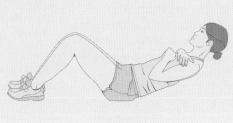

Abdominals
Lie down on your back, fold your arms over your chest and bend your knees, keeping your feet flat on the ground. Contract your abdominal muscles and slowly raise your shoulders, keeping your head in alignment with the rest of your body. Hold this position for 1 or 2 seconds, then slowly lower your shoulders back down. Repeat this 5–10 times.

Warning! If an exercise is painful, stop it immediately.

RELIEVING BACKACHES

- **STOP THE ACTIVITY THAT TRIGGERED THE PAIN**

- **SOOTHE THE PAIN**
  Soothe the pain by means of anti-inflammatories or analgesics if your state of health allows, and be sure to follow the dosage indicated.

- **APPLY COLD, THEN HEAT**
  During the first 48 hours, apply cold to the pain, to reduce the inflammation, in alternating periods of 15 minutes with, then without, ice. After 48 hours, apply heat to the painful area, to relax the muscles and encourage healing.

- **LIE DOWN ON A HARD SURFACE**
  Lie down on your back, either directly on the floor or on a firm mattress, with a pillow under your knees. If you have major pain, you can stay lying down, although it is preferable to try to get up and walk around for a few minutes every hour.

- **DO NOT STAY IN BED**
  Do not stay in bed more than two or three days. As soon as you can, do moderate exercise like walking, cycling, or swimming.

  Warning! Talk to a doctor if you have major pain or if the pain persists.

PREVENTING BACKACHES

- **BREATHE**
  Relax and breathe correctly, that is, slowly and from the abdomen. Stress and tension contribute to backache.

- **LIFT OBJECTS CORRECTLY**
  Avoid carrying overly heavy loads, and lift objects by bending your knees and keeping your back straight, with the items held close to your body. Do not twist your back suddenly or awkwardly. Use your leg muscles, not your back muscles.

- **AVOID SLEEPING ON YOUR STOMACH OR ON AN OVERLY SOFT MATTRESS**

- **MOVE**
  Walk and stretch regularly. Avoid standing or sitting for extended periods of time.

- **WEAR COMFORTABLE SHOES**

- **MAINTAIN GOOD POSTURE**
  Maintain good posture, especially at work and behind the wheel of your car: back and head held straight, elbows naturally bent. Your work chair and the seat of your car should provide support to your lower back (add an orthopedic support, if needed).

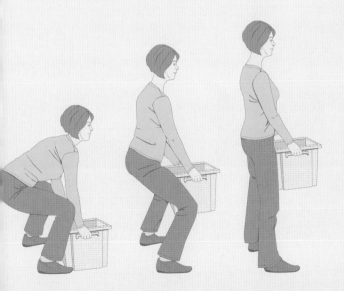
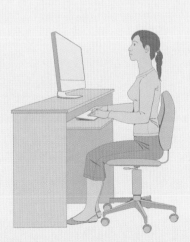

The bones, joints, and muscles | Joint diseases

RHEUMATISM

The joints can suffer from a number of **inflammatory** or **degenerative** diseases, which are given the generic name of rheumatism. Arthrosis is a degenerative disease, while arthritis designates all of the inflammatory joint diseases: rheumatoid arthritis, ankylosing spondylitis, gout. Rheumatism causes pain, stiffness, and, in some cases, swelling and deformation. These troublesome symptoms can be limited or prevented by following certain recommendations.

RELIEVING RHEUMATISM

■ SOOTHE THE PAIN

Soothe the pain by means of antirheumatics prescribed by your doctor. Some doctors advise patients with arthrosis to take glucosamine and chondroitin sulfates. These substances are thought to lubricate the joints and reduce the inflammation causing the pain. Furthermore, they are believed to contribute to the regeneration of the damaged joint cartilage.

■ LOSE YOUR EXCESS WEIGHT

Excess weight increases the pressure on your joints, particularly your knees and hips.

■ WEAR COMFORTABLE SHOES

■ WATCH YOUR DIET

Eat foods rich in calcium and Vitamin D (or take these in the form of dietary supplements) to prevent the degeneration of the articular cartilage.

Calcium... page 95

■ DO MODERATE EXERCISE ON A REGULAR BASIS

Exercise like walking, cycling, yoga, and swimming can reduce joint stiffness. Swimming is particularly beneficial because it is a no-impact way to increase muscle strength and joint flexibility.

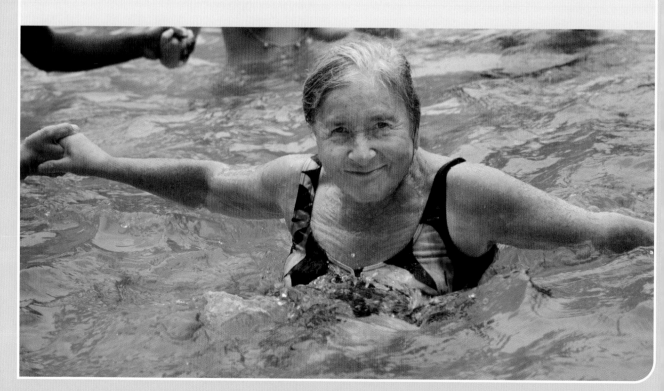

ARTHROSIS

Arthrosis is a **degenerative** disease characterized by the gradual wearing away of the cartilage in the joints. It is very common after the age of 60, but can also appear earlier in the case of joint injury (torn meniscus, sprain). This disease is also furthered by excess weight, intense physical activity, bad posture, and hereditary factors. Arthrosis causes localized pain triggered by excess strain on a joint. It develops in spurts, during which the affected joint becomes more painful and may swell. With time, the joint stiffens and may become deformed and lose its mobility. The joints most often affected are the knees, hips, fingers, cervical vertebrae, and lumbar vertebrae.

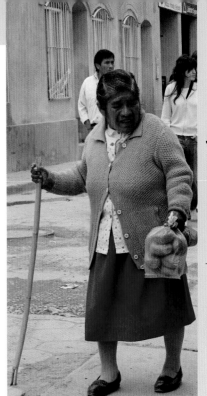

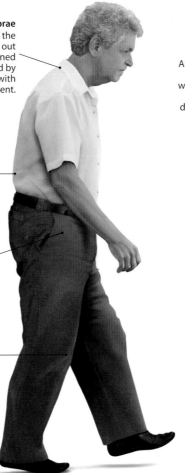

Cervical vertebrae
Cervical arthrosis causes pain at the nape of the neck (possibly radiating out to the shoulder and arm), combined with gradual stiffening. It is caused by spending extended periods of time with the neck bent.

Lumbar vertebrae
Lumbar arthrosis is very common and is often the result of damage to an intervertebral disk, repeated strain on the spinal column, at work or during physical activity (bad posture, continuous repetition of the same movement). Lumbar arthrosis causes pain in the lower back, which can extend to the lower limbs.

Hip
Hip arthrosis, common after age 50, can considerably decrease the patient's mobility. In very advanced cases, the joint may be replaced with a **prosthesis**.

Knee
Arthrosis of the knee is the most common form of arthrosis. **Trauma** (like sprains), misalignment (deformities), and excess weight can all contribute to its onset.

Thumb
Arthrosis of the base of the thumb primarily affects women. It causes a gradual deformation, resulting in difficulty handling objects.

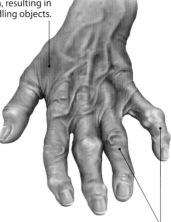

Fingers
Arthrosis of the fingers results in swelling, pain, deformations, and loss of mobility in the fingers.

Locations of arthrosis

117

THE **DEVELOPMENT** OF **ARTHROSIS**

Arthrosis develops slowly, generally appearing at the age of 40 or later. The first symptoms (effort-related pain and stiffness in the morning) often remain subtle for several years, and the disease does not always reach the most severe stage.

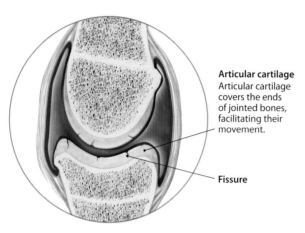

Articular cartilage
Articular cartilage covers the ends of jointed bones, facilitating their movement.

Fissure

1. Formation of fissures
With age, the renewal of articular cartilage is less effective, leading to the formation of fissures.

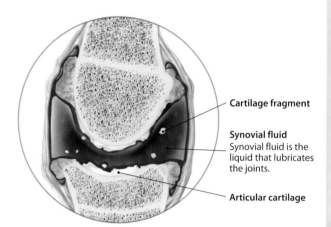

Cartilage fragment

Synovial fluid
Synovial fluid is the liquid that lubricates the joints.

Articular cartilage

2. Degradation of the cartilage
Cartilage degradation causes the bone surfaces to be uncovered, after which they start to rub against one another. Fragments of cartilage immersed in the synovial fluid can lead to inflammation.

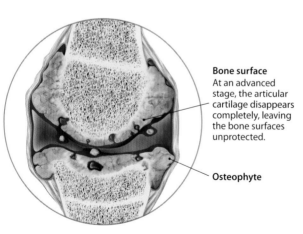

Bone surface
At an advanced stage, the articular cartilage disappears completely, leaving the bone surfaces unprotected.

Osteophyte

3. Degeneration of bone surfaces
The surfaces of the bone then begins to degenerate. Painless bony outgrowths (osteophytes) develop, gradually restricting the joint's mobility.

ARTHROSIS

SYMPTOMS:

Effort-related pain and stiffness in the morning, which develops in spurts. Deformation of certain joints (particularly the fingers). One or more joints may be affected.

TREATMENTS:

Analgesics, nonsteroidal anti-inflammatories (NSAIDs) and rest during attacks. Injection of corticosteroids in the case of very serious inflammation. Wearing an orthosis. Replacement of the joint with a prosthesis (hip, knee).

PREVENTION:

Moderate exercise on a regular basis. For people who are obese, weight loss.

Rheumatism... page 116

RHEUMATOID ARTHRITIS

Rheumatoid arthritis is an **inflammatory** joint disease. Fairly common, it affects 0.5%–1% of the population, two to three times more often women than men. This **chronic** disease appears as stiffness in the morning, and pain and swelling in several joints, particularly the feet, hands, and wrists. Over time, rheumatoid arthritis can lead to deformation, loss of mobility, and, in the most serious cases, disability. It is incurable, but there are treatments that can control its development and prevent the aggravation of injuries.

Rheumatism... page 116

Rheumatism... page 116

THE **DEVELOPMENT** OF **RHEUMATOID ARTHRITIS**

Rheumatoid arthritis is caused by an autoimmune response of an unknown cause. It typically starts between the ages of 35 and 50, and its evolution is characterized by unpredictable flare-ups, interspersed with periods of remission of varying lengths. The chronic inflammation leads to the gradual destruction of the articular cartilage and neighboring tissues (ligaments, tendons, and bones). After a few years, the inflammation and erosion of the joint's surfaces can result in deformation and blockage of the joint.

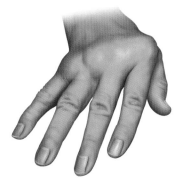

Affected hand
At an advanced stage, chronic inflammation deforms joints, which can lead to disability.

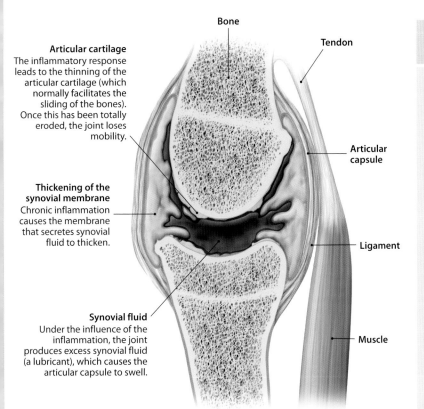

Bone

Tendon

Articular cartilage
The inflammatory response leads to the thinning of the articular cartilage (which normally facilitates the sliding of the bones). Once this has been totally eroded, the joint loses mobility.

Articular capsule

Thickening of the synovial membrane
Chronic inflammation causes the membrane that secretes synovial fluid to thicken.

Ligament

Synovial fluid
Under the influence of the inflammation, the joint produces excess synovial fluid (a lubricant), which causes the articular capsule to swell.

Muscle

RHEUMATOID ARTHRITIS

SYMPTOMS:
Pain, hot sensation and swollen joints, most often symmetrical. Joint stiffness in the morning, fatigue, weight loss, sometimes fever during flare-ups. Lumps under the skin (rheumatoid nodules) are sometimes observed.

TREATMENTS:
Disease-modifying drugs: antirheumatics, immunosuppressants, biotherapy. During flare-ups: rest, nonsteroidal anti-inflammatories (NSAIDs), antirheumatics, corticosteroids. Moderate exercise during periods of remission. Surgery in advanced cases.

PREVENTION:
Early detection improves the efficacy of treatments.

ANKYLOSING SPONDYLITIS

Ankylosing spondylitis is a **chronic inflammatory** disease that primarily affects the joints in the spinal column and pelvis. It causes pain, stiffness, and a gradual decline in the mobility of the diseased joints, resulting in the deformation of the spinal column. Ankylosing spondylitis mainly affects men. Its onset occurs between the ages of 15 and 35. The cause of the disease is unknown, although there is a **genetic** predisposition. Treatment essentially consists in reducing the symptoms and maintaining mobility.

THE **DEVELOPMENT** OF **ANKYLOSING SPONDYLITIS**

Ankylosing spondylitis typically starts with pain and stiffness in the buttocks and lower back. These appear towards the end of the night and in the morning when rising. Over time, the symptoms spread upward along the spinal column, which stiffens and deforms (kyphosis). The progression of ankylosing spondylitis continues over a period of 10–20 years, in successive flare-ups. The end result is ankylosis, that is, the decline, or even complete disappearance, of mobility in the affected joints.

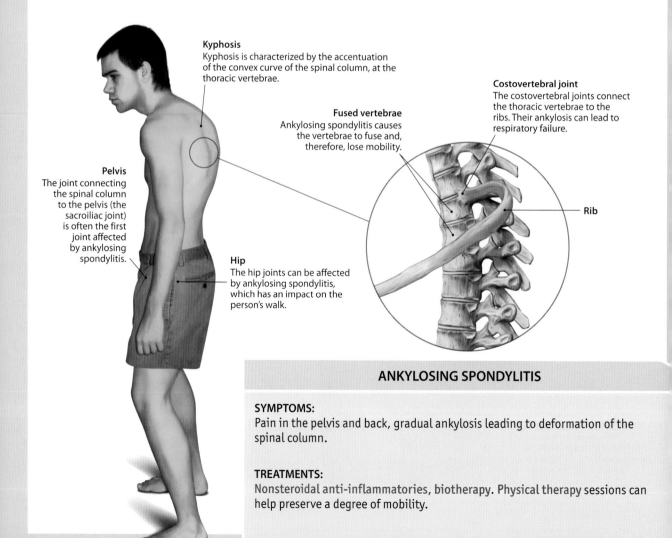

Kyphosis
Kyphosis is characterized by the accentuation of the convex curve of the spinal column, at the thoracic vertebrae.

Costovertebral joint
The costovertebral joints connect the thoracic vertebrae to the ribs. Their ankylosis can lead to respiratory failure.

Fused vertebrae
Ankylosing spondylitis causes the vertebrae to fuse and, therefore, lose mobility.

Pelvis
The joint connecting the spinal column to the pelvis (the sacroiliac joint) is often the first joint affected by ankylosing spondylitis.

Rib

Hip
The hip joints can be affected by ankylosing spondylitis, which has an impact on the person's walk.

ANKYLOSING SPONDYLITIS

SYMPTOMS:
Pain in the pelvis and back, gradual ankylosis leading to deformation of the spinal column.

TREATMENTS:
Nonsteroidal anti-inflammatories, biotherapy. Physical therapy sessions can help preserve a degree of mobility.

GOUT

Gout (or gouty arthritis) is caused by excess uric acid in the body, leading to the formation of crystallized deposits in the joints. The vast majority of gout patients are middle-aged men. The disease appears as sudden, intense flare-ups of joint **inflammation**, especially in the big toe. Gout is most often linked to eating habits (excessive intake of alcohol and certain meats). It can also be associated with hereditary factors or certain medications, or may be secondary to another disease.

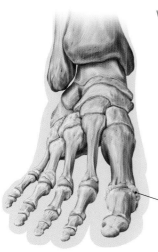

Crystallized deposits of uric acid

GOUT

SYMPTOMS:
Intense pain, swelling, redness and shiny appearance of the joint. Sudden flare-ups that become more frequent over time. Tophi (small, whitish masses of hardened uric acid) may appear under the skin at different places on the body.

TREATMENTS:
Colchicine, allopurinol, anti-inflammatories.

PREVENTION:
Avoid eating game meat, offal, shellfish and certain fish (anchovies, sardines, herring). Drinking lots of water and avoiding alcohol.

BURSITIS

Bursitis is the inflammation of a bursa (a small sac). It appears as the swelling and thickening of the affected tissues. Because it is typically caused by a physical impact, excessive pressure, or repeated rubbing against a bursa, bursitis is often linked to a professional or sporting activity. Bursitis mainly occurs in the elbows, knees, shoulders, hips, and ankles.

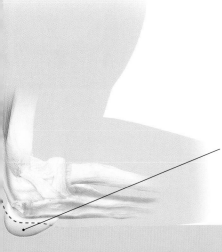

Bursa
A bursa is a sac filled with synovial fluid (joint lubricant). When inflamed, the bursa fills with blood or excess synovial fluid, leading to swelling that may, in some cases, be staggering. The fluid causing the swelling is usually reabsorbed within a few weeks, although a bacterial **infection** can also develop in the bursa.

BURSITIS

SYMPTOMS:
Pain, local swelling that may be very significant. Redness, heat, fever in the event of infection.

TREATMENTS:
Rest, bandaging, anti-inflammatories in benign cases. **Antibiotics** in the event of infection. Aspiration of the content of the bursa if the swelling does not go down on its own. In some severe cases, ablation of the bursa may be necessary.

PREVENTION :
Better posture when working can prevent recurrences. Protection of the elbows and knees when performing high risk sports or jobs.

MUSCLE PAIN

Muscle pain is a symptom that appears frequently after intense, sustained muscular effort. This pain, called myalgia, can also be caused by bad posture, contracture (cramp, torticollis), muscle injury (tears), an **infection**, a **metabolic** or **autoimmune** disease, or an unidentified cause.

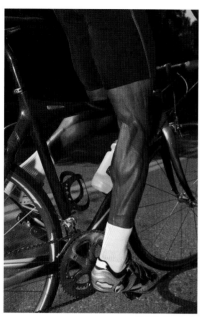

TEMPORARY MUSCLE PAINS
AND **ACHES**

Temporary muscles pains, which gradually fade once the muscle is at rest, are differentiated from aches, which appear several hours after the effort. These two types of pain require no special treatment, although taking analgesics can help reduce their intensity.

Temporary muscle pain
During intense, sustained effort, the oxygen supply to the body is no longer sufficient to meet the needs of the muscle fibers. This oxygen deficiency leads to the increased production of an organic substance, lactic acid. Its accumulation in the muscles is the source of temporary muscle pain. Good hydration (drinking water during physical effort) allows the body to better evacuate lactic acid.

FIBROMYALGIA

Fibromyalgia, which mainly affects women, is characterized by diffuse muscle pain combined with pain in specific regions of the body (neck, chest, shoulders, buttocks, elbows, knees). Other symptoms may appear in addition to this muscle pain: headache, fatigue, sleep disorders, and sometimes depression. Because fibromyalgia is difficult to diagnose, in the past, it was placed in the same category as psychiatric disorders. It has now been recognized by the World Health Organization as a disease of the osteoarticular, muscle, and connective tissue system, although its precise cause is still under debate (disorder of certain neurotransmitters, abnormal blood supply to the brain, autoimmune disease). The suggested treatments aim to alleviate discomfort, increase pain tolerance, and improve sleep quality.

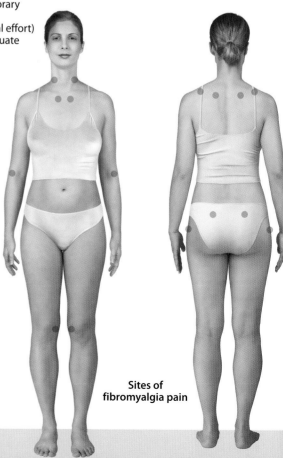

Sites of fibromyalgia pain

CONTRACTURE

A contracture is the involuntary contraction of a muscle or of the muscle fibers. This contraction, which can be long or short in duration, can lead to pain and localized motor problems. Most often, these are harmless (cramps, torticollis), caused by excessive strain on a muscle or poor posture. Rest, muscle relaxants, anti-inflammatories, and analgesics can relieve painful contractures within a few days.

CRAMPS

Cramps are sudden, painful muscle contractures, most often localized in a lower limb. Cramps typically appear during sustained physical effort, although they can also occur while at rest. This means that a foot or calf muscle can suddenly contract during the night (night cramps), especially in pregnant women (pregnancy cramps). The causes of these cramps remain relatively unknown, but they are believed to be linked to a mineral deficiency (calcium, sodium, potassium, or magnesium), poor blood circulation, or the accumulation of lactic acid in the muscles. When a cramp occurs, stretching the contracted muscles can make it disappear. Athletes often have leg cramps, particularly in very hot weather. Drinking water regularly can often prevent cramps.

SPASMS

A spasm is a contracture that can appear in an isolated or repetitive manner. It can affect the skeletal muscles, although it involves the smooth muscles of the internal organs in particular. Spasms can be caused by digestive disturbances (intestinal cramps, stomach cramps), a neurological disease, or nerve irritation (such as hiccups).

Smooth muscles... page 98

TORTICOLLIS

Torticollis is a lasting, painful contracture that chiefly involves the sternocleidomastoid muscles in the neck. It causes the neck to twist and restricts head motion. Torticollis is common and benign, occurring as the result of a forced movement, a chill, or bad posture, especially during sleep. Rest is usually sufficient to make the symptoms disappear after a few days.

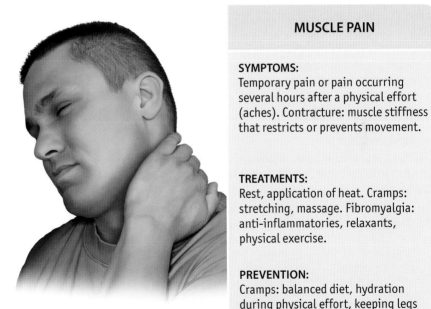

MUSCLE PAIN

SYMPTOMS:
Temporary pain or pain occurring several hours after a physical effort (aches). Contracture: muscle stiffness that restricts or prevents movement.

TREATMENTS:
Rest, application of heat. Cramps: stretching, massage. Fibromyalgia: anti-inflammatories, relaxants, physical exercise.

PREVENTION:
Cramps: balanced diet, hydration during physical effort, keeping legs slightly raised at night, warm-ups before exercising, gradual training, appropriate equipment.
Torticollis: bedding that provides for a good head position.

Relieving and preventing muscle pain... page 124

TETANY

Tetany is a rare syndrome characterized by fits of contractures mainly involving the hands (the fingers tense and bend in towards the wrist). Less frequently, tetany can also affect the feet or the mouth. This condition affects children and young women in particular. A calcium, magnesium, or potassium deficiency may be the cause.

RELIEVING AND PREVENTING MUSCLE PAIN

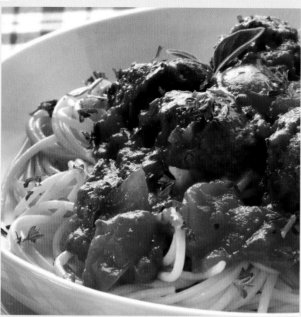

PREFER COMPLEX CARBOHYDRATES AND PROTEINS

Eat food rich in complex carbohydrates before and after playing sports. Complex carbohydrates, found in cereal products and legumes, provide the energy that your muscles need and limit aches. Also eat protein-rich food (meat, fish, eggs, dairy products, nuts, legumes). Proteins are essential to muscle fiber regeneration and repair.

DRINK WATER

Drink a lot of water while engaging in physical activity. Water helps to prevent muscle exhaustion, cramps, and aches.

EAT SIMPLE CARBOHYDRATES DURING PHYSICAL EFFORT

During physical activity (especially long and intense activities), eat simple carbohydrates. These can be found in fruit (especially dried fruit) and in sugary foods and beverages. Simple carbohydrates provide a fast supply of energy to working muscles and prevent or limit their exhaustion.

WARM UP

Warm up before starting a physical activity. Stretching allows the muscles, tendons, and ligaments to be activated gradually. Afterward, they are better able to absorb impacts.

MASSAGE YOUR MUSCLES

Massage and gently stretch your muscles after exercising. This will reduce the risk of cramps and aches.

REST

When you have aches, rest your sore muscles to allow them to recuperate. Take anti-inflammatories for particularly painful aches.

STRETCH THE CONTRACTED MUSCLE

If you have a muscle cramp, stretch and rub the painful muscle, then apply heat to it. Avoid uncomfortable positions, which can also trigger cramps.

AVOID OVEREXERTION

When engaged in sports or work activities (handling boxes, computer transcription, etc.), avoid overexerting your muscles and tendons by excessively repetitive movements. Take regular breaks to stretch and rest the muscles and tendons you are using.

Healthy bones, joints, and muscles... page 100

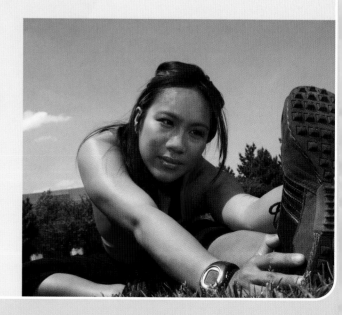

MUSCLE INJURIES

Muscles subjected to overworking or a direct impact can suffer a tear or **contusion**. These injuries usually occur while playing sports or in the event of an accident. In most cases, rest and treatment of the **inflammation**, especially through the application of ice, are sufficient to allow the muscle to heal rapidly. Complete recovery can take a few days to a few weeks, depending on the severity of the injury.

TORN MUSCLES:
PULLS OR STRAINS

A muscle tear is the rupture of a number of muscle fibers. It is typically caused by an overly intense effort or effort without sufficient warm-up, or by stretching the muscle beyond its elastic capacity. A pull is a benign tear, characterized by minor injuries affecting just a few of the muscle's fibers. The pain disappears after a few hours, although resting for 3–4 days is advised.
A strain is a more severe tear characterized by the rupture of multiple muscle fibers. The pain is intense and continuation of the effort is not possible. Several weeks of complete rest is required.

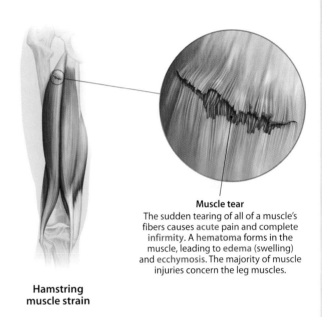

Muscle tear
The sudden tearing of all of a muscle's fibers causes acute pain and complete infirmity. A hematoma forms in the muscle, leading to edema (swelling) and ecchymosis. The majority of muscle injuries concern the leg muscles.

Hamstring muscle strain

MUSCLE INJURIES

SYMPTOMS:
Tears: acute pain, infirmity, swelling, ecchymosis.

TREATMENTS:
Reduction of the inflammation by applying ice, compression using a bandage, and raising the limb, partial or complete rest, nonsteroidal anti-inflammatory drugs, muscle relaxants, physical therapy for serious injuries. Surgery in rare cases. Return to the activity only after complete recovery.

First aid: Falls and traumas... page 552

PREVENTION:
Tears: gradual warm-up and stretching of the muscles and tendons before exercising, diet appropriate to the sport being played, hydration during physical exercise.

MUSCLE CONTUSIONS

Muscle contusions are injuries caused by a direct impact to a skeletal muscle, with no tearing of the skin or muscle. Contusions present themselves through muscle pain and the formation of a hematoma in the muscle, followed by swelling and bruising.

APPLICATION OF ICE

Thanks to its vasoconstricting effect, ice can reduce hemorrhaging in the injured muscle tissue. It also acts as an analgesic and reduces spasms. Ice should be applied immediately and not for longer than 15 minutes at a time.

TENDON INJURIES

The tendons play a vital role in the body's movements by anchoring the muscles to the bones. When the muscles are overworked, or in the event of a **trauma**, the tendons are subjected to pressure at a level greater than their resistance and may be injured. Treatment is primarily based on resting the damaged tendon and treating the **inflammation**.

TENDINITIS

Tendinitis is the inflammation of a tendon. This ailment affects the shoulders, elbows (epicondylitis), hips, knees, and ankles in particular. Tendinitis is caused by repeated, sports- or work-related microtraumas (work on a production line, computer work, inventory handling, etc.), more substantial trauma, an inflammatory joint disease, the aging of the tendons, or, less frequently, a bacterial infection. Tendinitis appears as localized pain, present at rest and accentuated during movement or when pressure is applied.

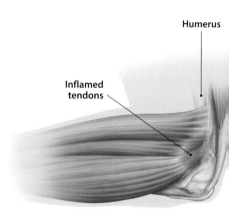

Epicondylitis
Epicondylitis (or tennis elbow) is a form of tendinitis that affects the tendons on the outside of the elbow (at the humerus). These tendons are placed under a lot of strain when playing tennis.

RELIEF AND PREVENTION OF REPETITIVE STRAIN INJURIES

Repetitive strain injuries (RSIs) cover all ailments involving the nerves, tendons, muscles, and certain other soft tissues, caused by repeating the same movements over and over. These injuries especially concern the upper limbs (wrists, hands, shoulders, and elbows), which are often affected by a repetitive exercise or manual work, such as extended use of a keyboard or mouse. Carpal tunnel syndrome, tendinitis, tenosynovitis, and bursitis are all examples of RSIs. To relieve or prevent them:

• Take regular breaks and consistently do warm-up exercises (rotating your wrists, stretching your arms, etc.).

• Correct your posture and opt for an ergonomic work environment that allows you to keep your arms and wrists relaxed.

• Soothe the pain by means of anti-inflammatories.

Warning! If the pain persists, stop the activity that caused the injury and consult a doctor.

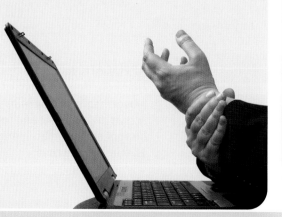

TENOSYNOVITIS

Tenosynovitis is the inflammation of the sheath around certain tendons, especially those attached to the extensor and flexor muscles in the hands and feet. It causes edema (swelling), which prevents the tendon from sliding correctly in its sheath. Tenosynovitis is caused by the overexertion of a joint (excessive repetition of a movement, improper position, vibrations) or by certain illnesses (rheumatoid arthritis, infections). It appears as pain when pressure is applied and when using the affected tendons.

PLANTAR FASCIITIS

Plantar fasciitis is the inflammation of the plantar fascia, the membrane that covers the sole of the foot. It is the most common cause of pain in the heel. Plantar fasciitis is often triggered by excess weight or by intense or repetitive sports involving running or jumping. The intermittent pain appears gradually and is usually localized in the heel, although it may radiate out to the sole of the foot.

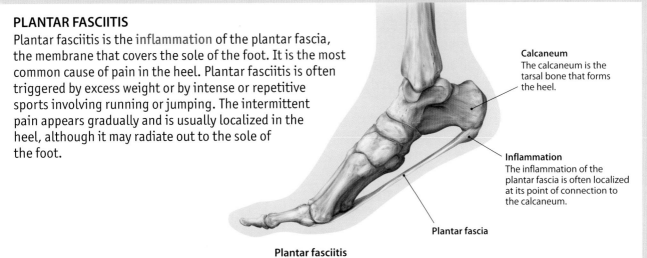

Calcaneum
The calcaneum is the tarsal bone that forms the heel.

Inflammation
The inflammation of the plantar fascia is often localized at its point of connection to the calcaneum.

Plantar fascia

Plantar fasciitis

Gastrocnemius

Achilles tendon
The Achilles tendon is the tendon that anchors the calf muscle (gastrocnemius) to the calcaneum (heel bone). It is the largest, most powerful tendon in the body.

Depression
A depression caused by the ruptured tendon appears above the heel, accompanied by ecchymosis and edema (swelling).

Calcaneum

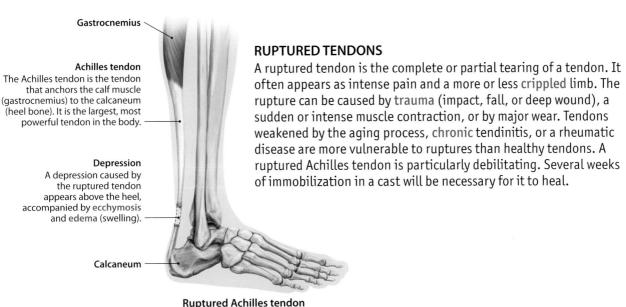

Ruptured Achilles tendon

RUPTURED TENDONS

A ruptured tendon is the complete or partial tearing of a tendon. It often appears as intense pain and a more or less crippled limb. The rupture can be caused by trauma (impact, fall, or deep wound), a sudden or intense muscle contraction, or by major wear. Tendons weakened by the aging process, chronic tendinitis, or a rheumatic disease are more vulnerable to ruptures than healthy tendons. A ruptured Achilles tendon is particularly debilitating. Several weeks of immobilization in a cast will be necessary for it to heal.

TENDON INJURIES

SYMPTOMS:
Localized or radiating pain, redness, heat, swelling. Ruptured tendon: cracking at the time of rupture, sharp pain, infirmity.

TREATMENTS:
Rest, support (bandage, splint, or cast), application of ice, nonsteroidal anti-inflammatories (NSAIDs), analgesics, physical therapy, cortisone injection (in the case of chronic pain). Severely ruptured tendon: surgery.
First aid: Falls and traumas... page 552

PREVENTION:
Warm-up, hydration, and stretching before each sports activity, gradual training, appropriate equipment (shoes). Plantar fasciitis: avoiding excess weight and standing for long periods.

The bones, joints, and muscles | Muscle diseases

127

DYSTONIA

Dystonia is a disease characterized by intense, sometimes painful contractures, which affect one or more muscle groups. These contractures are responsible for abnormal body positions, varying in duration. The source of dystonia may be **genetic**, although in most cases it is unknown. There are several forms of dystonia, which are differentiated according to the affected body part.

WRITER'S CRAMP

Writer's cramp is a form of dystonia mainly affecting the muscles in the hand and wrist. It appears as spasms (often painless) and locking of the fingers when flexed or extended, during certain precise, repetitive movements. This ailment is found in people who write regularly, as well as in musicians who play certain types of instruments. The symptoms appear at the start of the movement (from the first words written or first notes played), preventing its continuation. Physical therapy can help reduce the spasms, sometimes eliminating them permanently.

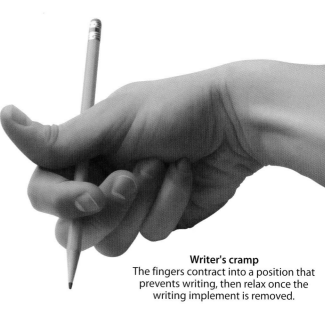

Writer's cramp
The fingers contract into a position that prevents writing, then relax once the writing implement is removed.

SPASMODIC TORTICOLLIS

Spasmodic torticollis (or cervical dystonia) is a form of dystonia characterized by the contracture of certain muscles in the neck. Its cause is usually unknown. It may be the result of improper functioning of the areas of the brain that control movement (e.g. the basal ganglia). Spasmodic torticollis differs from standard torticollis by the severity of the symptoms, which appear gradually, then tend to persist.
An abnormal position of the head is accompanied by potentially painful spasms and shaking. Spasmodic torticollis is most common in middle-aged adults. Physical therapy, combined with muscle relaxants, can relieve the symptoms, although the disease will generally persist throughout the patient's life.

DYSTONIA

SYMPTOMS:
Intense contractures that affect one or more muscle groups and cause abnormal postures.

TREATMENTS:
Muscle relaxants, injection of botulinum toxin in the contractured muscles, physical therapy, neurosurgery in severe cases.

DUPUYTREN'S CONTRACTURE

Dupuytren's contracture is characterized by the thickening of the palmar aponeurosis, a membrane located in the palm of the hand. This thickening gradually causes the fingers to bend. The origin of the disease remains unknown, although it is often hereditary. It occurs more often in men over 50 years of age and usually affects both hands. The disease may be combined with damage to the aponeurosis in the sole of the foot (Ledderhose's disease).

Nodule
The thickening of the palmar aponeurosis can be seen in the appearance of hard, palpable nodules in the palm of the hand and at the base of the fingers.

Ring finger and little finger
The ring finger and the little finger are the ones most commonly affected.

DUPUYTREN'S CONTRACTURE

SYMPTOMS:
Hard, painless nodules under the skin of the palms of the hands and at the base of the fingers. Gradual, irreducible bending of the fingers (most often the ring finger and the little finger).

TREATMENTS:
Surgical section of the aponeurosis using a needle inserted into the skin. In the event of failure or frequent recurrence: removal of the nodules and affected tissues, followed by rehabilitation with an orthosis.

MYASTHENIA

Myasthenia is a disease characterized by weak, easily fatigued skeletal muscles. Usually **autoimmune** in origin, it is caused by a blockage of communication between the motor neurons and muscle fibers. It is a rare ailment that can appear at any age, affecting women more than men. Its treatment aims to reduce the symptoms, but cannot cure the disease.

Muscle tissue... page 99

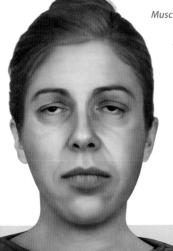

Symptoms of autoimmune myasthenia
In general, myasthenia first affects the muscles of the face (drooping eyelids, impaired vision, weak jaw, and throat muscles) before spreading to the limbs.

MYASTHENIA

SYMPTOMS:
Vision problems, joint impairment, difficulty chewing and swallowing, inexpressive face, weak limbs, general fatigue, respiratory problems during acute phases of the disease. Symptoms aggravated by physical effort. The disease develops in flare-ups.

TREATMENTS:
Medications that promote the presence of acetylcholine (which enables the transmission of nerve impulses to the muscles), removal of the thymus (which is abnormal in 75% of cases), immunosuppressants. Respiratory aid (acute phases of the disease).

MUSCULAR DYSTROPHY

Muscular dystrophy refers to a set of hereditary diseases characterized by the **degeneration** of the muscle fibers. The muscles gradually atrophy and weaken, potentially leading to major disabilities and affecting the vital functions. There has been much research on muscular dystrophy, but it remains incurable to this day. Its treatment consists of slowing the progression of the symptoms and improving the patient's quality of life.

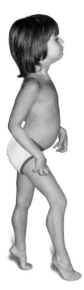

DUCHENNE MUSCULAR DYSTROPHY

Duchenne muscular dystrophy is characterized by the absence of the protein dystrophin in the muscles. Dystrophin ensures the cohesion of the muscle fibers, and its absence entails the weakening, then degeneration, of the muscles. Because it is transmitted by a recessive gene on the X chromosome, Duchenne muscular dystrophy only affects boys. It is the most common form of muscular dystrophy, affecting 1 boy in 3,500. The muscle weakness appears during infancy, and the disease evolves rapidly, to the point where walking becomes impossible around 10 years of age. The damage to the respiratory and heart muscles gradually endangers the vital functions. Multidisciplinary treatments can extend the patient's life expectancy.

Heredity... page 50

Heredity... page 50

OTHER FORMS OF MUSCULAR DYSTROPHY

Becker's muscular dystrophy is a less severe form of Duchenne muscular dystrophy, in which the symptoms are less pronounced or appear later. Landouzy-Dejerine muscular dystrophy, which affects both men and women, evolves slowly and mainly affects the muscles in the face and shoulder girdle (shoulder area). It can appear during childhood, adolescence, or young adulthood. Steinert's disease (or myotonic dystrophy) is the most common form of muscular dystrophy that appears during adulthood. It affects both men and women. The gradual weakening of the muscles leads to a loss of facial expressiveness and major or minor motor disability. One of the characteristic symptoms of the disease is myotonia, an anomaly characterized by the delayed relaxation of the muscles after a voluntary contraction (difficulty releasing an object).

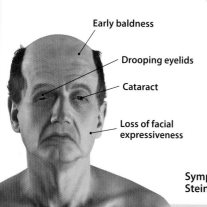

Early baldness

Drooping eyelids

Cataract

Loss of facial expressiveness

Symptoms of Steinert's disease

MUSCULAR DYSTROPHY

SYMPTOMS:
Symptoms appear after more or less time and gradually become aggravated: muscle weakening and atrophy, leading to abnormal posture, loss of facial expressiveness, and functional disabilities (difficulty walking or inability to walk, impaired motor coordination, speech impairment).

TREATMENTS:
No curative treatment. Treatments to slow the progression of the disease: corticosteroids, physical activity, physical therapy, orthopedics. Palliative treatments: respiratory or cardiac assistance.

PREVENTION:
In at-risk families, prenatal testing (amniocentesis) can allow for a decision to abort the pregnancy.

TETANUS

Tetanus is an **infectious** disease caused by the *Clostridium tetani* bacterium, which attacks the nervous system. It results in long, very painful muscle contractures. The infection can extend to the whole body, causing potentially fatal suffocation (asphyxia). Tetanus is virtually nonexistent in industrialized countries today, thanks to systematic **vaccination**. In developing countries, where vaccination is not sufficient, tetanus remains very widespread. It affects newborns in particular, through infection of the umbilical cord.

THE **DEVELOPMENT** OF **TETANUS**

Tetanus is caused by the penetration of *Clostridium tetani* into the body through a wound, even a very small one (injury with a rusty nail, prick from a rose thorn, splinter, bite, etc.). In rare cases, the disease remains limited to the area around the wound (localized tetanus), but most of the time, generalized tetanus breaks out after an incubation period of 4–20 days. Intense, painful, lasting contractures of the jaw muscles (trismus, or lockjaw) are the first symptom. One or two days later, the contractures spread to the muscles in the neck and torso. The risk of suffocation is high, making hospitalization in an intensive care unit necessary. The mortality rate varies between 20% and 90%, depending on the country and on access to treatment. Newborns and the elderly are the most vulnerable to the disease.

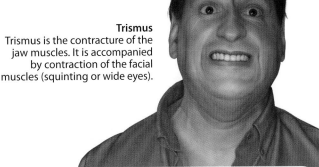

Trismus
Trismus is the contracture of the jaw muscles. It is accompanied by contraction of the facial muscles (squinting or wide eyes).

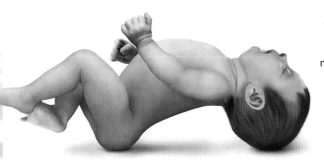

Opisthotonos
Opisthotonos is the strong arching of the back, characteristic of generalized tetanus, caused by the intense contracture of the muscles in the torso.

CLOSTRIDIUM TETANI

Clostridium tetani (or Nicolaier's bacillus) is the bacterium responsible for tetanus. It is found in a latent state in the ground and in the intestines of mammals. Once inside the human body, it secretes large quantities of toxins from the point of infection. These toxins enter the central nervous system and disrupt its functions. The result is muscle hyperactivity (twitching) and intense contractures.

TETANUS

SYMPTOMS:
Contractures of the muscles in the jaw (trismus), neck, torso, and limbs; fever; perspiration; rapid breathing; rapid heart rate.

TREATMENTS:
Injection of human antibodies against tetanus, treatment of the infected wound, antibiotics, muscle relaxants, respiratory aid.

PREVENTION:
Vaccination (with a booster every 10 years) is well-tolerated and effective, and is the only way to prevent the disease. Early booster in the case of an at-risk wound. Without vaccination, possible recurrence of the disease.

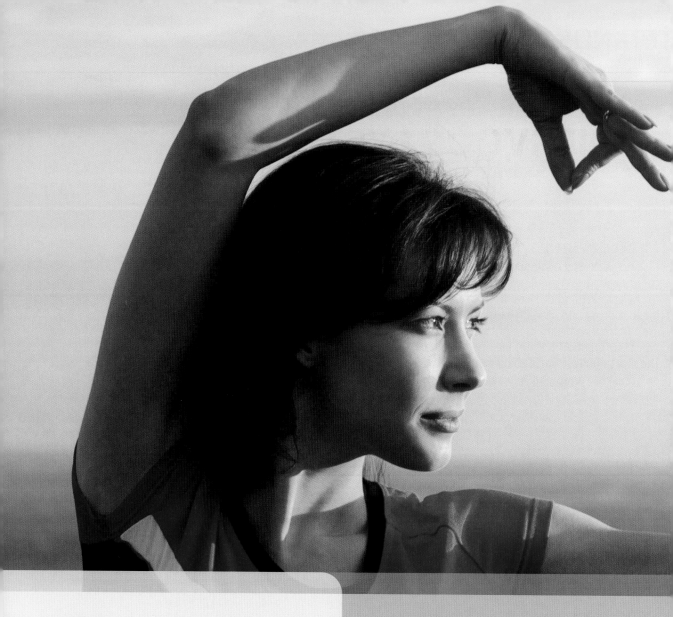

THE **NERVOUS SYSTEM**

Thinking, speaking, moving, feeling, and breathing: all of these functions are possible thanks to the nerve messages that are constantly traveling through our bodies. Composed of the brain, spinal cord and nerves, the nervous system ensures the psychological, sensory, motor, and autonomic functions of the body. The basis of this system is the neuron, a specialized cell that communicates with other neurons using electrical and chemical signals.

Injury to the nervous system can disrupt some functions that are dependent on it, such as movements, sensitivity, reasoning, and consciousness. An injury may be caused by an outside impact, tumor, cerebrovascular accident, **infection**, or **degenerative** disease like Alzheimer's. Mental illnesses, which disrupt thought, emotions, perceptions, and behaviors, include extremely varied disorders (neuroses, psychoses, affective disorders), and their causes remain relatively unknown today.

THE **STRUCTURE** OF THE **NERVOUS SYSTEM**

The nervous system allows our bodies to perceive sensations, to think, and to perform all of our movements, both voluntary and involuntary. It is composed of the brain, spinal cord, and nerves. This system functions mainly via the neurons, which are specialized cells that communicate with one another. Anatomically speaking, the nervous system is comprised of the central nervous system (the brain and spinal cord), which are the interpretation and command centers, and the peripheral nervous system, composed of the nerves (the transmission network).

Brain
Located in the cranium, the brain is responsible for our intellectual functions, our emotions, and most of our movement commands. It governs our vital functions in conjunction with the endocrine system.

Cranial nerves
The cranial nerves emerge from the brain and mainly innervate the neck and head.

Spinal cord
Located in the spinal column, the spinal cord transmits information between the spinal nerves and the brain. It is also responsible for certain reflex movements.

THE **CENTRAL NERVOUS SYSTEM**

The central nervous system, comprised of the brain and spinal cord, interprets the sensory information carried by the nerves and determines motor responses (movements).

THE **PERIPHERAL NERVOUS SYSTEM**

The peripheral nervous system is comprised of the cranial and spinal nerves. These subdivide into countless branches in order to innervate all of the parts of the body. The peripheral nervous system carries messages from the sensory receptors to the central nervous system and transmits motor commands from the central nervous system to the muscles and glands.

Spinal nerves
The spinal nerves radiate from the spinal cord. Their branches innervate all of the parts of the body, except the face.

■ The central nervous system

■ The peripheral nervous system

HOW THE NERVOUS SYSTEM WORKS

Functionally speaking, the nervous system is comprised of the somatic nervous system and the autonomic nervous system. The somatic nervous system, or voluntary system, makes it possible for the body to interact with its environment. It acts only on the skeletal muscles and governs voluntary movements, reflexes, semiautomatic movements (maintaining balance, posture, walking), as well as receives the sensory messages from the skin and the sensory organs. The autonomic nervous system regulates unconscious visceral functions: breathing, digestion, heart rhythm, blood circulation, excretion, etc. It acts on the smooth muscles (which enable the involuntary movements of the organs), certain glands, the vascular system, and the heart muscle.

The muscles… page 98

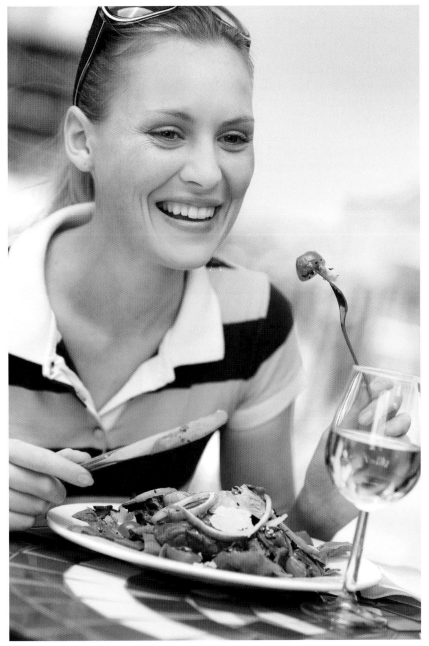

THE ANTAGONISTIC ACTIONS OF THE AUTONOMIC NERVOUS SYSTEM

The autonomic nervous system is made up of the sympathetic and parasympathetic nervous systems. These two systems generally perform antagonistic actions on the same organs, enabling precise control of their activities. The sympathetic nervous system prepares the body for action and allows it to respond to emergency situations. It is involved in the stress mechanism and in emotions such as anger and fear. The parasympathetic nervous system is responsible for resting the body. It reduces the energy consumed by the body while performing certain vital functions such as digestion and the elimination of waste.

Actions of the autonomic nervous system on digestion
The parasympathetic nervous system increases the secretion of digestive juices and allows food to travel through the digestive tract. At the same time, the sympathetic system slows the activity of the digestive tract so that the energy that it consumes can be devoted to other functions (physical activity, etc.).

THE **NEURON**

In the nervous system, information is carried in the form of electrical and chemical signals, by highly complex cells called neurons. The human body contains some 100 billion neurons, which form a part of the nervous tissue (the brain, spinal cord, and nerves). Although their shape can vary, all of the neurons have a similar structure: a cell body with extensions (dendrites and an axon), which provide for the reception and transmission of nerve messages. In the peripheral nervous system, these extensions form nerve fibers that make up the nerves. Neurons can only survive for a few minutes without oxygen, and most of them are unable to divide.

THE **TRANSMISSION** OF **MESSAGES** BY **NEURONS**

Nerve messages are transmitted from one part of the body to another via nerve impulses. These signals, which are initially electric, travel along a neuron's axon. When they reach the point of contact between the neuron and another cell (another neuron, a muscle fiber, or a secretory cell of an endocrine gland), they are converted into chemical signals. Neurotransmitters (chemical messengers) are released and attach to the receptors in the membrane of the other cell. The result is an excitatory or inhibitory response: creation of a new nerve impulse, muscle contraction, gland secretion, etc.

A LONG LIFE

The neurons differ from the other cells in the body by their exceptionally long life span. Even though, starting at birth, we lose many neurons every minute of our lives, some of them can, just like us, survive for more than 100 years!

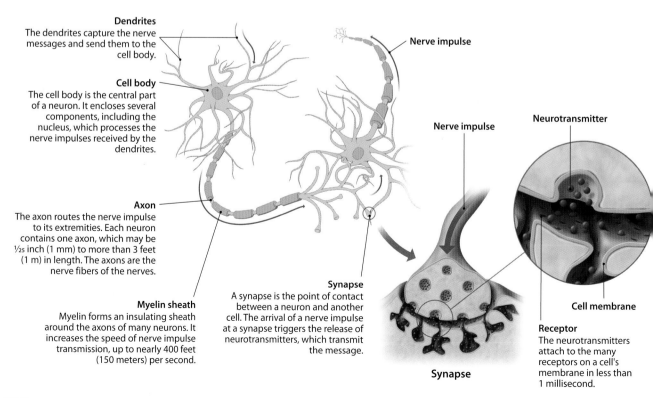

Dendrites
The dendrites capture the nerve messages and send them to the cell body.

Cell body
The cell body is the central part of a neuron. It encloses several components, including the nucleus, which processes the nerve impulses received by the dendrites.

Axon
The axon routes the nerve impulse to its extremities. Each neuron contains one axon, which may be ⅟₂₅ inch (1 mm) to more than 3 feet (1 m) in length. The axons are the nerve fibers of the nerves.

Myelin sheath
Myelin forms an insulating sheath around the axons of many neurons. It increases the speed of nerve impulse transmission, up to nearly 400 feet (150 meters) per second.

Nerve impulse

Synapse
A synapse is the point of contact between a neuron and another cell. The arrival of a nerve impulse at a synapse triggers the release of neurotransmitters, which transmit the message.

Synapse

Nerve impulse

Neurotransmitter

Cell membrane

Receptor
The neurotransmitters attach to the many receptors on a cell's membrane in less than 1 millisecond.

136

THE **NERVES**

The nerves are long cords formed of nerve fibers (axons) that carry sensory and motor messages between the central nervous system and the rest of the body. Sensory nerves carry sensations, and motor nerves trigger voluntary and involuntary movements. However, most nerves are mixed, meaning that they carry both types of information. Depending on the part of the central nervous system from which they emerge, the nerves are called either spinal or cranial.

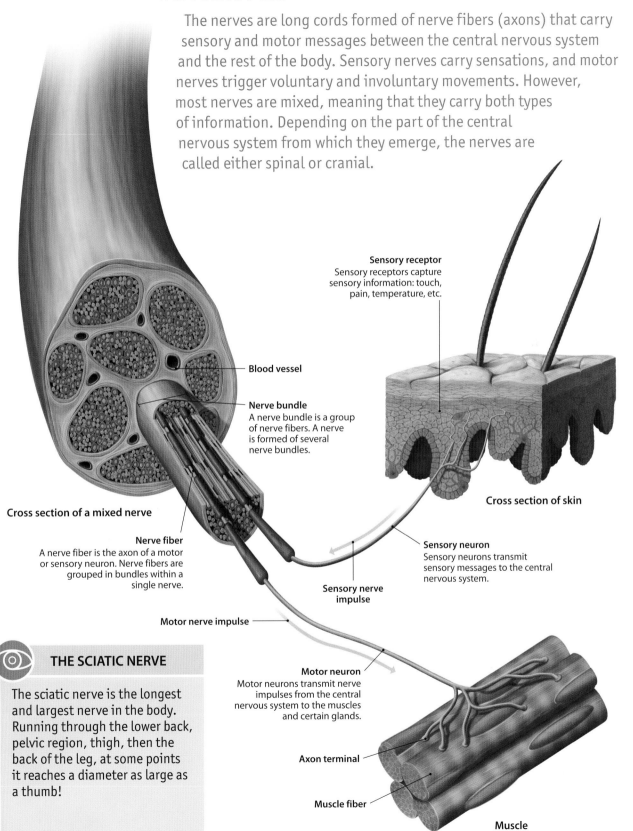

Sensory receptor
Sensory receptors capture sensory information: touch, pain, temperature, etc.

Blood vessel

Nerve bundle
A nerve bundle is a group of nerve fibers. A nerve is formed of several nerve bundles.

Cross section of skin

Cross section of a mixed nerve

Nerve fiber
A nerve fiber is the axon of a motor or sensory neuron. Nerve fibers are grouped in bundles within a single nerve.

Sensory neuron
Sensory neurons transmit sensory messages to the central nervous system.

Sensory nerve impulse

Motor nerve impulse

Motor neuron
Motor neurons transmit nerve impulses from the central nervous system to the muscles and certain glands.

THE SCIATIC NERVE

The sciatic nerve is the longest and largest nerve in the body. Running through the lower back, pelvic region, thigh, then the back of the leg, at some points it reaches a diameter as large as a thumb!

Axon terminal

Muscle fiber

Muscle

137

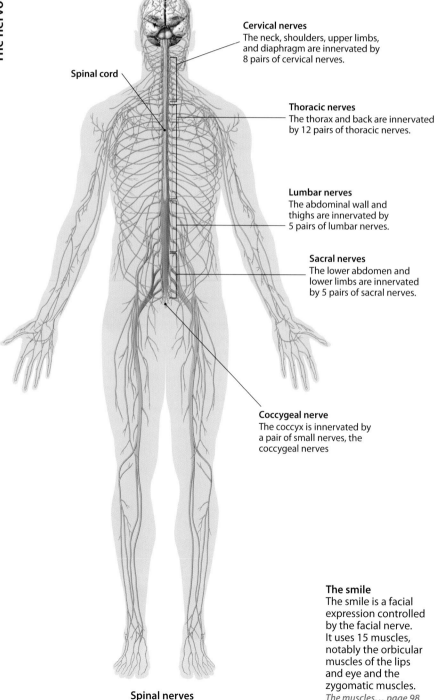

SPINAL NERVES

The 31 pairs of spinal nerves are mixed nerves emerging from the spinal cord and innervating all of the parts of the body, except the face. All muscles of the limbs and viscera are innervated by several spinal nerves, which reduces the risk of motor loss in the event of lesion.

Cervical nerves
The neck, shoulders, upper limbs, and diaphragm are innervated by 8 pairs of cervical nerves.

Spinal cord

Thoracic nerves
The thorax and back are innervated by 12 pairs of thoracic nerves.

Lumbar nerves
The abdominal wall and thighs are innervated by 5 pairs of lumbar nerves.

Sacral nerves
The lower abdomen and lower limbs are innervated by 5 pairs of sacral nerves.

Coccygeal nerve
The coccyx is innervated by a pair of small nerves, the coccygeal nerves

Spinal nerves

CRANIAL NERVES

The 12 pairs of cranial nerves come from the brain, mainly the cerebral trunk. Some among them are essentially motor nerves, such as the oculomotor nerve, responsible for certain eye movements. Others are uniquely sensitive, such as the olfactory and optical nerves, responsible respectively for smell and sight. Finally, some cranial nerves are mixed, such as the facial nerve. The facial nerve controls the movements of the face and plays a role in the sense of taste. The cranial nerves mainly serve the head and the neck, with the exception of the vagus nerve, associated with the parasympathetic nervous system, which regulates the heart rate, breathing, and activity of the digestive system.

The functioning of the nervous system… page 135

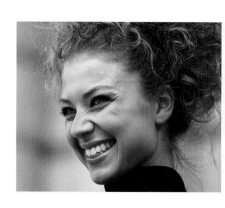

The smile
The smile is a facial expression controlled by the facial nerve. It uses 15 muscles, notably the orbicular muscles of the lips and eye and the zygomatic muscles.
The muscles… page 98

THE **SPINAL CORD**

The spinal cord is formed by a cord of nervous tissue more than 16 inches (40 cm) in length located in the vertebral canal, inside the spinal column. It spans from the spinal bulb to the second lumbar vertebra and is extended by a collection of nervous fibers, the cauda equina. Composed of motor and sensory neurons, the spinal cord ensures the transmission of messages between the spinal nerves and the brain, in addition to being a reflex center. Elastic, the spinal cord stretches during movements of the head and trunk. However, it is fragile and very sensitive to direct pressure. A lesion of the spinal cord leads to a function, motor or sensory loss, the extent of which depends on the location of the lesion.

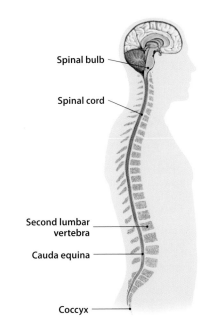

Spinal bulb

Spinal cord

Second lumbar vertebra

Cauda equina

Coccyx

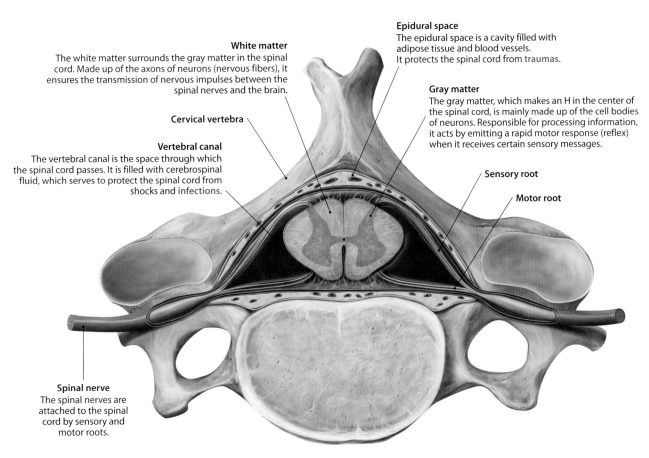

White matter
The white matter surrounds the gray matter in the spinal cord. Made up of the axons of neurons (nervous fibers), it ensures the transmission of nervous impulses between the spinal nerves and the brain.

Epidural space
The epidural space is a cavity filled with adipose tissue and blood vessels. It protects the spinal cord from traumas.

Gray matter
The gray matter, which makes an H in the center of the spinal cord, is mainly made up of the cell bodies of neurons. Responsible for processing information, it acts by emitting a rapid motor response (reflex) when it receives certain sensory messages.

Cervical vertebra

Vertebral canal
The vertebral canal is the space through which the spinal cord passes. It is filled with cerebrospinal fluid, which serves to protect the spinal cord from shocks and infections.

Sensory root

Motor root

Spinal nerve
The spinal nerves are attached to the spinal cord by sensory and motor roots.

Transversal cross section of the spinal column

139

THE **BRAIN**

The brain, or encephalon, is the part of the central nervous system contained in the skull. It includes the cerebrum, the cerebellum, the cerebral trunk, and the diencephalon, which notably includes the thalamus and the hypothalamus. Pink and gelatinous, the brain weighs approximately 3.3 lb (1.5 kg) and contains billions of neurons. It is protected by the skull and meninges and is surrounded by cerebrospinal fluid. Working with the endocrine system, the brain is responsible for perceptions, most movements, memory, language, reflection, hunger, emotions, and pain, and it also participates in controlling the vital functions: heart rate, arterial pressure, etc. Always active, even during sleep, the brain is irrigated by numerous blood vessels and consumes 20% of the oxygen of the resting organism. Like the spinal cord, the brain is composed of gray matter, which processes information, and white matter, responsible for transmitting this information. Gray matter is mainly formed by the cell bodies of neurons and makes up the exterior layer of the cerebellum and cerebrum, as well as several small internal masses (thalamus, hypothalamus, basal ganglia). White matter is made up of extensions of neurons.

The endocrine system… page 218

CEREBELLUM

The cerebellum is the part of the brain located under the cerebrum, behind the cerebral trunk. It ensures motor coordination as well as the maintenance of balance and posture. Made up of gray matter and white matter, it continuously analyzes the messages from the sensory receptors and adjusts muscle tension depending on the motor commands issued by the cerebrum. The cerebellum also allows for harmonious voluntary movements, without useless effort, without losing balance and without trembling.

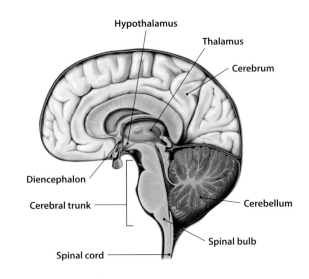

Lateral cross section of the brain

CEREBRAL TRUNK

The cerebral trunk is the part of the brain located in the extension of the spinal cord. It regulates numerous vital functions, plays a primordial role in sleep regulation, and carries out transmissions between the spinal cord, cerebrum and cerebellum. Ten of the twelve cranial nerves are directly attached to it. The cerebral trunk comprises the spinal bulb. It controls numerous vital functions (breathing, blood pressure, heart rate), participates in the maintenance of different physiological constants (body temperature, blood pressure, heart beat rhythm, etc.), and manages reflexes such as swallowing, vomiting, coughing, and sneezing.

MENINGES AND CEREBROSPINAL FLUID

Meninges are the three membranes (dura mater, arachnoidea, and pia mater) that envelop and protect the encephalon and spinal cord. Cerebrospinal fluid circulates between the meninges. Manufactured in the cerebral ventricles, cerebrospinal fluid is made up of water, proteins, and nutrients. In addition to protecting the central nervous system during trauma, it maintains intracerebral pressure, transports hormones, and eliminates waste from the metabolism.

CEREBRUM

The cerebrum is the most voluminous and most complex part of the brain. It is made up of two hemispheres subdivided into four cerebral lobes, which cover the diencephalon. The most complex functions are completed by the exterior layer of the brain, the cerebral cortex.

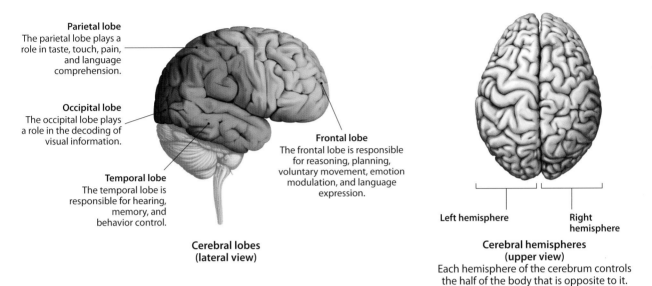

Parietal lobe
The parietal lobe plays a role in taste, touch, pain, and language comprehension.

Occipital lobe
The occipital lobe plays a role in the decoding of visual information.

Temporal lobe
The temporal lobe is responsible for hearing, memory, and behavior control.

Frontal lobe
The frontal lobe is responsible for reasoning, planning, voluntary movement, emotion modulation, and language expression.

**Cerebral lobes
(lateral view)**

Left hemisphere

Right hemisphere

**Cerebral hemispheres
(upper view)**
Each hemisphere of the cerebrum controls the half of the body that is opposite to it.

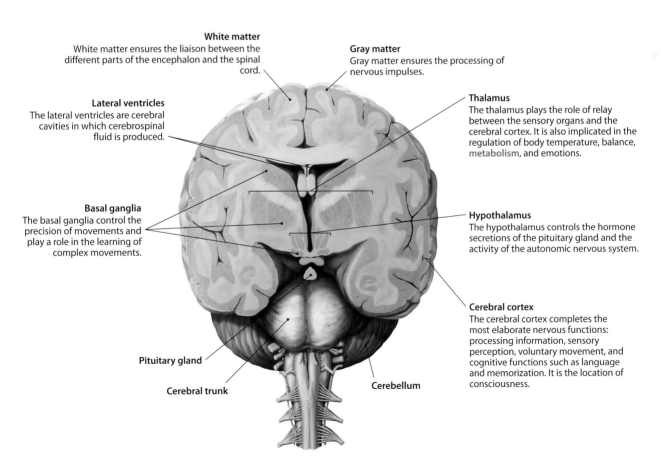

White matter
White matter ensures the liaison between the different parts of the encephalon and the spinal cord.

Gray matter
Gray matter ensures the processing of nervous impulses.

Lateral ventricles
The lateral ventricles are cerebral cavities in which cerebrospinal fluid is produced.

Thalamus
The thalamus plays the role of relay between the sensory organs and the cerebral cortex. It is also implicated in the regulation of body temperature, balance, metabolism, and emotions.

Basal ganglia
The basal ganglia control the precision of movements and play a role in the learning of complex movements.

Hypothalamus
The hypothalamus controls the hormone secretions of the pituitary gland and the activity of the autonomic nervous system.

Cerebral cortex
The cerebral cortex completes the most elaborate nervous functions: processing information, sensory perception, voluntary movement, and cognitive functions such as language and memorization. It is the location of consciousness.

Pituitary gland

Cerebral trunk

Cerebellum

Front cross section of the brain

The nervous system | The body

THE HEALTH OF THE BRAIN

With time, the brain becomes less and less able to perform, mostly due to the aging of the blood vessels that travel through it, but also to the natural progressive death of neurons (apoptosis), which accelerates after 40 years of age. Here is some advice to help you preserve your mind for a long time.

■ AVOID HARMFUL ELEMENTS

Sugar, saturated and trans fats, alcohol, tobacco smoke, and pollution, particularly that which is linked to heavy metals, are harmful elements for the brain. Avoid them as much as possible.

■ ADOPT A HEALTHY DIET

Some nutritious elements promote good blood circulation and proper functioning of the brain. This is particularly the case for antioxidants, present in tomato-based products, green tea, berries, dark legumes, etc. Unsaturated fatty acids like Omega 3 and Omega 6 are also beneficial. They are found in fatty fish, vegetable oil, avocados, nuts, and grains. Protein from eggs, meat, poultry, fish, legumes, and dairy products is also excellent, just like the vitamins present in dark vegetables, legumes, and eggs. Complex carbohydrates (whole cereal, legumes) provide energy to the brain.

Nutrition...page 11

■ EXERCISE

Physical activity stimulates blood circulation and oxygenation of the body, crucial factors for the proper functioning of the brain.

Exercise...page 22

■ GET ENOUGH SLEEP

While sleeping, certain neurons are regenerated by slowing down their activity. Others function actively, thus allowing the assimilation of information gathered during the day.

■ RELAX AND MEDITATE

Major pressure and stress are harmful for the brain. However, meditation and relaxation are beneficial and prevent its premature aging.

Stress control...page 28

■ STIMULATE YOUR BRAIN

Mental activities stimulate the creation of new nervous connections. Change your habits, learn new things, do intellectual exercises, such as jigsaw puzzles, while always increasing the difficulty.

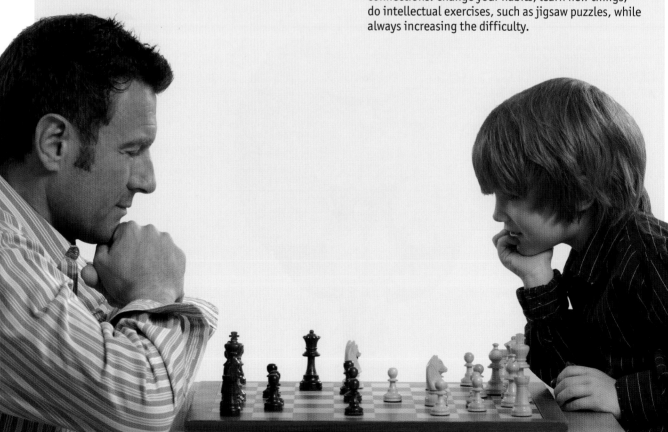

MOVEMENTS

Movements can be voluntary or involuntary. The commands that cause them are emitted by the central nervous system, then transmitted by the motor neurons, which trigger the contraction of muscles. As soon as the movement is carried out, sensory messages are sent to the brain, which then makes the necessary adjustments.

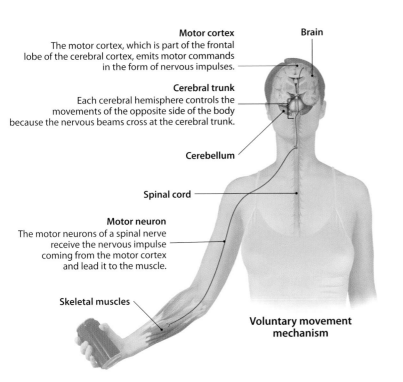

Motor cortex
The motor cortex, which is part of the frontal lobe of the cerebral cortex, emits motor commands in the form of nervous impulses.

Brain

Cerebral trunk
Each cerebral hemisphere controls the movements of the opposite side of the body because the nervous beams cross at the cerebral trunk.

Cerebellum

Spinal cord

Motor neuron
The motor neurons of a spinal nerve receive the nervous impulse coming from the motor cortex and lead it to the muscle.

Skeletal muscles

Voluntary movement mechanism

VOLUNTARY MOVEMENTS

A voluntary movement is an intentionally executed movement caused by the motor commands emitted by the motor cortex. These commands are transmitted to the skeletal muscles through the spinal cord and spinal nerves. The muscle contraction that results produces the desired movement. The cerebellum controls the precision and coordination of voluntary movements.

REFLEXES

A reflex is an instant, brief, and involuntary motor response to a stimulus. Sudden extension of the leg when the patellar tendon is hit, the closing of the eye to the sudden approach of an object, or letting go of a burning object are examples of reflexes. Some reflexes are produced without us realizing it, particularly those that run the activities of the internal organs. Therefore, there are two categories of reflexes: somatic reflexes, which activate the skeletal muscles, and autonomic reflexes, which activate the smooth muscles, cardiac muscle, and glands.

The muscles... page 98

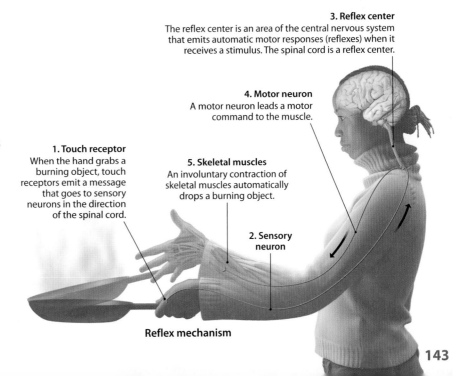

3. Reflex center
The reflex center is an area of the central nervous system that emits automatic motor responses (reflexes) when it receives a stimulus. The spinal cord is a reflex center.

4. Motor neuron
A motor neuron leads a motor command to the muscle.

1. Touch receptor
When the hand grabs a burning object, touch receptors emit a message that goes to sensory neurons in the direction of the spinal cord.

5. Skeletal muscles
An involuntary contraction of skeletal muscles automatically drops a burning object.

2. Sensory neuron

Reflex mechanism

CONSCIOUSNESS

Consciousness is the perception that an individual has of their environment and of themselves. It is a vital function that allows a person to react to the world that surrounds them and live there. It notably includes the sensations, movements, memory, judgment, and reasoning. Awakeness, or arousal, is the normal state of consciousness in which the brain is ready to consciously react to stimuli. During the day, it oscillates between two forms: active awakeness, characterized by very short reaction time, quick movements, desire to communicate, and the facility to learn, and passive awakeness, characterized by a desire to relax, less propensity to speak, and higher sensitivity to the cold. Awakeness is regularly and naturally altered by sleepiness and sleep. It can also be altered in an abnormal manner by the loss of consciousness or coma.

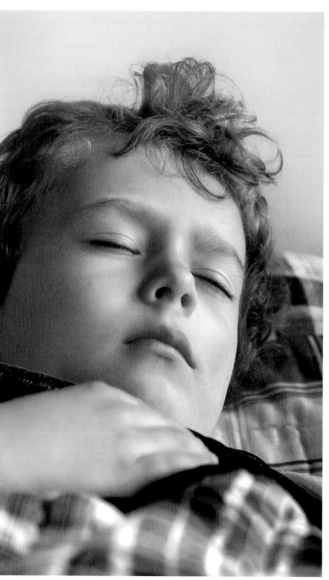

SLEEP

After approximately 16 hours of being awake, the need for sleep is felt. Temporary and immediately reversible, sleep (outside of REM periods of sleep) is characterized by the decrease in the ability to react to stimuli, change in metabolism and heart rate, lowering of arterial pressure and body temperature, and muscle relaxation. An optimal night of sleep lasts on average 7 hours for adults, but it may vary between 5 to 12 hours depending on age and individuals. Sleep performs a vital function of rest and regeneration of the body and plays a role in memory and the assimilation of knowledge.

SLEEP CYCLE

A night of sleep is characterized by the succession of four to six cycles. Each cycle lasts 90 to 120 minutes and has two phases: non-rapid eye movement sleep (NREM) and rapid eye movement sleep (REM). NREM sleep, which lasts 70 to 100 minutes, is marked by a slower and more deep breathing, slowing of cerebral waves, and lowering of heart rate and arterial pressure. REM sleep, which lasts approximately 20 minutes, is characterized by quicker and more irregular breathing as well as by intense cerebral activity accompanied by rapid eye movement. It is during this period that most dreams occur.

IMAGING OF THE NERVOUS SYSTEM

Several medical imaging techniques are used to visualize the interior of the brain or assess its functioning. These exams, rapid and painless, allow the detection of numerous problems: intracranial **hematoma**, cerebrovascular accident, multiple sclerosis, tumor, Alzheimer's, epilepsy, etc.

TOMODENSITOMETRY AND MAGNETIC RESONANCE IMAGING

Tomodensitometry uses an X-ray scan to obtain a section image of the internal organs, generally the brain, rib cage, abdomen, and bones. It emphasizes different densities by analyzing the absorption of X-rays by different tissues, which allows for the diagnosis of a tumor, internal bleeding, malformation, etc. Magnetic resonance imaging (MRI) is being used increasingly frequently over tomodensitometry. This technique uses an electromagnet that produces a very powerful magnetic field. It provides an image of the internal organs in two or three dimensions, using the magnetic properties of hydrogen atoms that make up the human body. An MRI allows for the visualization of damage that does not appear in a scan, ultrasound or X-ray. It can be used to diagnose a disease of the nervous system, for example.

ELECTROENCEPHALOGRAPHY

Electroencephalography is a technique that records the electrical activity of the brain (cerebral waves) using electrodes placed on the scalp. During the test, the patient is submitted to various stimulations to study the corresponding cerebral activity. The result is presented in the form of an electroencephalogram. Electroencephalography allows for the assessment of the brain function and the diagnosis of certain disorders, such as epilepsy, a tumor, or cerebrovascular accident. However, it does not reveal the cause of the disease.

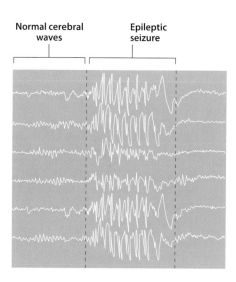

Normal cerebral waves   **Epileptic seizure**

Electroencephalogram
The electroencephalogram is a graphic plotting of the electrical activity of the brain, printed on paper or displayed on a computer screen. Anomalies of the plotting correspond to a change in frequency or amplitude of cerebral waves, or the appearance of abnormal patterns in the plotting.

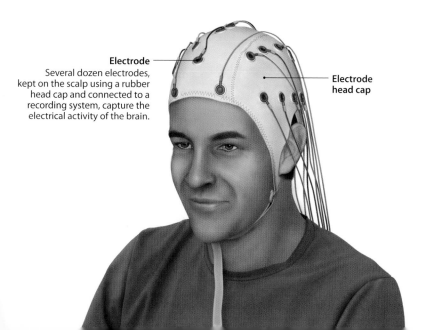

Electrode
Several dozen electrodes, kept on the scalp using a rubber head cap and connected to a recording system, capture the electrical activity of the brain.

Electrode head cap

NEURALGIA

Neuralgia is a pain caused by irritation or lesion of a mixed or sensory nerve. It is located on the nerve path or in the area that it innervates. Some cases of neuralgia are the consequence of a disease (herniated disk, arthrosis, herpes zoster, tumor, etc.), but the majority have an unknown cause. The pain, of a variable intensity, is sometimes very debilitating. Neuralgia is often located in the lower or upper limbs. This is the case in sciatica, which affects the thighs and legs, or cervicobrachial neuralgia, which attacks the lower part of the neck, shoulders, arms, and hands.

The nerves... page 137

SCIATICA

The irritation or lesion of the sciatic nerve causes a common neuralgia, sciatica. It is characterized by a pain in the posterior face of a lower limb, which can extend from the buttocks to the foot and is accentuated by the standing position. Sciatica, frequently preceded by a lumbago (pain in the lumbar region), may be caused by a herniated disk that compresses a root of the nerve. It can also be caused by arthrosis of the lumbar vertebrae, pelvic fracture, tumor, or even result from an injection that was poorly administered in the buttocks.

FACIAL NEURALGIA

Facial neuralgia is a pain that affects the face and that results from the irritation or lesion of the trigeminal nerve that irrigates it. It manifests itself through very violent and sudden attacks, comparable to electrical discharges. The pain is unilateral and disappears without leaving sequelae. It sometimes causes involuntary twitching of muscles, called a facial tic. The attacks can be triggered without any apparent reason or following the stimulation of a specific cutaneous area. Facial neuralgias most often affect women over 50 years of age. They generally are of an unknown origin, but compression of the trigeminal nerve by a blood vessel is sometimes the cause. Cases of facial neuralgia can also be side effects of a disease (tumor, infection, multiple sclerosis, herpes zoster, etc.).

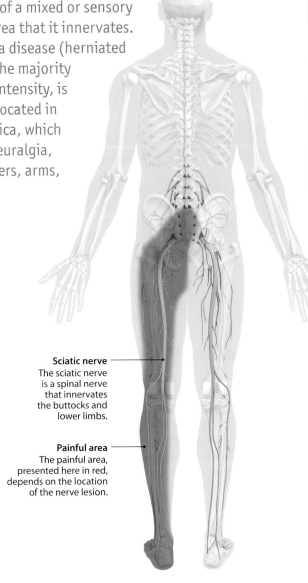

Sciatic nerve
The sciatic nerve is a spinal nerve that innervates the buttocks and lower limbs.

Painful area
The painful area, presented here in red, depends on the location of the nerve lesion.

NEURALGIA

SYMPTOMS:
Intense variable pain may appear in attacks and be located on the damaged nerve path and in the area that it innervates.

TREATMENT:
Temporary immobilization (bed confinement, splint, neck brace, etc.), analgesics, anti-inflammatories, physical therapy. The cause of neuralgia must also be treated if it is known. Surgical intervention is sometimes necessary to desensitize or decompress the nerve.

CANAL SYNDROME

In some places of the body, nerves pass through canals; their compression at one of these natural conduits can cause pain as well as sensory and motor problems. The symptoms, collectively known as canal syndrome, generally result from a hypertrophy of an element of the canal, following a **trauma**, **inflammation**, or disease. The most common canal syndrome is carpal tunnel syndrome.

CARPAL TUNNEL SYNDROME

Carpal tunnel syndrome is caused by the compression of the median nerve of the hand in the carpian canal, a space defined in part by the wrist bones and a ligament in the shape of a ring (annular carpal ligament). The syndrome is manifested by numbness, tingling, and pain in the hands, palm, and sometimes in the forearm. These symptoms are more acute at night and in the morning when waking up. They may be accompanied by sensory troubles at the fingertips, and a decrease in force of the thumb. Carpal tunnel syndrome especially affects women, notably during menopause and pregnancy, as well as people carrying out repetitive gestures for work (wrist extension, support, or pressure on the heel of the hand). Other causes are possible: rheumatoid arthritis, gout, fracture, paratenonitis, synovial cyst of the wrist.

ERGONOMIC OFFICE

Microtraumas and inflammation that cause carpal tunnel syndrome may be prevented by using work tools adequately, primarily the computer.

- Adapt your workspace. Your forearms must always be supported by armrests, your shoulders relaxed. Your arm must form a 90° angle with your forearm. Adjust the height of the table, keyboard, or chair as needed.

  Preventing backache... page 114

- Keep your forearms, wrists, and hands aligned and avoid extending, folding, or twisting the wrists. Adjust the inclination of the keyboard as needed or use a wrist rest.

- Use a mouse adapted to the size of your hand and place it at the same level and next to the keyboard. Use it in a relaxed manner.

- Place the documents that you use most often nearby.

- Periodically do some exercises to relax your joints such as rotating the shoulders and wrists.

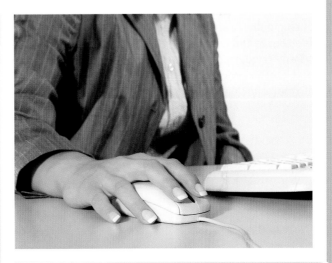

CANAL SYNDROMES

SYMPTOMS:
Sensory and motor coordination troubles, tingling sensation, numbness, pain.

TREATMENT:
Corticosteroid injections, immobilization by a splint. In case of failure, surgical release of the compressed nerve.

PREVENTION :
Avoiding repetitive movements. Ergonomic workplace.

HEADACHES AND MIGRAINES

Headaches are common and generally benign pains of variable causes: fatigue, stress, noise, polluted atmosphere, excess alcohol, irregular meals, excess or lack of sleep, periods, oral contraception, etc. A migraine is a type of intense headache that manifests itself in attacks. Headaches can last several hours to several days and recur. Their treatment depends on their cause. Some headaches are symptomatic of a disease: sinusitis, ophthalmological, dental, or rheumatological troubles, hypertension, depression, fever, meningitis, cranial **trauma**, cerebral tumor, etc.

MIGRAINE

A migraine manifests itself by attacks of variable intensity and duration, characterized by very painful headaches, often located on only one side of the head, in the forehead, or temples. Amplified by noise, light, and movement, the pain fluctuates in rhythm with the heart beat. It is often associated with digestive troubles (nausea, vomiting) and mood disorders. The first migraine attacks generally occur before 40 years of age.
Two to three times more frequent in women, migraines appear often during puberty and disappear at menopause and during pregnancies. The causes and mechanisms of the migraine are poorly known, but several triggering factors have been discovered: hormonal (periods, oral contraception), psychological (stress), and dietary (consumption of alcohol, chocolate, etc.).

WARNING SIGNS OF A MIGRAINE

Migraine attacks may be preceded by fatigue, mood disorders (irritability, euphoria, depressive state), or the craving for a specific food. They can also follow a series of symptoms collectively known as migraine aura: decrease in visual field, light spots before the eyes, blurred vision, impression that the body is distorted, tingling in the arms and face.

Warning! The first time that you experience these symptoms or if you don't know their cause, consult a doctor.

WHEN **TO CONSULT** A **DOCTOR**?

Some headaches should be taken seriously and require immediate medical attention. This is the case when they follow a cranial shock or when they are unusual, sudden, very intense, or continuous for 48 hours. Headaches accompanied by other symptoms such as fever, vision troubles, convulsions, loss of consciousness, neurological troubles (vertigo, loss of balance, numbness, mental confusion, difficulty speaking, etc.), vomiting, cutaneous eruptions, sleepiness, or neck stiffness (pain or stiffness in the nape of the neck) require medical attention.

PREVENTION AND ALLEVIATION OF HEADACHES

Of various origins, headaches are common and most often benign. Simple measures can alleviate them. If you are subject to headaches or migraines, find and avoid the factors that trigger them.

■ ADOPT A HEALTHY LIFESTYLE

Have a balanced diet and, at set hours, drink plenty of water (6 to 8 cups [1.5 to 2 liters] per day), get enough sleep, and exercise regularly. Avoid alcohol abuse.

■ AVOID AGGRAVATING FACTORS

If you are subject to headaches, avoid situations that encourage them: noisy or poorly ventilated environments, stress, overwork, conflict. Some foods with vasodilators or that are rich in histamine can aggravate a headache (e.g. chocolate, smoked food, fish, crustaceans, some fermented cheeses, fats, alcohol).

■ GET PLENTY OF REST

Treat headaches by isolating yourself in a calm, well-ventilated place with filtered lighting or totally sheltered from light. Lie down and sleep for a moment if you can.

■ APPLY A COOL OR WARM COMPRESS ON THE NAPE OF THE NECK OR ON THE PAINFUL AREA

The cold causes a decrease in diameter of the blood vessels, while the warmth has a relaxing effect on the muscles. These phenomena can ease your migraine.

■ DO RELAXING ACTIVITIES

Massage your shoulders, neck, face, and scalp. Practice relaxing sports such as yoga, walking, swimming, and biking.

■ TAKE MEDICATION

If your state of health allows it, take analgesics or nonsteroidal anti-inflammatories, medications that are generally effective in alleviating benign headaches. Follow the dosage indicated on the packaging and be careful not to abuse them, at the risk of increasing the frequency of headaches and causing other problems (renal, cardiovascular, gastrointestinal, etc.). Migraines must be treated by specific medications.

■ OTHER TIPS

Strong coffee and tea may ease headaches.

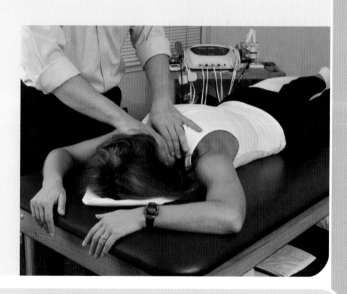

HEADACHES AND MIGRAINES

SYMPTOMS:
Headaches. Migraine attacks: pulsating pain that begins in a precise point then extends to the entire side of the skull, to the face and sometimes the entire head, nausea, vomiting, intolerance to light and noise. Absence of symptoms between attacks.

TREATMENT:
Analgesics and nonsteroidal anti-inflammatories. Migraine: anti-migraine medications (triptans, ergot derivatives).

PREVENTION :
Adopt a healthy lifestyle, avoid triggering factors (stress, fatigue, alcohol abuse, noise, poor air circulation, etc.). Migraine: when attacks occur several times per month, long-term medical treatment may be used to decrease their frequency and intensity.

CRANIAL TRAUMAS

A cranial **trauma** is a collection of lesions and disorders caused by a shock to the head. There are several types of them, of varying severity: skull fracture, cerebral commotion, cerebral **contusion**, intracranial **hematoma**. The symptoms of a trauma may appear immediately after the shock or manifest a few hours to several weeks later. It is recommended to call for medical assistance if the victim of a shock to the head presents one of the following symptoms: loss of consciousness, even brief, problems with balance or speech, bleeding from the ears, vomiting, abnormal behavior. Car accidents and sporting accidents are responsible for the majority of cranial traumas.

Fractures of the skull... page 103

CEREBRAL CONTUSION AND **INTRACRANIAL HEMATOMA**

A cerebral contusion is a bruise to the brain caused by a violent head injury. It is a serious cranial trauma, which results in the destruction of nerve cells and bleeding located at the point of impact or on the opposite side (contrecoup). Cerebral contusion causes neurological problems: loss of consciousness, motor and sensory deficiency, behavior disorders, convulsions, etc. These impairments are generally reversible, but they may lead to sequelae. Secondary complications are also likely to occur, such as intracranial hematoma (buildup of blood inside the skull). The hematoma exerts a more or less significant pressure on the surrounding cerebral areas (intracranial hypertension) and causes the destruction of nerve tissue. This results in headaches, consciousness problems, or even paralysis.

CEREBRAL CONCUSSION

The most common and most benign form of cranial trauma is cerebral concussion: a shaking of the brain, without any apparent organic lesion. It generally leads to a loss of consciousness and may temporarily cause headaches, nausea, vomiting, memory troubles, difficulty concentrating, and irritability. Recovery generally does not result in sequelae.

CRANIAL TRAUMAS

SYMPTOMS:
More or less brief loss of consciousness, coma, nose or ear bleeding, balance problems, nausea and vomiting, headaches, difficulty speaking, paralysis, sensory and vision troubles, abnormal behavior, convulsions.

TREATMENT:
Treatments (surgical intervention, medical treatment) prevent the spread of the lesions. Hospital monitoring allows for the detection of potential complications.

PREVENTION :
Wearing seat belts in vehicles. Wearing a helmet when participating in activities that risk leading to a shock to the head.

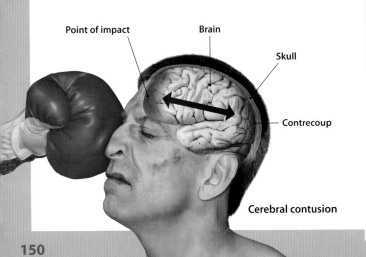

Point of impact   Brain

Skull

Contrecoup

Cerebral contusion

PARALYSIS

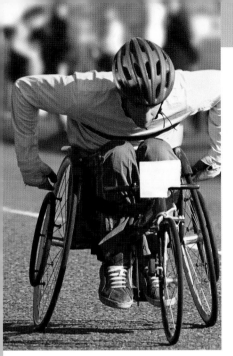

Paralysis is a temporary or permanent loss of motor function of a muscle, group of muscles, or part of the body, due to a lesion of the nervous system. It is sometimes associated with a total or partial loss of sensitivity in the affected region. Depending on the location of the lesion, paralysis may affect the face, half of the body, or the entire trunk in addition to the four limbs. Lesions at the origin of paralysis are often caused by a **trauma** (car or sporting accident) or a cerebrovascular accident (stroke). It can also be caused by multiple sclerosis, a tumor, or an **infection** such as diphtheria, poliomyelitis, or syphilis.

Cerebrovascular accidents... page 156

FACIAL PARALYSIS

Facial paralysis is a paralysis of face muscles innervated by the facial nerve. Generally unilateral (on one side), it can only affect the lower or upper part of the face. When it is caused by a cerebrovascular accident, facial paralysis is often accompanied by a hemiplegia (paralysis of half of the body). Facial paralysis may also result from an infection (otitis, herpes zoster, etc.) or tumor, but it occurs most often without any apparent cause. The symptoms vary depending on the lesion: inability to wrinkle the forehead, close eyelids, smile, whistle, yawn, or difficulty eating and speaking. Sometimes there is an exaggerated perception of sounds, loss of taste, and decrease in the secretion of saliva and tears. Facial paralysis can regress, but sequelae are frequent.

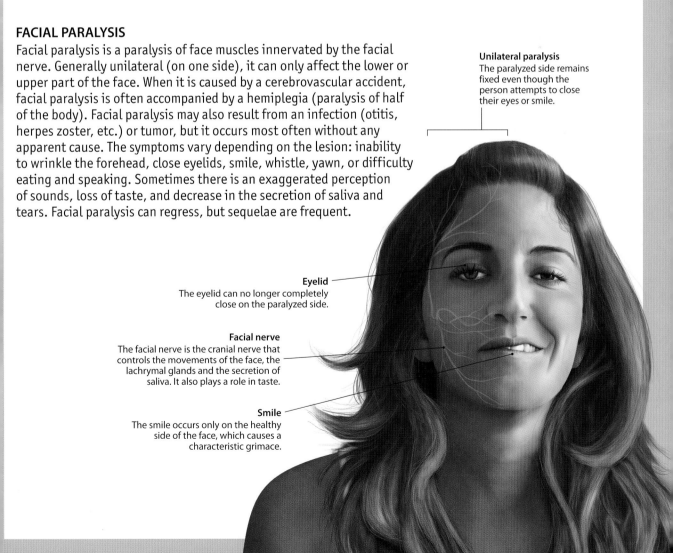

Unilateral paralysis
The paralyzed side remains fixed even though the person attempts to close their eyes or smile.

Eyelid
The eyelid can no longer completely close on the paralyzed side.

Facial nerve
The facial nerve is the cranial nerve that controls the movements of the face, the lachrymal glands and the secretion of saliva. It also plays a role in taste.

Smile
The smile occurs only on the healthy side of the face, which causes a characteristic grimace.

HEMIPLEGIA

Hemiplegia is a paralysis of the right or left half of the body, caused by a lesion to the encephalon. It can extend through the entire body or only affect one part (face, arm, leg). Hemiplegia can set in suddenly, like in the case of a cerebrovascular accident, or progressively, for example following a brain tumor. It can be associated with loss of language and partial blindness. Recovery is possible, but the victim often experiences sequelae.

PARAPLEGIA

Paraplegia is a form of paralysis that affects the two lower limbs and a part of the trunk. It is generally caused by a lesion to the spinal cord at the thoracic or lumbar vertebrae. The chances of recovery and the possibilities of treatment depend on the disorder responsible and the degree of deterioration of the nerve fibers; it is actually impossible to surgically recompose a severed spinal cord. The victim may be unable to walk and may suffer from incontinence or urinary retention. They may also have trouble exhaling or coughing if the lesion is high. Erection and ejaculation may also be affected. On the other hand, a female paraplegic may carry out a pregnancy, but forceps must be used during birth in the event of paralysis of the abdominal muscles.

TETRAPLEGIA

Tetraplegia, or quadriplegia, is a paralysis that affects the four limbs and trunk. It occurs generally from a lesion to the spinal cord at the cervical vertebrae, caused notably by arthrosis or a hyperextension-hyperflexion injury (rabbit punch). As with paraplegia, the chances of recovery depend on several factors, including the severity of the injury inflicted on the spine. The victim suffers from a loss of motor skills and sensitivity, urinary and anal incontinence, and breathing problems of a varying severity: difficulty exhaling and coughing, even inability to breathe without assistance.

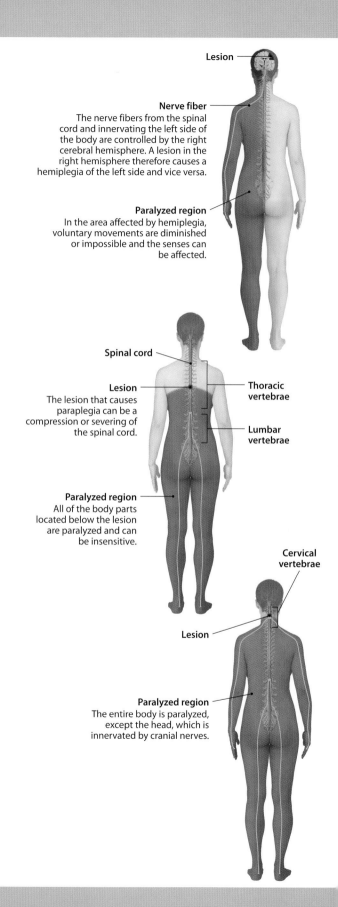

Lesion

Nerve fiber
The nerve fibers from the spinal cord and innervating the left side of the body are controlled by the right cerebral hemisphere. A lesion in the right hemisphere therefore causes a hemiplegia of the left side and vice versa.

Paralyzed region
In the area affected by hemiplegia, voluntary movements are diminished or impossible and the senses can be affected.

Spinal cord

Lesion
The lesion that causes paraplegia can be a compression or severing of the spinal cord.

Thoracic vertebrae

Lumbar vertebrae

Paralyzed region
All of the body parts located below the lesion are paralyzed and can be insensitive.

Cervical vertebrae

Lesion

Paralyzed region
The entire body is paralyzed, except the head, which is innervated by cranial nerves.

WHIPLASH

A whiplash, or hyperextension-hyperflexion injury, is a trauma to the cervical column caused by a sudden extension and flexion of the neck. It generally occurs during a car or sports accident. A whiplash can cause headaches, tinnitus, vertigo, and vision problems and lead to muscular lesions, a sprain, a spinal fracture, or a lesion to the spinal cord, depending on the severity of the trauma.

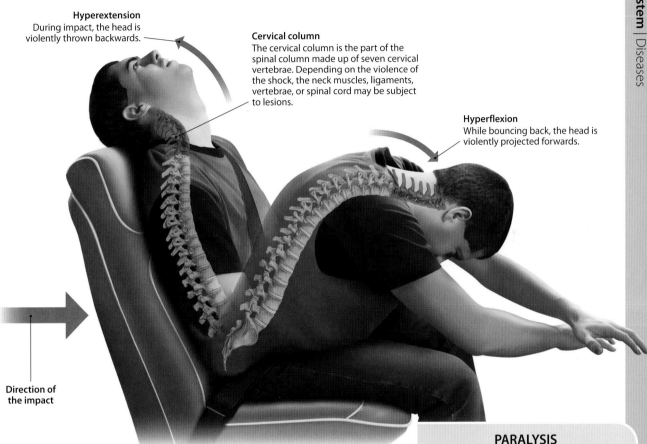

Hyperextension
During impact, the head is violently thrown backwards.

Cervical column
The cervical column is the part of the spinal column made up of seven cervical vertebrae. Depending on the violence of the shock, the neck muscles, ligaments, vertebrae, or spinal cord may be subject to lesions.

Hyperflexion
While bouncing back, the head is violently projected forwards.

Direction of the impact

Whiplash during a car accident

PARESIS

Paresis is a partial paralysis, meaning a decrease in the muscle strength of a body part linked to a lesion of the motor neurons. The muscles most affected are those of the limbs and eyes. Paresis is a symptom of different illnesses of the nervous system, particularly multiple sclerosis. It can also occur in the event of bone fracture. Depending on the cause and severity of the paresis, remission can be rapid, motor skills can be recovered by medical treatment, or the neurological impairment may be irreversible. In this last case, retraining lets the individual learn to use the remaining active muscles as best as possible. The recourse to physiotherapy also prevents atrophy of the affected muscles.

PARALYSIS

SYMPTOMS:
Inability to carry out voluntary movement, sometimes associated with a loss of sensitivity. Some paralysis is accompanied by an increase in muscle tone that can cause spasms and contractures.

TREATMENT:
There is no specific treatment for paralysis. The chances of recovery depend on the severity of the lesion and are improved by retraining.

LOSS OF CONSCIOUSNESS

Loss of consciousness, or fainting, is a partial or total interruption of consciousness, which can occur suddenly or progressively. When it is of short duration (**syncope** or fainting), it can be due to a cardiovascular problem or result from a temporary malfunctioning of the autonomic nervous system. When the loss of consciousness is extended, this is called a coma. Loss of consciousness is a symptom of numerous diseases and **traumas**. It is therefore important to consult a doctor to determine its cause and to implement treatment accordingly.

First aid: Malaise and loss of consciousness... page 559

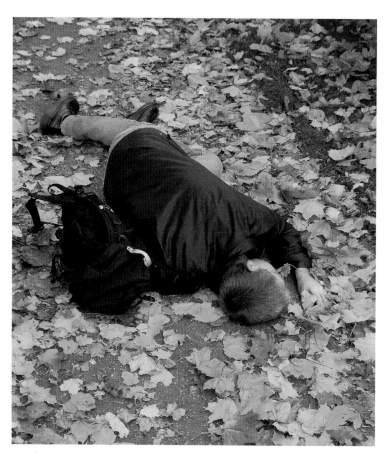

SYNCOPE

Syncope is a complete loss of consciousness for a short duration of time, following a sudden decrease in the oxygen or blood supply in the brain. This decrease is most often due to a transitory malfunctioning of the autonomic nervous system (vasovagal syncope), but can also result from a cardiovascular malfunctioning, pulmonary embolism, asphyxia, electrocution, decrease of potassium levels in the blood, etc. Victims collapse, remain unconscious for a few moments (generally less than 1 minute), then come to, without remembering their fall. While passed out, they do not react to pinching or noise. Sometimes convulsions and a release of urine are observed. Syncope can occur while resting or active.

VASOVAGAL SYNCOPE AND VAGAL MALAISE

Vasovagal syncope is caused by excessive activity of the vagus nerve, which plays an important role in the slowing of the heart and breathing rate. Most of the time, it is not serious and can affect young people in good health without heart problems. Vasovagal syncope sometimes follows a sudden change from sitting or lying down to standing. It can also follow vagal malaise. This is a state of discomfort (pallor, sweating, blurred vision, humming in the ears, slowing of the heart rate) accompanied by an impression of imminent fainting. Vagal malaise is due to excess activity of the vagus nerve on the cardiovascular system, generally linked to a strong emotion or intense pain.

COMA

A coma is a prolonged interruption of consciousness, characterized by an absence or quasi-absence of reaction to external stimuli, but with a relative conservation of circulatory and respiratory functions. It can result from a cranial trauma, cerebrovascular accident, hypoglycemia, poisoning, or various diseases: tumor, meningitis, epilepsy, hepatitis, diabetes, etc. A coma can last a few hours to several months, or several years. Its evolution essentially depends on its cause and the prognosis is extremely difficult to establish.

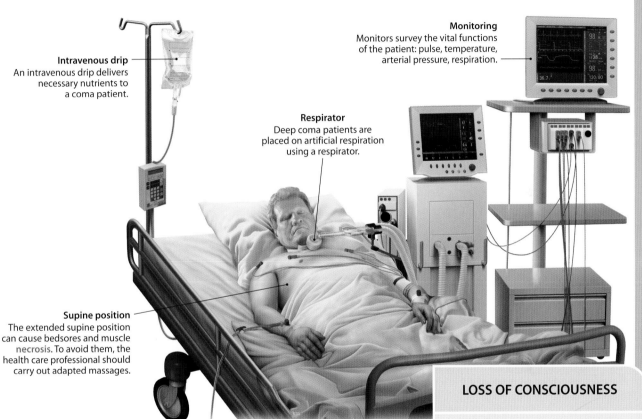

Intravenous drip
An intravenous drip delivers necessary nutrients to a coma patient.

Monitoring
Monitors survey the vital functions of the patient: pulse, temperature, arterial pressure, respiration.

Respirator
Deep coma patients are placed on artificial respiration using a respirator.

Supine position
The extended supine position can cause bedsores and muscle necrosis. To avoid them, the health care professional should carry out adapted massages.

STAGES OF A COMA

A coma can reach four stages of depth. The first stage (semi-comatose), the patient grunts when spoken to and reacts to pain. At the second stage (somnolent), the patient does not react to sounds but some reflexes persist. In the third stage (deep coma), the patient does not react to stimuli and presents a complete muscle relaxation and vegetative problems, particularly breathing problems. The fourth stage is the state of being brain dead. Brain death is the stoppage of all brain activity and all spontaneous respiratory activity, with a temporary persistence of cardiac activity. It is considered being legally dead in many countries.

LOSS OF CONSCIOUSNESS

SYMPTOMS:
Partial or total interruption of consciousness, of a variable duration.

TREATMENT:
A person in a coma requires specific care, particularly to maintain vital functions.

PREVENTION :
Lying down as soon as the first signs of vagal malaise are experienced to avoid injury while falling.

CEREBROVASCULAR ACCIDENTS

A cerebrovascular accident, or stroke, is a sudden alteration in the blood circulation of the brain, due to the obstruction of an artery or the rupture of its walls. In Western countries, strokes are the third greatest cause of death and the greatest cause of acquired handicaps (motor coordination, sensory and intellectual deficiencies). They affect all ages, but the risk increases after 60 years of age and in the event of arterial hypertension, atherosclerosis, diabetes, or aneurysm. Smoking, alcoholism, and family history also increase the risk. A stroke requires emergency hospitalization. Immediate treatment diminishes the risk of irreversible neurological lesions and death. Recurrence is frequent and 75% of people who survive have sequelae of varying severity.

SYMPTOMS OF A STROKE

The symptoms of a stroke appear suddenly and can differ depending on the nature and site of the lesion: paralysis, vision and language problems (indistinct speech, difficulty finding words, or understanding others), sensitivity (numbness) or coordination (trembling, clumsiness) problems, vertigo, loss of consciousness, violent headache, convulsions, etc. When the symptoms of a stroke disappear spontaneously in less than 24 hours, it is a transitory ischemic accident. This type of accident, caused by a brief interruption of the blood irrigation of the brain, constitutes a warning signal since it often precedes cerebral infarction. It requires an emergency medical consultation.

CEREBRAL INFARCTION

Cerebral infarction represents 80% of strokes. It follows the obstruction of a cerebral artery by embolism or thrombosis. In the case of thrombosis, the obstruction is caused by a blood clot (thrombus) that forms directly in a cerebral artery, at an atheromatous plaque. It is the most common cause of cerebral infarction. In the case of embolism, the obstruction is created by a foreign body having migrated to the brain, often a blood clot that formed in the heart or detached itself from an atheromatous plaque. The infarction causes the interruption of the blood flow to the brain, and, to a varying extent, the destruction of its tissues. It can also cause the formation of a cerebral edema or develop into intracerebral hemorrhage.

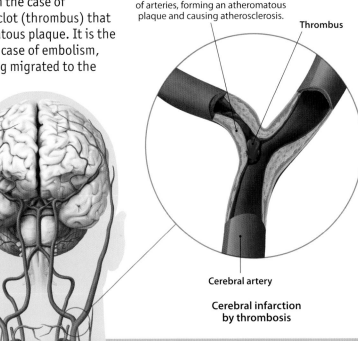

Atheromatous plaque
In the case of excess cholesterol, lipids can attach to the internal wall of arteries, forming an atheromatous plaque and causing atherosclerosis.

Thrombus

Cerebral artery

Cerebral infarction by thrombosis

Atherosclerosis... page 256

CEREBRAL HEMORRHAGE

Cerebral hemorrhage, which represents 20% of strokes, often takes the form of blood effusion inside the brain (intracerebral hemorrhage), caused by the rupture of a cerebral artery. It results in the destruction of nerve cells as well as the formation of a hematoma and sometimes edema. The main cause of intracerebral hemorrhage is arterial hypertension, which weakens the blood vessels. The blood effusion may not occur in the brain, but between the meninges that cover it (meningeal bleedings). More frequent in women, meningeal bleeding is generally caused by the rupture of an aneurysm.

Aneurysm… page 270

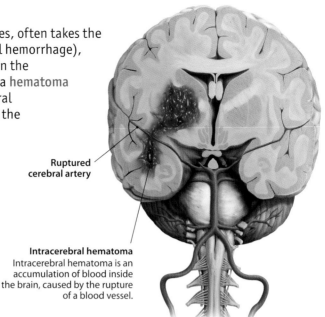

Ruptured cerebral artery

Intracerebral hematoma
Intracerebral hematoma is an accumulation of blood inside the brain, caused by the rupture of a blood vessel.

Intracerebral hemorrhage

CEREBRAL EDEMA

A cerebral edema is an accumulation of fluid in the tissues of the brain. Its causes are varied: cerebrovascular accident, cranial trauma, tumor, etc. Cerebral edema leads to headaches and neurological problems (language problems, hallucinations, blindness, amnesia, decrease in strength and sensitivity, loss of consciousness). It may cause intracranial hypertension as well as compression of the brain and is a common cause of death.

PREVENTING CEREBROVASCULAR ACCIDENTS

Preventing cerebrovascular accidents lies mainly in detecting warning signs, obtaining rapid medical attention, and reducing risk factors.

■ ADOPT A HEALTHY LIFESTYLE

A poor diet (excessive consumption of salt and saturated fats), lack of exercise, stress, smoking and alcoholism are all other factors that predispose an individual to stroke by increasing the risk of arterial hypertension, atherosclerosis, hypercholesterolemia, diabetes, etc. It is important to monitor these problems and treat them by adopting a healthier lifestyle. People who have already suffered from a transitory ischemic accident should be particularly careful.

■ CONSULT A DOCTOR AS SOON AS THE FIRST SYMPTOMS APPEAR

CEREBROVASCULAR ACCIDENTS

SYMPTOMS:
Paralysis, sensitivity problems, vision, language and coordination problems, loss of consciousness, vertigo, violent headache, convulsions. Symptoms arise suddenly.

TREATMENT:
Treatment (surgery, thrombolysis, anticoagulants) aims to prevent the extension of lesions to avoid death and limit sequelae. Functional recovery is variable and rests on retraining.

PREVENTION:
Reducing risk factors (arterial hypertension, hypercholesterolemia, atherosclerosis, etc.). Consultation with a doctor as soon as the first signs appear (transitory ischemic accident).

TUMORS OF THE NERVOUS SYSTEM

In adults, primitive tumors of the nervous system are most often located within the cerebrum. In children, they appear more frequently on the cerebellum and cerebral trunk. The nervous system is also the site of secondary tumors, caused by metastases of other cancers. Tumors of the nervous system, even benign, can compress the brain or spinal cord and cause neurological problems: paralysis, muscular weakness, epileptic attacks, balance problems.

Cancer... page 55

TYPES OF TUMORS OF THE NERVOUS SYSTEM

There are mainly three types of tumors affecting the nervous system: neurinoma, meningioma, and glioma. Neurinoma is a benign tumor that grows slowly and that affects the cranial or spinal nerves. Meningioma develops in the meninges that envelop the brain and spinal cord. It is most often benign and develops slowly, but there are invasive forms that produce metastases. Glioma, which can be benign or malignant (glioblastoma), develops in the central nervous system in the glial cells (cells that support, nourish, and protect neurons). Almost half of the tumors located within the brain are gliomas.

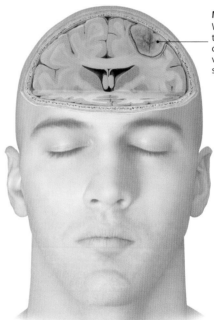

Meningioma
When it is located in the skull, meningioma can cause headaches, vomiting, epileptic seizures, and paralysis.

GLIOBLASTOMA

Glioblastoma is a malignant brain tumor, caused by the proliferation of glial cells, which form a part of the nerve tissue. Generally located in one of the two cerebral hemispheres, glioblastoma causes intracranial hypertension and lesions of the nerve cells that lead to neurological deficiencies: paralysis, sensory problems. It must be treated as quickly as possible because its volume increases quickly. Recurrences are frequent and this tumor is often fatal in the year that follows its diagnosis.

TUMORS OF THE NERVOUS SYSTEM

SYMPTOMS:
Headaches, nausea and vomiting, convulsions, vision troubles, behavior disorders, disturbance of intellectual functions, hallucinations, vertigo, neurological deficiencies (muscular weakness, paralysis, sensory problems). The symptoms depend on the location of the tumor.

TREATMENT:
Radiation therapy, chemotherapy, surgery. Medication to treat the symptoms of the tumor. If a tumor grows very slowly and does not cause symptoms, it is possible that no treatment will be implemented (the side effects of treatment can be more harmful than the tumor itself). Regular monitoring is therefore necessary.

ENCEPHALITIS

Encephalitis is the **inflammation** of the brain, most often caused by a viral **infection** or an **autoimmune** reaction. More rarely, encephalitis is caused by a cranial **trauma**, poisoning, bacterial infection, or tumor. In moderate forms, the disease manifests itself by somnolence, flu-like syndrome, and headaches, sometimes resulting in slight sequelae like slowing of thought process and speech or abnormal behavior (change in mood, agitation). Severe forms of encephalitis are at the origin of major neurological problems: **convulsions**, mental confusion, memory troubles, sensory and motor troubles. They can leave irreversible sequelae (paralysis, sensory and motor disorders, lowering of cognitive faculties, epilepsy, coma) and lead to death.

Flu-like syndrome... page 320

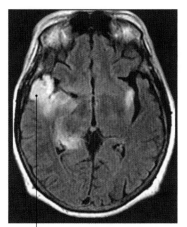

Herpetic encephalitis

Temporal lobe
The temporal lobe is the area most frequently affected by herpetic encephalitis. Its inflammation often causes language problems and convulsions.

VIRAL ENCEPHALITIS

Most cases of encephalitis are caused by a virus that directly infects the encephalon. The virus can be transmitted by mosquitoes (Japanese encephalitis, West Nile encephalitis), ticks (tick meningoencephalitis), or a mammal bite (rabies). However, the most common form of viral encephalitis is herpetic encephalitis, caused by the *Herpes simplex* virus. Herpes simplex, responsible for labial herpes and genital herpes, is transmitted by direct contact with herpetic lesions or with a contaminated object (utensils, towels, etc.). Herpetic encephalitis is one of the rare forms to benefit from a specific treatment, acyclovir. It especially affects children younger than 3 years of age and adults between 40 and 50 years of age. Mortality is elevated and the sequelae, if the disease is not treated in an early stage, are often severe. Thus, as soon as viral encephalitis is suspected, it is treated by acyclovir even before the diagnosis of herpetic encephalitis is confirmed.

Labial herpes... page 86
Genital herpes... page 447

POST-INFECTIOUS ENCEPHALITIS

Post-infectious encephalitis is caused by an autoimmune reaction following an infection not directly affecting the encephalon. Viruses like those of the flu, measles, rubella, poliomyelitis, or AIDS can trigger the disease. Infrequently, encephalitis can be triggered by the administration of a vaccine.

ENCEPHALITIS

SYMPTOMS:
Moderate forms: flu-like syndrome, headaches, memory troubles, confusion, abnormal behavior, drowsiness.
Severe forms: sensory and motor disorders (photophobia, coordination problems, paralysis), language problems.

TREATMENT:
Antivirals (acyclovir), antibiotics, treatment of symptoms.

PREVENTION :
Vaccination against rabies, rubella, poliomyelitis, influenza, measles. Protection against mosquitoes.

RABIES

Known of for several millenia, rabies is a viral disease that affects the nervous system and causes a fatal **inflammation** of the brain (encephalitis). It is transmitted to people by infected animals, particularly foxes, bats, raccoons, and stray dogs. Contamination occurs through saliva following a bite or licking of a wound. Rabies has a global presence, except in a few countries (United Kingdom, Ireland, Japan, Iceland, Australia, New Zealand, Norway, Sweden). **Vaccination** prevents contamination for people at risk and treats those that have been exposed to the virus by a bite. Once the disease is confirmed, death is rapid and inevitable.

SYMPTOMS OF RABIES

Symptoms of rabies appear in a few days to several months after contamination. The incubation period is shorter when the bite is located in richly innervated areas or near the head. The patient starts feeling pain at the site of the bite, and can present difficulties swallowing and mood disorders: despondency, anxiety, excitation, crying fits, fear of water. The disease can then evolve into two different clinical forms. In the furious form (80% of cases), the patient becomes aggressive and violent. In the paralytic form, general paralysis sets in within a few days. In both cases, the disease evolves quickly into coma or death, often by asphyxia.

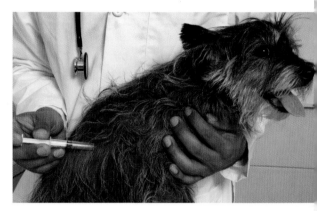

Rabies in animals
When the disease is confirmed, the rabid animal displays excessive salivation and abnormal behavior: disorientation, agitation or, on the contrary, lethargy, difficulty walking. An animal appearing healthy can nevertheless be a carrier of the disease and transmit it to humans because the virus is present in saliva before the appearance of symptoms. Any non-vaccinated mammal is susceptible to infection. Vaccination of domestic animals is therefore essential.

RABIES

SYMPTOMS:
Fever, mood disorders, excessive salivation, hallucinations, fear of water, contractures, paralysis.

TREATMENT:
Immediate vaccination after exposure to the virus, serotherapy. There is no specific treatment once the disease has been confirmed.

Serotherapy... page 286

PREVENTION :
Vaccination (humans and animals). Immediately consult a doctor in the case of a bite by an unknown animal or one that is suspected of having rabies to initiate treatment before the disease develops.

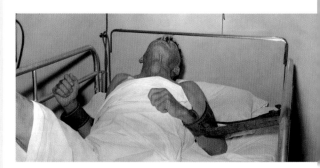

Furious rabies
In the furious form of rabies, the individuals present motor hyperexcitation (**convulsions**, contractures) and excessive salivation. Anxious, agitated, and aggressive, they are the victims of hallucinations and suffer from a pathological fear of water (hydrophobia).

MENINGITIS

Meningitis is an **inflammation** of the meninges (membranes enveloping the brain and spinal cord) caused most often by an **infection**. The most common forms, caused by parasitic viruses in the intestine, are generally benign and resolve spontaneously in a few days. However, some forms of meningitis caused by bacteria (pneumococcus, streptococcus, *Haemophilus influenzae, Listeria monocytogenes, Escherichia coli*, meningococcus), fungi, and certain viruses (herpes, varicella) can be very serious, notably in children and older people or the **immunodeficient**. It must be treated rapidly with **antibiotics** because it can lead to neurological sequelae (loss of motor coordination, hearing loss, learning disabilities), even death. Meningitis caused by meningococcus in particular is very contagious, virulent, and sometimes sudden. It particularly affects children and adolescents and can cause epidemics. Thanks to **vaccination**, cases of meningitis have become quite rare in Western countries.

SYMPTOMS OF MENINGITIS

Meningitis is characterized by a collection of symptoms (meningeal syndrome): high fever, headaches, intolerance to light, vomiting, irritability, stiffness of the nape of the neck, convulsions. The appearance of small red marks on the skin is a sign of severity and requires emergency hospitalization. In newborns, the diagnosis of the disease is more difficult because the symptoms are not specific: crying, gray complexion, lack of muscle tone, drowsiness, round fontanel, convulsions, etc.

LUMBAR PUNCTURE

A lumbar puncture consists in introducing a needle between two lumbar vertebrae, up to the subarachnoid space (located between two meninges), to remove a sample of cerebrospinal fluid or introduce medication (antibiotic, chemotherapy, etc.). The sampling of cerebrospinal fluid allows for the diagnosis of meningeal bleeding or meningitis. It also allows for the evacuation of an overflow of cerebrospinal fluid (e.g. in the case of intracranial hypertension). A lumbar puncture is carried out in the hospital, under local anesthesia or without anesthesia. It is safe and can be done on patients of any age, including newborns.

Meninges and cerebrospinal fluid... page 140

Point of puncture
A lumbar puncture is generally carried out between the fourth and fifth lumbar vertebrae.

MENINGITIS

SYMPTOMS:
Fever, headaches, intolerance to light, vomiting, stiffness in the nape of the neck, convulsions. Meningococcus meningitis: red spots on the skin.

TREATMENT:
Antibiotics.

PREVENTION:
There are vaccines against certain forms of bacterial meningitis (pneumococcus, meningococcus A and C, *Haemophilus influenzae*). Antibiotics are administered in a preventive manner to people who were in contact with an individual infected by meningococcus.

HERPES ZOSTER

The varicella-zoster virus is present in a latent state in the nerve ganglions of anyone who has suffered from chickenpox. It can be reactivated in the form of herpes zoster, or shingles, when the immune defenses are weakened by factors such as stress, **infection**, or cancer. Herpes zoster is characterized by a very painful skin eruption located on the path of a sensory nerve, particularly the intercostal nerves, ophtalmic nerve, and cervical nerves. The disease can be transmitted by contact with the vesicles and cause chickenpox in people who never contracted it.

Chickenpox... page 519

SYMPTOMS OF HERPES ZOSTER

Manifestations of herpes zoster are unilateral and located on the path of the affected nerve, because the virus travels the length of the nerve up to the skin. Symptoms begin with a burning sensation followed by the appearance of rashes and vesicles on the skin. Generally, the pain that accompanies these is very intense. Recovery happens in 2–6 weeks, but the pain can persist for several years. Recurrence is rare. In people that are severely immunodeficient (e.g. suffering from AIDS or cancer), there is a risk that the infection becomes generalized and attacks the viscera, meninges, or brain and causes hemorrhage.

OPHTHALMIC HERPES ZOSTER

When herpes zoster affects the ophthalmic nerve, it manifests itself by a rash and vesicles located on the forehead, perimeter of the eye, and the cornea. It can cause lesions in the eye and lead to a decrease in visual acuity, even blindness. It is therefore systematically treated with antivirals.

Spinal ganglion
The varicella virus remains latent in the spinal ganglions, sometimes for dozens of years, before being reactivated and causing herpes zoster.

Intercostal nerve
Herpes zoster often affects an intercostal nerve, causing skin lesions on the nerve path.

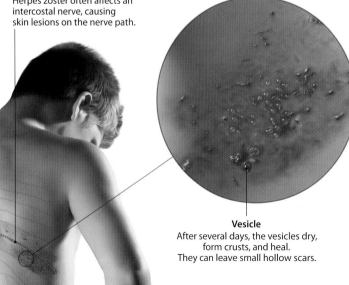

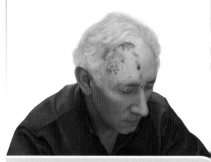

Vesicle
After several days, the vesicles dry, form crusts, and heal. They can leave small hollow scars.

HERPES ZOSTER

SYMPTOMS:
Burning sensation, or skin rash, and vesicles along the nerve path. Intense pain. Sometimes, slight fever and headaches.

TREATMENT:
Disinfection of lesions, analgesics. Antivirals are prescribed to immunodeficient individuals and in the case of ophthalmic herpes zoster.

POLIOMYELITIS

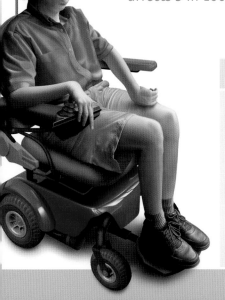

Poliomyelitis, or polio, is an **infection** of the nervous system by the poliovirus, a virus that is transmitted by contact with secretions (coughing, sneezing, droplets of saliva) or with contaminated water and food. When the disease sets in, it causes fever, headaches, back pain, and stiffness in the neck. In some cases, the disease leads to an often irreversible paralysis of certain muscles, causing their atrophy and sometimes very debilitating deformities. Poliomyelitis essentially affects children. Today, while it is decreasing thanks to the **vaccine**, it remains endemic in some countries in Africa and Asia.

POLIOMYELITIS

SYMPTOMS:
Fever, vomiting, headaches, back pain, stiffness in the neck, pain in the limbs. Sometimes, paralysis of certain muscles.

TREATMENT:
No treatment.

PREVENTION:
Vaccination, hygienic measures.

AMYOTROPHIC LATERAL SCLEROSIS

Amyotrophic lateral sclerosis, or Lou Gehrig's disease, is a **degenerative** disease of an unknown cause that affects the motor neurons innervating the skeletal muscles. It first manifests itself by muscle weakness in the hand and forearm and by the progressive atrophy of the hand muscles. The impairment then spreads to all of the voluntary muscles, developing into paralysis. The aggravation of symptoms can be very rapid or extend over several years and death is usually caused by respiratory failure or a pulmonary infection. The disease generally begins around 60 years of age and affects 5 in 100,000 people in the world.

AMYOTROPHIC LATERAL SCLEROSIS

SYMPTOMS:
Muscular dysfunction (paralysis, muscle atrophy, excessive muscle stiffness, cramps, spontaneous and irregular contractions), respiratory, speech and swallowing problems. Related symptoms: trouble sleeping, constipation, weight loss.

TREATMENT:
Treatment of symptoms: gastric catheter, respiratory assistance, etc. Medication (riluzole) slows the development of the disease.

MULTIPLE SCLEROSIS

Multiple sclerosis is an **autoimmune** disease that leads to the destruction of the myelin sheath of the axons of the central nervous system. It causes neurological problems of varying severity. The disease generally begins between 20 and 40 years of age and often evolves in spurts punctuated by periods of remission and the regression of symptoms. It affects approximately 2.5 million people worldwide, the majority of which are women (a ratio of three women to every man).

The neuron... page 136

DEMYELINATION

Demyelination is the destruction of the myelin sheath that encircles and isolates the axons of neurons. It causes a disturbance or interruption in the conduction of nerve impulses and can result in irreversible lesions of neurons. It leads to various neurological problems, depending on the location of lesions. The demyelination of axons can be caused by an autoimmune disease (multiple sclerosis, systemic lupus erythematosus) or by an infection (Lyme disease, AIDS).

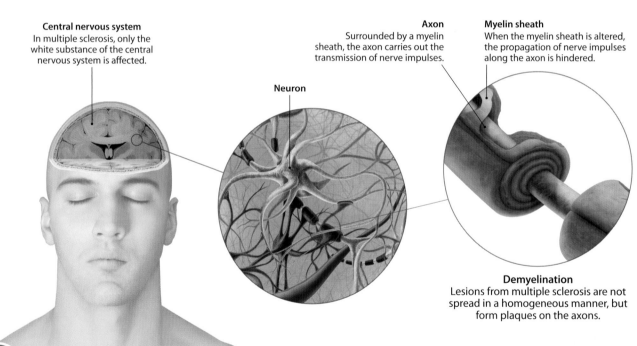

Central nervous system
In multiple sclerosis, only the white substance of the central nervous system is affected.

Neuron

Axon
Surrounded by a myelin sheath, the axon carries out the transmission of nerve impulses.

Myelin sheath
When the myelin sheath is altered, the propagation of nerve impulses along the axon is hindered.

Demyelination
Lesions from multiple sclerosis are not spread in a homogeneous manner, but form plaques on the axons.

CAUSES OF MULTIPLE SCLEROSIS

The factors responsible for multiple sclerosis are still poorly known and may have various origins. The disease particularly ravages Northern Europe, Canada, and the northern United States, which suggests the existence of an environmental or genetic factor in its appearance. The disease can also be triggered by a virus (flu, herpes) in vulnerable people. Several research teams are opposed to the idea of a hypothetical link between the appearance of multiple sclerosis and vaccination against hepatitis B. The World Health Organization also rejects this idea and insists on the great benefit of the vaccine.

EVOLUTION OF MULTIPLE SCLEROSIS

The evolution of multiple sclerosis can take several forms. In most cases, the symptoms appear in flare-ups that alternate with periods of complete remission. After several years, the neurological state is gradually aggravated by the flare-ups. In other forms of the disease, the impairment develops progressively and continuously, without periods of remission. Multiple sclerosis causes various neurological problems that depend on the location of demyelination plaques: problems with vision, sensitivity, balance, walking, urinating, mood, etc. After several years, the disease can generate severe impairment (paralysis, blindness) and cause an individual's loss of autonomy.

MULTIPLE SCLEROSIS

SYMPTOMS:
Motor, sensory, and psychological problems. Acute and chronic pains, severe fatigue. The symptoms generally appear in spurts. After several years, they are aggravated and become permanent.

TREATMENT:
Corticosteroids during flare-ups. Disease-modifying therapy between flare-ups: interferon, immunosuppressants in severe cases. Incurable disease.

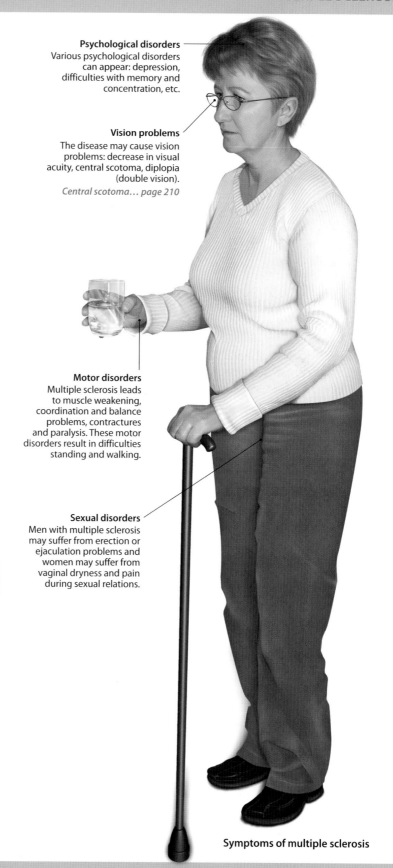

Psychological disorders
Various psychological disorders can appear: depression, difficulties with memory and concentration, etc.

Vision problems
The disease may cause vision problems: decrease in visual acuity, central scotoma, diplopia (double vision).
Central scotoma... page 210

Motor disorders
Multiple sclerosis leads to muscle weakening, coordination and balance problems, contractures and paralysis. These motor disorders result in difficulties standing and walking.

Sexual disorders
Men with multiple sclerosis may suffer from erection or ejaculation problems and women may suffer from vaginal dryness and pain during sexual relations.

Symptoms of multiple sclerosis

EPILEPSY

Epilepsy is a neurological disease that manifests itself in recurring attacks resulting in a sudden and temporary malfunctioning of electrical activity of the brain. Epilepsy can result from a **genetic** anomaly, **infection**, or lesion of the brain. However, in half of all cases, its cause cannot be established. The diagnosis of epilepsy, based on the repetition of attacks, is confirmed using electroencephalography. The attacks can lead to cerebral lesions. In addition, alcoholic intoxication, as well as the sudden stoppage of medications, risk causing an attack or a series of abnormally long tonic-clonic seizures (longer than 30 minutes) in epileptics, which can cause respiratory failure, neurological and intellectual sequelae, even death.

EPILEPTIC ATTACKS

Epileptic attacks occur most often in an unpredictable manner even if there are triggering factors in some cases: stress, fatigue, strong emotion, flashing light (television, computer, video game), alcohol. When they are caused by a localized malfunctioning of the electric activity of the brain, the attacks, said to be partial, can cause localized motor or sensory problems and psychological problems (hallucinations, change in behavior) for several minutes. Generalized attacks, which affect the entire body, are caused by a diffuse electrical discharge in the cortex. There are two types of generalized epileptic attacks: absences (minor, or petit mal, epilepsy) or tonic-clonic seizures (grand mal).

ABSENCES

An absence is a brief interruption of consciousness. It is manifested by a stoppage of speech and a fixed look for several seconds, sometimes accompanied by automatic movements (swallowing, chewing, etc.). In an epileptic, absences can repeat themselves several times a day.

EPILEPSY

SYMPTOMS:
Generalized epilepsy: convulsions, absences. Partial epilepsy: localized motor or sensory problems, psychological problems.

TREATMENT:
Antiepileptic medications, surgical ablation of the implicated area of the cortex. Some cases of partial epilepsy in children subside or disappear spontaneously.

PREVENTION:
Antiepileptic medications, together with a healthy lifestyle (sufficient and regular sleep, moderation in alcohol consumption, limitation of light stimulations), often help prevent epileptic attacks.

Tongue
During epileptic seizures, patients sometimes bite their tongue. Despite everything, do not attempt to slide something between their teeth or block their movements.

Convulsions
Convulsions are sudden and involuntary muscle contractions of the entire body, interrupted by intervals of muscle relaxation. Symptomatic of epilepsy, they can also have other origins: cranial trauma, cerebrovascular accident, infection (meningitis), tumor, poisoning, and febrile seizures caused by dehydration or fever in young children.

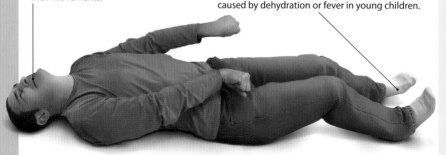

Tonic-clonic seizure
Tonic-clonic seizures are characterized by a loss of consciousness and convulsions lasting 5 to 10 minutes, followed by an unconscious recovery phase.

PARKINSON'S DISEASE

Parkinson's disease is a **degenerative** neurological disease characterized mainly by motor problems collectively known as parkinsonian syndrome. It results from the degeneration of neurons located on the cerebral trunk that are responsible for the production of dopamine, a neurotransmitter implicated in the control of voluntary movements. The cause of this degeneration is unknown. Parkinson's disease occurs progressively, generally around 55 years of age, and affects 1% to 2% of the population older than 65 years of age. It is incurable, but there are treatments available that reduce the symptoms and provide a satisfying quality of life for the afflicted individual.

PARKINSONIAN SYNDROME

Parkinsonian syndrome is a collection of symptoms characteristic of Parkinson's disease: resting tremors, akinesia, bradykinesia, plastic hypertonia, problems with posture and balance. Diagnosis of the disease lies in the identification of these symptoms because no medical test can test for it. Parkinsonian syndrome can also be accompanied by amimia, fatigue, depression, and sometimes memory and concentration problems. Other diseases can cause the appearance of parkinsonian syndrome (cerebrovascular accident, poisoning, etc.).

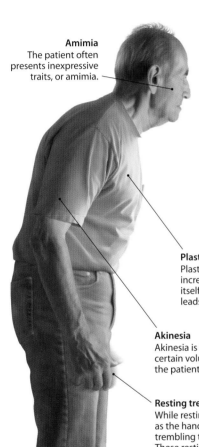

Amimia
The patient often presents inexpressive traits, or amimia.

Plastic hypertonia
Plastic hypertonia is the abnormal increase in muscle tone. It manifests itself by excessive muscle stiffness and leads to a change in posture.

Akinesia
Akinesia is the inability to carry out certain voluntary movements. It gives the patient a fixed look.

Resting tremors
While resting, certain parts of the body such as the hand, chin, or foot are affected by a trembling that reduces voluntary movements. These resting tremors constitute the first symptom in many affected individuals.

Bradykinesia
Bradykinesia is an abnormal slowing of voluntary movements.

PARKINSON'S DISEASE

SYMPTOMS:
Resting tremors, akinesia, bradykinesia, plastic hypertonia, resulting in a loss of dexterity, trouble walking, change in posture. A decrease, generally slight, in intellectual faculties. Symptoms and development vary depending on the individual.

TREATMENT:
Treatment aims to alleviate symptoms: medication, physical therapy, surgery (implantation of electrodes in the mesencephalon).

ABNORMAL MOVEMENTS

Involuntary muscle contractions can cause abnormal movements (tics, tremors, chorea). They are often a symptom of a neurological affection such as Tourette's syndrome or Huntington's disease, but they can also appear without any apparent reason.

TOURETTE'S SYNDROME

Tourette's syndrome, named after the neuropsychiatrist who published the first description of the disease in 1885, is a rare neurological disease characterized by motor or vocal tics. The repetition of words or phrases or even the exclamation of obscenities can sometimes be observed. The disease mostly affects men and generally sets in before the age of 10. It is sometimes accompanied by other problems: obsessive compulsive disorders, hyperactivity, learning disabilities, etc.

HUNTINGTON'S DISEASE

Huntington's disease, or Huntington's chorea, is a hereditary genetic disease that generally becomes noticeable between 30 and 50 years of age. It causes the degeneration of certain areas of the brain, which leads to chorea, psychological disorders such as depression or psychosis, as well as language, attention, or memory disorders that can evolve into dementia. The disease is fatal after 10 to 20 years.

TICS

Tics are involuntary, sudden, and intermittent movements that can be temporarily stopped by choice. They often occur in the face (blinking eyes, contraction of cheeks), the neck (rotation of the head), or shoulders. Frequent in children, they are often linked to anxiety, fatigue, or emotions and most often resolve spontaneously after a few years.

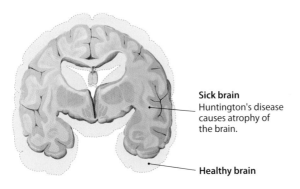

Sick brain
Huntington's disease causes atrophy of the brain.

Healthy brain

CHOREA

Chorea is a syndrome characterized by involuntary, sudden, and anarchical movements, accompanied by motor coordination problems that particularly affect walking. The movements, present during rest and sometimes while sleeping, are particularly marked in the limbs, face, and neck. Chorea can notably be caused by poisoning (carbon oxide, alcohol), certain medications, and Huntington's disease.

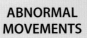

ABNORMAL MOVEMENTS

SYMPTOMS:
Involuntary muscle contractions causing tics, tremors, chorea, etc.

TREATMENT:
Medication can make some abnormal movements disappear. Tics: behavior therapy. If the symptoms are very debilitating, they can be eased by the implantation of microelectrodes in certain structures of the brain.

AMNESIA

Amnesia is the total or partial loss of memory, in a temporary or permanent manner. It can be caused by lesions to the brain caused by cerebrovascular accident, cranial **trauma**, a disease such as Alzheimer's or encephalitis, or by poisoning (medication, alcohol, drugs). It can also be caused by a psychological trauma or by a mental disease such as psychosis.

TYPES OF AMNESIA

There are different types of amnesia that can affect memory: anterograde amnesia, which results in the inability to form new memories; retrograde amnesia, which is characterized by the inability to remember past events; lacunar amnesia, which is the forgetting of events surrounding a trauma; and psychogenic amnesia, which is manifested by the inability to remember personal information.

MEMORY

The ability of the brain to save the trace of a past experience and to bring it to consciousness is memory. This faculty allows individuals to place themselves in a temporal continuity and accomplish their present and future activities, which rely on memorized knowledge. Memory is a three-phase process: encoding, storing, and recovering information. Encoding, meaning the transformation of perceptions into memory, is a personal process that is carried out depending on the centers of interest and prior knowledge of each person. It can be voluntary or involuntary. Storing can have a variable duration, from several seconds (short-term memory) to the entire life (long-term memory). It depends on the quality of encoding. Recovery is the return of memorized information to consciousness.

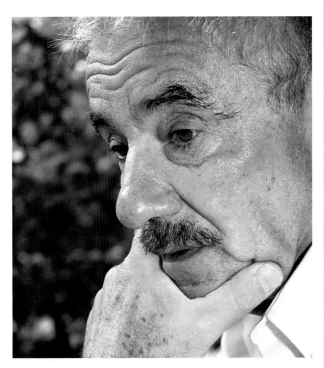

Psychogenic amnesia
Psychogenic amnesia is a rare type of amnesia that arises in the case of violent emotional shock (aggression, rape, accident) and is characterized by the inability to remember personal information (name, age, address). Psychogenic amnesia can last from several hours to several months. It is sometimes accompanied by fugue.

AMNESIA

SYMPTOMS:
Partial or total disappearance, temporary or permanent, of old memories or of the ability to acquire new memories.

TREATMENT:
Therapeutic measures aim to give amnesia patients a certain autonomy, notably due to particular learning techniques.

ALZHEIMER'S DISEASE
AND OTHER FORMS OF **DEMENTIA**

Dementia is the progressive and irreversible deterioration of intellectual faculties due to lesions in the brain. Some forms of dementia are the consequence of a clearly identified disease, such as cerebrovascular accident or syphilis, while others, such as Alzheimer's, are due to a **degeneration** of neurons, the cause of which is unknown. Dementia is characterized by various problems that in the long term lead to a loss of autonomy of the afflicted individual.

ALZHEIMER'S DISEASE

Alzheimer's disease is the primary cause of dementia in Western countries. It affects approximately 5% of the population over 65 years of age and 10% to 20% of people in their eighties. It is a degenerative neurological disease characterized by a decrease in the number of neurons in the brain and by cerebral atrophy, which inevitably leads to dementia. The patient suffers from cognitive problems (aphasia, problems with memory, organization, recognizing people and things, etc.) and behavior disorders (aggressiveness, delirium, anorexia, etc.). These troubles increase progressively, over several years, until the patient is no longer capable of completing the slightest activity alone. The causes of Alzheimer's disease are not yet established, but several elements could represent a risk factor, including age, family history, obesity, smoking, and environmental factors (exposure to heavy metals).

APHASIA

Aphasia is the difficulty of expression and comprehension of written or spoken language, which results from a cerebral lesion. It may first occur with difficulty in finding one's words. Later, the patient may totally lose the signifiance of words and become mute.

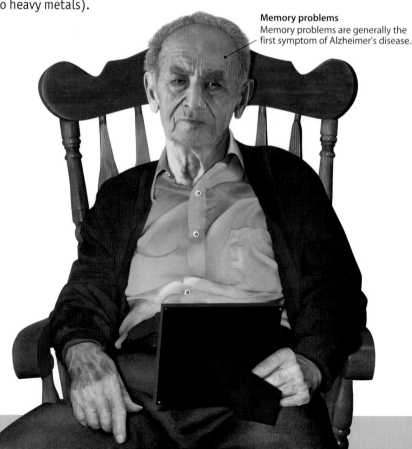

Memory problems
Memory problems are generally the first symptom of Alzheimer's disease.

VASCULAR DEMENTIA

Vascular dementia is caused by the repetition of cerebrovascular accidents. It is the second greatest cause of dementia in Western countries, after Alzheimer's disease. Vascular dementia evolves in stages, with periods of stability, and is often characterized by mood problems such as hyperemotivity and apathy.

Cerebrovascular accidents...page 156

PRECURSORS TO ALZHEIMER'S DISEASE

It is normal to have isolated and remediable losses of memory, particularly when aging. Also, the symptoms associated with Alzheimer's disease can be present in anyone. Nevertheless, they multiply and are emphasized when someone has the disease. Pay attention to precursors and consult a specialist if you have the slightest doubt. The earlier the diagnosis, the more effective treatment can be in slowing the development of the disease.

Precursors:

- Memory problems: forgetfulness or difficulty retaining events or recent information, difficulty recognizing people, loss of distant memories.

- Difficulty completing familiar tasks: preparing a meal, taking medication, etc.

- Language problems: difficulty expressing oneself, tendency to search for words and replace them with other inadequate words.

- Difficulty establishing a schedule.

- Progressive loss of sense of direction in space and time.

- Loss of judgment, adoption of behavior that is unadapted to a situation.

- Difficulty assimilating abstract notions such as calculations, numbers, etc.

- Tendency to misplace objects and place them in inappropriate places.

- Mood or behavioral changes that are very sudden or without any apparent reason.

- Change in personality: confusion, suspicion, apathy, etc.

- Particular lack of enthusiasm.

ALZHEIMER'S DISEASE AND OTHER FORMS OF DEMENTIA

SYMPTOMS:
Cognitive problems (memory, language, reasoning, attention), behavior disorders (confusion, agitation, apathy, aggressiveness, anxiety, eating disorders, wandering, hallucinations, compulsions, hyperemotivity, etc.), sleeping problems, depression.

TREATMENT:
Most forms of dementia are incurable. Some symptoms can be reduced (anxiety, depression, sleeping problems) and there are treatments that can slow the development of the disease.

PREVENTION:
Vascular dementia: prevention of cerebrovascular accidents.

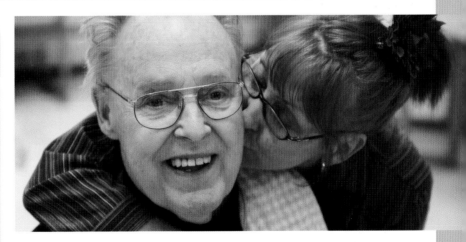

HOW TO HANDLE ALZHEIMER'S DISEASE

There is no treatment for Alzheimer's disease. Only some medication and approaches such as relaxation techniques can limit certain symptoms and improve the quality of life of patients. It is important to offer support to afflicted individuals, visit them regularly, and communicate with them and make their daily environment safe so as to avoid accidents and infections. Providing a reminder and creating a stable, calm, and ritualized life can also combat Alzheimer's disease. The regular practice of physical activity can also be beneficial: it provides an objective, maintains physical abilities, and has a calming effect on people while stimulating their brains.

PSYCHOSIS

A person suffering from psychosis presents a disorganized personality as well as problems with perception, judgment, reasoning, and behavior of which they are not aware. Psychotic episodes can be interspersed with lucid periods. Psychosis groups together several mental diseases, including schizophrenia and paranoia. They are presumably caused by several factors: malfunctioning of neurotransmitters in the brain, **genetic** factors, hypersensitivity to stress, etc. The first symptoms generally appear between 16 and 30 years of age. Some psychotic individuals can be dangerous to themselves and others.

SCHIZOPHRENIA

Schizophrenia is a form of psychosis that manifests itself by a withdrawal into oneself, incoherent thoughts, and contradictory feelings (great ambivalence). It results in various symptoms: delirium, hallucinations (often auditory), disorganized thought, catatonia, apathy, unmotivated laughter, soliloquy (talking to oneself), etc. These symptoms are often accompanied by anxiety and depression. Schizophrenia affects 1% of the population and is characterized by alternating periods of remission and relapses.

CATATONIA

Catatonia is characterized by different symptoms: immobility, absence of reaction to external stimulations, or, on the contrary, automatic obedience, repetition of words or phrases, or refusal to speak or eat. In the case of schizophrenia, it can manifest itself through the maintenance of an unusual and uncomfortable position for a very long duration.

PARANOIA

Paranoia is a psychosis characterized by a systemized and generally well-constructed delirium (development of false conclusions from real events). Paranoid delirium can take several forms: delirium of interpretation (everything takes a personal significance), delirium of persecution, delirium of claims, jealousy, illusion of being loved by others. Paranoia generally begins between 30 and 45 years of age in a person with a personality that has a paranoid tendency (suspicion, pride, overestimation of self, sensitivity, false judgment, inflexibility). Aggressive reactions can be frequent and violent; hospitalization is sometimes necessary.

DELIRIUM

Delirium is the loss of a sense of reality and results in false and unshakable convictions. The afflicted individual can, for example, feel persecuted, have the impression of being manipulated by an external force, or have excessive ambition. Delirium can be sudden and unexpected or develop progressively. It is more or less coherent and can be transitory or irreversible. Delirium manifests itself in a number of mental problems.

PSYCHOSIS

SYMPTOMS:
Problems with perception, judgment, reasoning, and behavior.

TREATMENT:
The treatment of psychoses combines psychotherapy and medications (antipsychotics, lithium).

NEUROSIS

People suffering from neurosis have abnormal behavior of which they are conscious, but they cannot change. This psychological disorder, due to an imbalance in the release of neurotransmitters, disturbs affective life without compromising intellectual faculties. Contrary to psychosis, there is no loss of contact with reality. Neurosis is specific to each afflicted individual, but there are characteristic symptoms allowing its diagnosis: relational difficulties, anxiety, sense of ill-being, compulsions, obsessions, phobias, sexual disorders, etc. Certain forms of neurosis constitute a severe social handicap and can cause depression, even suicide.

Neurons... page 136
Depression and other affective disorders... page 179

OBSESSIVE COMPULSIVE DISORDER

Obsessive compulsive disorder (OCD), or obsessional neurosis, is a neurosis characterized by the presence of obsessions and compulsions. These symptoms exert a strong constraint on afflicted individuals, who dedicate a lot of energy to them. They recognize the absurd nature of their behavior, but cannot change it. OCD generally begins during adolescence and is frequently associated with other mental disorders such as depression, phobias, anorexia, schizophrenia, or affective dependence.

OBSESSION

Obsession is an intrusive thought that imposes on the mind in a repetitive, persistent, and irrational manner. It generally results from a fear finding its origin in a past experience. There are numerous types of obsessions: error obsession (fear of forgetting something, getting something wrong), misfortune obsession (superstition), soil obsession (getting dirty), etc. Generating from anxiety, obsessions can hinder intellectual tasks and influence professional, social and family activities. The afflicted individual fights them through compulsive behaviors.

COMPULSION

Compulsion is a ritualistic behavior or mental act (repetition of formulas) that afflicted individuals cannot stop from accomplishing, under penalty of feeling an intolerable anguish and guilt. Compulsions are a response to obsessions. They have the objective of preventing or reducing anxiety; afflicted individuals feel that these actions allow them to avoid a feared situation. There are numerous types of compulsions: washing, verification, eating disorders such as bulimia and anorexia, uncontrollable and excessive shopping, stealing, repetition of mathematical formulas, etc. Some individuals pull out locks of hair while others bite their nails.

Eating disorders... page 527

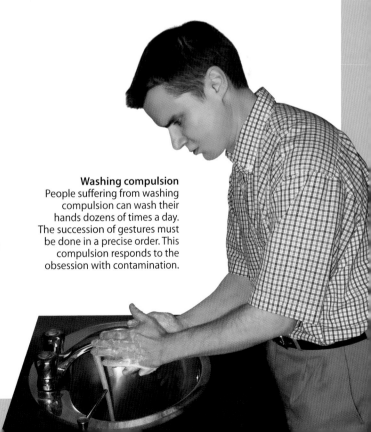

Washing compulsion
People suffering from washing compulsion can wash their hands dozens of times a day. The succession of gestures must be done in a precise order. This compulsion responds to the obsession with contamination.

The nervous system | Diseases

GENERALIZED ANXIETY DISORDER

Generalized anxiety disorder, or anguish neurosis, is a form of neurosis characterized by permanent anxiety (constant worry and alarm, preparation for the worst). In addition, sometimes there can be sudden attacks, during which the afflicted individual has the impression of becoming crazy or dying and presents physical symptoms: intestinal spasms, acceleration of heart rate, sweating, sensation of oppression, tremors, drying of mucous membranes. Generalized anxiety disorder most often affects women and young adults.

PHOBIAS AND PHOBIC NEUROSIS

A phobia is an intense fear triggered by an object or situation which is not, objectively, dangerous in itself. There are several types: phobias related to space (agoraphobia, claustrophobia), social phobias (fear of situations in which one is observed or judged), specific phobias such as a fear of certain animals, transportation, natural elements, blood, certain situations, etc. A phobia is a symptom of numerous psychiatric diseases and is the dominant symptom of phobic neurosis. Afflicted individuals experience a paralyzing, uncontrollable, and incoercible fear facing the object of the phobic situation. In a constant state of alarm, they devise ways to avoid being in contact with the object of their phobia. They can also use fetish objects that, by their presence, allow them to reduce their anxiety and confront the phobic situation.

THE MOST COMMON PHOBIAS

The most common phobias are social phobias and those related to spaces: fear of speaking or blushing in public (ereutophobia), fear of empty or extended spaces and crowds (agoraphobia), fear of enclosed spaces (claustrophobia). Other specific phobias are also widespread, such as the fear of spiders (arachnophobia), dogs (cynophobia), snakes (ophiophobia), water (aquaphobia), strangers (xenophobia), flying (pteromerhanophobia or aviophobia), heights (acrophobia), etc.

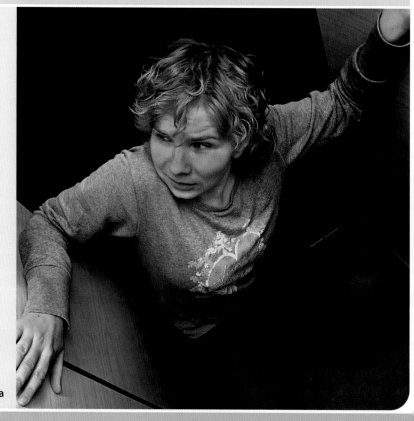

Claustrophobia

PSYCHOTHERAPY

Psychotherapy is a non-medicated technique used to treat mental disorders. There are many types, such as psychoanalysis, behavioral therapy and cognitive therapy. It is common that, in practice, several approaches are combined by psychotherapists.

COGNITIVE AND BEHAVIORAL THERAPY

In behavioral therapy, patients must detect and then abandon their psychopathological behavior by replacing it with a more adapted behavior, allowing them to adequately function in society. This technique is notably used in the case of phobias, obsessive compulsive disorders, depression, and sexual disorders. Cognitive therapy aims to first recognize the erroneous psychological mechanisms resulting in irrational beliefs, such as drawing false conclusions, exaggerating failures, self attribution of responsibility for independent events, etc. It then consists of correcting these ways of thinking and acting, particularly by practical exercises.

PSYCHOANALYSIS

Psychoanalysis aims to discover the unconscious significance of psychological phenomena at the origin of a neurosis. Once brought to the consciousness, these phenomena stop having an effect. The main technique consists in analyzing comments freely expressed by patients as well as their dreams and by proposing an interpretation. This work can only be accomplished by a practitioner (psychoanalyst) having themselves undergone psychoanalysis. To be deemed a success, psychoanalysis necessitates the total engagement of the patient for a long duration.

NEUROSIS

SYMPTOMS:
Very variable depending on the type of neurosis and the individual: obsession, compulsion, phobia, anxiety, sexual disorders, relational difficulties, etc.

TREATMENT:
Combination of medication (anxiolytics, antidepressants) and psychotherapy.

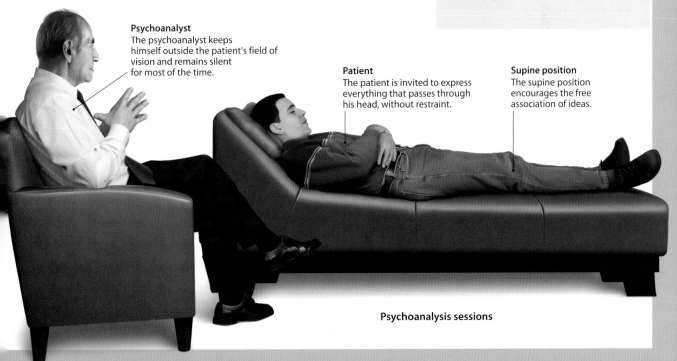

Psychoanalyst
The psychoanalyst keeps himself outside the patient's field of vision and remains silent for most of the time.

Patient
The patient is invited to express everything that passes through his head, without restraint.

Supine position
The supine position encourages the free association of ideas.

Psychoanalysis sessions

SLEEP DISORDERS

Sleep disorders are common and affect all age groups. They can have several forms: insomnia, excess sleep, narcolepsy, sleepwalking, bruxism (teeth grinding), involuntary urinating (enuresis), night terrors, etc. These disorders generally have significant repercussions on academic, professional, family, or affective life and can cause drowsiness during the day, causing accidents. Sleep disorders can often be symptoms of a physical or psychological disturbance (stress, anxiety, mental disease). They can also be linked to an inadequate sleep environment (temperature, noise, etc.) or an unhealthy lifestyle: irregular sleep hours, consumption of stimulants in the evening.

Stress control... page 28

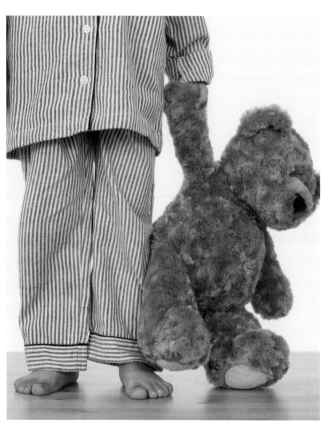

SLEEPWALKING

A person suffering from sleepwalking unconsciously sleepwalks during the night, without having any memory of it. This sleep disorder mainly affects children and generally disappears during adolescence. Of neurological origin, it occurs during deep sleep and does not last more than 30 minutes. Sleepwalking can have several causes: genetic predisposition, stress, lack of sleep, migraine, diseases (Tourette's syndrome, epilepsy), or consumption of alcohol, drugs, or psychotropic medication (in adults), etc. If necessary, sleepwalking is treated by taking benzodiazepines or by hypnosis.

Sleepwalker
With open eyes and an inexpressive look, sleepwalkers may be seated on their bed or walking around, talking, and making generally dexterous gestures. They have the tendency to become easily irritated and may display violent behavior. Their moving about may put them in danger. It is best to calmly lead them back to bed, without speaking to them, and ensure their safety if they are agitated (block access to stairs, remove any dangerous objects, etc.).

NIGHT TERRORS

Night terrors, a sleep disorder close to sleepwalking, can affect children until adolescence. It generally manifests itself at the beginning of the night by attacks that last a maximum of 20 minutes. The sleeping child seems to be awake and in a state of panic. He is red, sweating, his heart rate and breathing are accelerated, he yells, cries and struggles. The child does not recognize his parents and does not react to any attempts to calm him down. He falls asleep spontaneously and has no memory of the episode. Night terrors are not pathological. Their frequency can increase with the lack of sleep or with stress (move, divorce, etc.). In the case of an attack, it is advised to not wake the child, watch him to make sure he does not hurt himself, and do not speak of the event the next morning.

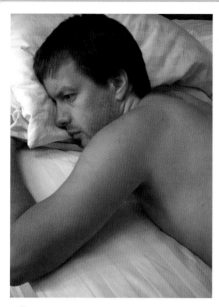

INSOMNIA

Insomnia is the difficulty falling asleep and having a satisfying quantity and quality of sleep. It can be caused by a disturbance in the biological rhythm (jet lag, night shift) or by an unhealthy lifestyle (consumption of stimulants, intense night activities). It can also be secondary to a psychological disorder such as stress, anxiety, depression, or psychosis. Finally, insomnia is sometimes the consequence of a physical disorder causing pain, fever, involuntary movements, or even respiratory problems (sleep apnea). The lack of sleep can cause fatigue, affective problems such as depression, deregulation of hormonal secretions, difficulty concentrating, and memory problems. Children who suffer from prolonged insomnia can develop a speech delay and psychomotor development delay.

PREVENTING INSOMNIA

■ ADOPT A REGULAR SLEEP SCHEDULE

Go to bed and get up at regular hours. If you cannot fall asleep after about 30 minutes, get up and do something relaxing such as reading.

■ SLEEP IN A HEALTHY ENVIRONMENT

Your room must be a place that is conducive to sleep. It must be orderly, quite cool (around 65°F [18°C]), isolated from noise and light, and devoid of electronic devices such as a television or computer. The mattress should be firm and your pajamas comfortable. Essential oils such as lavender promote sleep.

■ RELAX BEFORE GOING TO BED

Adopt a ritual for preparing for sleep by practicing relaxing activities such as listening to music, reading, or taking a bath. Empty your head.

■ PAY PARTICULAR ATTENTION TO YOUR EVENING MEAL

In the evening, your meal should contain less proteins and simple carbohydrates (sugared foods) and more complex carbohydrates (cereal, bread, pasta, rice, corn, legumes, potatoes). Balancing the level of sugar in the blood promotes sleep. In the evening, avoid consuming stimulants such as chocolate, tea, coffee, nicotine, and soda. Rather, drink milk with honey, or herbal tea with chamomile, lemon balm, or valerian.

■ EXERCISE

Regular physical activity promotes sleep due to its relaxing effect on the body. Physical exercise, however, must be practiced at least 3 hours before going to bed to avoid excessive agitation.

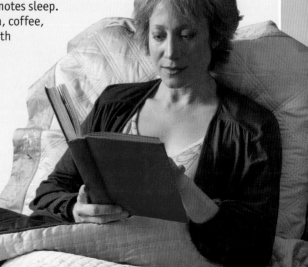

BED-WETTING

Bed-wetting, or enuresis, is characterized by involuntary urination while asleep. It affects young children and may, in some cases, continue through adolescence. Bed-wetting can occur after a period of several months of being dry and may have a variety of causes: heredity, immature bladder, hormonal disorders, affective disorders, urinary infection, diabetes, constipation, etc. To correct it, a doctor may suggest medication, bladder control exercises, behavioral therapy through motivation (rewards), or the installation of a nighttime alarm system that wakes the child upon urination.

NARCOLEPSY

Narcolepsy is a condition characterized by sudden sleeping fits during the day and drops in muscle tone (cataplexy). It affects men slightly more often than women and may start at any age, following an episode of major stress. On average, these sleeping fits last from a few minutes to just under an hour and are often accompanied by hallucinations when falling asleep or waking up. Daytime sleeping fits are separate from episodes of cataplexy.

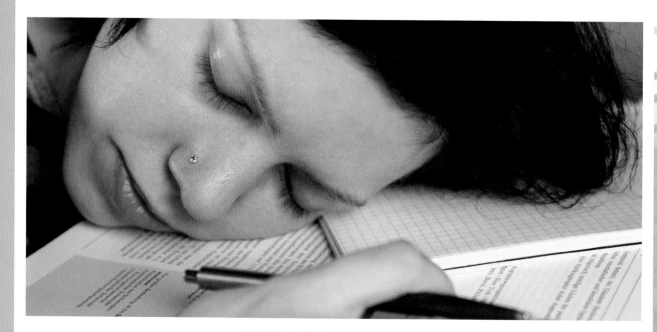

CATAPLEXY

Cataplexy is the sudden, more or less complete loss of muscle tone, without losing consciousness. It may be localized within one muscle group (neck, hands, etc.) or may affect the whole body. The person collapses to the ground but remains conscious. Cataplexy is generally caused by intense emotion.

SLEEP DISORDERS

SYMPTOMS:
Fatigue, mood disorders. Narcolepsy: daytime sleeping fits, cataplexy.

TREATMENTS:
Insomnia: treatment of the cause of the insomnia, sleeping pills.
Narcolepsy: medication, naps in the afternoon.

PREVENTION:
Insomnia: healthy lifestyle (relaxation exercises, regular sleep schedule, a sufficient dinner, restriction of stimulants, regular exercise), a sleep-conducive environment (silence, darkness, cool temperature).

DEPRESSION
AND OTHER AFFECTIVE DISORDERS

Affective disorders, or mood disorders, are psychological ailments characterized by changing or unstable moods, shifting towards either elation or despondency. They are usually accompanied by a change in the person's pace of activities. These disorders tend to be recurrent and related to stressful events. They notably include depression, bipolar affective disorder, seasonal affective disorder, and postpartum depression. Mood disorders can be a severe social handicap, leading to risky behavior, or even suicide.

BIPOLAR AFFECTIVE DISORDER

Bipolar affective disorder, or manic depression, is a mood disorder characterized by alternating periods of depression and mania. These periods may last from a few days to a few months. Sometimes, they can even alternate during a single day. For certain people, they are accompanied by hallucinations or delirium, particularly delusions of persecution or of grandeur (exaggerated feelings of physical strength, power, or wealth). Between episodes, the person may present no symptoms. Cyclothymia is a mild form of bipolar affective disorder, characterized by rapidly alternating phases of moderate elation and moderate despondency. In one-third of affected people, it may worsen, becoming a true bipolar disorder.

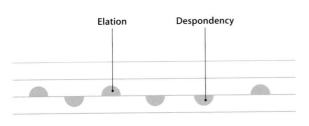

Normal mood fluctuations
People's moods normally undergo occasional fluctuations (elation or despondency) over time, depending on events in their lives.

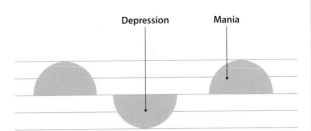

Bipolar affective disorder
In bipolar affective disorder, manic and depressive episodes alternate one after the other.

MANIA

Mania is a state of agitation, accompanied by constant psychomotor hyperexcitation. It is characterized by an overabundance of ideas and words (possibly to the point of incoherence), euphoria, a feeling of power, and exuberant—although usually ineffectual—activity. Some behaviors may pose a high risk of negative consequences, such as overconsumption (food, extravagant purchases, alcohol, drugs, etc.) or out-of-control sexuality. Mania is characteristic of bipolar affective disorders. It can also appear in the case of a neurological ailment (e.g. a tumor or head trauma) or an endocrine disease (e.g. hyperthyroidism).

SEASONAL AFFECTIVE DISORDER

Seasonal affective disorder, or seasonal depression, is a form of depression that typically starts in autumn or early winter and disappears in the spring. In addition to symptoms of depression, there may be a strong inclination to sleep and overeat, particularly sweets. This form of depression primarily affects women, who account for 75% of cases, and it is more common in the northern regions. It is believed to be caused by the lack of light associated with the winter season, and by a drop in the secretion of certain substances in the body (serotonin and melatonin). Its treatment is based on phototherapy, which involves exposure to an intense light source.

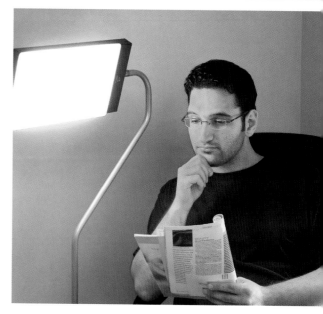

Phototherapy

DEPRESSION

Depression is a pathological mental condition characterized by a feeling of profound sorrow and despair, accompanied by emotional suffering and the inability to function normally in everyday life. Depression involves factors that may be hereditary, physiological (dysfunction of certain neurotransmitters), family-based, or environmental (unhealthy lifestyle, negative external events, job burnout, etc.). It should be differentiated from depressive reactions, which are states of temporary despondency arising as a response to certain events in life. Depression is a more and more common condition, currently affecting 5–8% of the populations of Western countries. It is expected to become the second leading cause of disability (after cardiovascular disease) by 2020.

ANTIDEPRESSANTS

Used to treat depression, antidepressants are drugs that act on the body's neurotransmitters. Within a few weeks, they can alleviate the symptoms of depression and provide the patient with renewed energy and positive thoughts. These medications are prescribed for several months, usually in combination with psychotherapy. Depending on the specific antidepressant, different side effects may be experienced: drowsiness, dizziness, blurred vision, dry mouth, shaking, change in the libido or sexual performance, digestive disturbances, weight gain, excessive perspiration, nightmares, etc. They must not be used in combination with alcohol, and their consumption must be tapered off gradually.

Neurons... page 136

DEPRESSION OR JOB BURNOUT?

The difference between depression and burnout can sometimes be difficult to discern. These two conditions are, in fact, very closely related and present a number of similar symptoms: fatigue, discouragement, difficulty concentrating, lack of efficiency at work, feeling of failure, etc. However, they are two separate disorders. Depression affects all spheres of one's life, and its source may be found in any of these areas. Job burnout is directly related to the stress of the workplace environment. In addition, most scientists agree that depression may follow after burnout, but that the opposite is not possible.

Burnout... page 182

SYMPTOMS OF DEPRESSION

Depression is expressed as a set of physical and psychological disorders. If you experience more than one of these symptoms at the same time, make an appointment with your doctor as soon as possible. He or she may prescribe antidepressants for you and may suggest that you undergo psychotherapy or participate in a support group.

The symptoms:

- Feelings of sorrow, discouragement and helplessness
- Self-depreciation and feeling of guilt
- Lack of enthusiasm and loss of interest in one's normal activities
- Thoughts of death or suicide
- Anxious, aggressive, highly emotional state, with crying
- Difficulty concentrating and making decisions

- Loss of appetite and weight loss
- Disturbed sleep and intense fatigue
- Headache, drop in libido, palpitations, vertigo

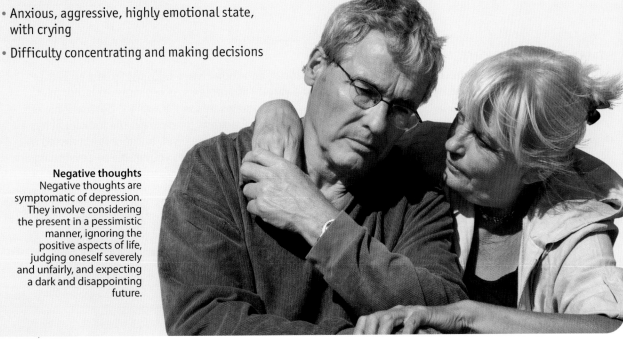

Negative thoughts
Negative thoughts are symptomatic of depression. They involve considering the present in a pessimistic manner, ignoring the positive aspects of life, judging oneself severely and unfairly, and expecting a dark and disappointing future.

SUICIDE

Mood disorders such as depression and bipolar affective disorder can lead afflicted individuals to take their lives voluntarily. Suicide is also a possible consequence of certain mental illnesses, such as schizophrenia. It is the expression of a desire to put an end to a situation considered to be intolerable. Suicide is the cause of 1 million deaths each year around the world, while the number of attempted suicides is 10–20 times higher. These attempts are considered to be cries for help. The risk of recurrence is high.

DEPRESSION AND OTHER AFFECTIVE DISORDERS

SYMPTOMS:
Despondency and negative thoughts (depression) or, on the contrary, extreme elation and euphoria (mania). Impaired sleep, appetite and sexuality, fatigue, anxiety, agitation.

TREATMENTS:
Combination of medication (antidepressants, neuroleptics) and psychotherapy.

BURNOUT

Burnout, or job burnout, is a form of physical, emotional, and mental exhaustion that arises in conditions of lasting, intense stress at work. It takes hold gradually and more or less quickens, depending on the individual's ability to withstand stress. The process starts with an enthusiastic, very energetic attitude, and very high goals as well as a high level of personal investment in the job. When the efforts made do not meet one's personal demands and those of one's employer, the individual doubles his or her efforts, but does not receive the expected recognition. Disillusionment and a strong feeling of frustration then follow, expressed as a loss of motivation and of prospects, as well as a multitude of negative sentiments. The afflicted person ends up being extremely discouraged, loses all interest in his or her work, family and friends, becomes aggressive, and is no longer able to work.

Stress control… page 28

SYMPTOMS OF BURNOUT

Burnout manifests itself through different physical, emotional, and cognitive symptoms. From a physical standpoint, it is characterized by continuous fatigue and a variety of problems, often stress-related: pain, gastrointestinal disturbances, persistent viral infections, skin problems, insomnia, weight fluctuations, etc. Emotionally, job burnout can cause a loss of motivation, frustration, anxiety, or despair. The individual has a negative attitude towards him or herself and towards others. At the cognitive level, burnout is expressed in particular as memory loss and difficulty concentrating. The person also becomes vulnerable to developing an addiction (alcohol, drugs, etc.). Just a few of these symptoms can serve as a warning and prompt a request for the aid of a health-care professional or a psychologist, in order to reassess personal and professional priorities, and to then take appropriate action.

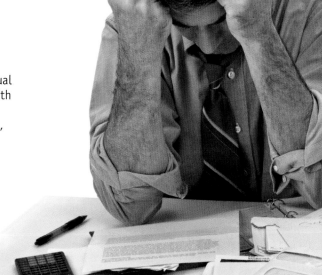

FACTORS THAT CONTRIBUTE TO JOB BURNOUT

Burnout can happen to any worker. It is the result of individual factors and work-related problems. Perfectionists, people with a high level of professional conscience or who are unable to delegate, along with introverts, people with low self-esteem, and the emotionally unstable are all at particular risk of burnout. At work, several factors can lead to burnout: intense stress, work overload, lack of independence, poorly-defined responsibilities, imbalance between the effort made and the recognition received (pay, esteem, respect, etc.).

PREVENTING BURNOUT

In a company, the prevention of burnout is the responsibility of both the employees and the employer. This can be achieved primarily by reducing stress factors.

◼ AS AN EMPLOYEE

- Surround yourself with supportive people and discuss your problems with friends and family.

- Watch out for stress-related symptoms, identify their causes, and find solutions.

- Do not let frustrations build up; discuss the organization of work with your colleagues and superiors, in order to define changes that would be helpful to you (more realistic and more gratifying objectives, list of priority tasks, etc.).

- Learn to say no to excessive tasks, and learn to delegate.

- Take your mind off things during lunch and for a few minutes each hour of work (music, stretching, meditation, etc.).

- Set hours during which you are available for work and stick to them, especially by cutting off means of communication (Internet, cellphone, etc.).

- Analyze your lifestyle and eliminate those habits that contribute to stress, such as the overconsumption of stimulants in food and drink (coffee, tea, sugar, chocolate, soft drinks, alcohol, tobacco, etc.).

- Exercise regularly.

- Take the time to enjoy life. Devote some time to recreation.

◼ AS AN EMPLOYER

- Define the roles and responsibilities of your employees clearly and fairly, show confidence in them, and include them in decision-making.

- Show your recognition with marks of appreciation: respect, encouragement, possibility of promotion, a pay raise, etc.

- Encourage communication and mutual aid, and settle conflicts quickly by discussing them openly.

- Do not create inequalities or too much competition between employees.

- Be available to listen, and pay attention.

- Create pleasant working conditions that are compatible with personal life: reasonable, flexible hours, well-organized workspaces, appropriate tools, childcare service, etc.

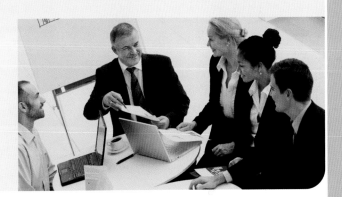

BURNOUT

SYMPTOMS:
Insomnia, hormone imbalances, persistent fatigue, stress-related physical ailments (back, muscle, head, and stomach pain, skin problems, hypertension). Emotional issues: discouragement and negative feelings (feeling of incompetence, guilt, impatience, distrust, aggressiveness, cynicism, etc.). Cognitive problems: difficulty concentrating and making judgments, inability to perform simple tasks, etc.

TREATMENTS:
Rest, and a change in work environment, lifestyle and philosophy. Consultation with a psychotherapist, potentially involving antidepressants or medical leave from work.

PREVENTION:
Detect early-warning signs and reduce stress factors at the workplace. Assert yourself, manage your stress and your time effectively, taking into account your limitations and needs. Clearly separate your professional life from your personal life.

DRUG ADDICTION

Drug addiction is the **chronic**, out-of-control use of substances that are potentially toxic to the body, such as alcohol, tobacco, drugs, and medications. These substances, used for their **psychotropic** effects (well-being, altered state of consciousness, hallucinations, disappearance of inhibitions, euphoria, stimulation, etc.), encourage the action of a neurotransmitter (dopamine) in the areas of the brain responsible for the emotions and for pleasure. The repeated stimulation of these areas leads more or less rapidly to addiction, depending on the individual, the type of substance, and the frequency of consumption. This dependence appears as abusive consumption that is harmful to the health.

Neurons... page 136

DOPAMINE

Dopamine is a neurotransmitter that plays a role in motor activities, learning, mood, alertness, behavior, management of certain emotions (such as desire, pleasure, and pain), etc. When released at the end of a neuron (at the synapse), it attaches to a specific receptor (the dopaminergic receptor) on another neuron, which causes a feeling of pleasure or a decreased sensitivity to pain. The dopamine is then either destroyed or recovered by the neuron that produced it. By stimulating the release of dopamine, decreasing its recovery, or reducing its degradation, certain substances (drugs and alcohol) disrupt this mechanism and are involved in the development of dependence.

DEPENDENCE

Dependence is a physical and psychological condition characterized by the regular, irrepressible desire to consume a drug. It is usually caused by the repeated use of substances that increase the quantity of dopamine in the system. An imbalance occurs, which can only be maintained by constant—and often increasing—consumption of the drug (habituation). Stopping this intake results in a withdrawal syndrome, a set of symptoms that vary based on the the drug consumed: aggressiveness, insomnia, anxiety, pain, hallucinations, etc.

Nicotine addiction... page 338
Alcoholism... page 358

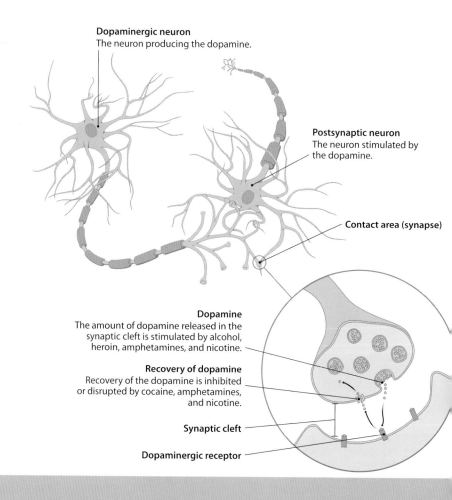

Dopaminergic neuron
The neuron producing the dopamine.

Postsynaptic neuron
The neuron stimulated by the dopamine.

Contact area (synapse)

Dopamine
The amount of dopamine released in the synaptic cleft is stimulated by alcohol, heroin, amphetamines, and nicotine.

Recovery of dopamine
Recovery of the dopamine is inhibited or disrupted by cocaine, amphetamines, and nicotine.

Synaptic cleft

Dopaminergic receptor

DRUGS

A drug is a natural or artificial chemical substance that changes the brain's activity and produces a psychotropic effect. There are many types, which are differentiated by their chemical composition, their mechanism of action, their method of administration, and their effects: alcohol, nicotine, heroin, cocaine, amphetamines, cannabis, benzodiazepines, LSD, etc.

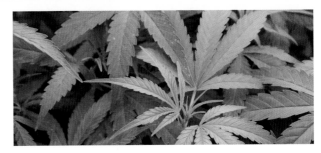

Cannabis

COCAINE

Cocaine is a drug extracted from coca, a plant native to South America. It comes in the form of a whitish powder, usually mixed with other substances. It can be inhaled through the nose, smoked, or injected intravenously. Cocaine produces a sense of euphoria, a feeling of power, and indifference to pain, fatigue, and hunger. It also causes vasoconstriction, arrhythmia and, in some cases, psychological disturbances (delusions, panic). Cocaine, like crack (a derivative), quickly instills a strong level of dependence, and overdosing on either can be fatal.

CANNABIS

Cannabis, or Indian hemp, is a plant consumed by inhaling the smoke from burning its leaves and dried female buds (marijuana) or its resin (hashish). At low doses, it causes euphoria and peacefulness, followed by drowsiness. Higher doses can lead to impaired speech and motor coordination, anxiety, dry mouth, an accelerated heart rhythm, and, sometimes, vomiting.

AMPHETAMINES

Amphetamines are synthetic chemical compounds. The many derivatives are used, in tablets or capsules, as medications (for attention disorders, narcolepsy, asthenia, and obesity) or as drugs (speed and ecstasy). Amphetamines cause increased endurance, reduced fatigue and hunger, a feeling of power, euphoria, and the disappearance of inhibitions. At high doses, amphetamines can produce hallucinations or a severe depressive state and can lead to death.

HEROIN

Heroin is a drug obtained from morphine, a plant substance extracted from the poppy. It comes in the form of a brown or white powder, most often injected intravenously after having been diluted and heated. The fast-acting, powerful psychotropic effects (euphoria, feeling of ecstasy, relaxation, and peacefulness) is accompanied by physical effects: hypothermia, nausea, vertigo, slowed heart rhythm, and shallower breathing. Heroin dependence is strong and can set in rapidly. Habituation can lead to overdosing and to death by respiratory arrest.

BENZODIAZEPINES

Benzodiazepines are medications used to reduce anxiety or to treat sleep disorders. They can produce a number of side effects: memory impairment, confusion, reduced alertness, and reduced muscle tone. The consumption of benzodiazepines causes dependence, more or less quickly, and a withdrawal syndrome in the case of sudden stoppage.

DRUG ADDICTION

SYMPTOMS:
Euphoria, depressive condition, confusion, memory impairment, indifference to pain, to fatigue and to hunger, disappearance of inhibitions, hallucinations, arrhythmia, nausea, hypothermia, vertigo, increased endurance, and decreased muscle tone.

TREATMENTS:
Withdrawal by stopping consumption and temporarily administering replacement medications. Psychological support.

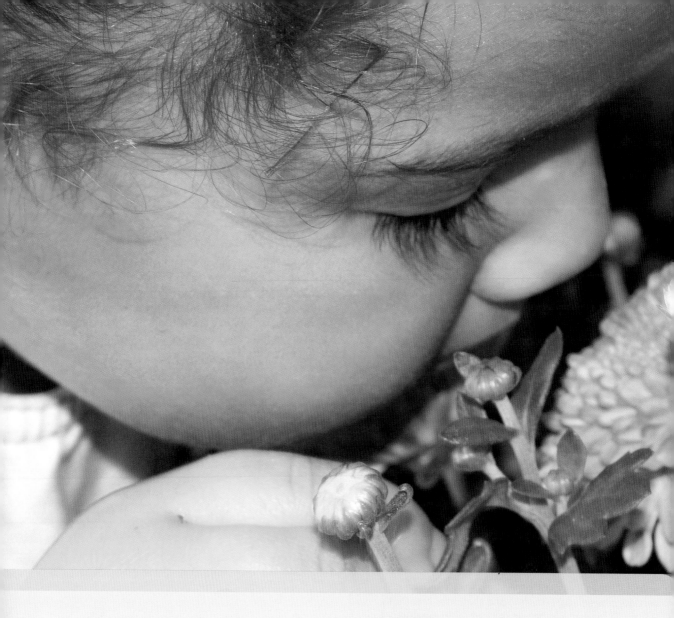

THE BODY

THE **SENSES**

The senses allow the nervous system to perceive and analyze the outside world. Sight, hearing, touch, smell, and taste make it possible to analyze the physical and chemical stimuli emanating from our environment: light, sound, pressure, temperature, odorous, and gustatory molecules, which can be smelled and tasted, etc.

Sight is our most highly developed sense, but also our most fragile one. Its deterioration is primarily the result of aging, which reduces visual acuity (presbyopia, cataracts, etc.). Other disorders like myopia (nearsightedness), color blindness, and conjunctivitis are the result of malformations of the eye, **genetic** diseases, and **infections.** Deafness and hearing problems, which are also common, often stem from **inflammation** of the ear (otitis), hereditary problems, and acoustic **trauma**, especially exposure to overly loud noise. Anomalies in smell, taste, and touch are less frequent and fewer in number.

THE **SENSORY ORGANS**

The sensory organs capture the physical and chemical signals from our environment. These signals are transformed into nerve impulses by specialized tissues: touch receptors for touch, the retinas for sight, the cochleae for hearing, the taste buds for taste, and the olfactory cells for smell. The nerve impulses are then analyzed in the zones of the brain specific to each sense. Injury of a sensory organ can seriously affect its operation.

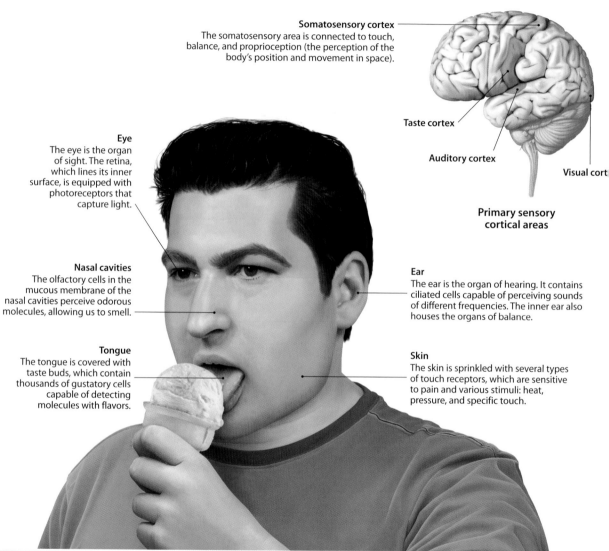

Somatosensory cortex
The somatosensory area is connected to touch, balance, and proprioception (the perception of the body's position and movement in space).

Taste cortex

Auditory cortex

Visual cort

Primary sensory cortical areas

Eye
The eye is the organ of sight. The retina, which lines its inner surface, is equipped with photoreceptors that capture light.

Nasal cavities
The olfactory cells in the mucous membrane of the nasal cavities perceive odorous molecules, allowing us to smell.

Tongue
The tongue is covered with taste buds, which contain thousands of gustatory cells capable of detecting molecules with flavors.

Ear
The ear is the organ of hearing. It contains ciliated cells capable of perceiving sounds of different frequencies. The inner ear also houses the organs of balance.

Skin
The skin is sprinkled with several types of touch receptors, which are sensitive to pain and various stimuli: heat, pressure, and specific touch.

THE SENSES ON ALERT

The sensory organs of human beings are relatively well-developed. The eye can distinguish an object measuring ½ inch (1 cm) at a distance of 130 feet (40 m). The ear can detect close to 400,000 sounds. The nose can perceive up to 10,000 odors, although the human sense of smell remains limited, especially when compared to that of a number of other living beings. For example, a dog's sense of smell is thought to be thousands of times more sensitive than ours, allowing it to sense pheromones from miles away.

SIGHT

Colors, shapes, distances, and the speed of objects are perceived thanks to sight (or vision), the most developed sense in human beings. The eye captures light via the photoreceptors in the retina. These cells, on the inner surface of the eye, transform light into nerve impulses, which are carried by the optical nerves to the brain. This mechanism is extremely fragile. Even tiny eye deformations and lesions can lead to visual impairment.

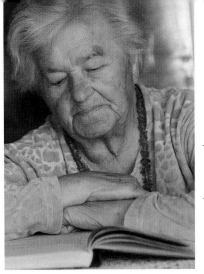

THE **VISIBLE PART** OF THE **EYE**

The visible part of the eye is composed of the pupil, the iris, and the conjunctiva. It is protected by the eyelids, the eyelashes, the eyebrows, and tears.

THE EYELIDS

The eyelids are thin folds of skin that cover and protect the surface of the eye. They also maintain the eye's hydration, by spreading tears across its surface. The upper eyelid is larger and more mobile than the lower eyelid.

Eyelashes
The eyelashes prevent foreign bodies from coming into contact with the eye. Their hair follicles have highly sensitive nerve endings that, when stimulated, cause the eyelids to close.

Lower eyelid

Pupil

Eyebrow
The eyebrow protects the eye from light and sweat.

Upper eyelid

Conjunctiva

Iris
The color of the iris is a hereditary feature.
Heredity... page 50

TEARS

Tears are a liquid secreted by glands attached to the eyeball, the lachrymal glands and the Meibomian glands. Spread by the blinking of the eyelids, they play a protective, lubricating, and cleansing role at the surface of the eye. Tears are evacuated towards the nasal cavities via the lachrymal canal.

Lachrymal gland
The lachrymal gland sits within the eye socket, above the eye.

Meibomian gland
The Meibomian gland is located in the epidermis, on the edge of the eyelid.

Tears
Tears contain **antiseptic** molecules that protect the eye against **infection**.

Lachrymal canal
The lachrymal canal is the conduit by which the tears are evacuated towards the nasal cavities.

IN THE BLINK OF AN EYE

Blinking the eyelids occurs very frequently. On average, we blink our eyes 5,400 times a day, equivalent to a total of around 30 minutes with our eyes shut.

THE **EYE**

The eye, or eyeball, is a sphere 1 inch (2.5 cm) in diameter set in the eye socket. It is formed of multiple layers of tissues surrounding a transparent, gelatinous substance called the vitreous body.

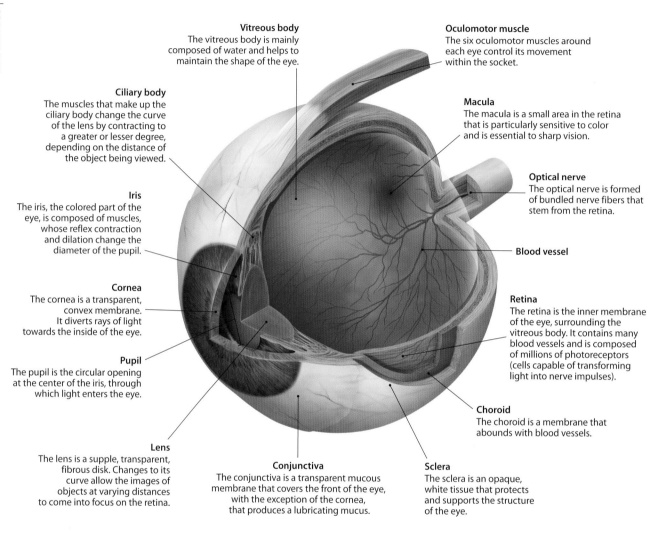

Vitreous body
The vitreous body is mainly composed of water and helps to maintain the shape of the eye.

Oculomotor muscle
The six oculomotor muscles around each eye control its movement within the socket.

Ciliary body
The muscles that make up the ciliary body change the curve of the lens by contracting to a greater or lesser degree, depending on the distance of the object being viewed.

Macula
The macula is a small area in the retina that is particularly sensitive to color and is essential to sharp vision.

Iris
The iris, the colored part of the eye, is composed of muscles, whose reflex contraction and dilation change the diameter of the pupil.

Optical nerve
The optical nerve is formed of bundled nerve fibers that stem from the retina.

Blood vessel

Cornea
The cornea is a transparent, convex membrane. It diverts rays of light towards the inside of the eye.

Retina
The retina is the inner membrane of the eye, surrounding the vitreous body. It contains many blood vessels and is composed of millions of photoreceptors (cells capable of transforming light into nerve impulses).

Pupil
The pupil is the circular opening at the center of the iris, through which light enters the eye.

Choroid
The choroid is a membrane that abounds with blood vessels.

Lens
The lens is a supple, transparent, fibrous disk. Changes to its curve allow the images of objects at varying distances to come into focus on the retina.

Conjunctiva
The conjunctiva is a transparent mucous membrane that covers the front of the eye, with the exception of the cornea, that produces a lubricating mucus.

Sclera
The sclera is an opaque, white tissue that protects and supports the structure of the eye.

THE PUPIL

The contraction and dilation of the smooth muscles of the iris increase or reduce the diameter of the pupil, thus regulating the amount of light entering the eye. This mechanism optimizes visual perception, based on light levels in the environment.

The muscles... page 98

Low light
When there is not much light, the diameter of the pupil expands.

Bright light
When there is a lot of light, the diameter of the pupil shrinks.

THE **MECHANISM** OF **SIGHT**

The mechanism of sight involves several steps. The eye's lenses (the cornea and the lens) deflect the image of the viewed object, so as to project a clear image of it onto the retina. The photoreceptors in the retina then transform the light signal into a nerve impulse, which is carried to the brain by the optical nerve. The visual cortex (the region of the brain involved in sight) then analyzes the nerve impulses, allowing us to perceive the shape, color, depth, distance, and movement of objects.

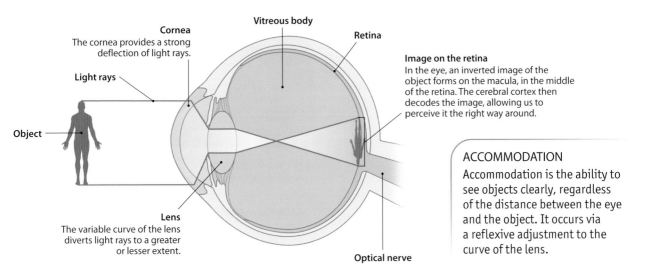

Cornea
The cornea provides a strong deflection of light rays.

Vitreous body

Retina

Light rays

Image on the retina
In the eye, an inverted image of the object forms on the macula, in the middle of the retina. The cerebral cortex then decodes the image, allowing us to perceive it the right way around.

Object

Lens
The variable curve of the lens diverts light rays to a greater or lesser extent.

Optical nerve

ACCOMMODATION
Accommodation is the ability to see objects clearly, regardless of the distance between the eye and the object. It occurs via a reflexive adjustment to the curve of the lens.

STEREOSCOPIC VISION

Stereoscopic vision is the ability to perceive three-dimensional objects, that is, to grasp the depth and contours of the visual environment. This is possible thanks to the perception of two slightly different images by the two eyes, and their combination into a single image by the brain.

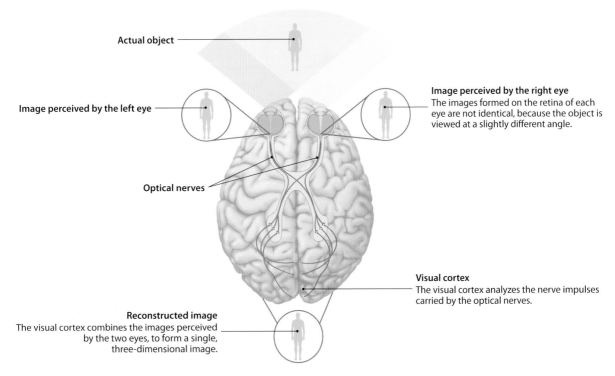

Actual object

Image perceived by the left eye

Image perceived by the right eye
The images formed on the retina of each eye are not identical, because the object is viewed at a slightly different angle.

Optical nerves

Visual cortex
The visual cortex analyzes the nerve impulses carried by the optical nerves.

Reconstructed image
The visual cortex combines the images perceived by the two eyes, to form a single, three-dimensional image.

PREVENTING VISION PROBLEMS AND DISORDERS

■ **PAY ATTENTION TO WARNING SIGNS AND HAVE REGULAR SCREENINGS**

If you experience impaired vision, such as blurred vision, the appearance of spots in your visual field, or a change in your perception of colors, consult an ophthalmologist. After the age of 40, most people's sight deteriorates due to the aging process. As a result, it is strongly advised that you have your eyesight examined every other year and, if necessary, to correct your sight by means of glasses or contact lenses. Preventive examinations are also recommended for young children, because visual impairment can lead to developmental lags.

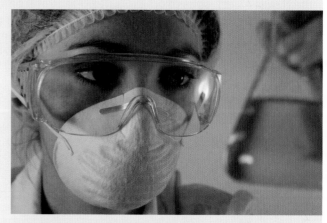

■ **AVOID EXPOSURE TO OVERLY BRIGHT LIGHT**

Solar rays and certain other sources of intense light can cause ocular lesions. Protect your eyes, particularly by wearing tinted UV-blocking lenses and a hat with a visor.

■ **AVOID SMOKING**

Smoking can cause vascular accidents and contribute to macular degeneration and cataracts.

■ **HANDLE HAZARDOUS PRODUCTS WITH CARE AND WEAR PROTECTIVE GOGGLES**

If you handle chemicals or perform manual labor like carpentry or welding, wear protective goggles. Chemical substances or foreign bodies that come into contact with your eyes can lead to serious injury and impair your vision. In the case of an accident, see a doctor quickly.

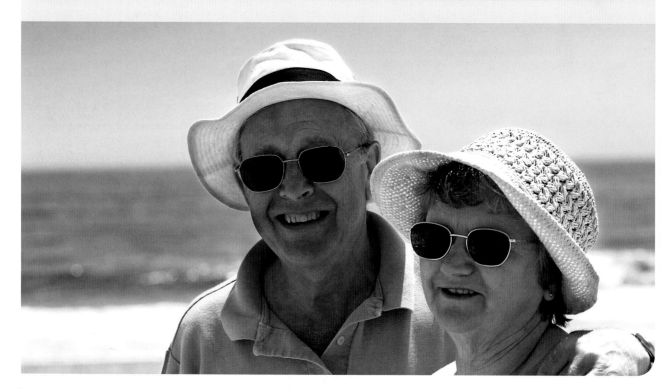

EYE EXAMINATIONS

There are several types of examinations that test the different aspects of the eye's functions. These tests are used to detect visual impairments and eye diseases and to monitor their development.

THE VISUAL FIELD

The visual field is the extent of space that the eye can perceive when at rest. The visual field can be evaluated using simple vision tests that require little equipment, like the Amsler grid, or by means of techniques that need more complex instruments, such as the Goldmann perimeter. The Goldmann perimeter is a device that can establish a precise graph of the field of vision and highlight any gaps (scotomas) or shrinking of the visual field.

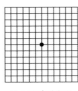 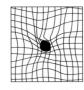

Normal vision   **Defective vision**

Amsler grid

The Amsler grid is a test used to detect any anomalies in the central part of the visual field. The test, which can easily be performed at home, consists in focusing on the central point in a grid and then drawing any anomalies observed with each eye. This exam can reveal blind spots (areas on the retina that are not sensitive to light stimulation) and distortions, particularly in the case of age-related macular degeneration.

OPHTHALMOSCOPY

Ophthalmoscopy (examination of the inside of the eyeball) can detect damage to the retina or the choroid, along with any anomalies in its vascularization. The inspection is performed using an optical device, the ophthalmoscope, after dilating the pupils using special drops (mydriatics). The examination lasts a few minutes and may cause blurred vision for a few hours afterward. Retinal angiography is a medical imaging technique used to examine the blood vessels in the retina and the choroid, by making them visible by means of an intravenous injection of fluorescent dye (the effects of which wear off after a few hours).

VISUAL ACUITY

The smaller or the further away an object is, the more difficult it is for the eye to distinguish it. The eye's ability to distinguish objects in its visual field is called visual acuity. It can be measured based on the distance of an object (e.g. using the Snellen chart).

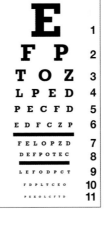

Snellen chart

The Snellen chart is composed of high-contrast letters of decreasing size, laid out on several lines. The lowest line that a person, placed at a certain distance from the chart, can read corresponds to his or her level of visual acuity. This test can reveal a number of visual impairments, such as myopia (nearsightedness).

Ophthalmoscope

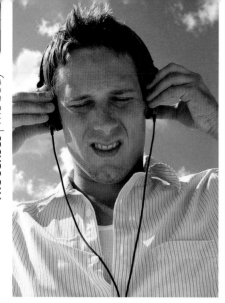

HEARING AND BALANCE

Hearing is the perception of sound by the ears and its interpretation by the brain. The structures of the outer ear capture sound vibrations and direct them towards the middle ear. The middle ear amplifies the vibrations and transmits them to the sensory organs in the inner ear, which detect the frequency and intensity of the sound. The ear is also home to the balance organs, which perceive the movement of the head and its position in space.

THE EAR

The ear has three parts: the outer ear, the middle ear, and the inner ear. The outer ear is composed of the pinna and the external auditory meatus (ear canal). The middle ear, set into the temporal bone, contains the three ossicles and is separated from the external auditory meatus by the eardrum. The inner ear, also set in the temporal bone, holds the sensory organs for hearing (cochlea) and balance (semicircular canals and vestibule).

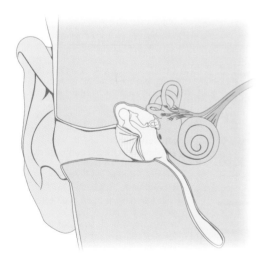

Outer ear

Middle ear

Inner ear

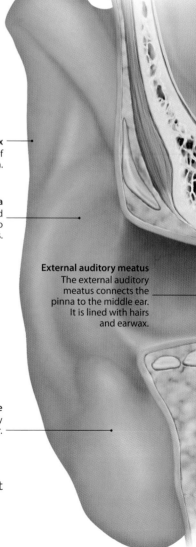

Helix
The helix is the rim of the ear's pinna.

Pinna
The pinna captures sound vibrations and directs them to the external auditory meatus.

External auditory meatus
The external auditory meatus connects the pinna to the middle ear. It is lined with hairs and earwax.

Earlobe
The earlobe is the fleshy extremity of the outer ear.

EARWAX

Earwax, or cerumen, is the yellowish, oily substance secreted by the sebaceous glands in the external auditory meatus. It provides lubrication and protection against infectious agents and foreign bodies. Earwax can accumulate inside the ear, forming a plug that can cause irritation or even lead to hearing loss.

TINY BONES

At just a few millimeters long, the ossicles are the smallest bones in the human body.

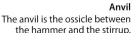

Stirrup
The stirrup is the ossicle in contact with the inner ear.

Anvil
The anvil is the ossicle between the hammer and the stirrup.

Hammer
The hammer is the ossicle in contact with the eardrum.

Semicircular canals
The semicircular canals are bony conduits filled with fluid and arranged according to the three dimensions of space. They control balance while the head is in motion.

Ossicles
The ossicles are three small bones located inside the middle ear cavity. They are responsible for amplifying sound vibrations.

Auditory nerve

Vestibular nerve
The vestibular nerve is the branch of the auditory nerve responsible for balance. It carries messages to the central nervous system from the semicircular canals and the vestibule.

Cochlear nerve
The cochlear nerve is the branch of the auditory nerve responsible for hearing. It carries nerve impulses from the cochlea to the brain.

Temporal bone

Cochlea
The cochlea is a spiraled tube of bone filled with fluid. It contains the sensory receptors for hearing.

Vestibule
The vestibule is a bony chamber filled with fluid. Responsible for the perception of static equilibrium (balance at rest), it informs the central nervous system of the head's position in space.

Eustachian tube
The eustachian tube is a narrow canal that connects the middle ear to the pharynx (the section of the alimentary canal located in the upper part of the throat). It serves to balance the pressure on either side of the eardrum.

Eardrum
The eardrum is a thin, elastic membrane that closes off entry to the middle ear. It carries sound vibrations from the external auditory meatus to the ossicles.

Tympanic cavity
The tympanic cavity is the cavity of the middle ear.

THE **HEARING MECHANISM**

Sounds travel through the air in the form of vibrations in the molecules of the air. These vibrations are captured by the pinna (the outer ear), which directs them towards the external auditory meatus (ear canal), where they cause the eardrum to vibrate. The three ossicles amplify the vibrations in the eardrum and transmit them to the cochlea, which transforms them into nerve signals. Sound vibrations are also conducted by the bones of the skull, particularly the temporal bone, which surrounds the cochlea. A sound can therefore be perceived by the inner ear despite injury to the middle ear (ossicles). In this case, however, the quality of conduction is diminished.

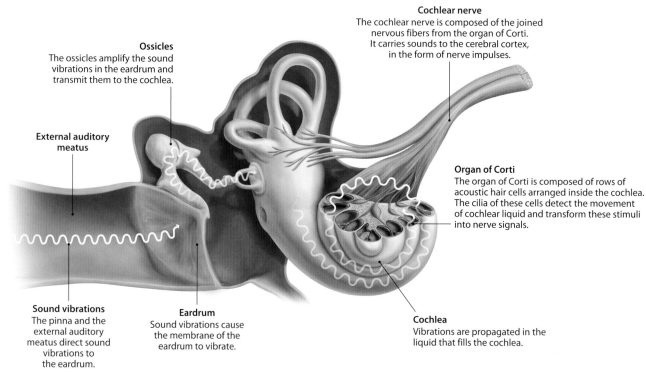

Cochlear nerve
The cochlear nerve is composed of the joined nervous fibers from the organ of Corti. It carries sounds to the cerebral cortex, in the form of nerve impulses.

Ossicles
The ossicles amplify the sound vibrations in the eardrum and transmit them to the cochlea.

External auditory meatus

Organ of Corti
The organ of Corti is composed of rows of acoustic hair cells arranged inside the cochlea. The cilia of these cells detect the movement of cochlear liquid and transform these stimuli into nerve signals.

Sound vibrations
The pinna and the external auditory meatus direct sound vibrations to the eardrum.

Eardrum
Sound vibrations cause the membrane of the eardrum to vibrate.

Cochlea
Vibrations are propagated in the liquid that fills the cochlea.

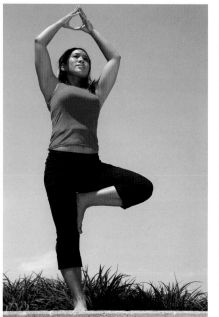

TINNITUS

Tinnitus is an abnormal auditory sensation perceived by the brain. Its symptoms are whistling or ringing sounds that do not come from an external sound stimulation. Tinnitus can have a multitude of causes, including injury to the middle or inner ear, but it is most often the result of injury to the cochlea, arising with age or due to exposure to excessively loud noise, or infection.

BALANCE

Balance is a sense that allows us to perceive and control the position of our bodies in space. It is provided in part by the organs located in the inner ear, in conjunction with the cerebellum. The body's position is also estimated through sight, which gives us our bearings in relation to our surroundings, and through our perception of our muscles stretching and the position of our joints (proprioception).

The cerebellum... page 140

PREVENTING HEARING PROBLEMS AND DISORDERS

■ AVOID EXPOSURE TO
EXCESSIVELY LOUD NOISE

Repeated exposure to loud noise, like that of jackhammers, airplane engines, and amplified concerts, can injure the cochlea and lead to hearing disorders. Prolonged, high-volume use of personal stereo systems can also increase the risk of acoustic trauma. Lower the volume of your personal equipment and restrict your listening time. Also, distance yourself from sources of intense noise or protect your ears with protective earphones or suitable earplugs.

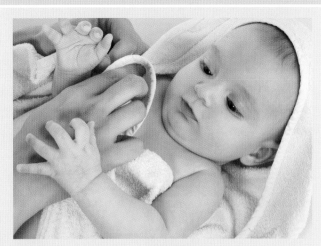

■ DO NOT LEAVE THE EAR CANAL WET
AND DO NET INSERT OBJECTS INTO IT

The presence of objects or moisture in the external auditory meatus can cause infection (otitis) or hearing problems. Some objects may even pierce the eardrum. To remove moisture, gently wipe the ear using a towel, particularly after taking a bath or swimming.

■ TREAT EAR INFECTIONS RAPIDLY

Poorly treated ear infections (otitis) can lead to serious complications (spread of infection, injury of the eardrum and ossicles, deafness).

■ REMOVE EARWAX PLUGS USING EARDROPS

It is usually not necessary to clean the ear canal. However, an accumulation of earwax can create a plug that may cause irritation or reduce your hearing. Do not try to get rid of it with a cotton swab, because this can push it deeper inside. To remove it, use special drops instead (cerumenolytics), which will help to dissolve it. If the earwax plug is not reabsorbed within a few days, see your doctor, who will remove it with a probe.

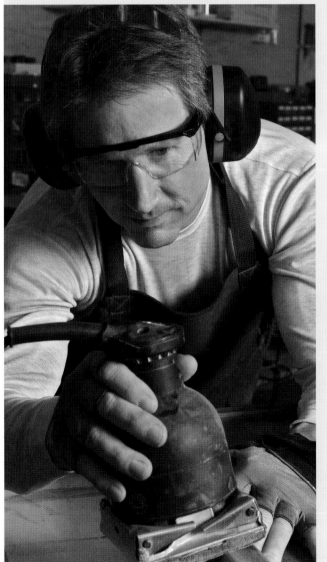

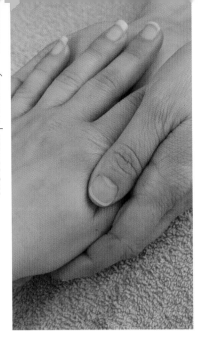

TOUCH

Touch is the sense that allows us to perceive certain physical properties of objects and our environment: pressure, temperature, texture, etc. These stimuli are captured by the touch receptors in the skin. The receptors generate nerve signals, primarily directed towards a zone of the brain's parietal lobe, the somatosensory cortex, where they are interpreted. Touch, which is responsible for superficial and conscious sensibility, is complemented by deep sensibility (usually unconscious), provided by receptors located in the viscera, the muscles, and the bones (proprioception). With respect to pain, it is felt when a specialized receptor, the nociceptor, is stimulated by injury.

TOUCH RECEPTORS IN THE SKIN

Touch receptors are sensory neuron endings embedded more or less deeply in the skin. There are several different types, usually specialized in perceiving a specific type of stimulus. Once stimulated, the touch receptors emit nerve signals that are carried to the somatosensory cortex, which interprets them and orders the appropriate responses.

Neurons... page 136

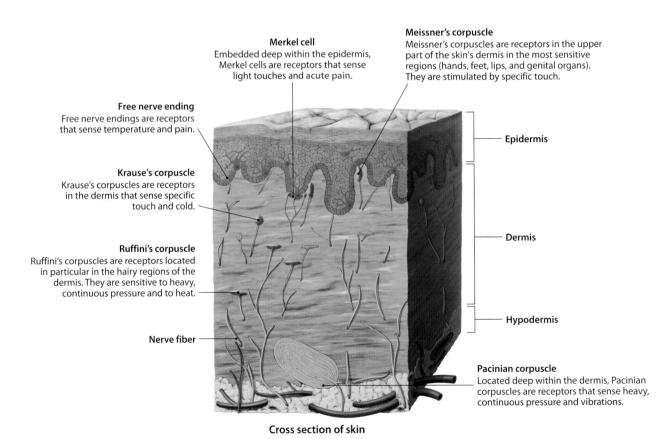

Merkel cell
Embedded deep within the epidermis, Merkel cells are receptors that sense light touches and **acute pain**.

Meissner's corpuscle
Meissner's corpuscles are receptors in the upper part of the skin's dermis in the most sensitive regions (hands, feet, lips, and genital organs). They are stimulated by specific touch.

Free nerve ending
Free nerve endings are receptors that sense temperature and pain.

Krause's corpuscle
Krause's corpuscles are receptors in the dermis that sense specific touch and cold.

Ruffini's corpuscle
Ruffini's corpuscles are receptors located in particular in the hairy regions of the dermis. They are sensitive to heavy, continuous pressure and to heat.

Nerve fiber

Epidermis

Dermis

Hypodermis

Pacinian corpuscle
Located deep within the dermis, Pacinian corpuscles are receptors that sense heavy, continuous pressure and vibrations.

Cross section of skin

198

PAIN

Tissue injury is usually accompanied by a sensation of pain, induced by the stimulation of specialized receptors called nociceptors. The majority of nociceptors are free nerve endings located in the epidermis. They are also present in the muscles, tendons, joints, and viscera. Pain is highly subjective and is tolerated differently from one person to the next. Acute, rapid, intense pain is a warning system that alerts and protects the body against aggression, particularly trauma (blows, burns, cuts, stings, etc.) and diseases (inflammation, tumors, etc.).

ANALGESICS

Analgesics, also called antalgics or painkillers, are medications designed to relieve pain. Administered orally, commonly used analgesics such as paracetamol, aspirin, and ibuprofen act peripherally and are recommended in the case of mild to moderate pain. Administered orally, intravenously, or by epidural, analgesics that act on the central nervous system, such as morphine, are used to relieve severe pain. Their use is strictly controlled, as they can lead to confusion, dependence, and respiratory arrest.

Structure of the nervous system... page 134

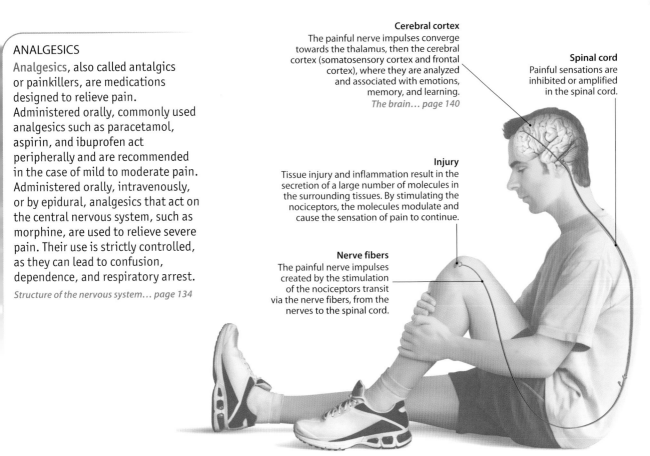

Cerebral cortex
The painful nerve impulses converge towards the thalamus, then the cerebral cortex (somatosensory cortex and frontal cortex), where they are analyzed and associated with emotions, memory, and learning.
The brain... page 140

Spinal cord
Painful sensations are inhibited or amplified in the spinal cord.

Injury
Tissue injury and inflammation result in the secretion of a large number of molecules in the surrounding tissues. By stimulating the nociceptors, the molecules modulate and cause the sensation of pain to continue.

Nerve fibers
The painful nerve impulses created by the stimulation of the nociceptors transit via the nerve fibers, from the nerves to the spinal cord.

Pain mechanisms

ANESTHESIA

Used in potentially painful medical interventions, anesthesia temporarily suppresses the sensibility of all or part of the body. The substances used and techniques of administration vary depending on the type of anesthesia. Local anesthesia, used when only a small area needs to be anesthetized (e.g. to treat a cavity) does not alter the patient's consciousness. It can be administered by injection under the skin or by surface application of an anesthetic agent. Locoregional anesthesia is used to anesthetize a larger portion of the body, such as for childbirth. It is administered by injecting an anesthetic agent into the cerebrospinal fluid, the epidural space, or close to one or more nerves. Finally, for general anesthesia, a combination of anesthetic agents is administered by inhalation or intravenously, in order to cause the temporary suppression of consciousness and of the body's sensitivity.

Local anesthesia

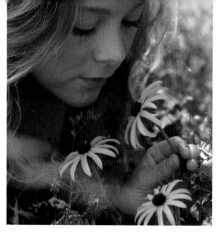

SMELL

Smell (or olfaction) is the brain's perception and interpretation of odors. Relatively undeveloped in human beings, smell is closely related to taste: certain stimuli activate taste and smell receptors at the same time. As a result, our sense of smell helps us to better appreciate the flavors of the food that we eat.

THE **NASAL CAVITIES**

The nasal cavities are located inside the nose. They connect to the outside via the nostrils and to the mouth via the nasopharynx. Each nasal cavity encloses an olfactory epithelium, whose stimulation by odorous molecules generates nerve signals. These are routed to the brain, where the odors are analyzed and associated with emotions and memories.

The upper respiratory tract... page 311

Nasal cavity
The walls of the nasal cavities are covered with a mucous membrane that produces nasal mucus. The odorous molecules dissolve in the nasal mucus of the olfactory epithelium (or olfactory mucous membrane).

Olfactory epithelium
The olfactory epithelium (olfactory mucous membrane) covers approximately one square inch (2.5 cm²) of the roof of the nasal cavities. It contains millions of extremely sensitive olfactory cells (olfactory neurons), whose stimulation by odorous molecules generates nerve impulses. There are hundreds of types of specialized olfactory neurons, thanks to which we can detect thousands of different smells.

Ethmoid bone
Olfactory nerves (bundles of olfactory cell nerve fibers) run through the ethmoid bone.

Olfactory bulb
Located above the nasal cavity and the ethmoid bone, the olfactory bulb collects the nerve signals carried by the olfactory nerves and redirects them towards the brain's olfactory centers.

Nostril
Carried by the air, odorous molecules enter the nasal cavities through the two nostrils during inhalation.

Nasopharynx
The nasal cavities communicate with the mouth via the nasopharynx (the upper part of the pharynx, or retronasal passage), which allows for the perception of the aromas of the food being ingested.

IMPAIRED SENSE OF SMELL

A decrease in our capacity to smell, or anosmia, can occur during inflammation of the mucous membrane in the nose (due to colds or allergies). It can also arise when the nasal cavities are obstructed by nasal polyps. This is a temporary, harmless condition. However, full or partial loss or absence of smell due to aging or a congenital factor is usually permanent. A viral infection or injury to the olfactory nerves (often following a head trauma) can also cause the complete disappearance of our sense of smell.

REGENERATING NEURONS

The olfactory cells are thought to be the only neurons in the human body that can regenerate. Their life span is around 60 days.

TASTE

The flavor of substances is perceived by our sense of taste, which involves thousands of sensory receptors throughout the mouth, especially on the tongue. The main functions of taste are to inform us about the quality of our food and drink, and to trigger the secretion of digestive juices. Nerve and touch receptors also tell us about the temperature, the consistency, and even the spiciness of our food, giving us a complete taste sensation.

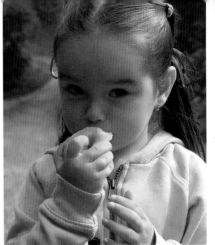

THE **TONGUE** AND THE **TASTE BUDS**

The tongue, which is involved in taste, chewing, and speech, is composed of muscle tissue covered with a mucous membrane. This membrane is formed of thousands of small protuberances (papillae) and a connective tissue that supports them by providing blood irrigation and innervation. Some papillae (the taste papillae) contain taste buds, tiny organs that perceive taste sensations. When a taste bud comes into contact with a sapid substance (that has a flavor) dissolved in the saliva, the cells that form the bud generate nerve signals. Sensory nerves route these to the cerebral cortex, where the conscious perception of flavor occurs.

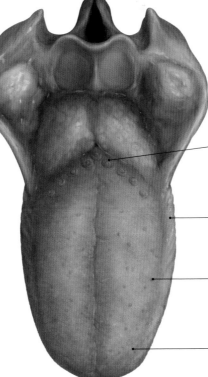

View of the tongue from above

Circumvallate papilla
The circumvallate papillae are large taste buds located at the back of the tongue.

Foliate papilla
Foliate papillae are striated taste buds located on the sides of the tongue.

Fungiform papilla
Fungiform papillae are round, red taste buds on the upper surface of the tongue.

Mucous membrane
The surface of the tongue's mucous membrane is mainly composed of filiform papillae, which give it its smooth appearance. The conical filiform papillae have no taste buds, and so play no role in sense of taste.

THE BASIC TASTE SENSATIONS

The taste buds can only differentiate five basic sensations: sweet, salty, sour (e.g. lemon, vinegar), bitter (e.g. beer, coffee, and endives), and savory (e.g. soy sauce, tomatoes, and asparagus). Sensitivity to the basic taste sensations varies by person and with age. For example, children are more sensitive to bitterness than adults.

TASTE IMPAIRMENT

The complete or partial disappearance of taste, called ageusia, may be linked to nerve injury (like facial paralysis), certain medications, psychiatric disorders, or aging. It can also be due to a shortage of saliva, infection of the taste papillae (taste buds), or poor oral hygiene.

A MATTER OF TASTE

A food's "taste" is, quite often, just its aroma, that the olfactory receptors in our nasal cavity perceive while we chew. If you pinch your nose while eating, the aroma will disappear, leaving only the more limited, basic taste sensations. The sensation created by the combination of the aroma and the taste is called the flavor.

AMETROPIA

Ametropia, which is often caused by a **congenital** malformation, refers to vision disorders characterized by the eye's inability to correctly focus the images of objects on the retina. Its forms include myopia (nearsightedness), hyperopia (farsightedness), and astigmatism. Strictly speaking, presbyopia is not a form of ametropia, but rather a natural phenomenon associated with aging. Most cases of ametropia can be corrected, either by wearing glasses or contact lenses, or by surgery.

The mechanism of sight... page 191

MYOPIA

Myopia, or nearsightedness, is caused by an overly long eyeball, an overly curved cornea, or an anomaly in the lens. It causes blurred vision of faraway objects, but does not affect near vision. Myopia usually appears in early adolescence and stabilizes at adulthood. Very strong nearsightedness increases the risk of developing certain eye diseases, like cataracts and retinal detachment. As a result, myopic people should go for regular, routine checkups.

PRESBYOPIA

Presbyopia, or presbytia, is the lens's declining power of accommodation, associated with aging. It usually appears around the age of 40, as difficulty seeing clearly at short distances (e.g. for reading), while far vision usually remains intact. Presbyopia may be accompanied by headache and visual fatigue.

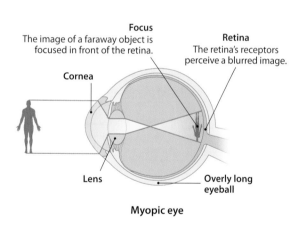

Focus
The image of a faraway object is focused in front of the retina.

Retina
The retina's receptors perceive a blurred image.

Cornea

Lens

Overly long eyeball

Myopic eye

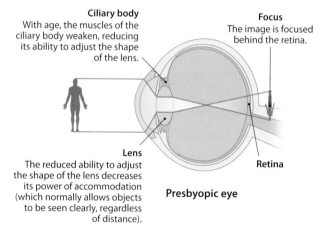

Ciliary body
With age, the muscles of the ciliary body weaken, reducing its ability to adjust the shape of the lens.

Focus
The image is focused behind the retina.

Lens
The reduced ability to adjust the shape of the lens decreases its power of accommodation (which normally allows objects to be seen clearly, regardless of distance).

Retina

Presbyopic eye

ASTIGMATISM

An astigmatism is the result of an irregularity in the curve of the cornea. It leads to deformed images and defective vision at all distances. Often hereditary, it can also be caused by injury or by surgical operation for cataracts or keratoconus (a **genetic** disease that entails the gradual deformation of the cornea).

HYPEROPIA

Hyperopia, or farsightedness, is caused by insufficient length of the eyeball, an overly flat cornea, or an anomaly in the lens. Images focus behind the retina, creating defective vision at short distances. The eye's lens naturally corrects moderate hyperopia, although it may still cause headache. In children, farsightedness can cause strabismus and may lead to a decrease in visual acuity.

GLASSES

Glasses are lenses attached to a frame, designed to correct a vision defect or to protect the eyes. The lenses may be concave for myopia, convex to treat hyperopia and presbyopia, or aspherical (nonspherical) with a curve adjusted to improve the focusing of rays in the eye and to correct astigmatism. Some lenses may have multiple curves (bifocal, trifocal, and progressive lenses). Often prescribed for presbyopic patients, these lenses are composed of different areas with different optical features. One area, often towards the bottom of the lens, is designed to improve near vision, while another, towards the top, is assigned to far vision. Wearing tinted glasses is recommended for diseases like keratitis and albinism, but also for everyday life, when in the presence of bright light.

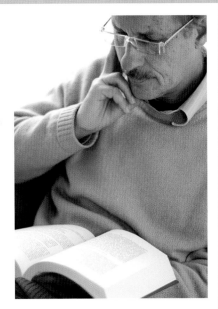

CONTACT LENSES

Contact lenses, or corneal lenses, are optical prostheses placed directly on the cornea to improve vision. They may be hard or soft and can easily correct myopia and hyperopia, but are less helpful for astigmatism and presbyopia. Compared with glasses, contact lenses provide the advantage of covering the entire field of vision and of being less visible. On the other hand, contact lenses require adaptation and may result in intolerance (dry eye, conjunctivitis, keratitis, etc.). Strict, regular care must be followed for contact lenses, to prevent the risk of infection.

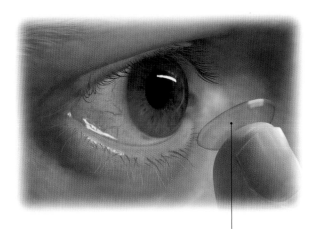

Contact lens
Contact lenses are placed directly over the cornea.

CORNEAL SURGERY

Myopy, mild hyperopia, and astigmatisms can be treated by corneal surgery, which involves reshaping the curve of the cornea. Corneal surgery uses a number of techniques, including photorefractive keratectomy (PRK) and LASIK. Photorefractive keratectomy is the microscopic abrasion of the cornea using a laser beam. LASIK, which also uses laser beams, abrades the cornea deeper inside. This surgery first requires the removal of the superficial layer of the cornea, which is put back in place at the end of the operation. In this way, LASIK can correct stronger forms of ametropia than photorefractive keratectomy. These simple, relatively nontraumatic corneal operations are now commonplace in industrialized countries.

AMETROPIA

SYMPTOMS:
Imperfect vision from afar (myopia), close up (hyperopia, presbyopia), or at all distances (astigmatism). Headache, eyestrain.

TREATMENTS:
Corrective lenses, contact lenses, corneal surgery.

INFLAMMATION OF THE EYE

The eye can be subject to attacks from many different sources: **infection**, **trauma**, allergies, and foreign bodies. The result is an **inflammation**, which can affect various parts of the eye. Some inflammations are benign and easy to treat, while others can persist and lead to a decrease in visual acuity, or even blindness.

INFLAMMATION OF THE EYELIDS

The eyelids are vulnerable to several types of benign inflammation, including styes, blepharitis, and chalazion. Styes are painful boils that form on the eyelid, caused by bacterial infection of the hair follicle of an eyelash. Blepharitis is an inflammation of the rim of the eyelid due to a bacterial infection or overproduction of sebum. It causes redness, tearing, and discomfort. Chalazion, whose origin is relatively unknown, is characterized by the inflammation of a sebaceous gland of the eyelid and the accumulation of its secretions in the eyelid. It appears as a small lump under the skin. It can be surgically removed if it is large or does not disappear on its own. Inflammation of the eyelid caused by infection can be treated using an antibiotic ointment.

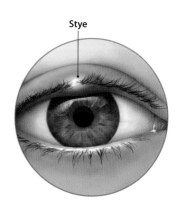
Stye

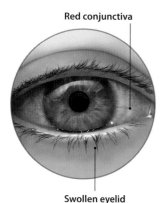
Red conjunctiva

Swollen eyelid

CONJUNCTIVITIS

Conjunctivitis is an inflammation of the conjunctiva, caused by allergy, infection (viral or bacterial), or the presence of a foreign body. It causes redness of the conjunctiva, swollen eyelids, watery eyes, stinging, and, in the case of a bacterial infection, highly contagious purulent secretions. The irritation can push the patient to rub the eye, at the risk of causing keratitis. Conjunctivitis is treated with anti-inflammatories, antibiotics, or antiallergics, depending on the cause.

UVEITIS

Uveitis is an inflammation of the vascularized casing of the eye (the uvea), which is composed of the iris, the ciliary body, and the choroid. The different types include iridocyclitis (inflammation of the iris and the ciliary body), choroiditis (inflammation of the choroid), and panuveitis, which affects all of these tissues. Iridocyclitis, whose precise cause can be difficult to identify, leads to redness around the cornea, deformation of the pupil, decrease in visual acuity, pain, and light sensitivity. Choroiditis appears as a whitish patch that is visible during ophthalmoscopy (inspection of the back of the eye) that impairs vision. Often associated with an infectious disease, it can cause a severe inflammation of the retina (retinitis).

The eye... page 190
Retinitis... page 208

KERATITIS

Keratitis is an inflammation of the cornea that can be caused by infection, allergy, trauma, burn, or exposure to bright light. It is characterized by decreased visual acuity, red, watery eyes, pain, and increased sensitivity to light. Keratitis must be treated rapidly to prevent perforation of the cornea.

COLLYRIUM

Collyria are medicinal solutions administered drop by drop onto the surface of the eyes. Depending on the disease being treated, they will contain different active ingredients: anti-inflammatories, antiseptics, antibiotics, antifungals, antivirals, anesthetics, decongestants, or antiallergics. Applied to the inside of the lower eyelid, collyrium drops are rapidly spread to all of the front structures of the eye, but they are not very effective for the treatment of problems behind the lens.

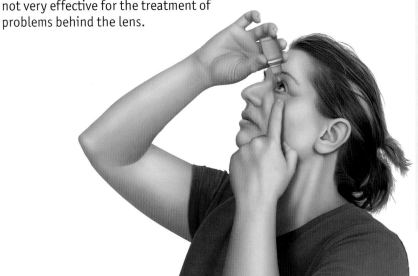

DRY EYE

Dry eye is characterized by an insufficient amount of tears or by a defect in their composition. A dry eye is painful and more vulnerable to **infection**, and vision may be impaired. Dry eye is mainly due to a dysfunction of the lachrymal gland, associated with aging. It may also be the result of an **inflammation**, a dry or polluted environment, taking certain medications, working on monitors, or an **autoimmune** disease affecting certain secretory glands. Treatment focuses on the use of eye drops as a replacement for tears.

Tears... page 189

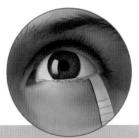

Schirmer's test
A diagnosis of dry eye is mainly based on Schirmer's test, which measures the amount of tears in the eye, using a strip of absorbent paper placed on the inside of the lower eyelid.

DRY EYE

SYMPTOMS:
Feeling of discomfort, burning, or stinging. If the cause is inflammatory, the eye will be red.

TREATMENTS:
Artificial tears in eye drops, treatment of the inflammation if applicable. In some cases, temporary or permanent sealing of the lachrymal canals, through which the tears drain, to preserve moisture on the surface of the eye.

PREVENTION:
Humidification of the air. Not wearing contact lenses or working for long periods in front of a monitor.

CATARACTS

Cataracts are a common age-related eye disease. They are characterized by the gradual opacification of the eye's lens, which is normally transparent. Most people over the age of 65 have lenses that have some level of opacity. Other types of cataracts are hereditary or the result of a **trauma**, a disease (like diabetes or hyperthyroidism), or an **infection** occurring during pregnancy. Cataracts may affect one or both eyes. If they are not operated on, they will lead to blindness.

EFFECTS OF CATARACTS

The lens comprises a fibrous core enveloped in a capsule. The fibers of the core are usually arranged so that the lens is transparent. The effect of a cataract is to disarrange these fibers, leading to opacification of the lens, which can no longer fulfill its role. Only part of the light then reaches the retina, and vision becomes cloudy.

CATARACTS

SYMPTOMS:
Decrease in visual acuity, especially at a distance. Cloudy vision.

TREATMENTS:
Surgical ablation (removal) of the lens, usually replaced by an artificial lens.

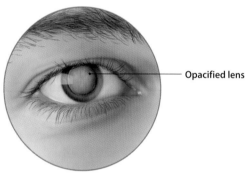

Opacified lens

TREATMENT OF CATARACTS

The only effective treatment of cataracts is to surgically remove the affected lens, using an ultrasonic probe. The operation, usually performed under local anesthesia, takes about half an hour. Destruction of the lens causes extreme hyperopia (farsightedness), which is typically corrected by the implantation of a soft artificial lens. Vision improves rapidly, although it is often necessary for the patient to wear glasses or contact lenses to make up for the residual lack of focus.

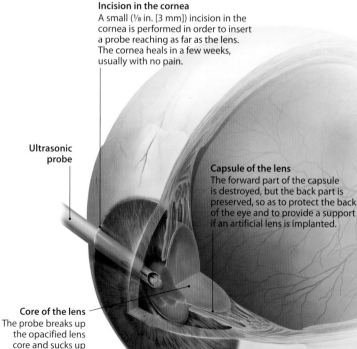

Incision in the cornea
A small (⅛ in. [3 mm]) incision in the cornea is performed in order to insert a probe reaching as far as the lens. The cornea heals in a few weeks, usually with no pain.

Ultrasonic probe

Capsule of the lens
The forward part of the capsule is destroyed, but the back part is preserved, so as to protect the back of the eye and to provide a support if an artificial lens is implanted.

Core of the lens
The probe breaks up the opacified lens core and sucks up the debris.

Surgical ablation of the lens

GLAUCOMA

Glaucoma is characterized by increased pressure within the eye, most often the result of an accumulation of fluid (aqueous humor) between the cornea and the lens. The disease causes **degeneration** of the optical nerve and can lead to blindness. There are several forms of glaucoma, which affect 1%-2% of the population. Its treatment involves reducing the pressure in the eye by means of collyria (drops). Surgery may also be performed, to restart drainage of the aqueous humor.

TYPES OF GLAUCOMA

There are two main forms of glaucoma. Open-angle glaucoma, or chronic glaucoma, is the most common form (80% of cases). Caused by an obstruction of the aqueous humor's drainage point (the trabeculum), it appears progressively, most often after the age of 45, and usually affects both eyes. At first asymptomatic, open-angle glaucoma then gradually reduces visual acuity and can even lead to blindness, if left untreated. The more rare narrow-angle glaucoma, or acute glaucoma, appears suddenly and only affects one eye. It is caused by an abnormally narrow angle between the iris and the cornea, which prevents drainage of the aqueous humor. Triggered by an innocuous factor, such as dilation of the pupil, narrow-angle glaucoma poses a threat to the optical nerve in just a few hours, and so must be treated immediately.

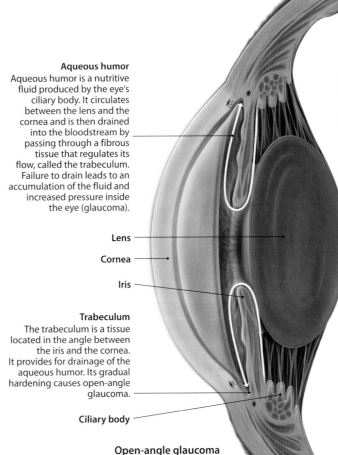

Aqueous humor
Aqueous humor is a nutritive fluid produced by the eye's ciliary body. It circulates between the lens and the cornea and is then drained into the bloodstream by passing through a fibrous tissue that regulates its flow, called the trabeculum. Failure to drain leads to an accumulation of the fluid and increased pressure inside the eye (glaucoma).

Lens

Cornea

Iris

Trabeculum
The trabeculum is a tissue located in the angle between the iris and the cornea. It provides for drainage of the aqueous humor. Its gradual hardening causes open-angle glaucoma.

Ciliary body

Open-angle glaucoma

GLAUCOMA

SYMPTOMS:
Chronic glaucoma: asymptomatic for a long period, followed by gradual decrease in visual acuity. Acute glaucoma: sudden sharp pain, red eye, decrease in visual acuity, sometimes nausea and vomiting.

TREATMENTS:
Collyria that reduce aqueous humor production or that stimulate its drainage through a parallel passageway, surgery to open a new drainage path.

PREVENTION:
Chronic glaucoma: systematic examinations starting at age 45. Acute glaucoma: preventive surgical treatment on the second eye after glaucoma in the first.

RETINOPATHY

Retinopathy covers a set of retinal diseases that may be hereditary, **infectious**, age-related, **trauma-related**, or associated with another disease such as diabetes. It often leads to a decrease in visual acuity and must be treated quickly, because it can lead to total blindness.

RETINAL DETACHMENT

Retinal detachment is characterized by the penetration of the vitreous body under the retina, most often caused by a torn retina. Its symptoms are the sudden appearance of floating spots and flashes, followed by a dark veil covering part of the visual field. Torn retinas are usually linked to the shrinkage of the vitreous body, which then separates from the retina and may cause a section to detach. This condition is caused by aging or strong myopia (nearsightedness). Retinal tears can also appear following a trauma to the eye, surgery, or illness (diabetic retinopathy). Retinal detachment is a serious disorder that can lead to blindness. It must be treated quickly by surgery or by the injection of gas to press the retina back against the wall of the eye.

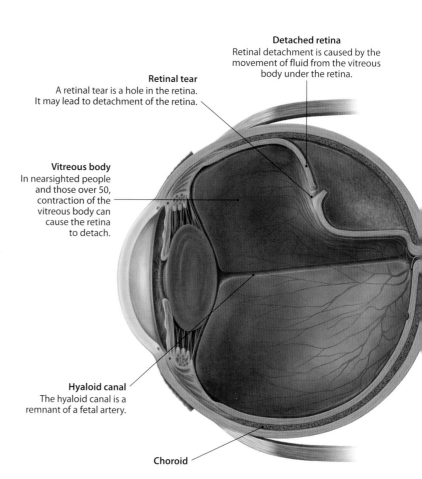

Detached retina
Retinal detachment is caused by the movement of fluid from the vitreous body under the retina.

Retinal tear
A retinal tear is a hole in the retina. It may lead to detachment of the retina.

Vitreous body
In nearsighted people and those over 50, contraction of the vitreous body can cause the retina to detach.

Hyaloid canal
The hyaloid canal is a remnant of a fetal artery.

Choroid

Retinal detachment

FLOATING SPOTS

Floating spots are dark or light dots, lines, or webs that appear to move around the visual field. They are caused by gelatinous masses in the vitreous body and are usually not serious. However, small black floating spots that appear suddenly are a sign of hemorrhaging in the vitreous body, due to rupture of a vessel during retinal detachment. These require immediate medical attention.

RETINITIS

Retinitis is an inflammation of the retina. It is often combined with inflammation of the choroid and usually originates from a congenital infection by the parasite responsible for toxoplasmosis. Less frequently, retinitis may be caused by a bacterium (tuberculosis), a virus (cytomegalovirus or rubella), or a fungus (candidosis).

Toxoplasmosis... page 478

DIABETIC RETINOPATHY

Diabetic retinopathy is characterized by the degeneration of the capillaries (very fine blood vessels) in the retina. Encouraged by high blood pressure, it affects diabetics whose hyperglycemia has not been under control for several years. The disease appears as different types of lesions (microaneurysms, hemorrhaging, cotton-wool spots, etc.) on the retina, which result in a decrease in visual acuity after a few years. Diabetic retinopathy is one of the leading causes of blindness in industrialized countries. Its treatment starts with getting arterial blood pressure and glycemia under control. Laser photocoagulation can be used to reduce certain lesions.

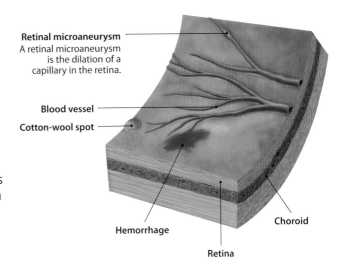

Retinal microaneurysm
A retinal microaneurysm is the dilation of a capillary in the retina.

Blood vessel

Cotton-wool spot

Hemorrhage

Choroid

Retina

LASER PHOTOCOAGULATION

Laser photocoagulation consists in projecting a laser beam onto the retina, to reduce certain lesions (retinal tears, microaneurysms, etc.) that could lead to retinal detachment. It may also be employed to treat open-angle glaucoma. Laser photocoagulation does not require hospitalization and is relatively painless. In some cases, this treatment may cause the retina to swell, but the swelling will be reabsorbed within a few days.

RETINITIS PIGMENTOSA

Retinitis pigmentosa, or pigmentary degeneration of the retina, is a hereditary genetic disease characterized by the gradual degeneration of the retina's photoreceptors. It appears during childhood, in the form of difficulty adjusting to darkness, reduction of the field of vision, and then decrease in visual acuity, potentially developing into blindness.

Heredity... page 50

Retinal tear

Retina

Choroid

Laser impact
The laser impacts around a retinal tear create adhesion between the retina and the choroid, to prevent retinal detachment.

Laser beam

Laser photocoagulation

RETINOPATHY

SYMPTOMS:
Decrease in visual acuity, reduced field of vision, floating spots, difficulty seeing in the dark.

TREATMENTS:
Retinitis: antibiotics, antivirals, antifungals, or antiparasitics, depending on the type of infection.
Retinal detachment: surgery, gas injections.
Retinitis pigmentosa: no treatment.

PREVENTION:
Retinal detachment: laser photocoagulation of retinal lesions.
Diabetic retinopathy: strict monitoring of blood pressure and glycemia.

MACULAR DEGENERATION

Macular **degeneration** is the gradual alteration of the macula (the part of the retina responsible for central vision). It is most often associated with aging, but it can also be hereditary and start during adolescence. Age-related macular degeneration, or ARMD, appears as problems with central vision. It can lead to blindness, of which it is a leading cause in industrialized countries. ARMD typically affects people over the age of 65 and often affects both eyes.

MACULAR DEGENERATION

SYMPTOMS:
Problems with central vision (central scotoma) and deformed vision, leading to difficulty reading and recognizing distant objects.

TREATMENTS:
No curative treatment. In some cases, degradation of the macula can be limited by various techniques: laser photocoagulation or injection of medications into the vitreous body.

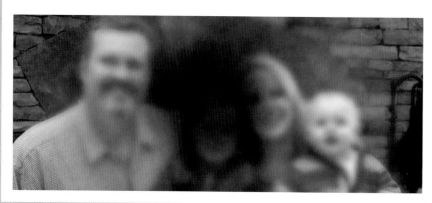

Central scotoma
A scotoma is a gap in part of the visual field. A central scotoma may lead to total central blindness, while peripheral vision remains intact.

COLOR BLINDNESS

Color blindness is a color visualization disorder caused by a recessive, gender-related (X chromosome), hereditary **genetic** anomaly. It affects 8% of men, but just 0.5% of women. In the color blind, certain color-sensitive photoreceptors in the retina are missing or deficient, which leads to defective perception of one or two of the basic colors in the visible light spectrum (red, green, and blue). The Ishihara test makes it possible to quickly diagnose color blindness, although there is no treatment for it.

Heredity... page 50

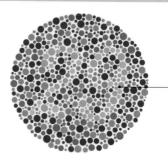

Color pattern
Patterns comprised of spots of similar colors stand out in the background to the normal eye, but are not perceived by color-blind people.

Ishihara plate
Ishihara plates are composed of a mosaic of colored spots.

COLOR BLINDNESS

SYMPTOMS:
Impaired vision of one or two primary colors (red, green, or blue) and their derivative colors.

TREATMENTS:
No treatment.

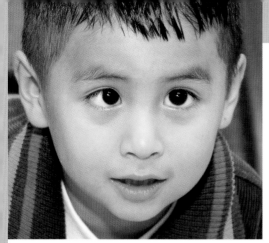

STRABISMUS

Common in children, strabismus is the defective parallelism of the visual axes, characterized by the deviation of one or both eyes. This deviation is usually horizontal, directed either inward or outward. Strabismus disrupts the perception of three-dimensional contours and may cause a decrease in visual acuity in young children.

TYPES OF STRABISMUS

The types of strabismus are differentiated according to the direction of deviation of the eye. Vertical strabismus is rare, and often combined with horizontal strabismus. Horizontal strabismus may be convergent or divergent. Convergent strabismus is the inward deviation of an eye. This is the most common form of strabismus, especially in young children. Sometimes hereditary, it can also be linked to ametropia (image focusing problems), the paralysis of an oculomotor muscle, a trauma, or a disorder of the eyeball, such as cataracts. In most cases, no cause can be identified. Divergent strabismus is the outward deviation of an eye. It usually appears after the age of one year and may be intermittent, appearing at times of fatigue or when focusing on a faraway object. It can also be a consequence of the surgical treatment of convergent strabismus.

Ametropia… page 202

TREATMENT OF STRABISMUS

Strabismus treatment consists of correcting the patient's ametropia by wearing glasses, then restoring the parallelism of the eyes and binocular vision through visual reeducation, particularly with the use of an occlusive dressing. Surgery may also be considered to treat a weakened oculomotor muscle. For the best results, strabismus treatments should start as early as possible.

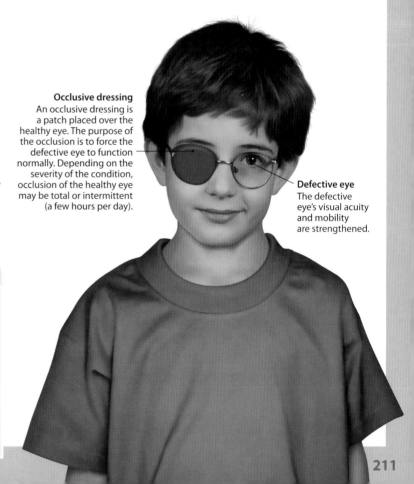

Occlusive dressing
An occlusive dressing is a patch placed over the healthy eye. The purpose of the occlusion is to force the defective eye to function normally. Depending on the severity of the condition, occlusion of the healthy eye may be total or intermittent (a few hours per day).

Defective eye
The defective eye's visual acuity and mobility are strengthened.

STRABISMUS

SYMPTOMS:
Deviation of one eye in comparison to the other, decrease in visual acuity, problems with three-dimensional vision.

TREATMENTS:
Glasses, visual reeducation, occlusive dressing, surgery.

DEAFNESS

Deafness, or hypoacusis, is hearing loss or decreased hearing, which can occur in one or both ears. It may be **congenital** or acquired (through **infection**, **trauma**, etc.), and affects more than 8% of the population worldwide. There are two major types of deafness: perceptive deafness and conduction deafness.

PERCEPTIVE DEAFNESS

Perceptive deafness, or nerve deafness, is linked to the incorrect functioning of the cochlea or of the nerve paths in the inner ear. It may or may not be congenital. The nerve paths can be damaged by a tumor, such as a neurinoma, an infection such as meningitis, or a vascular accident. The cochlea can be damaged by a disease such as Ménière's disease, a trauma, exposure to excessively loud sounds, or, most commonly, aging. The natural aging of the auditory system leads to a gradual decrease in hearing, called presbycusis. This is the leading cause of deafness in human beings. Perceptive deafness can sometimes be treated with surgery (removal of the neurinoma) or medication, but only the use of an audio prosthesis (hearing aid) can compensate for lost hearing.

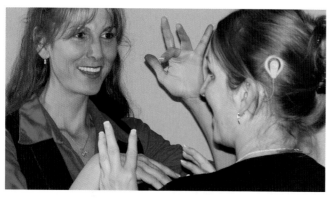

Sign language
Sign language is a means of communication employed by deaf people, who communicate using signs formed by the positions of their hands, movements, and facial expressions. Communication with signs is sometimes combined with lip-reading.

CONDUCTION DEAFNESS

Conduction deafness, or transmission deafness, is linked to damage to the outer or middle ear (eardrum, ossicles), which alters the conduction of sound vibrations. When it involves the outer ear, it is caused by an obstruction of the external auditory meatus (earwax plug, foreign body, boil). When it concerns the middle ear, its cause is otitis, congenital malformation, trauma such as a pierced eardrum, or a hereditary disease such as otospongiosis.

Heredity... page 50

OTOSPONGIOSIS

Otospongiosis is a hereditary genetic disease characterized by the gradual calcification and ankylosis of the stirrup, the third ossicle in the middle ear. Its treatment consists in the surgical removal of the stirrup, replacing it with a prosthesis.

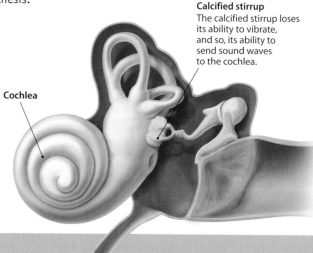

Calcified stirrup
The calcified stirrup loses its ability to vibrate, and so, its ability to send sound waves to the cochlea.

Cochlea

MEASUREMENT OF HEARING

There are several ways to measure hearing. Acoumetry uses simple clinical tests, such as the Rinne test, which helps to determine the nature of the patient's deafness. Audiometry uses more advanced instrumental techniques that provide a precise evaluation of the perception of different sound frequencies. The examination, performed using an audiometer, requires the conscious participation of the patient, who, wearing a headset, presses a button whenever he or she perceives a sound in either ear.

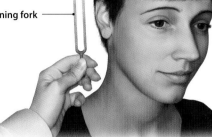

Tuning fork

Rinne test
The Rinne test consists in causing a tuning fork to vibrate, and then holding it successively behind and in front of the ear. When the tuning fork is placed behind the ear, against the temporal bone, the bone conducts the sound to the inner ear. When placed in front of the ear, the sound is conducted by air, moving through the external auditory meatus (ear canal) and the middle ear. Better perception of sound by bone transmission is a sign of conduction deafness.

AUDIO PROSTHESES

A number of audio prostheses can correct deafness. External prostheses (hearing aids) amplify sound via an electronic case containing a microphone, a receiver, and an amplifier. Of varying shapes and sizes, they are placed on the rim or in the hollow of the ear. Other audio prostheses, like cochlear implants, act directly on the inner ear. Their placement requires surgical intervention.

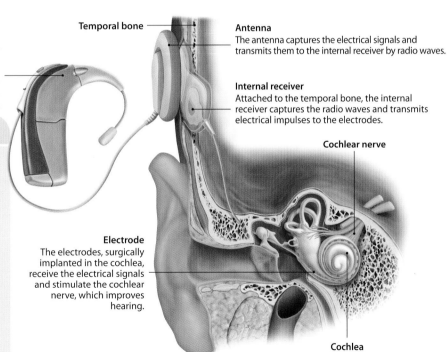

Temporal bone

Microphone
A microphone incorporated in an electronic case captures external sounds, transforms them into electrical signals, and transmits them to the antenna.

Antenna
The antenna captures the electrical signals and transmits them to the internal receiver by radio waves.

Internal receiver
Attached to the temporal bone, the internal receiver captures the radio waves and transmits electrical impulses to the electrodes.

Cochlear nerve

Electrode
The electrodes, surgically implanted in the cochlea, receive the electrical signals and stimulate the cochlear nerve, which improves hearing.

Cochlea

Cochlear implant
Cochlear implants are designed for people with profound or total deafness, for whom a hearing aid is not effective. They greatly improve their quality of life, in particular by allowing them to understand speech.

DEAFNESS

SYMPTOMS:
Hearing loss or reduction, possibly affecting certain frequencies only. Tinnitus.

TREATMENTS:
Depending on the cause: cleaning of the auditory meatus, antibiotic treatment of otitis, surgery. Audio prostheses can improve hearing.

PREVENTION:
Do not expose yourself to overly loud noise, treat otitis rapidly, do not insert anything into the ear canal.

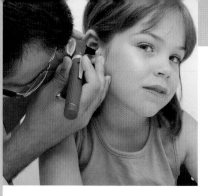

OTITIS

Otitis is an **inflammation** of the outer or middle ear. There are several forms, differentiated by their sources and the affected areas. The most common forms of otitis, especially in young children, affect the middle ear.

ACUTE OTITIS MEDIA

Acute otitis media is an inflammation of the middle ear caused by a viral or bacterial infection. It is often associated with rhinopharyngitis, whose infectious agents can easily spread from the throat via the eustachian tube. As this passageway is much shorter in children, they are more vulnerable to middle ear infections, up to 6 years of age. Acute otitis media appears as ear pain, fever, decrease in hearing, and increased irritability, sometimes accompanied by vomiting and diarrhea. In the case of a bacterial infection, pus may seep out of the ear, and rapid treatment is necessary (antibiotics, paracentesis). If not treated correctly, acute otitis media can lead to serious complications: spread of the infection (meningitis, labyrinthitis, or mastoiditis) and/or facial paralysis.

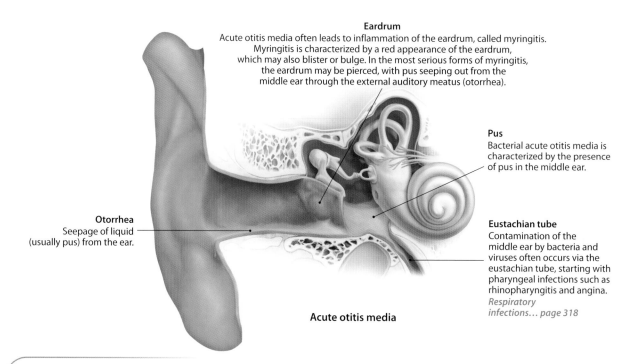

Eardrum
Acute otitis media often leads to inflammation of the eardrum, called myringitis. Myringitis is characterized by a red appearance of the eardrum, which may also blister or bulge. In the most serious forms of myringitis, the eardrum may be pierced, with pus seeping out from the middle ear through the external auditory meatus (otorrhea).

Pus
Bacterial acute otitis media is characterized by the presence of pus in the middle ear.

Otorrhea
Seepage of liquid (usually pus) from the ear.

Eustachian tube
Contamination of the middle ear by bacteria and viruses often occurs via the eustachian tube, starting with pharyngeal infections such as rhinopharyngitis and angina. *Respiratory infections... page 318*

Acute otitis media

OTITIS MEDIA SEROSA

Otitis media serosa, or seromucous otitis, is an inflammation of the middle ear caused by obstruction of the eustachian tube, preventing the drainage of secretions. The eustachian tube may be blocked by infection, allergic reaction, large adenoid vegetation (tonsils), or a congenital malformation. If the obstruction does not go away, otitis media serosa can become chronic and can permanently damage the hearing. Otitis media serosa can also develop into acute otitis media, if an infectious agent is introduced into the middle ear. Depending on the cause of the obstruction, the disease is treated using antibiotics or corticoids, or by surgery (paracentesis or adenoidectomy).

OTITIS EXTERNA

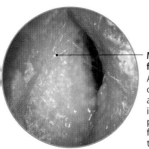

Microscopic fungus
A fungal infection of the external auditory meatus is shown by the presence of whitish filaments on the eardrum.

Fungal otitis externa

Otitis externa is an inflammation of the external auditory meatus (ear canal) or of the outer wall of the eardrum, most often caused by infection. The infection, caused by a microscopic fungus or a bacterium, is favored by moisture (swimming) and by irritants. Otitis externa appears as intense, shooting pains, itching, and discharge (otorrhea). Its treatment focuses on the use of antiseptic, antibiotic, or antifungal drops.

CHOLESTEATOMA

A cholesteatoma is a benign tumor that develops in the middle ear, starting at the eardrum or in the external auditory meatus (ear canal), due to injury to the eardrum or a congenital malformation. The cholesteatoma gradually expands, destroying the tissues of the middle ear, then those of the inner ear, and leading to chronic otitis, tinnitus, vertigo, and irreversible deafness. It is treated surgically by removing the tumor and reconstructing the eardrum and the ossicles.

PARACENTESIS

Paracentesis is a surgical incision in the eardrum to ventilate the middle ear or drain out the pus that it contains. Performed under local or general anesthesia, paracentesis is often followed by the installation of a transtympanic ventilator, a hollow tube creating a passage between the middle and outer ears. Recommended in the case of chronic otitis, particularly in children, the transtympanic ventilation tube remains in place for 8-12 months before being naturally expelled by the body.

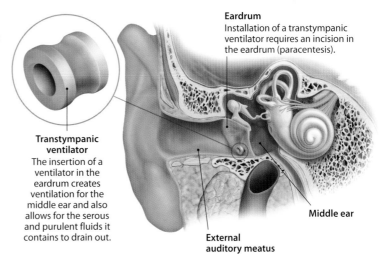

Eardrum
Installation of a transtympanic ventilator requires an incision in the eardrum (paracentesis).

Transtympanic ventilator
The insertion of a ventilator in the eardrum creates ventilation for the middle ear and also allows for the serous and purulent fluids it contains to drain out.

External auditory meatus

Middle ear

OTITIS

SYMPTOMS:
Pain, itching, decrease in hearing, tinnitus, sometimes fever, discharge from the ear, vomiting, diarrhea.

TREATMENTS:
Depending on the cause: antibiotics, anti-inflammatories, antifungals, paracentesis, implantation of a transtympanic ventilator, surgery (removal of adenoid vegetation or of the cholesteatoma).

PREVENTION:
Breast-feeding of newborns seems to prevent acute otitis. Preventive adenoidectomy. Allergy treatment. Not inserting objects into the ear canal and not leaving it wet, especially after swimming.

BALANCE DISTURBANCES

The balance organs normally serve to maintain the body in a stable position. Injury to these organs, or to the nerve paths connected to them, causes a loss of balance (vertigo), often accompanied by other symptoms: nausea, **tinnitus**, vomiting, deafness, anxiety, etc. The person may also suffer passing unsteadiness after a sudden movement or a loss of visual markers, without it being a true case of vertigo.

Hearing and balance... page 194

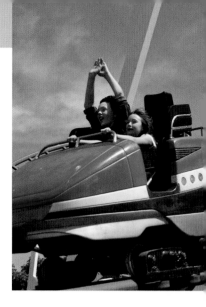

VERTIGO

Vertigo is the illusion of movement resulting from problems with the balance organs. The feeling of vertigo can be rotational (like on a carousel), linear (like in an elevator) ,or swaying (like on a ship's deck). It may be accompanied by nausea, deafness, tinnitus, and involuntary eye movements. Peripheral vertigo (associated with damage to the inner ear or the vestibular nerve) is differentiated from central vertigo (the consequence of an anomaly within the central nervous system). Vertigo often occurs in fits, triggered by sudden head movements, blowing one's nose, noise, or a particular position of the head.

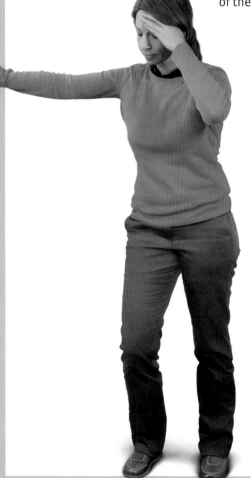

MÉNIÈRE'S DISEASE

Ménière's disease is a chronic disorder of the inner ear characterized by vertigo, deafness, and tinnitus. It affects adults and appears in spells that can last up to several hours. Ménière's disease, the cause of which is unknown, appears to be linked to excess pressure in the inner ear, due to poor reabsorption of the liquid it contains. With time, the associated deafness and tinnitus can become permanent. However, the dizzy spells will fade and evolve into permanent unsteadiness, due to loss of sensitivity of the balance organs.

BENIGN PAROXYSMAL POSITIONAL VERTIGO

Benign paroxysmal positional vertigo, or BPPV, is caused by calcium crystals that have detached from the wall of the vestibule in the inner ear—to which they are normally connected by sensory cilia—and that move around in the semicircular canals. This is the most common form of vertigo in adults and is displayed as transitory spells of unsteadiness (less than a minute) triggered by a change in position. The treatment of BPPV consists in shifting the crystals to a region of the inner ear where they will not cause vertigo, by means of head movements (Epley maneuver).

LABYRINTHITIS

Labyrinthitis is an inflammation of the inner ear cavity (the "labyrinth"), affecting one or both ears. It may be the result of an infection (acute otitis media, mumps, measles, flu, etc.), chronic otitis (cholesteatoma), a head injury, allergic reaction to a medication, etc. Labyrinthitis often appears as rotational (spinning) vertigo, sometimes accompanied by decrease in hearing. It may be cured spontaneously, but it is usually treated with antibiotics, antivirals, or surgery, depending on the cause. If not treated correctly, it could lead to total deafness or meningitis.

PREVENTING TRAVEL SICKNESS

Travel by car, train, airplane, or boat can be disorienting to the balance organs, causing travel sickness. This affects children ages 3-12 and women, in particular. It appears as sweating, nausea, and more or less intense vertigo, possibly to the point of vomiting. Here are a few recommendations for preventing travel sickness:

- Get enough rest before starting out on your trip.

- Before leaving, have a light meal that is easy to digest.

- Take antinausea or antihistamine medication before leaving (these may, however, lead to drowsiness and are not advised for some people, such as young children and pregnant women).

- In vehicles, sit in places that will be shaken the least, usually in the middle or in the front (avoid the back whenever you can).

- If possible, look at the horizon and focus on a fixed point.

- Do not read or drink alcohol.

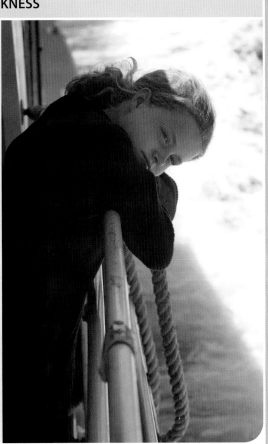

BALANCE DISTURBANCES

SYMPTOMS:
Loss of balance, nausea, vomiting, pale complexion, anxiety, partial deafness, tinnitus, uncontrolled eye movements.

TREATMENTS:
Rest and calm. After a dizzy spell, avoid darkness and prolonged time in bed. Depending on the cause: physical therapy, antivertigo drugs, antibiotics, antivirals, surgery.

PREVENTION:
Treating ear, nose and throat infections.

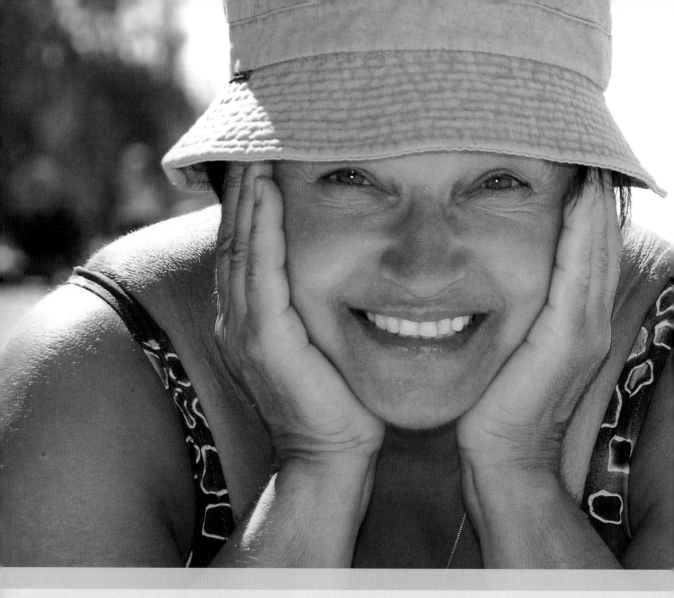

THE **ENDOCRINE SYSTEM**

The endocrine system regulates certain functions of our body through hormones released into the vascular network, specifically by the endocrine glands, and transported in the blood. Associated with the nervous system, it is a system of control and communication that enables the body to develop and function harmoniously: to maintain different physiological constants (such as body temperature or blood pressure), growth, sexual desire, reproduction, response to stress, etc.

An imbalance in hormonal secretions may cause a number of more or less serious problems, with very varied symptoms. The excess secretions are generally caused by a tumor affecting an endocrine gland. As for insufficiencies, such as diabetes, they may have diverse origins, including bad habits associated with modern lifestyles (obesity, physical inactivity, etc.). In case of removal or accidental destruction of an endocrine gland, a hormone replacement treatment must be administered for life, since the body cannot compensate for the absence of hormonal secretion.

THE **ENDOCRINE GLANDS** AND **HORMONES**

The endocrine system consists of an ensemble of cells and endocrine glands that release chemical substances, hormones, into the blood. By performing a precise action on a tissue or an organ, hormones make it possible to regulate certain functions of the body. The endocrine glands are, among others, the hypothalamus, the pituitary gland, the epiphysis, the thyroid, the parathyroids, the adrenals, the ovaries, and the testicles. There are also endocrine cells located in certain organs (kidneys, heart, liver, pancreas, gastric mucosa, intestines, placenta, etc.).

THE **EXOCRINE GLANDS**

Unlike the endocrine glands, the exocrine glands do not release their secretions into the blood, but on the surface of the skin or a mucous membrane. The sudoriparous glands, which secrete sweat, are exocrine glands. The pancreas is a mixed gland, in that its activity is both endocrine and exocrine.

The pancreas... page 350

Epiphysis
The epiphysis, a gland located in the brain, secretes melatonin, a hormone that has an influence on the formation of sperm, the menstrual cycle and the daily biological rhythm (circadian rhythm).

Hypothalamus
The hypothalamus is located in the median portion of the brain. It controls the hormonal secretions of the pituitary gland.

Pituitary gland
The pituitary gland secretes numerous hormones, some of which control the functioning of other endocrine glands.

Thyroid gland
The thyroid gland regulates metabolism and growth through the thyroid hormones. It also secretes calcitonin, a hormone that lowers the level of calcium in the blood.

Parathyroid glands
The parathyroids, located behind the thyroid, secrete parathormone, which increases the level of calcium in the blood.

Adrenal gland
Each adrenal gland has two parts: the adrenal cortex and the medulla. The adrenal cortex secretes hormones with varying effects (water and sodium retention, preparation for puberty, anti-inflammatories etc.). The medulla secretes adrenaline and noradrenaline in stressful situations.

Liver
Certain liver cells release hormones into the blood that play a role in growth.

Pancreas
The pancreas is the largest gland in the human body. Its endocrine part secretes insulin and glucagon, two hormones regulating the glucose level in the blood (glycemia).

Kidneys
Certain kidney cells produce hormones: erythropoietin, which stimulates the formation of red blood cells, and renin, which plays a role in controlling blood pressure.

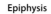

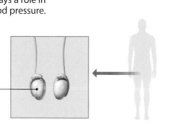

Testicle
In addition to manufacturing sperm, the testicles secrete the male sex hormones, specifically testosterone.

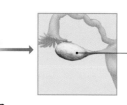

Ovary
The ovaries produce the ovules and secrete the female sex hormones: estrogen and progesterone.

Man   **Woman**

THE **ACTION** OF **HORMONES**

The hormones secreted by the endocrine glands are discharged into the bloodstream where they circulate as far as the cells on which they must act, the target cells. The hormones attach to them and modify their activity. A given hormone may have various effects on different target cells and a physiological process may be controlled by several hormones. Hormones regulate, among other things, growth, reproduction, and the body's response to different stimuli (to stress, for example). Hormonal disruptions may cause diseases such as diabetes and lead to various problems: menstrual cycle problems, sterility, lowered libido, acne, emotional problems, etc. More than one hundred hormones have been identified to date. Synthetic hormones, artificially manufactured, are used in the treatment of different disorders.

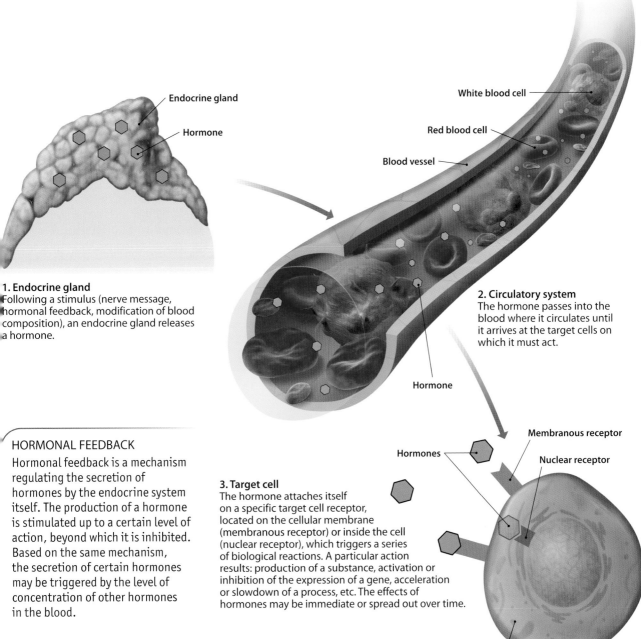

Endocrine gland

Hormone

White blood cell

Red blood cell

Blood vessel

Hormone

Hormones

Membranous receptor

Nuclear receptor

Target cell

1. Endocrine gland
Following a stimulus (nerve message, hormonal feedback, modification of blood composition), an endocrine gland releases a hormone.

2. Circulatory system
The hormone passes into the blood where it circulates until it arrives at the target cells on which it must act.

HORMONAL FEEDBACK

Hormonal feedback is a mechanism regulating the secretion of hormones by the endocrine system itself. The production of a hormone is stimulated up to a certain level of action, beyond which it is inhibited. Based on the same mechanism, the secretion of certain hormones may be triggered by the level of concentration of other hormones in the blood.

3. Target cell
The hormone attaches itself on a specific target cell receptor, located on the cellular membrane (membranous receptor) or inside the cell (nuclear receptor), which triggers a series of biological reactions. A particular action results: production of a substance, activation or inhibition of the expression of a gene, acceleration or slowdown of a process, etc. The effects of hormones may be immediate or spread out over time.

THE **THYROID GLAND**

The thyroid gland is an endocrine gland located under the larynx and in front of the trachea, in the back of the neck. It secretes hormones (calcitonin and thyroid hormones) which act on growth, the **metabolism** and the level of calciumin the blood.

CALCITONIN
AND THE **THYROID HORMONES**

The thyroid secretes calcitonin, a hormone that reduces the level of calcium in circulation in the blood and increases its concentration in the bones. The injection of synthetic calcitonin is prescribed in the treatment of certain bone diseases (osteoporosis, Paget's disease). The thyroid also secretes thyroid hormones (T3 and T4), which accelerate the general functioning of the body (basal metabolism), specifically by increasing the consumption of oxygen and the production of heat.

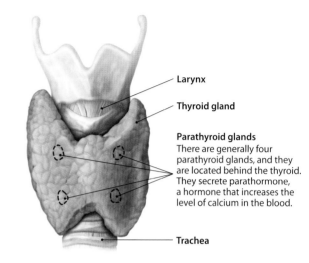

Larynx

Thyroid gland

Parathyroid glands
There are generally four parathyroid glands, and they are located behind the thyroid. They secrete parathormone, a hormone that increases the level of calcium in the blood.

Trachea

THE **ADRENAL GLANDS**

The adrenal glands are two endocrine glands located above the kidneys and consisting of two distinct parts: the medulla, the central part of the gland, and the adrenal cortex, the peripheral part. The medulla secretes adrenaline and noradrenaline, while the adrenal cortex secretes **corticosteroids** (aldosterone, cortisol, adrenal androgens). Synthetic corticosteroids are used as **anti-inflammatories** or **immunosuppressors**.

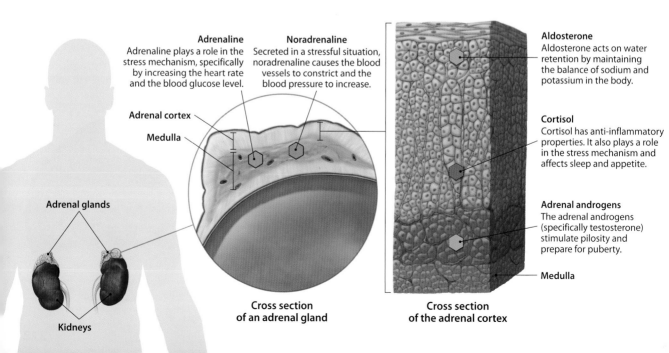

Adrenaline
Adrenaline plays a role in the stress mechanism, specifically by increasing the heart rate and the blood glucose level.

Noradrenaline
Secreted in a stressful situation, noradrenaline causes the blood vessels to constrict and the blood pressure to increase.

Aldosterone
Aldosterone acts on water retention by maintaining the balance of sodium and potassium in the body.

Cortisol
Cortisol has anti-inflammatory properties. It also plays a role in the stress mechanism and affects sleep and appetite.

Adrenal androgens
The adrenal androgens (specifically testosterone) stimulate pilosity and prepare for puberty.

Adrenal cortex

Medulla

Adrenal glands

Kidneys

Medulla

Cross section of an adrenal gland

Cross section of the adrenal cortex

THE PITUITARY GLAND

The pituitary gland is an endocrine gland located at the base of the brain. It is controlled in part by the hypothalamus, to which it is connected. The pituitary gland directly secretes six hormones, several of which govern the activity of the other endocrine glands. It also ensures the storage and the release of two hormones produced by the hypothalamus.

THE **STRUCTURE** OF THE **PITUITARY GLAND**

The pituitary gland consists of two lobes, the adenopituitary and the neuropituitary. These function independently from each other and according to different mechanisms. The adenohypophysis secretes the growth hormone and hormones performing a regulatory function on the other endocrine glands. These hormones are secreted in response to a hormonal stimulation that comes from the hypothalamus, connected to the pituitary gland by blood vessels. The neurohypophysis is connected to the hypothalamus by neurons. It stores two hormones (vasopressin and oxytocin) secreted by certain neurons of the hypothalamus and releases them into the bloodstream as needed.

Neurons... page 136

Pituitary gland
The pituitary gland is located in a cavity of the sphenoid bone.

Brain

Sphenoid bone

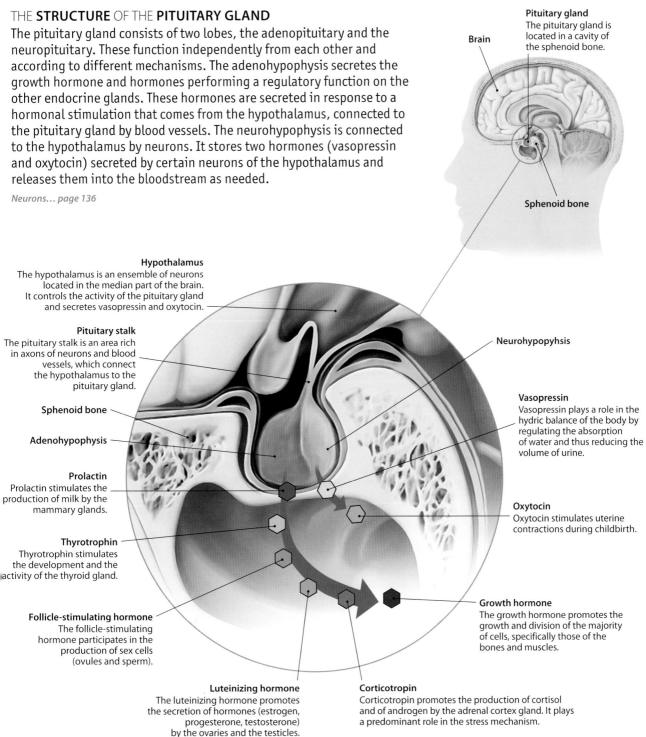

Hypothalamus
The hypothalamus is an ensemble of neurons located in the median part of the brain. It controls the activity of the pituitary gland and secretes vasopressin and oxytocin.

Pituitary stalk
The pituitary stalk is an area rich in axons of neurons and blood vessels, which connect the hypothalamus to the pituitary gland.

Sphenoid bone

Adenohypophysis

Prolactin
Prolactin stimulates the production of milk by the mammary glands.

Thyrotrophin
Thyrotrophin stimulates the development and the activity of the thyroid gland.

Follicle-stimulating hormone
The follicle-stimulating hormone participates in the production of sex cells (ovules and sperm).

Luteinizing hormone
The luteinizing hormone promotes the secretion of hormones (estrogen, progesterone, testosterone) by the ovaries and the testicles.

Corticotropin
Corticotropin promotes the production of cortisol and of androgen by the adrenal cortex gland. It plays a predominant role in the stress mechanism.

Neurohypopyhsis

Vasopressin
Vasopressin plays a role in the hydric balance of the body by regulating the absorption of water and thus reducing the volume of urine.

Oxytocin
Oxytocin stimulates uterine contractions during childbirth.

Growth hormone
The growth hormone promotes the growth and division of the majority of cells, specifically those of the bones and muscles.

STRESS

Stress is the body's response to physical and psychological attacks. It is a normal reaction that prepares the body to act by fight or flight. When the attacks are multiple and pronounced, the stress may become harmful and cause a state of excessive agitation, followed by physical and psychological exhaustion. In addition, stress decreases the body's immune defenses. Prolonged, it can promote the development of diseases and various disorders: psoriasis, eczema, endocrine, cardiovascular and digestive disorders, insomnia, depression, etc.

Stress management… page 28

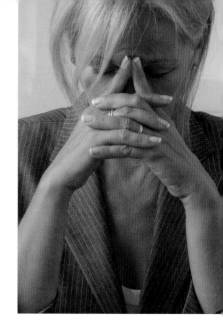

THE **MECHANISMS** OF **STRESS**

When the body is subject to a stress factor, the hypothalamus reacts so as to enable the body to respond to the attack by an immediate physical action (fight or flight). This reaction, both nervous and hormonal, acts on the metabolism and on different organs. Useful in case of physical danger, these biological reactions are, however, inappropriate for certain psychological attacks.

STRESS FACTORS

Stress factors are extremely varied external events, which can be negative or positive: accident, danger, disease, surgery, interpersonal conflict, intensive work, birth, promotion, marriage, moving, etc. The body's response (stress) to these events depends on the individual. Rest, playing a sport and relaxation make it possible to combat the harmful effects of prolonged stress.

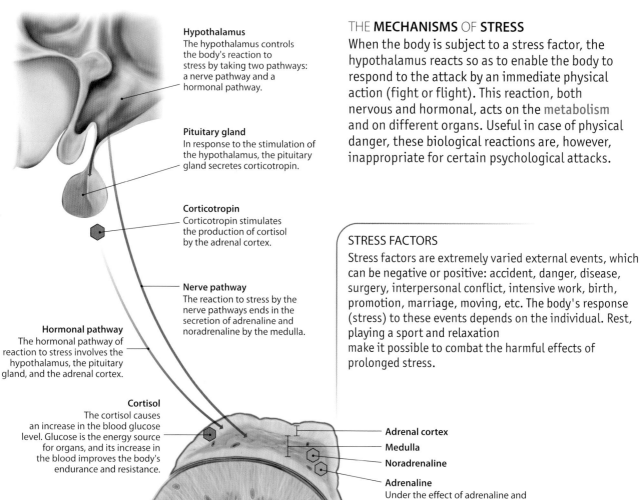

Hypothalamus
The hypothalamus controls the body's reaction to stress by taking two pathways: a nerve pathway and a hormonal pathway.

Pituitary gland
In response to the stimulation of the hypothalamus, the pituitary gland secretes corticotropin.

Corticotropin
Corticotropin stimulates the production of cortisol by the adrenal cortex.

Nerve pathway
The reaction to stress by the nerve pathways ends in the secretion of adrenaline and noradrenaline by the medulla.

Hormonal pathway
The hormonal pathway of reaction to stress involves the hypothalamus, the pituitary gland, and the adrenal cortex.

Cortisol
The cortisol causes an increase in the blood glucose level. Glucose is the energy source for organs, and its increase in the blood improves the body's endurance and resistance.

Kidney

Adrenal cortex
Medulla
Noradrenaline
Adrenaline
Under the effect of adrenaline and noradrenaline, the respiratory and cardiac rhythms accelerate, the cerebral activity intensifies, and the muscles are stimulated. The body is thus prepared for physical action.

THE **DISEASES** OF THE **THYROID GLAND**

Thyroid gland imbalances are expressed through either the excessive or insufficient functioning of the gland and result in serious **metabolic** problems. Women are more affected than men, and individuals whose diets are poor in iodine are particularly affected.

HYPERTHYRODISM

The excessive secretion of thyroid hormones, called hyperthyroidism, is manifested through various symptoms: goiter formation, excessive weakness, feeling of heat, weight loss, cardiac arrhythmia, insomnia, anxiety, excessive perspiration, trembling, diarrhea, etc. The most common causes of hyperthyroidism are Graves-Basedow disease, the presence of one or several thyroid nodules, and the **inflammation** of the thyroid.

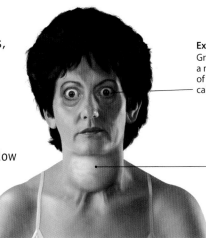

Exophthalmia
Graves-Basedow disease can cause a more or less marked protrusion of the eyes outside of the sockets, called exophthalmia.

Goiter
A goiter is the increase in thyroid gland volume. It can appear in connection with hypothyroidism or hyperthyroidism, be caused by a tumor, or develop for no known reason. Goiter affects 800 million people throughout the world.

Symptoms of Graves-Basedow disease
Graves-Basedow disease is an **autoimmune** disease resulting in hyperthyroidism.

THYROID NODULES

A thyroid nodule is a localized swelling of the thyroid gland. It may be a proliferation of cells (benign tumor, cancer of the thyroid) or a cyst. Thyroid nodules are common but benign in more than 90% of cases. Some nodules, called functional, secrete hormones and may cause hyperthyroidism.

THE DISEASES OF THE THYROID GLAND

SYMPTOMS:
Goiter, excessive weakness, weight gain or loss, feeling of cold or of heat, cardiac rhythm problems, trembling, change in the appearance of skin and hair, intestinal problems, etc.

TREATMENTS:
Hypothyroidism: hormonal treatment.
Hyperthyroidism: anti-thyroid drugs, partial or total removal of the thyroid gland, administration of radioactive iodine, hormonal treatment.

PREVENTION:
Adequate consumption of iodine (present in seafood products).

HYPOTHYRODISM

An insufficient secretion of thyroid hormones, called hypothyroidism, may result from a **congenital** anomaly, **chronic** thyroiditis, iodine deficiency, thyroid removal, treatment with radioactive iodine, or pituitary insufficiency. Hypothyroidism presents varied symptoms: **edema** of the face, sensitivity to the cold, bulging eyes, constipation, drying and thickening of the skin, hair loss, pallor, lethargy, decline in mental acuity, formation of a goiter (iodine deficiency), etc. If left untreated, serious hypothyroidism in newborns results in an irreversible delay in physical (small stature, abnormal proportions) and **psychomotor** development.

THE **DISEASES** OF THE **PITUITARY GLAND**

The most common pituitary gland disorders are tumors (adenomas), most often benign. They cause an increase or decrease in hormonal production. They may result, depending on the hormones in question, from growth problems, insipid diabetes, lactation problems, pituitary insufficiency, or a malfunction of the endocrine glands controlled by the pituitary hormones (adrenal cortex, sex and thyroid glands). By compressing the adjacent organs, the tumors may also cause headaches, intracranial hypertension and vision problems. In addition to drug treatment, the removal of the tumor, or even the pituitary gland, is sometimes necessary, together with a **radiation therapy** treatment.

THE **PITUITARY ADENOMA**

The pituitary adenoma is a benign tumor that develops in the front lobe of the pituitary gland (adenohypophysis) and disrupts its hormonal secretions. The adenoma causes a variety of problems depending on the hormones concerned: Cushing's disease, acromegaly, gigantism, pituitary insufficiency or galactorrhea (milky discharges that occur for no apparent reason). The surgical treatment of the pituitary adenoma consists in removing the tumor, taking care not to damage the pituitary gland. In certain cases, the pituitary gland must be removed with the adenoma. Treatment by hormone replacement therapy must then be followed.

DIABETES INSIPIDUS

Diabetes insipidus is a disease that is completely different from diabetes mellitus. It is characterized by the inability of the kidneys to concentrate urine, which causes abundant urination and intense thirst. Diabetes insipidus is caused by a vasopressin deficiency or a kidney's insensitivity to this hormone. Vasopressin is released by the pituitary gland and, normally, acts on the kidneys in order to cause the resorption of water in the blood.

CUSHING'S DISEASE

Cushing's disease is a rare disorder that primarily affects women between 20 and 40 years of age. It is caused by a pituitary adenoma which results in the excessive secretion of a hormone produced by the adrenal glands, cortisol. The disease is manifested through Cushing's syndrome, an ensemble of symptoms caused by the hypersecretion of cortisol: redistribution of fat in the face and the trunk, weight gain, weakness of the skin and capillaries, slow healing, muscular atrophy. Patients also suffer from high blood pressure and osteoporosis, and some develop diabetes.

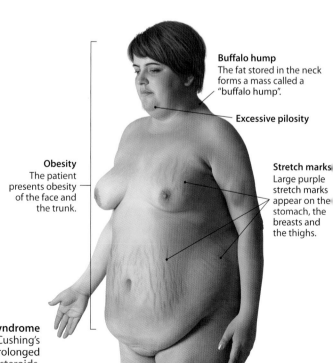

Buffalo hump
The fat stored in the neck forms a mass called a "buffalo hump".

Excessive pilosity

Obesity
The patient presents obesity of the face and the trunk.

Stretch marks
Large purple stretch marks appear on the stomach, the breasts and the thighs.

Cushing's syndrome
Cushing's syndrome may result from Cushing's disease, but also from a tumor or prolonged treatment with **corticosteroids**.

Bruising

ACROMEGALY

Acromegaly is a rare disorder that is found only in adults. It is characterized by an abnormal increase in the size of the nose, ears, chin, hands and feet compared with the rest of the body, as well as by hypertrophy of the heart and the thyroid gland. These permanent morphological changes result from an excessive secretion of growth hormone, most often due to a pituitary adenoma. Acromegaly may also result in a deformation of the spinal cord and osteoarthritis. In children, the hypersecretion of growth hormone causes gigantism.

PITUITARY INSUFFICIENCY

A pituitary tumor (adenoma) or a necrosis can cause a deficiency in pituitary hormones, or pituitary insufficiency. This results in a decrease in the activity of the glands controlled by the pituitary gland. The resulting problems occur progressively and vary depending on the hormone concerned: disappearance of body hair, weakening of hair, dry skin, decrease in intellectual capacities, memory problems, decrease in libido, amenorrhea, erectile dysfunction, growth stoppage in children, absence of puberty, etc.

Face
The morphology of the face changes: thickened features, detached ears, separated teeth, overhanging brows. The nose thickens while the lower jaw juts out.

Goiter
The development of a goiter (hypertrophy of the thyroid) is common.

Skin
The skin is thick, red and coarse. Perspiration is excessive.

Hand
The hands become large and thicken.

Foot
The feet are wider and bulkier. The big toe is abnormally enlarged.

Symptoms of acromegaly

THE DISEASES OF THE PITUITARY GLAND

SYMPTOMS:
The symptoms depend on the hormone affected: growth problems, lactation problems, diabetes, Cushing's syndrome, sexual problems, etc. Pituitary tumors (adenomas): headaches, intracranial hypertension, vision problems.

TREATMENTS:
Hormone replacement treatment. Pituitary adenoma: surgical removal, drug therapy, radiation therapy.

GIGANTISM

Gigantism is a rapid and exaggerated development of the skeleton, which may be constitutional or result from the hypersecretion of growth hormone before puberty. This growth problem results in excessive size without alteration of body proportions. Robert Pershing Wadlow (1918-1940), an American suffering from gigantism, measured 8 feet 11 inches (2.72 meters) at his death, almost the height of a bus. He is the tallest man that ever lived.

DIABETES

Diabetes, or diabetes mellitus, currently affects 200 million people and is the 5th cause of death throughout the world. This **chronic** disease, in constant increase, is characterized by an excess of glucose in the blood (hyperglycemia), which causes abundant urination and intense thirst. A distinction is made between type 1 and type 2 diabetes, which do not have the same cause, but can result in the same complications. These result from attacks on the blood vessels caused by the excess sugar: infarction, cerebral vascular accident, ulcer, gangrene, diabetic retinopathy, kidney failure, sensory problems, etc.

Diabetes insipidus… page 226

THE **NORMAL REGULATION** OF **GLYCEMIA**

Glycemia is the level of glucose in the blood. It is primarily regulated by two hormones produced by the pancreas, insulin and glucagon. These two hormones have antagonist effects: insulin lowers glycemia by promoting the use and the storage of glucose, while the glucagon causes its release into the blood by the liver. The blood glucose level, which is normally approximately 5 millimoles per liter (or 1 gram per liter), may be measured by blood analysis.

The pancreas… page 350

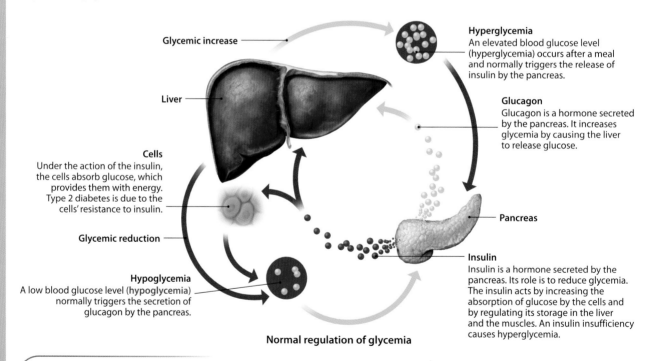

Glycemic increase

Liver

Cells
Under the action of the insulin, the cells absorb glucose, which provides them with energy. Type 2 diabetes is due to the cells' resistance to insulin.

Glycemic reduction

Hypoglycemia
A low blood glucose level (**hypoglycemia**) normally triggers the secretion of glucagon by the pancreas.

Hyperglycemia
An elevated blood glucose level (hyperglycemia) occurs after a meal and normally triggers the release of insulin by the pancreas.

Glucagon
Glucagon is a hormone secreted by the pancreas. It increases glycemia by causing the liver to release glucose.

Pancreas

Insulin
Insulin is a hormone secreted by the pancreas. Its role is to reduce glycemia. The insulin acts by increasing the absorption of glucose by the cells and by regulating its storage in the liver and the muscles. An insulin insufficiency causes hyperglycemia.

Normal regulation of glycemia

HYPOGLYCEMIA AND HYPERGLYCEMIA

Hyperglycemia is an increase in the blood glucose level, considered pathological beyond 7 mmol/l or 1.2 g/l. Significant and sustained hyperglycemia causes fatigue, increased appetite, and intense thirst. It is treated by an adapted diet, by hypoglycemic drugs, or by insulin injection. Hypoglycemia is a reduction in the blood glucose level (less than 3.5 mmol/l or 0.6 g/l), capable of causing a loss of consciousness. In diabetics, hypoglycemia can occur following an overdose of insulin, in case of hypoglycemic treatment, after a physical activity, or an insufficient meal. It is then treated through the administration of sugar.

TYPE 1 DIABETES

Type 1, or insulin-dependent diabetes, is an autoimmune disease that causes the destruction of the pancreatic cells producing the insulin, resulting in hyperglycemia. It accounts for 10% of cases of diabetes and generally appears before the age of 20, most often around the age of 12. Since the pancreas is unable to produce insulin in a quantity sufficient to prevent hyperglycemia, the treatment of type 1 diabetes requires the regular administration of insulin. It also requires an adapted diet and frequent self-testing of glycemia by capillary sampling. Left untreated, the disease can result in a coma, or even death.

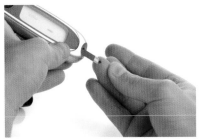

Capillary sampling
Self-testing of glycemia is done using a glucometer and a lancet device, which makes it possible to take a drop of blood from a fingertip.

THE SYMPTOMS OF TYPE 1 DIABETES

At the onset of the disease, the patient often does not feel any symptoms. When glycemia reaches very high values, the body tries to eliminate the excess glucose by increasing the frequency and abundance of urination, and by producing urine with a high sugar content. Dehydration follows, which causes intense thirst. Appetite increases, but this generally does not prevent weight loss. Type 1 diabetes also causes fatigue and headaches, and may promote repeated infections.

INSULIN INJECTION

Insulin injections are given from one to four times per day according to the individuals, by means of a single-use syringe, or with a reloadable insulin pen. They may also be given automatically and continuously using an insulin pump, a device worn at the waist and equipped with a catheter fixed under the skin. Insulin injections must be given in the subcutaneous tissue (hypodermis). An intra-muscular injection would cause the insulin to act too quickly, risking hypoglycemia, while too superficial an injection would cause the insulin to act too slowly, resulting in hyperglycemia.

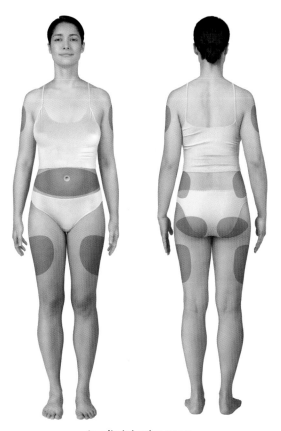

GESTATIONAL DIABETES

Gestational diabetes, or pregnancy diabetes, is an intolerance to glucose that occurs during pregnancy, generally during the 6th month. It may cause premature childbirth, as well as complications for the fetus (excess weight, heart malformation) and for the pregnant woman (gravidic hypertension). It generally disappears after childbirth. Women having suffered from gestational diabetes present an elevated risk for developing type 2 diabetes later.

Insulin injection areas
Many injection areas are possible and must be chosen on an alternating basis in the same day. Within the same area, each injection must be 1.2 inches (3 cm) away from the previous one.

LIVING WITH DIABETES

If you have diabetes, you must take a number of daily precautions in order to prevent the complications connected with the disease. The main recommendations consist of properly controlling your glycemia and adopting a healthy lifestyle.

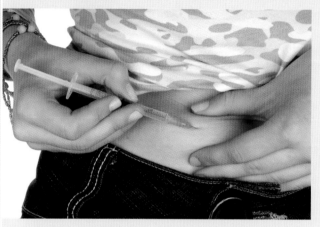

SCRUPULOUSLY FOLLOW YOUR TREATMENTS

Regularly monitor your glycemia and respect your medication by adapting it to different situations: sports, travel, diet, etc.

ADOPT PROPER ORAL HYGIENE

Diabetes promotes the production of dental plaque and thus the destruction of the support tissues of the teeth (periodontitis), specifically when glycemia is poorly controlled. In addition, a dental infection may, in turn, interfere with the regulation of glycemia. It is therefore important that you adopt good oral hygiene, in addition to controlling your glycemia.

TAKE CARE OF YOUR FEET

Diabetes promotes the development of ulcers. Clean and moisturize your feet regularly. Pumice callouses, file your nails. Avoid walking with bare feet. Wear clean and dry socks as well as comfortable shoes, being careful that they do not contain any harmful object (pebbles, twigs, etc.). Examine your feet daily and meticulously. In case of a minor lesion, wash, bandage and monitor it. If there is an infection (redness, swelling, presence of pus) or in case of a more serious injury, consult a doctor immediately.

HAVE EYE, BLOOD AND URINE TESTS ANNUALLY AND MONITOR YOUR BLOOD PRESSURE

Regular tests permit the immediate treatment of any damage.

ENGAGE IN A REGULAR PHYSICAL ACTIVITY

By engaging in a physical activity, particularly an endurance activity, you will be able to better control your glycemia. It is important, however, to pay particular attention to your feet by wearing the appropriate shoes. Also make sure to eat enough before and after the sport, to adapt your glycemic monitoring and your injections, and to have sugar on hand to counter hypoglycemia.

ADOPT A HEALTHY DIET

Have your meals and snacks at regular hours and maintain a healthy weight by eating in a balanced and diversified manner. Give preference to foods rich in fiber (vegetables, whole grains, legumes) and foods low in fats, salt and sugar.

LIMIT YOUR ALCOHOL CONSUMPTION TO ONE GLASS PER DAY, AT MEAL TIME

STOP SMOKING

PLAN AHEAD WHEN TRAVELING

Travel only if your diabetes is under control and if you are not suffering from any disabling complication. Prepare for your trip carefully, specifically by consulting your doctor and informing yourself about the health conditions and medical resources in your destination country. Be vigilant about your treatment, your diet, etc.

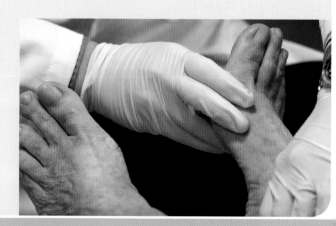

The endocrine system | Diseases

TYPE 2 DIABETES

Type 2, or non-insulin-dependent diabetes, is a chronic disease characterized by the resistance of the body's cells to the action of the insulin produced by the pancreas. The cells assimilate glucose poorly and it accumulates in the blood (hyperglycemia). As a result, the pancreas provides more and more insulin to lower glycemia, without effect. It becomes progressively exhausted, resulting in a decrease in insulin production that must be compensated for through injections. Type 2 diabetes is connected with aging, obesity, a sedentary lifestyle, as well as genetic factors that are poorly understood. It is increasing in industrialized countries and generally appears around age 50, but it is more and more common in younger people. It may remain asymptomatic for several years before revealing itself through a complication. Its treatment is based on reducing sugar and fats in the diet, increasing physical activity, and the administration of hypoglycemic drugs or insulin.

DIABETES

SYMPTOMS:
Onset often asymptomatic, thirst, frequent urination, loss of consciousness.
Type 1: weight loss.

TREATMENTS:
Type 1: administration of insulin and adapted diet.
Type 2: strict diet, physical activity, hypoglycemic drugs, insulin as needed.

PREVENTION:
Type 2: Weight loss (particularly in case of abdominal obesity), healthy lifestyle (balanced diet, physical activity). Diabetes complications can be limited by early screening and strict control of glycemia.

Eye disorders
Diabetes is responsible for diabetic retinopathy, which can cause blindness. It also promotes cataracts.

Cardiovascular diseases
The risk of cardiovascular diseases (myocardial infarction, cerebral vascular accident) is aggravated by excess cholesterol, high blood pressure, and abdominal obesity. Almost one half of all diabetics die from a coronary insufficiency.

Kidney disorders
Diabetes can cause diabetic neuropathy and kidney failure.

Sensitivity problems
Diabetes reduces sensitivity (particularly in the hands and feet), while preventing the proper healing of wounds, which increases the risk of ulcers. An ulcer can develop into gangrene. Thus, 5% to 10% of diabetics must undergo an amputation of a toe, a foot, or a leg.

Possible complications of diabetes
The complications of both types of diabetes are the same. They result from the alteration in the blood vessels caused by hyperglycemia.

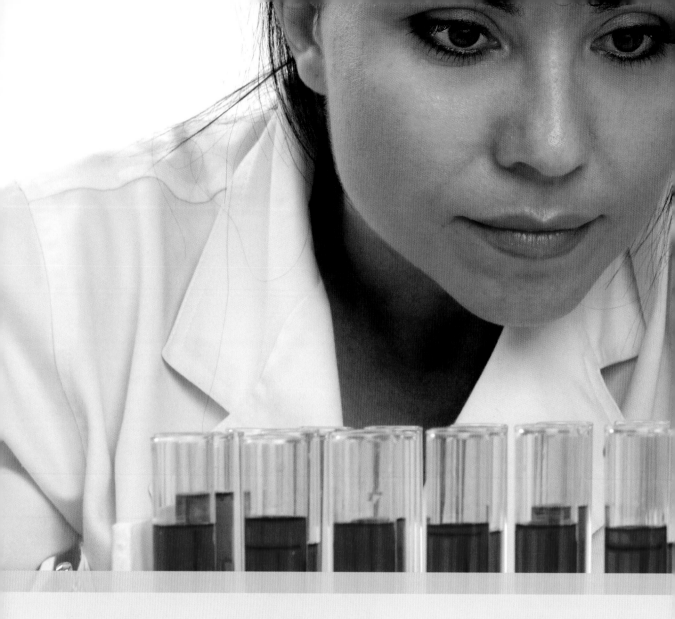

THE **BLOOD**

The proper functioning of our body is in large part ensured by the blood. This red liquid, pumped by the heart, circulates permanently from one end of the body to the other through the blood vessels. Blood has the fundamental role of distributing to the cells all of the elements that are indispensable for them (oxygen, nutritive substances, hormones, etc.) and of ensuring the evacuation of carbon dioxide and cellular waste. Blood also participates in the regulation of body temperature and the volume of bodily fluids. Furthermore, the white blood cells that it contains protect us from foreign agents such as germs.

Anomalies in the volume and the composition of blood result in problems that can more or less seriously affect the functioning of the body. Losses of blood (hemorrhages), normally quickly contained by the body itself, can be fatal if too profuse. Modifications in the number and appearance of different blood cells (red blood cells, white blood cells, etc.) are associated with diseases such as **anemia** and leukemia.Blood analyses, performed using blood samples, make it possible to diagnose these diseases.

THE **BLOOD**

Blood is a red, slightly viscous liquid that circulates in the blood vessels, pumped by the heart. Indispensable, it is responsible for transporting oxygen and nutritive substances to the cells and removing waste from them. The circulation of blood in the blood system participates in controlling body temperature as well as in regulating the volume of certain fluids in the tissues. In addition, the blood transports white blood cells, which defend our body against germs.

THE **COMPOSITION** OF **BLOOD**

Blood consists of a liquid element, the plasma, in which the blood cells bathe: red blood cells, white blood cells, and platelets. On average, plasma represents 54% of the total blood volume, the red blood cells 45%, the white blood cells, and platelets 1%. The red blood cells (or erythrocytes) transport oxygen from the lungs to the cells, and carbon dioxide from the cells to the lungs. The white blood cells (or leukocytes) have the ability to cross through the blood vessel wall and to penetrate the tissues in order to defend against pathogenic agents. There are three major categories of white blood cells: lymphocytes, monocytes, and granulocytes.

Granulocyte
Granulocytes are white blood cells that present granulations and whose nucleus consists of several lobes. There are three types: neutrophils, eosinophils and basophils. Neutrophils respond quickly in the inflammatory reaction by destroying bacteria. Eosinophils and basophils play a role in allergic reactions.
The immune system... page 278

Blood plasma
Blood plasma is a yellowish fluid, consisting of water, nutriments, minerals and proteins, in which blood cells are in suspension. Plasma performs numerous functions, specifically the transport of nutritive elements and hormones to the cells as well as the distribution of heat in the body.

Monocyte
Monocytes are the most numerous white blood cells. They migrate into the tissues during an inflammation and are transformed into macrophages, cells capable of surrounding and destroying bacteria and dead cells.

Blood vessel
Blood is transported throughout the body by the blood vessels.

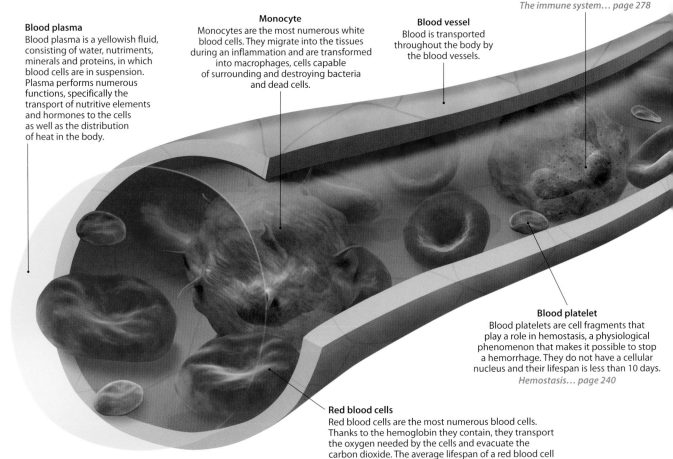

Blood platelet
Blood platelets are cell fragments that play a role in hemostasis, a physiological phenomenon that makes it possible to stop a hemorrhage. They do not have a cellular nucleus and their lifespan is less than 10 days.
Hemostasis... page 240

Red blood cells
Red blood cells are the most numerous blood cells. Thanks to the hemoglobin they contain, they transport the oxygen needed by the cells and evacuate the carbon dioxide. The average lifespan of a red blood cell is 120 days.

RED BLOOD CELLS BY THE BILLIONS

The adult body contains between 4.25 and 5.28 quarts (4 and 5 liters) of blood, in which circulate 25 trillion red blood cells, or 200 million in a single drop. Each red blood cell contains 250 million molecules of hemoglobin, which give blood its red color.

THE **FORMATION** OF **BLOOD CELLS**

The different blood cells are permanently formed in the red blood marrow in order to replace the millions that die each day. This process is called hematopoiesis. It is characterized by a type of cellular division that enables a stem cell to generate a cell different from itself. The most primitive stem cells (hemocytoblasts) give birth to two types of precursors: the lymphoid and myeloid stem cells. These, by dividing several times in turn, produce the white blood cells, the red blood cells and the platelets.

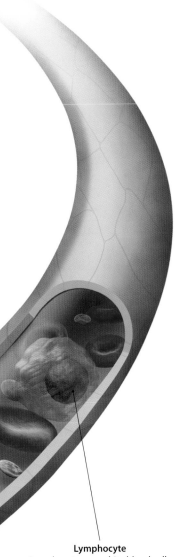

Lymphocyte
Lymphocytes are white blood cells that play an essential role in immunity, that is in defending the body against pathogenic agents. They produce antibodies and toxic substances that destroy germs. Stored in the lymphatic system, they are rapidly routed to the site of an infection by the blood circulation.
The lymphatic system… page 281

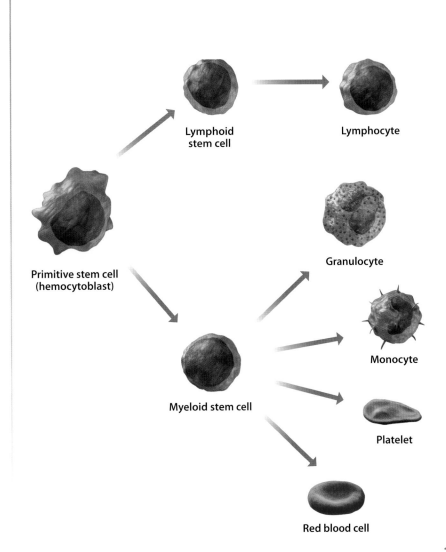

Lymphoid stem cell

Lymphocyte

Primitive stem cell (hemocytoblast)

Granulocyte

Monocyte

Myeloid stem cell

Platelet

Red blood cell

THE **BLOOD TRANSFUSION**

Without blood transfusion, significant losses of blood can be fatal. This consists of an injection of a concentration of red blood cells, platelets, or plasma. It may be done not only to compensate for a loss of blood (accident, surgery), but also to counter the side effects of heavy **chemotherapy** or to treat certain diseases such as **anemia**. The blood transfusion consists of several stages: the blood is first collected from voluntary donors, and then it is analyzed and processed before being injected in a receiver by intravenous drip.

THE **BLOOD DONATION**

A blood donation is a process by which a person (donor) voluntarily offers his blood or one of its components so that it can be used during blood transfusions. First, the donor is given a medical evaluation. The blood donation is completely harmless for a healthy person. Minor side effects, such as the appearance of an ecchymosis (or bruise), a swelling of the arm, a feeling of weakness and of nausea, or a reduction in iron level may sometimes temporarily occur following a donation. The blood collected is analyzed in order to make sure that it does not contain any infectious agent. It may be separated into platelets, plasma and red blood cells. These blood products have a lifespan of 5 to 35 days, with the exception of plasma, which can be frozen and stored for one year.

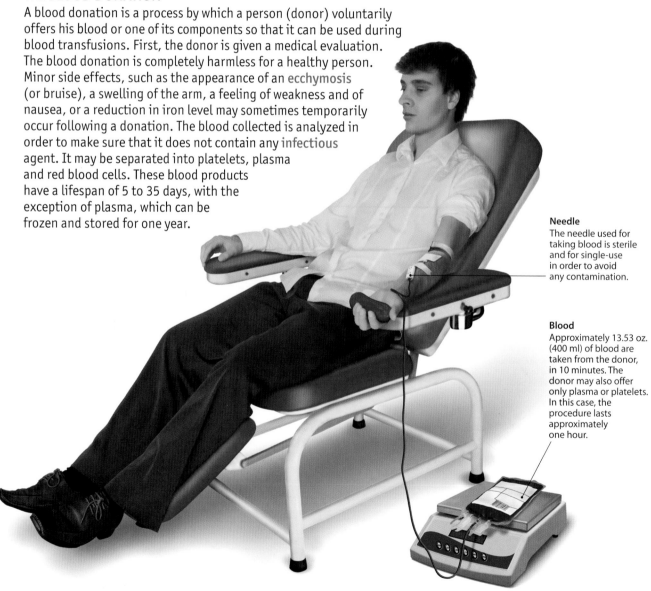

Needle
The needle used for taking blood is sterile and for single-use in order to avoid any contamination.

Blood
Approximately 13.53 oz. (400 ml) of blood are taken from the donor, in 10 minutes. The donor may also offer only plasma or platelets. In this case, the procedure lasts approximately one hour.

THE **BLOOD TYPES**

The blood transfusion must take into account the blood types of the donor and receiver in order to avoid the destruction of the transfused blood by the receiver's immune system. For a successful transfusion, the donor and the receiver must belong to the same blood type, that is to say their red blood cells must possess the same antigens. The antibodies present in the blood do not react to the antigens of the red blood cells from the same blood type. On the other hand, they destroy the foreign red blood cells, which have different antigens (rejection phenomenon). This immune reaction results in an anemia in the receiver and may even cause death. That is why the compatibility of blood types must be scrupulously respected. The blood types are combined into systems, of which the two main ones are the ABO system and the Rhesus system.

The immune system... page 278

THE ABO SYSTEM

The ABO system is based on the presence or the absence of A and B antigens. The A and B types include the individuals who are respectively the carriers of A and B antigens. People from the AB type carry both antigens. Those from the O type do not have any of them. The blood from type A contains antibodies against the B antigens and vice versa. The blood from type O has antibodies against both antigens, while the AB type does not have these antigens.

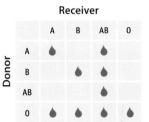

Compatibilities in the ABO system
The blood from type O can be transfused to individuals of all four types, but a type O subject can only receive blood belonging to his own type. Conversely, a person from the AB type can receive blood from the four types, but his blood is only transfused to individuals belonging to his own type.

THE RHESUS SYSTEM

The Rhesus system is based on the presence (Rh+) or the absence (Rh-) of the D antigen in the blood. Rh- individuals do not have antibodies against the D antigen. These can, however, appear following a blood transfusion from an Rh+ donor or after the birth of an Rh+ child. In the absence of appropriate treatment (vaccination), a subsequent pregnancy in an Rh- woman can have serious consequences for a newborn from the Rh+ type.

Rhesus incompatibility... page 480

Compatibilities in the Rhesus system
An Rh+ individual can receive the blood of an Rh+ or Rh- person, but his blood is only transfused to Rh+ individuals.

AUTOTRANSFUSION

Autotransfusion is the transfusion to an individual of his own blood, which was taken from him several days earlier. This type of procedure, practiced since the 1960s, makes it possible to avoid the incompatibilities between the blood of the donor and that of the receiver. It also makes it possible to avoid the transmission of contaminated blood (hepatitis, AIDS, malaria, syphilis), even though the risks today are very low due to the number of precautions taken. Autotransfusion can only be done if the need for blood is known in advance (scheduled surgery) and if the individual does not present any contraindication (infection, anemia). Autotransfusion is not always done for medical reasons. In fact, some athletes use it for a completely different reason: doping. The injection of a concentration of red blood cells, extracted from the blood taken a few days earlier, makes it possible to increase the transport of oxygen to the muscles, which also increases, in an illegal manner, endurance and performance.

THE **BLOOD SAMPLE**

Taking a sample of blood, or a blood sample collection, consists of taking a sample in order to perform blood analyses. The analyses make it possible to detect numerous disorders. These are manifested by the modification, in number or in appearance, of blood components (red blood cells, white blood cells, etc.) or by the presence of foreign bodies in the blood: bacteria, parasites, viruses.

THE **SAMPLING** OF **BLOOD**

The blood is collected from a vein or a capillary (very thin blood vessel) based on the volume needed and the type of test conducted. The venous sampling is most often done in the bend of the elbow. The capillary sampling consists of taking a drop of blood from a capillary, most often at the fingertip. It may be done at home using an easy-to-use lancet device, and specifically makes it possible for diabetics to check their blood glucose level.

Diabetes... page 228

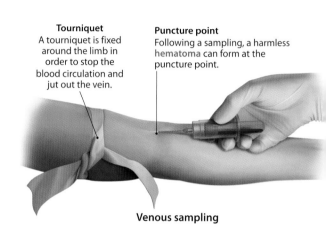

Tourniquet
A tourniquet is fixed around the limb in order to stop the blood circulation and jut out the vein.

Puncture point
Following a sampling, a harmless hematoma can form at the puncture point.

Venous sampling

BLOOD ANALYSIS TECHNIQUES

Diverse laboratory techniques make it possible to analyze blood. The blood smear is the examination of a drop of blood under the microscope. It makes it possible to study the morphological characteristics (shape, size, appearance) of red blood cells, white blood cells, and blood platelets in order to detect the presence of a parasite or possible anomalies, such as leukemia and anemia. The complete blood count (CBC) is an automated blood analysis that provides the breakdown per cubic millimeter of red blood cells, white blood cells, and platelets, as well as the percentage of each type of white blood cell. It makes it possible to detect various disorders: bacterial, viral or parasitic infection, anemia, leukemia, liver disorder, alcoholism, etc.

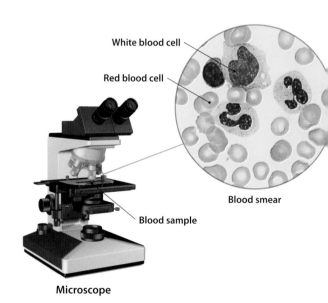

White blood cell

Red blood cell

Blood smear

Blood sample

Microscope

BLOOD SERUM ANALYSIS

The blood serum is a transparent, yellowish liquid. It is what remains of the plasma once the clotting factors, the proteins that enable the blood to coagulate, are removed. The serum analysis consists of finding different molecules (cholesterol, glucose, urea, proteins, antibodies, etc.) and in measuring their level. Excess cholesterol increases the risk of cardiovascular disease.
The presence of specific antibodies makes it possible to diagnose a bacterial, viral or parasitic infection. The accumulation of urea in the serum indicates a change in kidney functioning. The measurement of the glucose level specifically permits the diagnosis and monitoring of diabetes.

HEMORRHAGE

A hemorrhage is a more or less significant flow of blood outside of the blood vessels. The blood can flow inside or outside of the body. A hemorrhage is often caused by a wound or a violent shock, but the blood vessels may also burst spontaneously, as in the case of an aneurysm rupture. The seriousness of a hemorrhage varies according to the type of vessel affected and its location. The loss of a significant volume of blood can cause **hypovolemic shock**, or even death if it is greater than 30% of the total volume. An emergency blood transfusion must then be performed.

Aneurysm... page 270

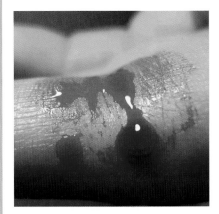

THE **EXTERNAL HEMORRHAGE**
The external hemorrhage is a flow of blood outside of the body, generally caused by a wound. It may affect an artery, a vein, or a capillary (small-diameter vessel). An arterial hemorrhage, characterized by a spasmodic squirting of bright red blood, can be dangerous because the blood is flowing rapidly. A venous hemorrhage is recognized by the dark red color of the blood and by its continuous flow. When the hemorrhage affects a capillary, the coagulation is quick and the losses of blood small.

Blood circulation and blood vessels... page 248

HYPOVOLEMIC SHOCK
Hypovolemic shock is a sudden weakening of the body's functioning (state of shock) due to a major reduction in blood volume. It most often occurs during a major hemorrhage, but it can also be caused by a massive loss of body fluids (very abundant diarrhea, serious burn, severe dehydration). Hypovolemic shock is expressed by cold and pale extremities, dizziness and vomiting, acceleration and weakening of the pulse, acceleration of respiration, intense thirst, and sometimes by loss of consciousness. The quantity of oxygen in the tissues decreases, which may result in serious functional problems. The body maintains the circulation in the most important organs (heart, lungs, brain) for as long as possible. When these are affected, death is imminent.

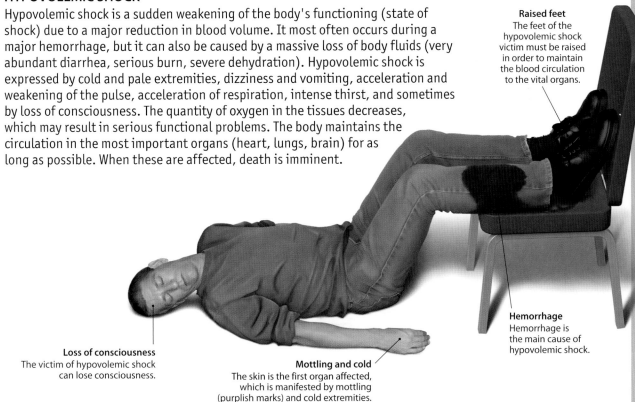

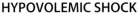

Raised feet
The feet of the hypovolemic shock victim must be raised in order to maintain the blood circulation to the vital organs.

Hemorrhage
Hemorrhage is the main cause of hypovolemic shock.

Loss of consciousness
The victim of hypovolemic shock can lose consciousness.

Mottling and cold
The skin is the first organ affected, which is manifested by mottling (purplish marks) and cold extremities.

HEMOSTASIS

When a wound causes blood to flow, the body quickly reacts by sealing off the opening by forming a blood clot. The ensemble of physiological phenomena that lead to the stopping of a hemorrhage and the repair of the damaged blood vessel is called hemostasis. It occurs in three successive stages: vasoconstriction, formation of a platelet plug, and coagulation.

1. Vasoconstriction

When a blood vessel is injured, the body immediately reacts by reducing the diameter of the vessel (vasoconstriction), which results in locally reducing blood circulation and limiting blood loss.

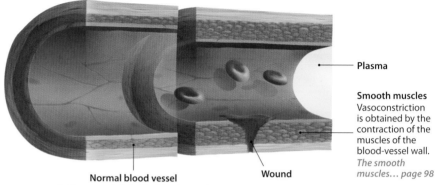

Plasma

Smooth muscles
Vasoconstriction is obtained by the contraction of the muscles of the blood-vessel wall. *The smooth muscles… page 98*

Normal blood vessel
In the normal state, the blood vessel muscles are slightly contracted.

Wound

2. Formation of a platelet plug

The platelet plug is an aggregate of blood platelets that form when a blood vessel is injured. The platelets swell and attach themselves to collagen, a type of protein present in the vessel wall. At the same time, they release substances promoting vasoconstriction and attracting new platelets.

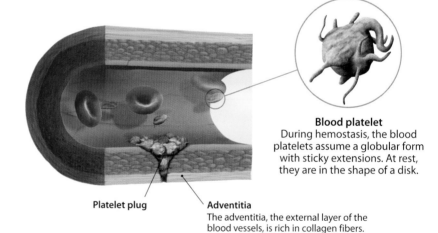

Blood platelet
During hemostasis, the blood platelets assume a globular form with sticky extensions. At rest, they are in the shape of a disk.

Platelet plug

Adventitia
The adventitia, the external layer of the blood vessels, is rich in collagen fibers.

3. Blood coagulation

Blood coagulation is the transformation of liquid blood into a semi-solid mass called a blood clot. This is composed of blood platelets, red blood cells, and fibrin (a protein). The fibrin, in the wound, acts as a kind of framework that reinforces the platelet plug and contains the red blood cells in order to form the blood clot. When the wound is healed, the clot dissolves.

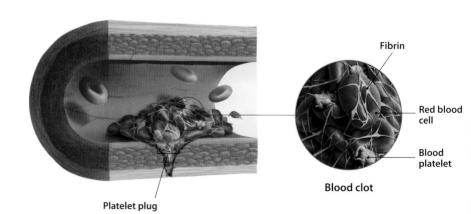

Fibrin

Red blood cell

Blood platelet

Blood clot

Platelet plug

THE **INTERNAL HEMORRHAGE**

The internal hemorrhage is a flow of blood inside a cavity, an organ or a tissue of the body. It may be caused by a more or less violent shock, an anomaly of the pregnancy, a cardiovascular problem, or by other disorders (cancer, hemophilia). An internal hemorrhage is sometimes expressed through a hematoma or through a discharge of blood through natural means: blood in the urine or in the stool, spitting or vomiting blood. It is not necessarily visible and may be expressed through indirect signs such as pains and functional problems. A significant outpouring of blood may result in hypovolemic shock, potentially fatal.

Abdominal hemorrhage
In case of abdominal hemorrhage, several quarts of blood may pour out into the abdomen, causing pain, swelling, and hypovolemic shock.

THE HEMATOMA

The hematoma is a mass of blood in a tissue or an organ that appears following an internal hemorrhage. The majority of hematomas are spontaneously resorbed, but some can cause pressure on the adjacent tissues and cause other dysfunctions. In case of voluminous and compressive hematoma, the blood may be evacuated by puncture or surgical incision of the skin. An ecchymosis (or bruise) is a subcutaneous hematoma, often caused by a shock. It is manifested by a blackish or bluish coloration of the skin and is resorbed in a few days.

Bruise
The bruise is resorbed taking on a yellowish color.

HEMORRHAGE

SYMPTOMS:
Internal hemorrhage: pain, swelling, loss of consciousness, discharge through natural means, hematoma.

TREATMENTS:
Wound compression (external hemorrhage), blood transfusion in case of significant loss of blood, suture of the injured vessels, puncture (internal hemorrhage). Capillary hemorrhages and bruises do not require treatment.

First aid: Hemorrhages… page 550

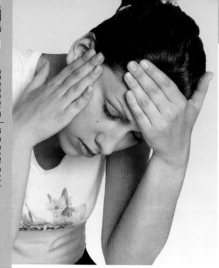

ANEMIAS

Anemia is an abnormal reduction of the hemoglobin level in the blood. Hemoglobin is the protein that allows the red blood cells to transport the oxygen that the body needs. Anemia thus results in a reduction in the blood's capacity to transport oxygen to the cells, which causes generally benign problems (pallor, fatigue, dizziness, shortness of breath, etc.). Several types of anemia can be distinguished based on their origin.

IRON-DEFICIENCY ANEMIA

The most common anemia is iron-deficiency anemia. It is caused by a deficiency in iron, a mineral element essential for the formation of hemoglobin. Iron-deficiency anemia appears most often in pregnant women or in children, whose iron needs are significant. It may also be caused by heavy periods or by a hemorrhage, such as digestive tract bleeding. Blood analysis reveals smaller and paler red blood cells.

PERNICIOUS ANEMIA

Pernicious anemia is caused by a deficiency in Vitamins B12 or B9, which prevents the normal formation of red blood cells. This deficiency may come from insufficient supply in the diet, but it most often results from poor absorption of these vitamins by the intestinal mucosa.

APLASTIC ANEMIA

Aplastic anemia is caused by the insufficient production of red blood cells by the red bone marrow stem cells. This rather rare form of anemia can be caused by toxic substances or by medical treatments (chemotherapy, radiation therapy). It can develop into leukemia.

HEMOLYTIC ANEMIA

Hemolytic anemia is caused by the abnormal and excessive destruction of red blood cells. It may be of autoimmune origin or result from an incompatible blood transfusion, from an infection (malaria) or a congenital disease such as sickle-cell anemia.

ANEMIAS

SYMPTOMS:
Pallor, fatigue, dizziness, shortness of breath, feeling of cold, palpitations, headaches. Slight anemias may be asymptomatic. Sickle-cell anemia: intense pain in the limbs and abdomen, icterus (jaundice).

TREATMENTS:
Based on origin: iron or Vitamin B9 supplements, intramuscular injection of Vitamin B12, stopping the hemorrhage, treatment of the infection, blood transfusion, bone marrow transplant.

PREVENTION:
Diet sufficiently rich in iron and in Vitamins B12 and B9 (meat, fish, seafood, etc.).

THE PREVENTION OF IRON-DEFICIENCY ANEMIA

You can prevent iron-deficiency anemia by adopting a diet sufficiently rich in iron, especially if you are a person at risk: growing children and adolescents, pregnant women, nursing women, or women with heavy periods. The following foods are rich in iron:

• Meat (specifically liver and blood sausage)

• Fish and shellfish

• Eggs

• Whole grain cereal products

• Dark green leafy vegetables (spinach, broccoli, kale, etc.)

• Soybeans and legumes

• Dry fruits, grains and nuts

Iron from an animal source is best absorbed by the body. It also allows for better absorption of iron from a plant source. Foods rich in Vitamin C (cabbage, cauliflower, citrus fruit, broccoli, pepper, tomato, strawberry, kiwi, etc.) also promote iron absorption. Conversely, the consumption of tea or coffee during meals is harmful to its absorption.

THALASSEMIA

Thalassemia is a hereditary disease characterized by defective hemoglobin production. It most often results in anemia. The most severe forms require regular blood transfusions. Thalassemia primarily affects the populations of the Mediterranean basin, the Middle East, India, Sub-Saharan Africa and Southeast Asia.

SICKLE-CELL ANEMIA

Sickle-cell anemia, or drepanocytosis, is a recessive hereditary disease characterized by the abnormal production of hemoglobin. The red blood cells, deformed and more rigid, obstruct the thinnest blood capillaries, which causes sudden and intense pain (hands, feet, abdomen, hips). The destruction of abnormal red blood cells by the spleen causes hemolytic anemia and a hypertrophy of the spleen. Patients suffer from a nutritional deficiency, which causes delayed growth, and are also more sensitive to infections, which reduces their life expectancy. Sickle-cell anemia exclusively affects ethnic groups of African origin and is manifested from six months of age. Frequent blood transfusions make it possible to fight against the anemia. The sole curative treatment is the bone marrow transplant.

Heredity... page 50

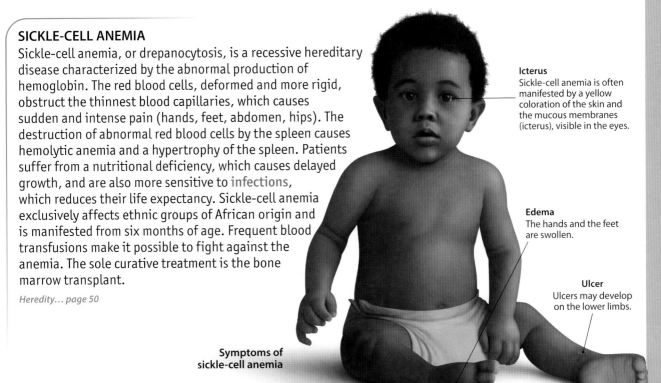

Icterus
Sickle-cell anemia is often manifested by a yellow coloration of the skin and the mucous membranes (icterus), visible in the eyes.

Edema
The hands and the feet are swollen.

Ulcer
Ulcers may develop on the lower limbs.

Symptoms of sickle-cell anemia

HEMOPHILIA

Hemophilia is a hereditary disease characterized by a blood coagulation problem that causes prolonged hemorrhages. It results from a **genetic** anomaly of the X chromosome, which causes a deficit of certain proteins, called coagulation factors, normally present in the blood plasma. The disease is manifested almost exclusively in men, but it is transmitted by women. Its treatment is based on the administration of coagulation factors to the patient.

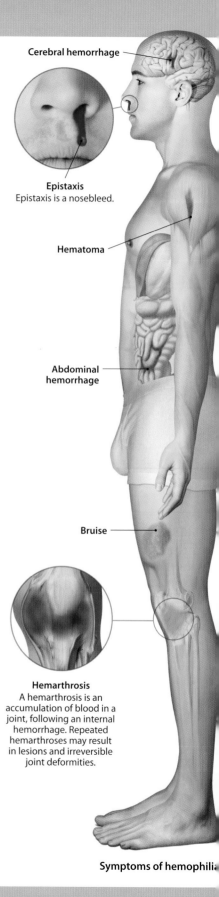

Cerebral hemorrhage

Epistaxis
Epistaxis is a nosebleed.

Hematoma

Abdominal hemorrhage

Bruise

Hemarthrosis
A hemarthrosis is an accumulation of blood in a joint, following an internal hemorrhage. Repeated hemarthroses may result in lesions and irreversible joint deformities.

Symptoms of hemophilia

THE **TYPES** OF **HEMOPHILIA**

There are two types of hemophilia. Hemophilia A, which represents 80% of cases, comes from a deficit in coagulation factor VIII. Hemophilia B, or Christmas disease, is caused by a deficit in factor IX. The symptoms are the same for types A and B: internal and external hemorrhages, hematomas, outpouring of blood into the joints. Hemophilias may also be classified according to their seriousness. In the mild form, hemorrhages are to be particularly feared during surgery. In the moderate form, hemorrhages are produced following falls or traumas. In the severe form, hemorrhages are spontaneously triggered.

THE TRANSMISSION OF HEMOPHILIA

Hemophilia is transmitted in a recessive mode connected with gender and with the X chromosome. A woman carrying the deficient gene does not develop the illness because she has a healthy copy of the gene on her second X chromosome. She has a 50-50 chance of transmitting the genetic anomaly to her children. Her affected daughters will be healthy carriers, while her affected sons will be hemophiliacs. A hemophiliac man transmits the deficient gene to all of his daughters, who are healthy carriers, but to none of his sons. If, however, both of the parents are carriers of abnormal X chromosomes, there is a 50-50 chance that their daughters will be affected and hemophiliac.

Heredity... page 50

HEMOPHILIA

SYMPTOMS:
Prolonged hemorrhages, which may be spontaneously triggered.

TREATMENTS:
Transfusions of concentrates of factors VIII or IX. Antibodies that destroy the coagulation factors are, however, capable of developing, which makes the treatment ineffective and aggravates the disease. The factor VIII can now be manufactured, which limits the risks of the transfusion.

LEUKEMIAS

Leukemia is a cancer of the bone marrow, the site of blood cell production. This disease is characterized by the development and the proliferation of abnormal or immature white blood cells, which progressively invade the bone marrow and prevent the manufacture of normal blood cells. Although leukemias represent almost half of the cancers in children, a large majority of them are triggered after age 50. The origin of the disease is most often unknown, but chemical substances and radiation have been implicated. The diagnosis is made from a blood analysis and a sample of bone marrow taken by tapping.

Cancers... page 55

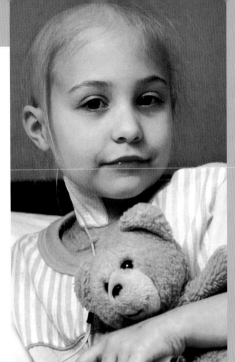

THE **TYPES** OF **LEUKEMIA**

Leukemia is said to be lymphoid or myeloid, according to the type of white blood cell affected. Lymphoid leukemia is characterized by a proliferation of abnormal lymphocytes, while myeloid leukemia is associated with a proliferation of abnormal granulocytes. A leukemia can also be chronic (slow-developing) or acute (quick-developing). The combination of these different characteristics makes it possible to distinguish four main types of leukemia: chronic myeloid, acute myeloid, chronic lymphoid, and acute lymphoid. The latter is the most common form of leukemia in children and the one that is most likely to be cured. Chronic lymphoid leukemia is the most common in adults. It affects twice as many men as women.

The blood... page 234

THE **TREATMENT** OF **LEUKEMIAS**

Intensive chemotherapy and radiation therapy treatments make it possible to destroy the patient's bone marrow and the cancerous cells that it contains. Once the diseased marrow is eliminated, a bone marrow transplant is then performed. Blood stem cells from a healthy and compatible donor (brother or sister of the patient if possible) then replace the destroyed, diseased marrow and begin to produce healthy blood cells within a few weeks. The autotransplant, done using the patient's own bone marrow, cleansed of cancerous cells, makes it possible to avoid rejection phenomena, but the risk of relapse is higher.

LEUKEMIAS

SYMPTOMS: ·
Fatigue, fever, bone pain, swelling of the spleen and the lymph nodes, sometimes skin lesions, anemia, bleeding gums, bruises, severe and repeated infections.

TREATMENTS:
Chemotherapy, radiation therapy, bone marrow transplant, according to the type of leukemia and the age of the patient. Long-term hospitalization necessary.

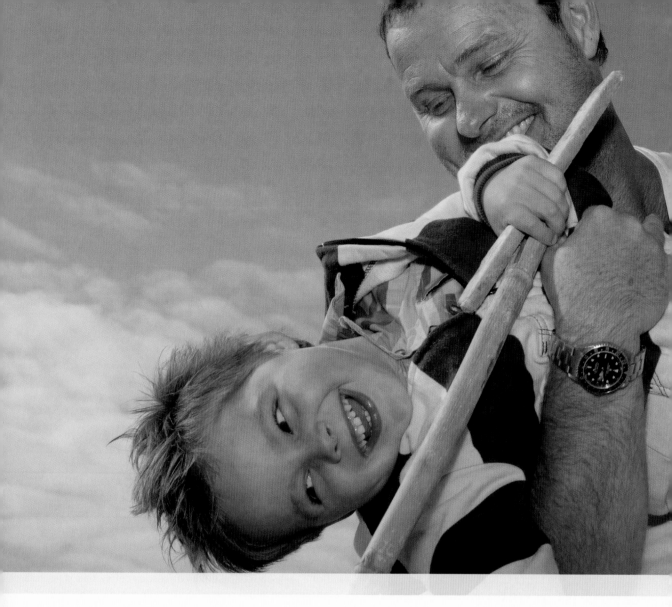

THE **CARDIOVASCULAR SYSTEM**

Thanks to the heart and the blood vessels, which constitute the cardiovascular system, the blood circulates throughout the body. The rhythmic contractions of the heart pump the red fluid into the arteries and then into the blood capillaries, which irrigate each cell of the body. The blood is then rerouted towards the heart by the veins.

Heart disorders and blood circulation problems can have serious consequences. Promoted by a sedentary lifestyle and overeating, high blood pressure and atherosclerosis are at the source of several cardiovascular diseases, specifically coronary heart disease, which can cause a myocardial infarction. Disorders of the heart (malformation, **infection**, arrhythmia) can prevent the efficient pumping of the blood. A cardiac insufficiency sets in, which, in the most severe cases, can lead to cardiac arrest. With regard to the blood vessels, they are sometimes subject to abnormal dilations (varicose veins, aneurysms) and to potentially dangerous obstructions (thromboses, phlebitis).

BLOOD CIRCULATION
AND **BLOOD VESSELS**

Pumped by the heart, the blood circulates throughout the body through a vast network of blood vessels. Three types of vessels transport blood: arteries, capillaries, and veins. Arteries carry the blood from the heart to all of the areas of the body. Capillaries, minuscule vessels, then permit the exchanges between the blood and the cells through their extremely thin walls. Finally, the blood returns to the heart through the veins.

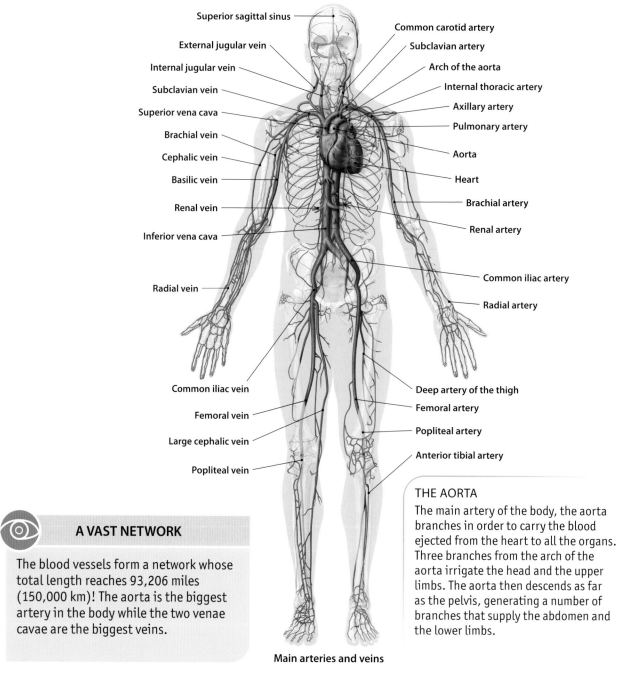

Superior sagittal sinus

External jugular vein

Internal jugular vein

Subclavian vein

Superior vena cava

Brachial vein

Cephalic vein

Basilic vein

Renal vein

Inferior vena cava

Radial vein

Common iliac vein

Femoral vein

Large cephalic vein

Popliteal vein

Common carotid artery

Subclavian artery

Arch of the aorta

Internal thoracic artery

Axillary artery

Pulmonary artery

Aorta

Heart

Brachial artery

Renal artery

Common iliac artery

Radial artery

Deep artery of the thigh

Femoral artery

Popliteal artery

Anterior tibial artery

Main arteries and veins

A VAST NETWORK

The blood vessels form a network whose total length reaches 93,206 miles (150,000 km)! The aorta is the biggest artery in the body while the two venae cavae are the biggest veins.

THE AORTA

The main artery of the body, the aorta branches in order to carry the blood ejected from the heart to all the organs. Three branches from the arch of the aorta irrigate the head and the upper limbs. The aorta then descends as far as the pelvis, generating a number of branches that supply the abdomen and the lower limbs.

248

THE **TWO CARDIOVASCULAR CIRCUITS**

The blood vessels separate into two distinct circuits: pulmonary circulation and systemic circulation. Pulmonary circulation is responsible for the gaseous exchanges between the blood and the air contained in the lungs. Systemic circulation is responsible for the blood irrigation of all organs and tissues. When the heart contracts, its two ventricles simultaneously eject blood into both circuits.

The heart... page 250
The respiratory tract... page 310

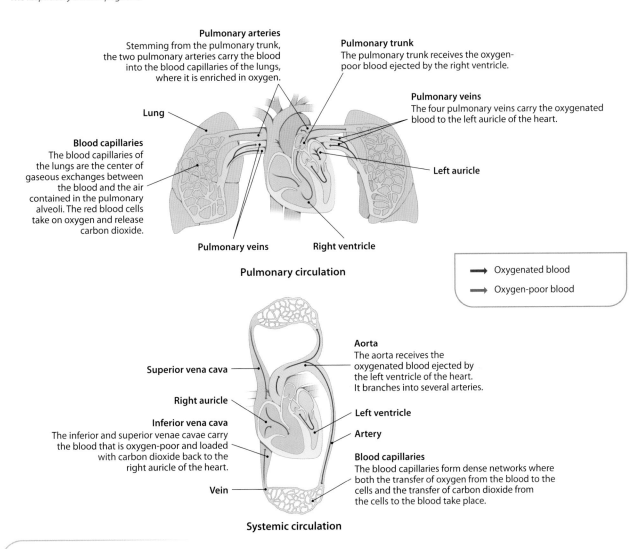

Pulmonary arteries
Stemming from the pulmonary trunk, the two pulmonary arteries carry the blood into the blood capillaries of the lungs, where it is enriched in oxygen.

Pulmonary trunk
The pulmonary trunk receives the oxygen-poor blood ejected by the right ventricle.

Pulmonary veins
The four pulmonary veins carry the oxygenated blood to the left auricle of the heart.

Lung

Blood capillaries
The blood capillaries of the lungs are the center of gaseous exchanges between the blood and the air contained in the pulmonary alveoli. The red blood cells take on oxygen and release carbon dioxide.

Left auricle

Pulmonary veins

Right ventricle

Pulmonary circulation

→ Oxygenated blood
→ Oxygen-poor blood

Aorta
The aorta receives the oxygenated blood ejected by the left ventricle of the heart. It branches into several arteries.

Superior vena cava

Right auricle

Inferior vena cava
The inferior and superior venae cavae carry the blood that is oxygen-poor and loaded with carbon dioxide back to the right auricle of the heart.

Left ventricle

Artery

Blood capillaries
The blood capillaries form dense networks where both the transfer of oxygen from the blood to the cells and the transfer of carbon dioxide from the cells to the blood take place.

Vein

Systemic circulation

VASOMOTRICITY

Vasomotricity is the ability of the blood vessels, specifically the arteries, to reduce their diameter (vasoconstriction) or to increase it (vasodilation) in order to regulate the blood flow: when the artery contracts, the arterial pressure increases and the blood flow decreases, while when it dilates, the pressure decreases and the flow increases. These are normal reactions controlled by the autonomic nervous system and the hormones. Adrenaline, for example, a hormone secreted during situations of stress, acts as a natural vasoconstrictor. Vasoconstriction and vasodilation may also be caused by diseases or certain drugs.

The functioning of the nervous system... page 135

THE **HEART**

The heart is a vital organ. As a powerful pump, it propels the blood and makes it circulate throughout all of the body's blood vessels. Located in the left center of the rib cage, between the lungs, the heart contracts an average of 70 times per minute, each day pumping 7,389 quarts (7000 liters) of blood through the vascular system. This organ is essentially formed by one muscle, the myocardium, which defines four cavities: two auricles and two ventricles.

THE **CAVITIES** OF THE **HEART**

The heart consists of two distinct parts, each containing an auricle and a ventricle. The right part of the heart is responsible for blood circulation towards the lungs. The left part is responsible for blood circulation to all of the other organs. The auricles receive the blood while the larger ventricles expel it. The ventricles are closed by cardiac valves, thin elastic structures that open to allow the passage of blood, then close to avoid its backflow.

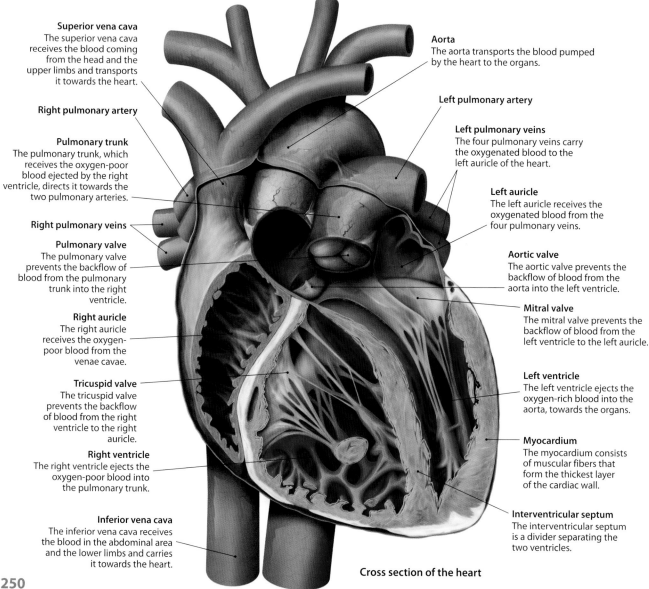

Superior vena cava
The superior vena cava receives the blood coming from the head and the upper limbs and transports it towards the heart.

Right pulmonary artery

Pulmonary trunk
The pulmonary trunk, which receives the oxygen-poor blood ejected by the right ventricle, directs it towards the two pulmonary arteries.

Right pulmonary veins

Pulmonary valve
The pulmonary valve prevents the backflow of blood from the pulmonary trunk into the right ventricle.

Right auricle
The right auricle receives the oxygen-poor blood from the venae cavae.

Tricuspid valve
The tricuspid valve prevents the backflow of blood from the right ventricle to the right auricle.

Right ventricle
The right ventricle ejects the oxygen-poor blood into the pulmonary trunk.

Inferior vena cava
The inferior vena cava receives the blood in the abdominal area and the lower limbs and carries it towards the heart.

Aorta
The aorta transports the blood pumped by the heart to the organs.

Left pulmonary artery

Left pulmonary veins
The four pulmonary veins carry the oxygenated blood to the left auricle of the heart.

Left auricle
The left auricle receives the oxygenated blood from the four pulmonary veins.

Aortic valve
The aortic valve prevents the backflow of blood from the aorta into the left ventricle.

Mitral valve
The mitral valve prevents the backflow of blood from the left ventricle to the left auricle.

Left ventricle
The left ventricle ejects the oxygen-rich blood into the aorta, towards the organs.

Myocardium
The myocardium consists of muscular fibers that form the thickest layer of the cardiac wall.

Interventricular septum
The interventricular septum is a divider separating the two ventricles.

Cross section of the heart

THE **CARDIAC CYCLE**

The cardiac cycle corresponds to the relaxation (diastole) then the contraction (systole) of the myocardium. It lasts an average of 0.8 seconds in adults and permits the expulsion of 2.37 oz (70 ml) of blood in the arteries.

1. Diastole

Diastole is the period of the cardiac cycle during which the myocardium relaxes, permitting the auricles and then the ventricles to fill with blood.

Superior vena cava

Left auricle

Pulmonary veins

Mitral valve
The mitral valve is open during diastole.

Right auricle

Tricuspid valve
The tricuspid valve is open during diastole.

Inferior vena cava

Left ventricle

Myocardium

Right ventricle

2. Auricular systole

At the end of diastole, the contraction of the auricles (or auricular systole) completes the filling of the ventricles. The closing of the mitral and tricuspid valves then produces a muffled sound.

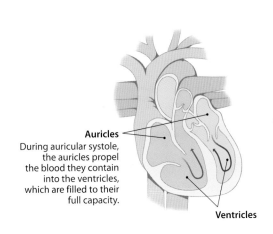

Auricles
During auricular systole, the auricles propel the blood they contain into the ventricles, which are filled to their full capacity.

Ventricles

3. Ventricular systole

Ventricular systole is the period of the cardiac cycle during which the ventricles of the heart contract, causing the expulsion of blood into the aorta and the pulmonary trunk. The closing of the aortic and pulmonary valves then produces a sharper beat than that of auricular systole.

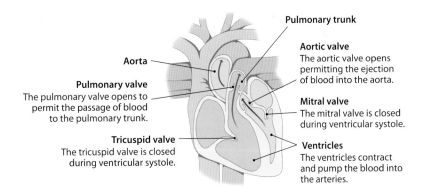

Pulmonary trunk

Aortic valve
The aortic valve opens permitting the ejection of blood into the aorta.

Aorta

Pulmonary valve
The pulmonary valve opens to permit the passage of blood to the pulmonary trunk.

Mitral valve
The mitral valve is closed during ventricular systole.

Tricuspid valve
The tricuspid valve is closed during ventricular systole.

Ventricles
The ventricles contract and pump the blood into the arteries.

CARDIAC RHYTHM AND THE PULSE

The cardiac rhythm is the number of cardiac cycles per minute. It can be measured by medical methods such as auscultation and electrocardiography, but also by the simple taking of the pulse. The pulse is a wave created each time the blood is expelled from the heart during its contraction (systole). It is perceptible upon palpation of an artery located near the surface of the skin. Its normal frequency is approximately 70 beats per minute at rest in adults, but it may exceed 100 beats per minute during physical exertion or following a strong emotion. The pulse is normally taken at the radial artery, on the inside of the wrist, or on the common carotid artery, on the side of the neck.

First aid: How to take a pulse... page 543

BLOOD PRESSURE

Arterial pressure, or blood pressure, is the force exercised by the blood on the wall of the blood vessels. It is measured in millimeters or in centimeters of mercury. Blood pressure varies during the cardiac cycle, reaching a maximum value at each contraction of the heart and a minimum value between the contractions. Age, sex, weight, and physical exertion normally influence blood pressure values. Poor lifestyle habits, **genetic** predispositions, and certain diseases, such as diabetes or kidney failure, can cause abnormally elevated blood pressure, or arterial hypertension.

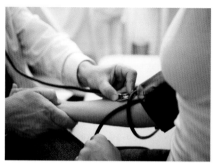

THE **MEASUREMENT** OF **BLOOD PRESSURE**

Blood pressure is measured using a sphygmomanometer, a medical device consisting of an inflatable cuff and a gauge. The cuff serves to control the blood flow in the brachial artery, which allows the gauge to measure the pressure that the blood is exercising on this artery. Blood pressure rises during the contraction of the heart (systole) and falls between the contractions (diastole).

SYSTOLIC BLOOD PRESSURE

The taking of systolic blood pressure makes it possible to measure the maximum force exercised by the blood on the walls of the arteries at the moment it is expelled from the heart. In order to obtain this measurement, the brachial artery is compressed using an inflatable cuff until the passage of blood is blocked (no pulse is then audible using a stethoscope). The cuff is then slowly deflated until it exercises a pressure just below that of the blood on the artery walls, which is signaled by the resumption of circulation (a pulse becomes perceptible using a stethoscope). The value read on the gauge at this moment corresponds to the systolic blood pressure. It is on average 120 mm (or 12 cm) of mercury.

DIASTOLIC BLOOD PRESSURE

The cuff continues to deflate and exercises less and less pressure on the artery, until the minimum pressure exercised by the blood between two heartbeats is greater than that exercised by the cuff (the pulse is perceived more and more faintly, then becomes inaudible). The artery is then no longer compressed and has resumed its normal diameter. The value read on the gauge at the moment the pulse disappears corresponds to the diastolic blood pressure. Its average value is 70 mm (or 7 cm) of mercury.

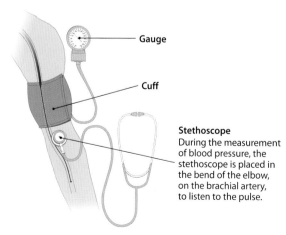

Gauge

Cuff

Stethoscope
During the measurement of blood pressure, the stethoscope is placed in the bend of the elbow, on the brachial artery, to listen to the pulse.

Systolic blood pressure

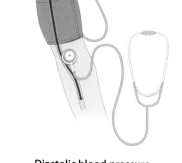

Diastolic blood pressure

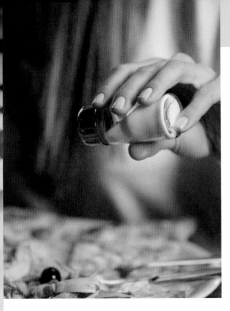

HIGH BLOOD PRESSURE

High blood pressure occurs when the blood pressure is maintained at a level higher than normal. It is often called the silent disease or silent killer because it is asymptomatic in most cases and can cause serious diseases such as the cerebral vascular accident (CVA) or myocardial infarction. High blood pressure affects approximately 15% of the population in industrialized countries.

THE **RISK FACTORS** OF **HIGH BLOOD PRESSURE**

Although the precise cause of high blood pressure is generally unknown, it is promoted or aggravated by several factors connected with the Western lifestyle: smoking, physical inactivity, stress, excessive consumption of salt, fats, and alcohol, etc. Men and people over 45 years of age or who have family histories are more likely to develop the disease.

DIET
The excessive consumption of salt is the main risk factor for high blood pressure. The absorbed salt causes water retention and an increase in blood flow aggravated by the vasoconstriction of the arteries.

Vasomotricity... page 249

TOBACCO
The consumption of tobacco causes a vasoconstriction of the blood vessels and an immediate and temporary elevation of the blood pressure.

Vasomotricity... page 249

OBESITY
Obesity, especially when it starts in childhood, increases the risks of high blood pressure. The concentration of fatty masses in the abdomen is associated with cardiovascular complications.

Obesity... page 355

DRUGS
The regular consumption of certain drugs may cause high blood pressure to appear in individuals predisposed to the disease. This is particularly the case of oral contraceptives containing estrogens and non-steroidal anti-inflammatories.

ALCOHOL
The regular consumption of alcohol in large quantities (more than two glasses of wine per day, for example) significantly increases blood pressure.

THE **CLASSIFICATION** OF **PRESSURE**

High blood pressure can be detected using a tensiometer. Blood pressure, measured in centimeters or millimeters of mercury, is expressed by two numbers: the systolic pressure and the diastolic pressure. A normal blood pressure at rest is below 130/85 (in millimeters) or 13/8.5 (in centimeters). It is possible to suffer from systolic hypertension and to have a normal diastolic pressure, and vice versa. It is also possible to suffer from hypotension, or low blood pressure. This is not treated if it is not accompanied by any symptoms. However, hypotension must be treated in case of dizziness, weakness, and loss of consciousness.

THE CLASSIFICATION OF PRESSURE		
Category	**Systolic pressure**	**Diastolic pressure**
Low blood pressure	less than 90 mm of mercury	less than 60 mm of mercury
Normal	from 90 to 129 mm of mercury	from 60 to 84 mm of mercury
At the limit of normal	from 130 to 139 mm of mercury	from 85 to 89 mm of mercury
High blood pressure - stage 1 (requires medical monitoring and lifestyle modifications)	from 140 to 159 mm of mercury	from 90 to 99 mm of mercury
High blood pressure - stage 2 (requires medical monitoring, lifestyle modifications and medication)	160 mm of mercury and more	100 mm of mercury and more

THE **CONSEQUENCES** OF **HIGH BLOOD PRESSURE**

High blood pressure causes premature aging of the vessels and the heart. Circulatory complications result in a number of organs (brain, heart, kidney, eye), which can be potentially serious, even fatal, if high blood pressure is not treated.

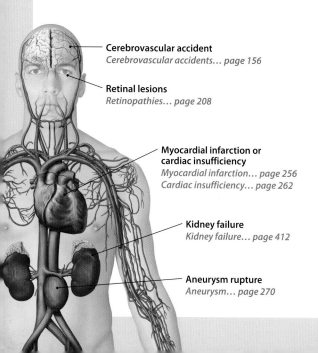

Cerebrovascular accident
Cerebrovascular accidents... page 156

Retinal lesions
Retinopathies... page 208

Myocardial infarction or cardiac insufficiency
Myocardial infarction... page 256
Cardiac insufficiency... page 262

Kidney failure
Kidney failure... page 412

Aneurysm rupture
Aneurysm... page 270

HIGH BLOOD PRESSURE

SYMPTOMS:
Most often asymptomatic. Headaches, loss of balance and loss of memory, eye problems.

TREATMENTS:
Antihypertensive drugs. Treatment of the cause when it is defined.

PREVENTION:
Limit consumption of salt, fats, alcohol, and tobacco. Avoid excess weight and stress. Regularly and moderately engage in endurance sports.

PREVENTION OF HIGH BLOOD PRESSURE

It is possible to control and to prevent high blood pressure by reducing certain risk factors and by following some recommendations, particularly if you are an elderly person or if you have family histories.

■ STOP SMOKING

The consumption of tobacco causes an acceleration of the cardiac rhythm, a reduction in blood vessel diameter (vasoconstriction), and a temporary elevation of arterial pressure.

Vasomotricity ... page 249

■ REDUCE YOUR CONSUMPTION OF ALCOHOL

Do not consume more than two glasses of alcohol per day.

Alcohol consumption, some facts... page 26

■ REDUCE YOUR CONSUMPTION OF SALT AND ADOPT A HEALTHY DIET

Give preference to fresh or frozen foods rather than to processed foods (canned, precooked, etc.), which often contain too much salt. When dining and when cooking foods, replace the salt with spices, herbs, lemon juice, or garlic. Foods rich in potassium can protect you against high blood pressure. Fruits, vegetables, and legumes (specifically bananas, oranges, melons, tomatoes, kiwis, potatoes, beans, and broad beans), as well as yogurt, milk, nuts, whole grain cereals, and fish are good sources of potassium.

■ MAINTAIN A HEALTHY WEIGHT

Engage in moderate and regular endurance exercise and adopt a low-fat diet.

■ AVOID THE CONSUMPTION OF CERTAIN DRUGS

Avoid consuming drugs such as oral contraceptives or non-steroidal anti-inflammatories if you are predisposed to high blood pressure.

■ HAVE YOUR BLOOD PRESSURE MEASURED REGULARLY

Measurement of your blood pressure must be done at least once a year by a doctor, more often if you already suffer from high blood pressure. Blood pressure is considered high when it is constantly greater than 140/99 mm (14/9 cm) of mercury.

■ COMBAT STRESS

Stress can increase and aggravate high blood pressure. Reduce the sources of stress, avoid working too much, rest, and get enough sleep. Try relaxation techniques such as yoga, meditation, or tai-chi.

The cardiovascular system | Diseases

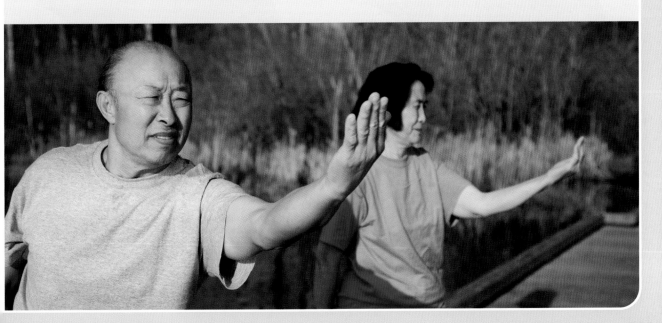

HEART DISEASE

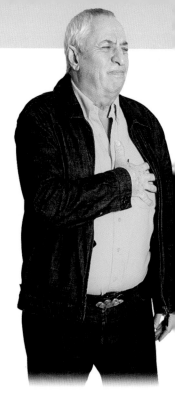

Heart disease constitutes the primary cause of death in Western countries. It occurs when the coronary arteries, that is, the vessels that nourish the heart, can no longer properly provide the blood irrigation of the heart muscle due to their narrowing or obstruction. Heart disease is manifested by painful attacks and, in its most serious form, by a myocardial infarction, or heart attack. This disorder primarily affects men over 45 years of age and menopausal women, as well as individuals with family histories. Excessive levels of cholesterol in the blood, high blood pressure, certain diseases (such as diabetes), and lifestyle factors such as physical inactivity, smoking, alcoholism, a diet rich in animal fats, and stress, heighten the risk for heart disease.

ATHEROSCLEROSIS

Atherosclerosis is the main cause of heart disease and of cardiovascular diseases in general. It is a disorder characterized by the growth of a plaque (atheroma) in the internal wall of the arteries, primarily those with a wide diameter. It is often associated with a thickening and a hardening of the arterial wall. Excess cholesterol in the blood contributes to the development of atherosclerosis, which is particularly widespread in Europe and in North America.

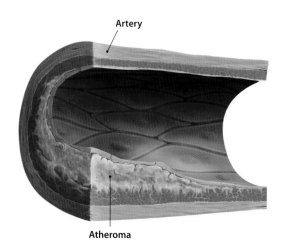

Artery

Atheroma

Atheroma
The atheroma is a fatty deposit, rich in cholesterol, that forms a plaque in the wall of an artery. It appears during adolescence and progressively increases in volume. The atheroma can cause a narrowing of the artery and lead to painful attacks known as angina pectoris.

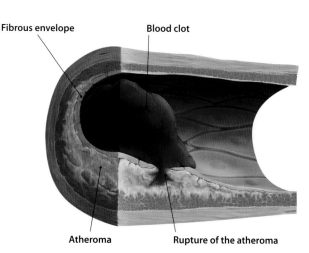

Fibrous envelope

Blood clot

Atheroma

Rupture of the atheroma

Rupture of the atheromatous plaque
In the advanced stage, the atheromatous plaque is covered by a fibrous envelope that separates it from the blood. If this envelope breaks, a blood clot forms very quickly at the opening. In less than five minutes, this clot can obstruct the vessel and prevent the passage of blood. The rupture of the atheromatous plaque can have serious consequences, such as myocardial infarction or cerebral infarction, depending on the location of the clot.
Cerebral vascular accidents... page 156

ANGINA PECTORIS

Angina pectoris, or angina, is a chest pain that is manifested by a crushing and burning feeling behind the sternum, in the middle of the chest. This pain may irradiate in the neck and in the left arm. It is caused by a lack of oxygen in the heart muscle, usually due to the narrowing of a coronary artery by an atheroma. Angina pectoris occurs in attacks that last several minutes. The pain is quickly calmed by immediately taking drugs (trinitrin). Stable angina is characterized by recurrent attacks most often occurring during physical exertion, exposure to cold, emotional shock, or during digestion. Unstable angina, due to the partial and sudden obstruction of a coronary artery, may occur at any time. It constitutes a serious problem that can develop into a myocardial infarction in a few hours.

THE MYOCARDIAL INFARCTION

Myocardial infarction, or heart attack, is the death (necrosis) of a portion of the heart muscle caused by the interruption of its blood irrigation. It is most often due to the formation of a blood clot in a coronary artery following the rupture of an atheromatous plaque. The disruption of the cardiac rhythm caused by the myocardial infarction may lead to cardiac insufficiency, even to cardiac arrest, and thus to death, in the hours or days following the infarction. The myocardial infarction requires emergency hospitalization. Fifty percent of the time, it occurs in individuals who suffer from angina pectoris. The symptoms are similar but more intense and long-lasting. The pain appears suddenly, generally at rest or during the night. It may be accompanied, in the days preceding it, by various symptoms: generalized weakness, breathing difficulty, nausea, vertigo, digestive problems, profuse perspiration.

Cardiac insufficiency... page 262

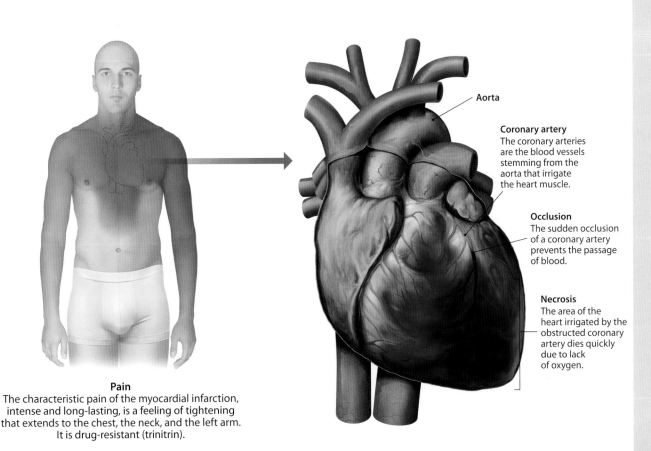

Pain
The characteristic pain of the myocardial infarction, intense and long-lasting, is a feeling of tightening that extends to the chest, the neck, and the left arm. It is drug-resistant (trinitrin).

Aorta

Coronary artery
The coronary arteries are the blood vessels stemming from the aorta that irrigate the heart muscle.

Occlusion
The sudden occlusion of a coronary artery prevents the passage of blood.

Necrosis
The area of the heart irrigated by the obstructed coronary artery dies quickly due to lack of oxygen.

GOOD AND BAD CHOLESTEROL

Cholesterol is a fatty substance naturally produced by the liver and indispensable for the proper functioning of the body. It enters into the make-up of our cells, permitting the development of certain hormones, and contributes to the proper functioning of our nervous system. To circulate in the blood, cholesterol combines with proteins, lipoproteins, of which there are various types. The name "good cholesterol" is given to high density lipoproteins (HDL) and "bad cholesterol" to low density lipoproteins (LDL). The HDLs take care of the excess cholesterol in our blood and carry it to the liver where it is eliminated. The LDLs carry the cholesterol from the liver to our cells. An excessive level of LDLs in the blood, called hypercholesterolemia, promotes atherosclerosis, that is the formation of fatty plaques in the walls of the arteries.

HYPERCHOLESTEROLEMIA

Hypercholesterolemia is a risk factor for a number of cardiovascular diseases: angina pectoris, myocardial infarction, cerebral vascular accident, phlebitis, ruptured aneurysm. Asymptomatic, it can only be diagnosed by a blood analysis. Hypercholesterolemia may be hereditary or result from a disease, such as diabetes or kidney failure. However, it most often occurs in individuals whose diet is rich in saturated and trans fatty acids: fatty meat, offal, prepared meat or pork products, butter, margarine based on partially hydrogenated or hydrogenated oil, egg yolks, milk fat products, palm or coconut oil, pastries, fried foods, and other foods containing hydrogenated oil. These foods promote "bad cholesterol", which tends to block the arteries. On the other hand, the fat contained in nuts, almonds, avocados, vegetable oils (such as olive oil and canola oil), and fatty fish (such as salmon, sardines, and herring) indirectly increases the level of "good cholesterol" in the blood and contributes to cleaning the arteries.

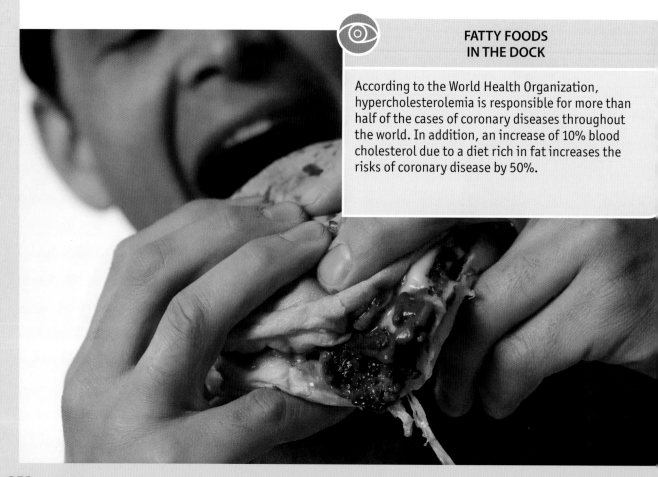

FATTY FOODS IN THE DOCK

According to the World Health Organization, hypercholesterolemia is responsible for more than half of the cases of coronary diseases throughout the world. In addition, an increase of 10% blood cholesterol due to a diet rich in fat increases the risks of coronary disease by 50%.

THE PREVENTION OF HEART DISEASES

Certain heart disease risk factors such as age, gender or heredity are non-modifiable. However, you can considerably reduce your risks of contracting a heart disease by adopting a healthy way of life. Here are some basic rules to keep your heart healthy.

■ MONITOR YOUR DIET AND CONTROL YOUR WEIGHT

Overeating is a significant risk factor for heart disease. A diet rich in saturated and trans fatty acids promotes the development of hypercholesterolemia. Salt, consumed in excess, contributes to high blood pressure, a major risk factor for cardiovascular diseases. The excessive consumption of sugar and alcohol as well as an insufficient amount of fruits and vegetables also contributes to increasing the risks. Eat less meat and more foods rich in fiber: vegetables, legumes, fruits, and whole-grain products. Give preference to lean meats, poultry, fish, low-fat milk products, and fat-free cooking methods. Choose food that have undergone the least processing.

Nutrition... page 11

■ HAVE YOUR BLOOD PRESSURE TAKEN

By increasing pressure on the walls of the arteries, high blood pressure promotes heart disease. The evaluation of your blood pressure by a doctor will enable you to take the necessary measures in case of high blood pressure.

High blood pressure... page 253

■ HAVE YOUR BLOOD TESTED

A blood analysis makes it possible to detect and possibly to control hypercholesterolemia or an elevated blood glucose level (diabetes), two important risk factors for cardiovascular diseases.

Diabetes... page 228

■ AVOID SMOKING

Tobacco, even consumed in moderation, is at the origin of cardiovascular complications, specifically when it is combined with the taking of oral contraceptives in women.

Smoking... page 338

■ EXERCISE

Engage in physical activities regularly and moderately, at least 30 minutes per day. Choose activities that make you breathe more quickly and cause your heart to beat faster (though not excessively): fast walking, dancing, bicycling, swimming, etc. In this way, your heart will become stronger and more efficient. A sedentary lifestyle, particularly common in the West, promotes obesity, hypercholesterolemia, diabetes, and high blood pressure, which are many of the risk factors for heart disease.

Exercise... page 22

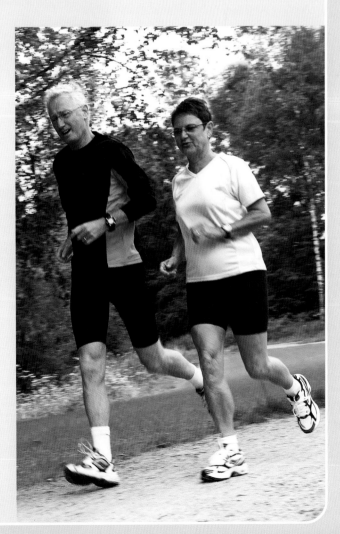

THE **TREATMENT** OF **HEART DISEASE**

Heart disease may be treated using drugs such as beta blockers or trinitrin. It sometimes requires emergency surgery (angioplasty, coronary bypass) in order to quickly reestablish blood circulation, after a myocardial infarction, for example. Coronarography (X-ray examination of the coronary arteries) makes it possible to detect and to locate the obstruction or the arterial constriction.

ANGIOPLASTY

Angioplasty is a procedure intended to reestablish the diameter of a blood vessel, generally an artery. Surgical angioplasty is performed by replacing the diseased portion with a segment of healthy vein. Transcutaneous angioplasty is performed using a catheter equipped with a balloon. It is only applied to constrictions located in coronary arteries affected by atherosclerosis. The artery is therefore not totally blocked.

1. Introduction of catheter
During a transcutaneous angioplasty, a catheter is introduced through the skin into a peripheral blood vessel and brought to the site of the arterial constriction.

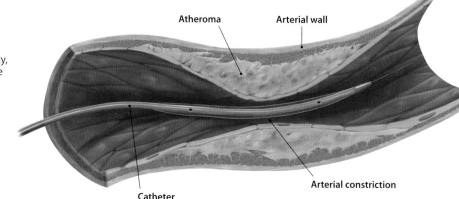

Atheroma   Arterial wall

Catheter

Arterial constriction

2. Inflating of the balloon
Once the catheter is in place, the balloon that it contains is inflated. This pushes the atheroma back on the arterial wall, which dilates.

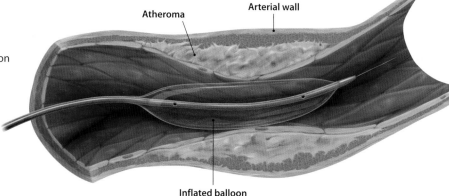

Atheroma   Arterial wall

Inflated balloon

3. Inserting a stent
Once the artery is dilated, the catheter and the balloon are withdrawn. The angioplasty is often accompanied by the insertion of a stent (expandable metal prosthesis), which averts a new constriction of the artery.

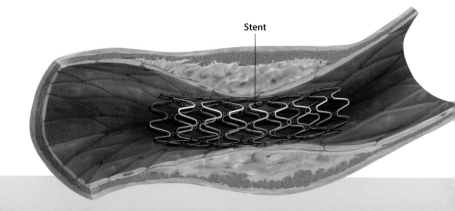

Stent

CORONARY BYPASS

The coronary bypass is a surgical operation that seeks to circumvent the constriction or obstruction of a coronary artery and to reestablish the blood irrigation of the myocardium. It consists in creating a bridge between the healthy portion of the blocked coronary artery and the aorta using a mammalian artery, or with a segment of the large saphenous artery taken from the leg. The operation, which lasts several hours, often requires open-heart surgery, involving the opening of the rib cage, stopping the heart, and diverting the blood circulation to an artificial external pump.

TRINITRIN AND THE BETA BLOCKERS

Trinitrin is a drug used to treat angina pectoris. It causes the dilation of the coronary arteries. Beta blockers are drugs that make it possible to reduce the strength and the frequency of heartbeats. They are particularly prescribed in the case of cardiac arrhythmia, heart disease, high blood pressure, migraine, facial neuralgia, and glaucoma.

HEART DISEASE

SYMPTOMS:
Atherosclerosis: asymptomatic.
Angina pectoris: radiating chest pain.
Myocardial infarction: very intense and persistent chest pain.

TREATMENTS:
Emergency anticoagulants, beta blockers, trinitrin, angioplasty, coronary bypass.

PREVENTION:
Limit consumption of saturated and trans fatty acids, salt, sugar, alcohol, and tobacco. Regularly engage in physical activities adapted to your state of health. Screening for hypercholesterolemia (blood analysis) and high blood pressure.

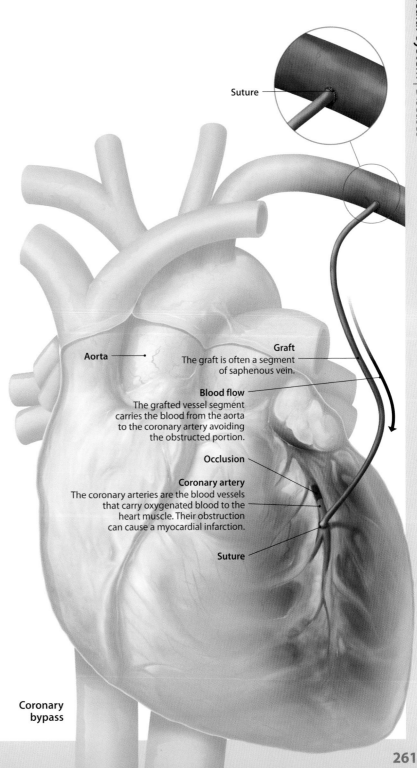

Suture

Aorta

Graft
The graft is often a segment of saphenous vein.

Blood flow
The grafted vessel segment carries the blood from the aorta to the coronary artery avoiding the obstructed portion.

Occlusion

Coronary artery
The coronary arteries are the blood vessels that carry oxygenated blood to the heart muscle. Their obstruction can cause a myocardial infarction.

Suture

Coronary bypass

CARDIAC INSUFFICIENCY

Cardiac insufficiency is the inability of the heart to propel the blood effectively in order to meet the needs of the body. It is most often the consequence of a cardiovascular disease, such as heart disease or high blood pressure. Cardiac insufficiency is a serious weakness that may affect one or both sides of the heart and can lead to cardiac arrest, and then to death. It is manifested by fatigue, significant respiratory difficulty, cardiac arrhythmia, and **edemas**. Its development may be stopped by early medical treatment. When the illness is very advanced, a heart transplant sometimes makes it possible to extend life expectancy.

LEFT CARDIAC INSUFFICIENCY

Left cardiac insufficiency is connected with the inability of the left ventricle to adequately contract or relax. Blood from the lungs is no longer normally ejected into the aorta. Blood flow decreases and the blood tends to stagnate in the left side of the heart and in the lungs, increasing the risks of a pulmonary edema. With time, the left cardiac insufficiency may also cause high blood pressure in the pulmonary artery, which can cause a right cardiac insufficiency. Left cardiac insufficiency most often occurs with the development of heart disease, either suddenly following an infarction, or progressively by a modification of the structure of the cardiac muscle.

Pulmonary edema... page 335

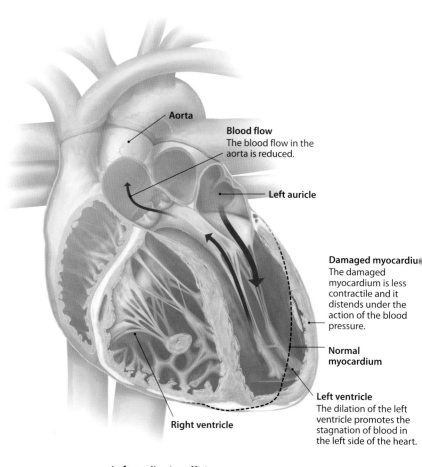

Aorta

Blood flow
The blood flow in the aorta is reduced.

Left auricle

Damaged myocardium
The damaged myocardium is less contractile and it distends under the action of the blood pressure.

Normal myocardium

Left ventricle
The dilation of the left ventricle promotes the stagnation of blood in the left side of the heart.

Right ventricle

Left cardiac insufficiency

RIGHT CARDIAC INSUFFICIENCY

Right cardiac insufficiency is the inability of the right ventricle to supply sufficient blood flow to the lungs. It may be due to a weakness of the right ventricle, to a chronic lung disease, or even to high blood pressure in the pulmonary artery, often following a left cardiac insufficiency. Right cardiac insufficiency causes the blood pressure in the vena cava to increase, resulting in the stagnation of the blood in the liver as well as the swelling of the jugular veins and lower limbs.

Edema... page 53

HEART TRANSPLANT

Cardiac transplantation, or heart transplant, is open-heart surgery, which consists of replacing a diseased heart with the healthy heart of a donor. It is used as a last recourse in people suffering from terminal cardiac insufficiency, when the risk of death by pulmonary edema or by cardiac arrest is very great. Blood circulation is diverted to an artificial external pump and the diseased heart is removed and then replaced by the heart of a donor. This is then sutured to the auricles, the aorta, and the pulmonary trunk, before blood circulation is reestablished. After the operation, the patient is kept under surveillance in an intensive care unit for several days. The risks of transplant rejection and death of the recipient in the following year are 20%.

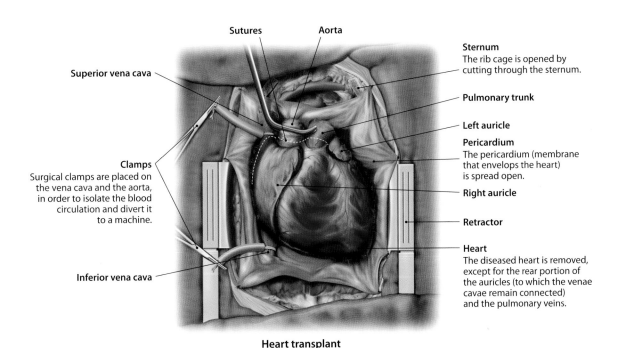

Sutures

Aorta

Superior vena cava

Sternum
The rib cage is opened by cutting through the sternum.

Pulmonary trunk

Left auricle

Pericardium
The pericardium (membrane that envelops the heart) is spread open.

Clamps
Surgical clamps are placed on the vena cava and the aorta, in order to isolate the blood circulation and divert it to a machine.

Right auricle

Retractor

Heart
The diseased heart is removed, except for the rear portion of the auricles (to which the venae cavae remain connected) and the pulmonary veins.

Inferior vena cava

Heart transplant

OPEN-HEART SURGERY

Open-heart surgery is surgery taking place directly on the heart. It requires opening the rib cage at the sternum, stopping the heart, and diverting the blood circulation towards an external device that oxygenates the blood during the operation. Open-heart surgery makes it possible to treat a number of cardiac diseases: heart disease, valvulopathy, heart failure, heart malformations.

CARDIAC INSUFFICIENCY

SYMPTOMS:
Left cardiac insufficiency: respiratory problems, fatigue.
Right cardiac insufficiency: swelling of the neck veins, edema of the lower limbs, liver enlarged and painful with exertion, digestive problems.
Cardiac insufficiency is often accompanied by arrhythmia.

Cardiac arrhythmia... page 264

TREATMENTS:
Beta blockers, vasodilators, diuretics, anticoagulants, digitalis. Treatment of the disease in question. Cardiac rehabilitation. Insertion of a pacemaker or defibrillator. Heart transplant as a last recourse.

PREVENTION:
Prevention of heart disease and high blood pressure.

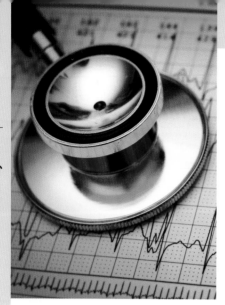

CARDIAC ARRHYTHMIA

Cardiac arrhythmia is a change in heart rhythm. It may take the form of a slow-down (bradychardia), an acceleration (tachycardia), an irregularity (extrasystole), or a disorganization (fibrillation). The causes of heart rhythm problems are multiple: heart disease, aging, consumption of drugs or of stimulants. Their seriousness varies. Some are harmless, while others may result in cardiac arrest.

PALPITATIONS

Palpitations are a feeling of very strong and very rapid heartbeats. Palpitations are not always symptomatic of a heart disease. Thus, they often appear in an individual with a healthy heart who suffers from anxiety or who has absorbed a stimulant, such as alcohol or caffeine.

ELECTROCARDIOGRAPHY

Electrocardiography, or ECG, is a medical exam that makes it possible to measure the heart's electrical activity. The electrical inflow that occurs within each cardiac cycle is captured by the electrodes and recorded in the form of a tracing, the electrocardiogram. When it is done on a person at rest, electrocardiography makes it possible to detect cardiac rhythm problems (extrasystole, tachycardia, bradycardia). These problems are revealed by irregularities or anomalies of the tracing. Electrocardiography may also be done on a person subject to a physical exercise (stress test). In this case, it makes it possible to evaluate the heart's resistance to stress and to diagnose a coronary disease.

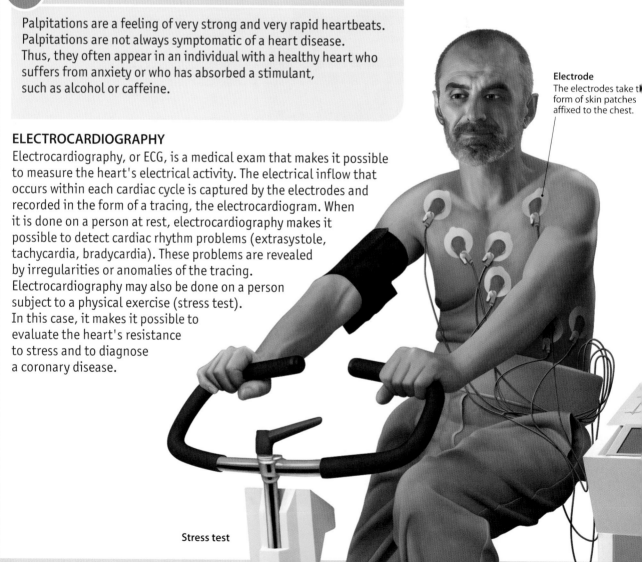

Electrode
The electrodes take the form of skin patches affixed to the chest.

Stress test

BRADYCARDIA

Bradycardia is a slowing of the heart rhythm to below 60 beats per minute. It may be due to an anomaly in the heart's electrical activity, a disease (hypothyroidism, myocardial infarction), or the taking of certain drugs. Normal bradycardia is observed in some individuals, specifically athletes and the elderly.

TACHYCARDIA

Tachycardia is the acceleration of the heart rhythm beyond 100 beats per minute in adults. Sometimes asymptomatic, it frequently appears as palpitations. Tachycardia may be normal, specifically when it follows physical exercise, an emotion, or the absorption of a stimulant such as caffeine. It may also arise from problems of the heart's electrical activity. Ventricular tachycardia is a serious form of tachycardia that may be the cause of a ventricular fibrillation.

THE EXTRASYSTOLE

The extrasystole is the premature occurrence of a cardiac contraction. Extrasystoles are generally manifested by palpitations. When they are less frequent, the extrasystoles are often not serious. When their frequency increases, they may be the sign of an underlying heart disease. Some extrasystoles sometimes develop into tachycardia.

FIBRILLATION

Fibrillation is a succession of rapid and disorganized contractions of the cardiac muscle. Auricular fibrillation is a frequent problem characterized by the irregular contraction of the auricles. It is sometimes accompanied by an irregular and faster contraction of the ventricles and is generally manifested by palpitations, as well as by a feeling of suffocation and shortness of breath. Auricular fibrillation may be transitory or become permanent, specifically in the elderly. Ventricular fibrillation, for its part, is a serious cardiac arrhythmia characterized by the anarchic contraction of the ventricles, unable to effectively pump the blood. It may be caused by a myocardial infarction, a heart disease, or an electric discharge. Ventricular fibrillation causes cardiac arrest and may result in death in a few minutes unless emergency treatment using electric shock (defibrillation) is given.

The heart... page 250

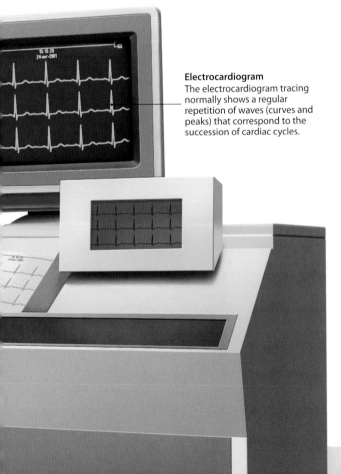

Electrocardiogram
The electrocardiogram tracing normally shows a regular repetition of waves (curves and peaks) that correspond to the succession of cardiac cycles.

CARDIAC ARREST

Cardiac arrest, or cardiorespiratory arrest, is the sudden stopping of heart contractions. It causes a loss of consciousness and respiratory arrest. Cardiac arrest is manifested by an absence of pulse. As it can cause death in a few minutes, it requires emergency resuscitation (heart massage, breathing assistance, use of an external defibrillator).

First aid: Cardiopulmonary arrest... page 544

THE **PACEMAKER**

The pacemaker, or artificial cardiac stimulator, is an electronic implant that sends electrical impulses causing the rhythmic contraction of the heart. The pacemaker is primarily used in the treatment of bradycardia. It consists of a box, inserted under the skin of the thorax, and of one to three sensors implanted in the right cavities of the heart. The sensors monitor and control the cardiac rhythm and transmit regular electrical pulses to the heart generated by the box. The insertion of a pacemaker requires a surgical procedure under local anesthesia.

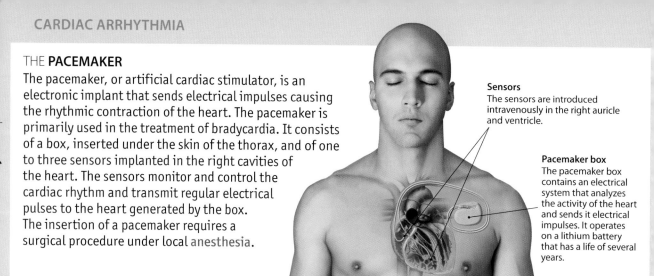

Sensors
The sensors are introduced intravenously in the right auricle and ventricle.

Pacemaker box
The pacemaker box contains an electrical system that analyzes the activity of the heart and sends it electrical impulses. It operates on a lithium battery that has a life of several years.

DEFIBRILLATION

Defibrillation is an emergency treatment for serious cardiac arrhythmias. It consists in administering an electrical shock to the heart that reestablishes the normal cardiac cycle. Defibrillation is performed using an implantable or external defibrillator. The implantable defibrillator is an electronic device similar to a pacemaker that makes it possible to instantly send an electrical shock to the heart when the latter presents a serious arrhythmia. It is implanted under the skin in people who have suffered cardiac arrest or suffer from ventricular tachycardia that risks evolving into fibrillation. The external defibrillator is a medical device that administers an electrical shock to the heart by means of electrodes placed on the thorax. The shock must be administered in the minutes following the loss of consciousness. The speed of the intervention determines the chances of survival and the risks of cerebral after-effects.

CARDIAC ARRHYTHMIA

SYMPTOMS:
Palpitations, fatigue, shortness of breath, complete and sudden loss of consciousness, feeling of suffocation.

TREATMENTS:
Drugs (antiarrhythmics, beta blockers, digitalis) and electrical (defibrillation, pacemaker). Sometimes, surgery.

PREVENTION:
Prevention of heart disease and of cardiac insufficiency.

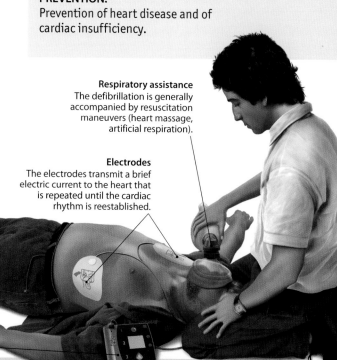

Respiratory assistance
The defibrillation is generally accompanied by resuscitation maneuvers (heart massage, artificial respiration).

Electrodes
The electrodes transmit a brief electric current to the heart that is repeated until the cardiac rhythm is reestablished.

External defibrillator
The defibrillator makes it possible to both measure the electrical activity of the heart and to generate an electrical current.

CARDIAC MALFORMATIONS

Heart malformations are relatively common **congenital** ailments. Several types exist, of variable seriousness. The benign forms do not require any treatment, but the most severe malformations require surgical treatment from childhood because they may lead to cardiac insufficiency.

INTERVENTRICULAR COMMUNICATION

Interventricular communication is the most frequent cardiac malformation. It is characterized by the presence of an opening in the interventricular septum (wall separating the two ventricles). This causes abnormal blood flow from the left ventricle to the right ventricle, which produces a characteristic sound perceptible on examination: the heart murmur. The quantity of blood ejected into the aorta by the left ventricle becomes insufficient to irrigate the entire body, while that moving towards the lungs from the right ventricle is increased. The excess blood in the lungs increases the pressure in the capillaries, which damages the lungs and creates irreversible lesions in the bronchial tubes and the vessels. Most of the time, the opening closes spontaneously during childhood. In the most severe forms, a significant quantity of blood passes into the right ventricle. The heart, abnormally stressed, tires and a cardiac insufficiency is established.

Cardiac insufficiency... page 262

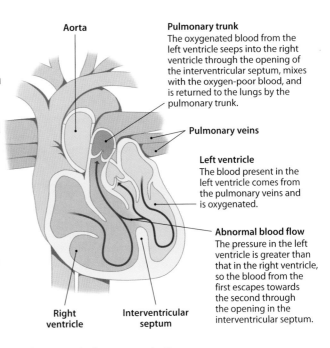

Aorta

Pulmonary trunk
The oxygenated blood from the left ventricle seeps into the right ventricle through the opening of the interventricular septum, mixes with the oxygen-poor blood, and is returned to the lungs by the pulmonary trunk.

Pulmonary veins

Left ventricle
The blood present in the left ventricle comes from the pulmonary veins and is oxygenated.

Abnormal blood flow
The pressure in the left ventricle is greater than that in the right ventricle, so the blood from the first escapes towards the second through the opening in the interventricular septum.

Right ventricle

Interventricular septum

Interventricular communication

THE **TETRALOGY OF FALLOT**

The tetralogy of Fallot results from the combination of four malformations: narrowing of the pulmonary trunk, interventricular communication, overriding of the aorta on the two ventricles, and thickening of the right ventricle. The non-oxygenated blood coming from the veins mixes with the oxygenated blood that is ejected into the aorta, causing poor oxygenation of the body's tissues. The latter is manifested by a delay in growth and by a blue coloration of the skin, particularly visible in the lips.

INTERAURICULAR COMMUNICATION

Interauricular communication is characterized by the presence of an opening between the two auricles, which allows the oxygenated blood to pass from the left auricle to the right auricle. This blood then returns to the lungs through the pulmonary trunk. Often asymptomatic during childhood, it manifests itself in adults as shortness of breath and may lead to cardiac arrhythmia, even cardiac insufficiency.

Bluish lips

CARDIAC MALFORMATIONS

SYMPTOMS:
Heart murmur, blue coloration of the skin, growth problems, shortness of breath. The most benign forms are sometimes asymptomatic.

TREATMENTS:
Surgery.

VALVE DISEASE

Valve disease is a disorder that affects a cardiac valve. It may be caused by a malformation, an **infection**, an **inflammation**, or a **degeneration** of the tissues. All four cardiac valves may be subject to valve disease, but the aortic and mitral valves are the most frequently affected. Valve diseases are detected by a typical sound during cardiac auscultation, the heart murmur. More or less severe, they generally contribute to the appearance of an arrhythmia or a cardiac insufficiency. There are two main types of valve disease: valve stenosis and valve insufficiency.

The heart... page 250

VALVE STENOSIS

Valve stenosis slows down blood flow. The valve is not sufficiently open during the passage of blood.

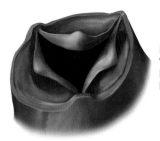

Healthy open valve
When it opens to let the blood pass, the edges of a healthy valve fold.

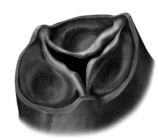

Valve stenosis
The thickening of the edges of the valve contributes to reducing the opening and to the slowing down of the blood flow.

VALVE INSUFFICIENCY

Valve insufficiency is a defect in the tightness of a heart valve. The valve does not close completely and the blood flows back.

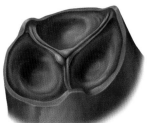

Closed healthy valve
The edges of a healthy valve, elastic and thin, close hermetically.

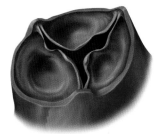

Valve insufficiency
The valve edges do not come together upon closing, which causes blood leakage.

VALVULOPLASTY

Valvuloplasty is a procedure intended to repair an abnormal heart valve. The thickened valve can be dilated using an inflatable balloon mounted on a catheter. The latter is introduced under local **anesthesia** in a superficial vessel then pushed as far as the damaged valve where the balloon is inflated. Valve insufficiency requires more serious surgery during which the valve is reshaped. In severe cases, the valve must be replaced by a **prosthesis**.

VALVE DISEASE

SYMPTOMS:
Shortness of breath, sometimes loss of consciousness, thoracic pain, palpitations.

TREATMENTS:
Prevention of infectious endocarditis. Advanced stage: valvuloplasty, valvular prosthesis.

HEART INFLAMMATIONS

The different tissues that make up the heart may be subject to **inflammations**. These often mean the presence of an **infection**, but their cause is not always defined. The inflammations can cause serious lesions and disrupt the functioning of the heart.

INFECTIOUS ENDOCARDITIS

Infectious endocarditis is an infection of the heart valves and the membrane that lines the inside of the heart, the endocardium. It is most often caused by a bacterium (streptococcus, staphylococcus) or, more rarely, by a fungus (*Candida albicans*). Endocarditis particularly affects those with valvular prostheses as well as individuals whose valves are weakened by a congenital malformation or by a disease such as atherosclerosis or acute rheumatic fever. The infectious agents reach the heart through the blood circulation, often following a minor infection (cavity, boil, otitis). They induce a growth of vegetation on the valves, excrescences that can cause valve diseases or cardiac insufficiency.

The heart... page 250

Aorta

Aortic valve
The aortic and mitral valves are the valves most affected by infectious endocarditis.

Vegetation

Reverse blood flow
When the aortic valve is altered by vegetation, it loses its impermeability and the blood flows back from the aorta to the left ventricle, which may cause a cardiac insufficiency.

Infectious endocarditis

ACUTE RHEUMATIC FEVER

Acute rheumatic fever is an inflammatory disease that affects the large joints (knees, elbows) and the heart. It often follows an untreated strep throat. Thanks to antibiotic treatments, the disease has practically disappeared from developed countries.

Angina... page 319

HEART INFLAMMATIONS

SYMPTOMS:
Fever. Infectious endocarditis: intense fatigue, perspiration, weight loss, pallor, joint and muscle pains.
Myocarditis: respiratory problems, cardiac arrhythmia.
Pericarditis: thoracic pain, respiratory problems.

TREATMENTS:
Antibiotics, anti-inflammatories, rest, sometimes surgery.

PREVENTION:
Infectious endocarditis: preventive antibiotic therapy in individuals at risk before surgery or dental care.

MYOCARDITIS AND PERICARDITIS

Myocarditis is the inflammation of the heart muscle (myocardium) while pericarditis is the inflammation of the membrane that covers it (pericardium). These two disorders are most often caused by a viral or bacterial condition: angina (inflammation of the throat), Lyme disease, tuberculosis, etc. Acute pericarditis is often accompanied by the effusion of a fluid between the superimposed leaflets of the pericardium. The fluid that accumulates may compress the heart and prevent it from filling with blood. It must then be subject to emergency tapping. Chronic constrictive pericarditis is a serious disorder characterized by the thickening and the hardening of the pericardium.

ANEURYSM

An aneurysm is the abnormal dilation of the arterial wall or, more rarely, of a vein or of the heart. We distinguish between different types of aneurysms based on their location (cerebral, aortic, cardiac aneurysm), their form (fusiform, saccular), and their cause. An aneurysm may be **congenital** or appear on a wall weakened by a **trauma**, an **infection** (syphilis), or atherosclerosis. Asymptomatic, it only reveals its presence when it ruptures. It then causes an internal hemorrhage that requires emergency surgery, specifically when it involves an aortic or cerebral aneurysm.

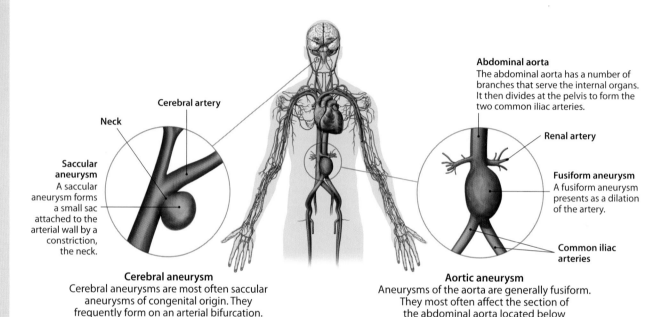

Cerebral artery

Neck

Saccular aneurysm
A saccular aneurysm forms a small sac attached to the arterial wall by a constriction, the neck.

Cerebral aneurysm
Cerebral aneurysms are most often saccular aneurysms of congenital origin. They frequently form on an arterial bifurcation.

Abdominal aorta
The abdominal aorta has a number of branches that serve the internal organs. It then divides at the pelvis to form the two common iliac arteries.

Renal artery

Fusiform aneurysm
A fusiform aneurysm presents as a dilation of the artery.

Common iliac arteries

Aortic aneurysm
Aneurysms of the aorta are generally fusiform. They most often affect the section of the abdominal aorta located below the renal arteries.

ANEURYSM RUPTURE

Aneurysms tend to dilate with time, under the pressure of the blood. They may bleed slightly or break suddenly. The aneurysm rupture is promoted by the aging of the arterial walls, by atherosclerosis, and by high blood pressure. The aortic aneurysm rupture causes a very extensive, often fatal, internal hemorrhage. It primarily affects men over 55 years of age. The cerebral aneurysm rupture generally occurs after age 35 and most often affects women. It causes a cerebral hemorrhage, which may lead to neurological complications: paralysis, memory problems, speech problems.

Cerebral vascular accidents... page 156

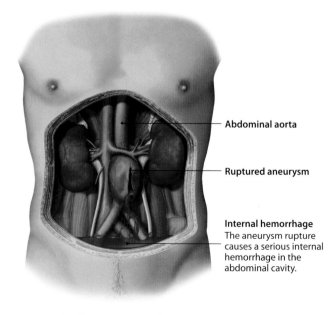

Abdominal aorta

Ruptured aneurysm

Internal hemorrhage
The aneurysm rupture causes a serious internal hemorrhage in the abdominal cavity.

Aortic aneurysm rupture

THE **TREATMENT** OF **ANEURYSMS**

The treatment of aneurysms calls on a number of surgical techniques (clamping, embolization, vessel graft) that are performed preventively on large aneurysms presenting risks of rupture, or on an emergency basis in order to repair a ruptured aneurysm. Small aneurysms are subject to regular monitoring that make it possible to check their diameter and to surgically intervene if this becomes critical.

EMBOLIZATION

Embolization consists of closing up an artery that has an aneurysm or that feeds a pathological structure, such as a fibroma or a tumor. It may be done using a balloon, synthetic particles, or a metallic filament. The obstruction of an aneurysm prevents the blood from circulating there and from causing its rupture.

CLAMPING

Clamping consists of stapling a blood vessel with the goal of stopping a hemorrhage or isolating an aneurysm. In the case of aneurysms with a wide neck, clamping permits better occlusion than embolization. This technique also involves less risk of thrombosis (formation of a blood clot).

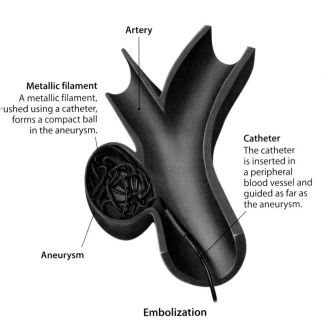

Artery

Metallic filament
A metallic filament, pushed using a catheter, forms a compact ball in the aneurysm.

Catheter
The catheter is inserted in a peripheral blood vessel and guided as far as the aneurysm.

Aneurysm

Embolization

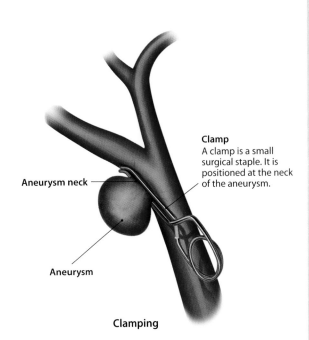

Clamp
A clamp is a small surgical staple. It is positioned at the neck of the aneurysm.

Aneurysm neck

Aneurysm

Clamping

ANEURYSM

SYMPTOMS:
Asymptomatic before the rupture. Ruptured aneurysm: pain, generalized discomfort, swelling in the case of an aneurysm affecting a superficial artery.

TREATMENTS:
Surgery (clamping, embolization, vascular graft, endovascular prosthesis). Infectious aneurysm: surgery and antibiotics.

PREVENTION:
Early diagnosis and regular monitoring. Prevention of high blood pressure and of atherosclerosis.

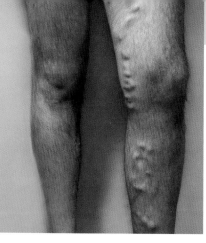

VARICOSE VEINS

Varicose veins are permanently dilated and deformed veins. They most often affect the legs, specifically the superficial vessels, that is, the vessels located under the skin. This very common problem affects one out of three individuals in Western countries, primarily women.

THE CAUSES OF VARICOSE VEINS

Varicose veins form following a venous insufficiency: an improper functioning of the venous circulation that occurs when the wall of the veins lacks tone and their valves do not function properly. Blood then tends to stagnate in the veins, which causes their abnormal dilation. Varicose veins develop slowly. They form blue cords that become increasingly more visible under the skin, becoming more prominent over the years if no treatment is sought. Treatments not only make it possible to eliminate the varicose veins, but also to avoid certain complications such as phlebitis and ulcers.

Ulcers... page 76
Phlebitis... page 274

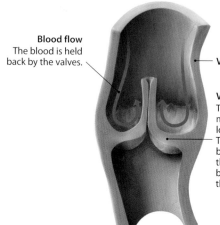

Blood flow
The blood is held back by the valves.

Vein

Valve
The valves are membranous folds located inside the veins. They form impermeable barriers that prevent the blood from flowing back downwards under the pull of gravity.

Dilated vein
The accumulation of blood in the vein causes its swelling.

Defective valve
The valve is pulled backwards by the weight of the blood that accumulates.

Reverse blood flow
When the valve is defective, the blood tends to flow back downwards and to stagnate in the vein.

Normal venous circulation

Abnormal venous circulation

VENOUS INSUFFICIENCY

Venous insufficiency is manifested by a heavy feeling in the legs, specifically at the end of the day, which may be accompanied by edema (swelling). Chronic venous insufficiency is manifested by the development of varicose veins.

THE DOPPLER ULTRASOUND TEST

The Doppler ultrasound test makes it possible to measure the speed of the blood using ultrasound and to diagnose the blood circulation anomalies. This medical test is often combined with an ultrasound echography, which makes it possible to obtain a two- or three-dimensional image of the blood vessels (or the heart cavities) examined. These two techniques specifically make it possible to locate the varicose veins and to evaluate their condition.

THE **TREATMENT** OF **VARICOSE VEINS**

The treatment of varicose veins consists of compensating for the venous insufficiency or by removing the affected veins by different methods: compression stockings, sclerotheraphy, stripping, laser. Compression stockings are elastic stockings designed to help the venous circulation. They apply pressure, which progressively decreases from the foot towards the thigh. Sclerotherapy consists in injecting an atrophying agent into the varicose veins intended to make them disappear. Stripping is the surgical extraction of superficial varicose vein, generally the large saphenous vein. After the removal of a superficial vein, blood circulation naturally flows back to other, deeper veins.

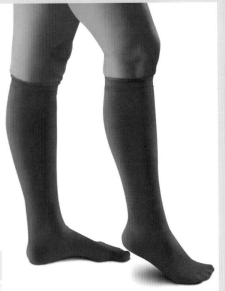

Compression stockings
Compression stockings are elastic stockings intended to relieve venous insufficiency by applying pressure that decreases from the foot to the thigh. There are different types, adapted to the seriousness of the venous insufficiency.

PREVENTING VARICOSE VEINS

Numerous factors promote the weakening of the wall of the veins and their dilation: family history, hormonal fluctuations in women, taking oral contraceptives, pregnancy, excess weight, sedentary lifestyle, prolonged standing, heat, aging. While heredity, age, and gender are factors that cannot be changed, certain measures may help you to prevent the appearance or the aggravation of varicose veins.

■ MOVE
Engaging in physical exercise such as walking, swimming, or bicycling promotes blood circulation. On the other hand, prolonged standing and sitting contribute to the stagnation of the blood.

■ MAINTAIN A HEALTHY WEIGHT
Excess weight makes the return of the blood to the heart difficult.

■ AVOID WEARING SOCKS AND CLOTHES THAT ARE TOO TIGHT
Pants, socks, stockings, and shoes that are too tight can act as a tourniquet and prevent proper venous circulation.

■ WEAR COMPRESSION STOCKINGS IN THE DAY
Regularly wearing compression stockings makes it possible to avoid the formation of new varicose veins and to limit the aggravation of those already formed. Ideally, you must put on the stockings before you get up in the morning.

■ ELEVATE YOUR LEGS AT NIGHT
The return of blood towards the heart will be facilitated if you sleep with pillows under your legs or if the foot of your bed is elevated.

■ AVOID EXPOSING LEGS TO THE HEAT
Very hot showers or baths as well as saunas and sunbathing promote the dilation of the veins.

VARICOSE VEINS

SYMPTOMS:
Dilated veins forming blue cords under the skin, which become prominent over time. Venous insufficiency: heavy swollen legs at the end of the day, painful veins, tingling, nocturnal cramps.

TREATMENTS:
Sclerotherapy, stripping, laser, compression stockings.

PREVENTION:
Engage in physical exercise promoting blood circulation (walking, swimming, bicycling). Elevation of the legs at night and wearing compression stockings during the day.

THROMBOSIS

Thrombosis is the formation of a blood clot in an artery or a vein. When a thrombosis occurs in a deep vein, it may cause serious complications, specifically a pulmonary embolism. Many factors can increase the risk of venous thrombosis, including prolonged immobilization (bed rest, wearing a cast, airplane travel), obesity, pregnancy, family history, smoking, taking oral contraceptives, and certain diseases (venous or cardiac insufficiency, certain cancers, etc.). When a thrombosis occurs in an artery, it prevents the blood irrigation of a region to a varying extent, which can cause gangrene or infarction and be life-threatening for the patient. Arterial thrombosis is promoted by smoking, diabetes, and atherosclerosis. Thrombosis, along with its complications, are serious conditions that require quick medical treatment, based on **anticoagulants**.

DEEP VEIN THROMBOSIS

Deep vein thrombosis is the formation of a blood clot, called a thrombus, in a deep vein, generally located in the lower limbs. It causes a phlebitis, an inflammation of the vein. This is accompanied by an inflammation of the adjacent tissues and sometimes by an edema (swelling), but the symptoms may be discreet, even non-existent. Venous thrombosis may result in serious complications, specifically when the clot detaches and migrates towards the lungs, causing a pulmonary embolism.

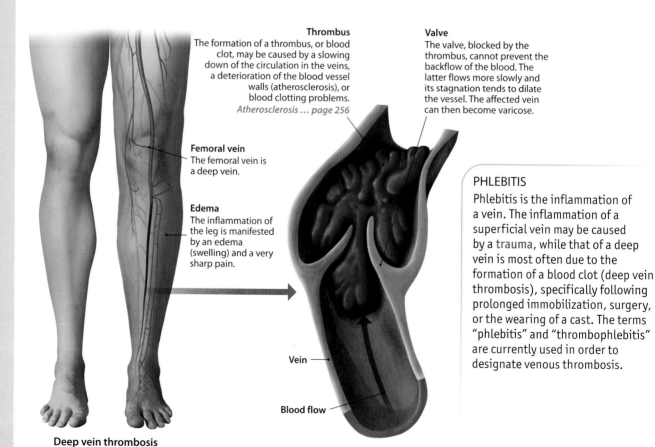

Thrombus
The formation of a thrombus, or blood clot, may be caused by a slowing down of the circulation in the veins, a deterioration of the blood vessel walls (atherosclerosis), or blood clotting problems.
Atherosclerosis ... page 256

Valve
The valve, blocked by the thrombus, cannot prevent the backflow of the blood. The latter flows more slowly and its stagnation tends to dilate the vessel. The affected vein can then become varicose.

Femoral vein
The femoral vein is a deep vein.

Edema
The inflammation of the leg is manifested by an edema (swelling) and a very sharp pain.

PHLEBITIS
Phlebitis is the inflammation of a vein. The inflammation of a superficial vein may be caused by a trauma, while that of a deep vein is most often due to the formation of a blood clot (deep vein thrombosis), specifically following prolonged immobilization, surgery, or the wearing of a cast. The terms "phlebitis" and "thrombophlebitis" are currently used in order to designate venous thrombosis.

Vein

Blood flow

Deep vein thrombosis

EMBOLISM

An embolism is a sudden obstruction of a blood vessel by an embolus, that is, a body of varied nature carried by the circulation of the blood. Embolisms most often affect an artery and prevent the blood irrigation of a tissue or an organ. An embolism is a serious, potentially fatal problem. It requires emergency medical treatment, specifically when it affects the vital organs such as the lungs (pulmonary embolism) or the brain (cerebral embolism).

Cerebrovascular accidents... page 156

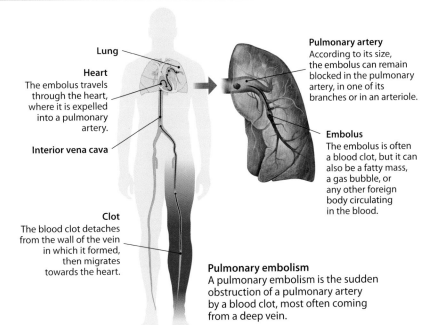

Lung

Heart
The embolus travels through the heart, where it is expelled into a pulmonary artery.

Interior vena cava

Clot
The blood clot detaches from the wall of the vein in which it formed, then migrates towards the heart.

Pulmonary artery
According to its size, the embolus can remain blocked in the pulmonary artery, in one of its branches or in an arteriole.

Embolus
The embolus is often a blood clot, but it can also be a fatty mass, a gas bubble, or any other foreign body circulating in the blood.

Pulmonary embolism
A pulmonary embolism is the sudden obstruction of a pulmonary artery by a blood clot, most often coming from a deep vein.

THE PREVENTION OF VENOUS THROMBOSIS

Prolonged immobility is among the main risk factors of venous thrombosis and phlebitis because it causes a stagnation of the blood in the veins. Limit, if possible, the duration of bed rest following surgery or childbirth and avoid staying in the same position for several hours. If you are restricted (for example during a flight lasting more than six hours) follow the next few recommendations:

- Drink lots of water and avoid consuming dehydrating beverages (coffee, alcohol). Dehydration promotes venous insufficiency.

- Stretch your legs regularly (flexing and extending the ankles) and take a few steps, ideally every two hours, in order to stimulate the blood circulation. When you take a plane, avoid taking a sleeping pill, which promotes immobility.

- Wear comfortable clothing and shoes. When they are too tight, they interfere with the blood circulation. For the same reason, do not cross your legs.

- If you already suffer from venous insufficiency (heavy legs, varicose veins), wear your compression stockings and take the anticoagulant drug your doctor prescribes. Elevate the legs when space permits it.

THROMBOSIS

SYMPTOMS:
Arterial thrombosis: pain, pallor, absence of pulse. Venous thrombosis: inflammation, edema (swelling), fever, sharp pain, sometimes asymptomatic. Pulmonary embolism: thoracic pain, feeling of suffocation, accelerated breathing, bluish coloration of the skin, heavy sweating.

TREATMENTS:
Anticoagulants, dissolving of of the thrombus (thrombolysis), anti-inflammatories, compression stockings, sometimes removal of the thrombus (thrombectomy). Arterial thrombosis: angioplasty.

PREVENTION:
Reduce immobility and bed rest after surgery or childbirth, physical exercise, preventive administration of anticoagulants.

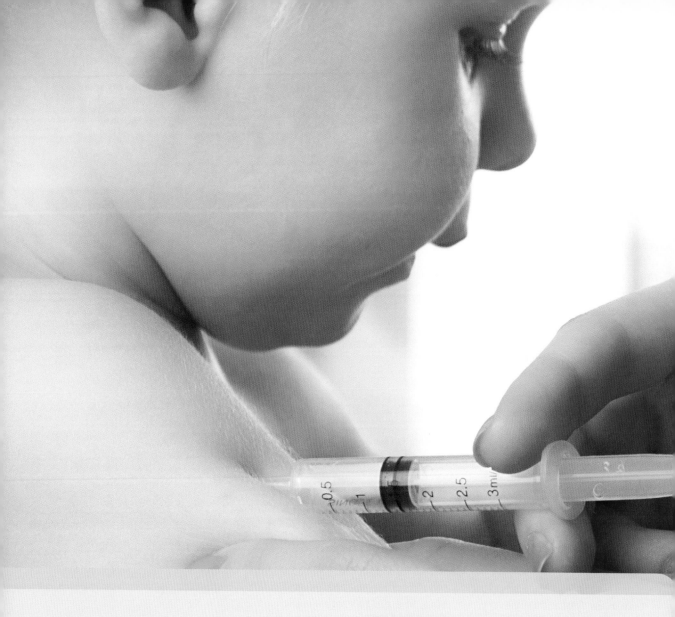

THE BODY

THE **IMMUNE SYSTEM**

At every moment, our body is in contact with microorganisms (viruses, bacteria, parasites, fungi) capable of causing **infectious** diseases. In order to protect us, our body can count on a very effective defense system, the immune system. It consists of various elements that, in collaboration with the lymphatic system, are responsible for detecting and destroying these harmful agents when they enter into the body. Fever, **inflammatory** reaction, and the production of antibodies are some of the manifestations of the immune system.

Thanks to the action of the immune system, a number of infectious diseases are spontaneously cured, but the most serious ones require medical treatment. Furthermore, disruptions of this system occur, causing allergies, immunodeficiency, or **autoimmune** diseases. The organs of the lymph system may also be the site of infections and tumors that promote the accumulation of lymph and the swelling of tissues.

DISEASES

THE **IMMUNE SYSTEM**

The immune system is all of the defense mechanisms which, with the lymph system, make it possible for the body to combat external attacks such **infectious** diseases. This system also ensures the elimination of potentially cancerous abnormal cells. The immune defense is based on physical barriers such as the skin, as well as on mechanisms such as fever, **inflammation**, and the action of cells and of specialized proteins (lymphocytes, antibodies). The immune system may be subject to disruptions, which result in allergies, immunodeficiency, or **autoimmune** diseases. Various medical and surgical treatments make it possible to strengthen this system and control its disruptions: **vaccines**, **antibiotics**, **immunosuppressors**, bone marrow transplant, etc.

THE **PHYSICAL BARRIERS**

The external surface of the body is covered with skin while mucous membranes cover its internal cavities. This protection is reinforced by various secretions (mucus, tears, sweat, sebum, saliva, gastric juices, etc.), by bacterial flora, and by the hair located near natural pathways. These elements form a physical barrier that prevents infectious agents from penetrating into the body.

BACTERIAL FLORA

A multitude of bacteria live naturally on the skin and in the internal cavities of the body such as the intestines or the vagina. These bacterial flora are not harmful to the body; on the contrary, they promote immunity and fight foreign microorganisms and pathogens.

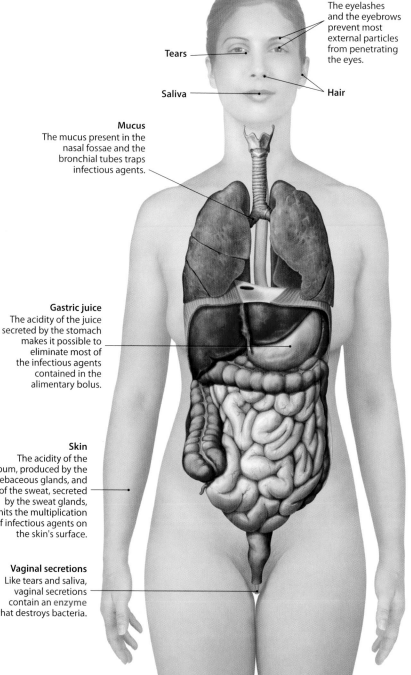

Eyelashes and eyebrows
The eyelashes and the eyebrows prevent most external particles from penetrating the eyes.

Tears

Saliva

Hair

Mucus
The mucus present in the nasal fossae and the bronchial tubes traps infectious agents.

Gastric juice
The acidity of the juice secreted by the stomach makes it possible to eliminate most of the infectious agents contained in the alimentary bolus.

Skin
The acidity of the sebum, produced by the sebaceous glands, and of the sweat, secreted by the sweat glands, limits the multiplication of infectious agents on the skin's surface.

Vaginal secretions
Like tears and saliva, vaginal secretions contain an enzyme that destroys bacteria.

INFLAMMATION

Faced with an external attack such as an infection or an injury, the body reacts first with an inflammation. This may occur in any of the tissues and organs. The inflammatory reaction is expressed as a rash (redness), an edema (swelling), or a feeling of heat and pain. It sometimes results in discomfort or in a functional disturbance, which may be reduced through the local application of cold compresses and the taking of anti-inflammatories.

1. Penetration of infectious agents
A skin wound allows infectious agents to penetrate the body. Specialized cells present under the skin react by secreting chemical messengers such as histamine.

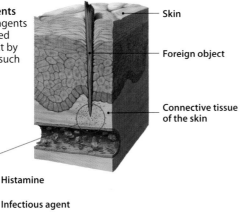

Skin

Foreign object

Connective tissue of the skin

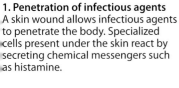

Histamine

Infectious agent

2. Appearance of an edema and of a rash
The infectious agents multiply locally in the connective tissue. Histamine causes the dilation of the blood capillaries, which become more permeable, which results in the appearance of a rash (redness on the skin) and of an edema. An edema is an effusion of fluid in the tissue, which is manifested by a swelling. When it is large, it compresses the adjacent nerves and causes pain as well as itching.

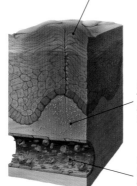

Edema and rash

Site of infection
The site of infection is the area of tissue where the infection develops.

Dilated blood capillary
Histamine makes the wall of the blood capillaries more permeable.

3. Digestion of infectious agents
Chemical messengers attract a large number of white blood cells (macrophages, neutrophils), which actively participate in the digestion of infectious agents.

Neutrophil
Neutrophils pass through the wall of the dilated blood capillaries in order to reach the site of infection.

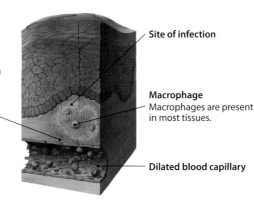

Site of infection

Macrophage
Macrophages are present in most tissues.

Dilated blood capillary

FEVER
Fever is an elevation of body temperature caused, most often, by the inflammatory reaction. It is generally manifested by a feeling of discomfort and of heat as well as shivering. A moderate fever, from 100°F (37.8°C) to 101.3°F (38.5°C), is beneficial because it promotes the destruction of certain infectious agents. On the other hand, a high fever, above 102.2°F (39°C), can cause feverish convulsions in children and behavior problems in the elderly. It therefore helps to bring it down using tepid baths, cold compresses, or antipyretics.

ANTI-INFLAMMATORIES
An anti-inflammatory is a drug that makes it possible to reduce certain symptoms of the inflammation (pain, edema), without, however, treating the cause. Steroidal anti-inflammatories are derivatives of corticosteroids, hormones secreted by the adrenal glands. Very powerful, they cause numerous side effects (dryness of the skin, weakness of the bones, etc.). More commonly used, the non-steroidal anti-inflammatories include a broad range of substances such as aspirin or ibuprofen.

LYMPHOCYTES AND ANTIBODIES

After the inflammatory reaction caused by an infection, the body puts a slower immune response into action involving specialized cells, the lymphocytes, and complex proteins, the antibodies. A lymphocyte is a type of white blood cell of which there are two major strains: T lymphocytes and B lymphocytes. During an infection, T lymphocytes migrate towards the site of the infection. They divide and participate in the immune response by destroying the cells recognized as foreign or abnormal. B lymphocytes, on the other hand, are transformed, in organs such as the lymph nodes or the spleen, into plasmacytes, antibody-producing cells.

The production of antibodies is due to the presence of an antigen (foreign molecule) in the body. An antigen can be an element of the infectious agent or a bacterial toxin, but also a harmless substance or an element of the body recognized as abnormal or foreign (allergy, autoimmune disease, rejection phenomenon). In all cases, the antibodies are developed by the plasmacytes in order to promote the specific recognition of the antigen in question and to neutralize it. When an antigen is covered with antibodies, other cells, such as the white blood cells (neutrophils, macrophages), proceed to destroy it. Once the antigens are destroyed and the infection beaten, the body retains a portion of its antibodies. By doing so, it stores the appropriate immune response against the beaten antigen in its memory for a certain time, facilitating its rapid elimination in the event of a recurrence.

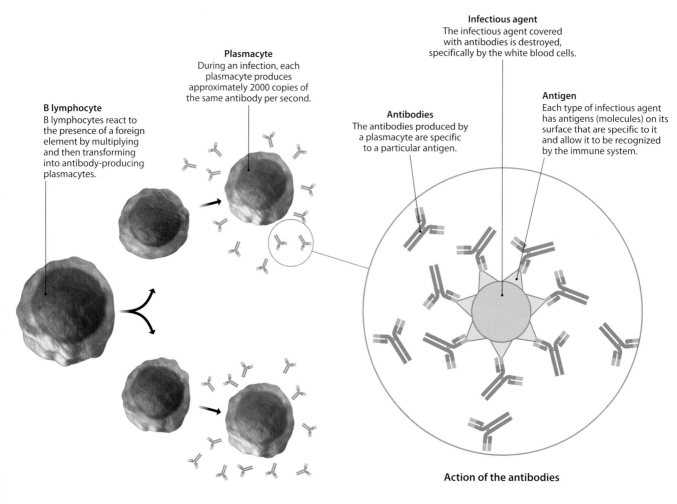

Plasmacyte
During an infection, each plasmacyte produces approximately 2000 copies of the same antibody per second.

Infectious agent
The infectious agent covered with antibodies is destroyed, specifically by the white blood cells.

B lymphocyte
B lymphocytes react to the presence of a foreign element by multiplying and then transforming into antibody-producing plasmacytes.

Antibodies
The antibodies produced by a plasmacyte are specific to a particular antigen.

Antigen
Each type of infectious agent has antigens (molecules) on its surface that are specific to it and allow it to be recognized by the immune system.

Action of the antibodies

THE LYMPHATIC SYSTEM

The lymphatic system consists of a combination of vessels and organs closely connected to the immune and cardiovascular systems. It carries lymph, a clear yellow fluid originating in the tissues of the body. The lymphatic system removes **infectious** agents from the lymph before releasing it into the blood. It also prevents the accumulation of fluid in the tissues, maintains a constant blood level, and plays a major role in immunity, specifically by ensuring the production and the circulation of lymphocytes.

THE **LYMPHATIC VESSELS**

The lymphatic vessels run alongside the blood vessels. They transport the lymph originating from the interstitial fluid, that is the fluid in which all of the cells of the body are bathed. The lymph circulates slowly under the action of the interstitial fluid pressure, muscular contractions, and respiratory movements. It passes through one or several lymph nodes before pouring into the cardiovascular system through subclavian veins.

Subclavian veins
The lymph pours into the subclavian veins.

Tonsils
The tonsils are irregularly shaped lymphoid organs, located on the perimeter of the pharynx. Rich in lymphocytes, they protect the body against the infectious agents that penetrate by the upper airways (nose, mouth).

Thymus
The thymus is a gland located in front of the trachea, between the lungs. This lymphoid organ contains T lymphocytes in various degrees of maturation. Its activity is particularly important in children. From puberty, the thymus atrophies, then maintains a reduced size in adults.

Spleen
Located in the abdomen, between the stomach and the left kidney, the spleen contains lymphocytes that proliferate and produce antibodies. This lymphoid organ, highly vascular, is also a site of blood storage and filtration. That is where the macrophages destroy the worn-out blood cells.

Lymph node
Located on the path of the lymphatic vessels, the numerous lymph nodes filter and clean the lymph by removing infectious agents from it. These small organs, rich in lymphocytes, form clusters in different parts of the body, specifically under the armpits, in the neck, in the groin, and in the intestines. During an infection, the lymphocytes, activated by contact with the antigens, multiply in the nodes, which increase in volume.

Bone marrow
The bone marrow is the site where blood cells, including the lymphocytes, are produced.

THE **LYMPHOID ORGANS**

The lymphoid organs are the organs in which the lymphocytes are produced and stored. The lymph nodes, the spleen, the tonsils, the thymus, and the bone marrow are lymphoid organs.

Lymphatic vessel
The interstitial fluid that accumulates in the tissues passes through the thin permeable wall of the lymphatic vessels, where it becomes lymph.

281

INFECTIOUS AGENTS

An **infectious** agent is an organism, most often microscopic, that causes an infection when it penetrates and multiplies in the body. Bacteria, viruses, microscopic fungi, and parasites are infectious agents. All of these microorganisms may exist in a latent state in the environment or be transmitted by carriers: flea, tick, mosquito, etc. Their presence in the body triggers an immune reaction that seeks to eliminate them. Specific drugs (**antibiotics**, antivirals, **antifungals**, antiparasitics) can destroy most infectious agents.

BACTERIA

A bacterium is a unicellular organism. That is, it consists of a single cell. It is surrounded by a wall and reproduces by simple cellular division. Bacteria present in different forms: rods, spheres, spiral filaments. Some are equipped with a flagella, a long filament that enables them to move. Most bacteria are not harmful and some are even needed for the proper functioning of the body, such as those that make up the skin, intestinal or vaginal flora. Preventive vaccination, hygiene measures and antibiotics make it possible to combat pathogenic bacteria or the toxins they produce.

PARASITES

A parasite is an organism that lives and develops at the expense of another. Some, called protozoa, consist of a single cell. Others consist of several cells such as certain worms, insects, or mites. Parasites generally enter the body through the ingestion of contaminated foods or through insect bites. They cause parasitoses, infections more common in tropical countries.

Filaria
The filaria is the parasitic worm responsible for filariasis.
Lymphatic filariasis... page 306

MICROSCOPIC FUNGI

A microscopic fungus is invisible to the naked eye, pathogenic or not. Such fungi include yeasts, consisting of a single cell, and molds, consisting of several filamentous cells. Microscopic fungi may be at the origin of infections called mycoses: tinea, athlete's foot, vaginal mycosis, aspergillosis, etc.

VIRUSES

A virus is an infectious agent of very small size (100 to 1000 times smaller than a cell), consisting of a capsule of proteins containing a nucleic acid. In order to multiply, the virus depends on the host cell it infects. The virus may be at the origin of benign (cold, warts), serious (rabies, hepatitis B), or sometimes epidemic (flu, meningitis, AIDS) diseases. Vaccination and antivirals make it possible to prevent or to treat certain viral diseases.

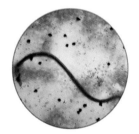

Nucleic acid
Nucleic acid is the genetic material of the virus. It is injected into the host cell whose structures it uses in order to multiply.
Lymphatic filariasis... page 306

Protein capsule

THE **INFECTION SITES**

The entry of an infectious agent into the body can take place through the skin, following, for example, a cut, a bite, an open fracture, or a burn. However, it most often takes place through the mucous membranes, since they cover the digestive, respiratory and urogenital tracts. Sometimes the pathogenic agent is introduced accidentally into the body during a blood transfusion or surgery.

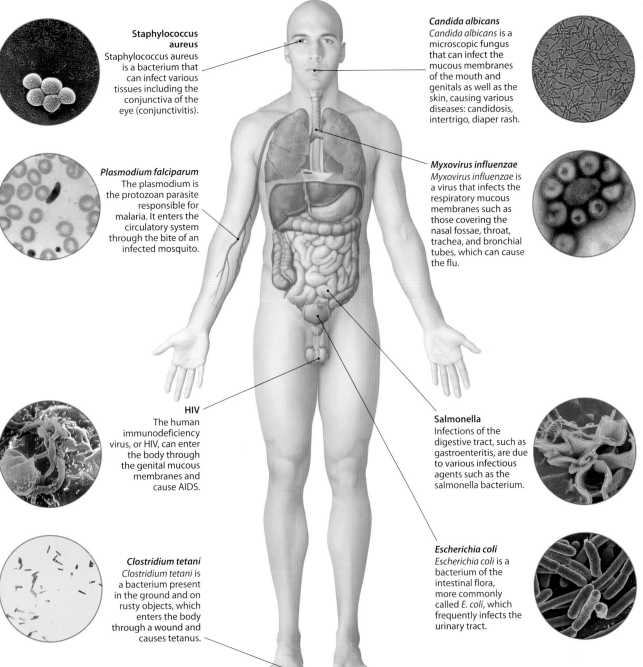

Staphylococcus aureus
Staphylococcus aureus is a bacterium that can infect various tissues including the conjunctiva of the eye (conjunctivitis).

Plasmodium falciparum
The plasmodium is the protozoan parasite responsible for malaria. It enters the circulatory system through the bite of an infected mosquito.

HIV
The human immunodeficiency virus, or HIV, can enter the body through the genital mucous membranes and cause AIDS.

Clostridium tetani
Clostridium tetani is a bacterium present in the ground and on rusty objects, which enters the body through a wound and causes tetanus.

Candida albicans
Candida albicans is a microscopic fungus that can infect the mucous membranes of the mouth and genitals as well as the skin, causing various diseases: candidosis, intertrigo, diaper rash.

Myxovirus influenzae
Myxovirus influenzae is a virus that infects the respiratory mucous membranes such as those covering the nasal fossae, throat, trachea, and bronchial tubes, which can cause the flu.

Salmonella
Infections of the digestive tract, such as gastroenteritis, are due to various infectious agents such as the salmonella bacterium.

Escherichia coli
Escherichia coli is a bacterium of the intestinal flora, more commonly called *E. coli*, which frequently infects the urinary tract.

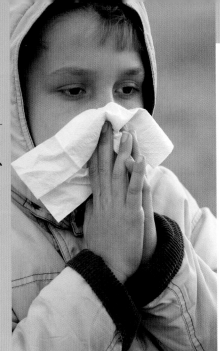

INFECTIOUS DISEASES

An **infectious** disease is the invasion of the body by an infectious agent. The infection, or contamination, can occur by direct or indirect contact with an infected person, or an animal carrying the infectious agent (carrier), or accidentally during a medical or surgical procedure. The transmission method, the incubation period, the symptoms, and the affected tissues depend on the infectious agent and the means of infection. Different laboratory techniques make it possible to identify the microorganisms at the origin of the disease and thus to adapt the treatment.

Respiratory infections... page 318
Infectious diseases in childhood... page 519

CONTAGION

Contagion is the transmission of an infectious disease to a healthy individual. It occurs by direct contact (skin, blood, semen, saliva, mucus) or through a dissemination agent (air, water) or a contaminated object. Certain diseases are more contagious than others, according to the nature of the infectious agent. The contagion period is the period during which the disease is capable of transmitting the infectious agent to other individuals.

ANIMAL TRANSMISSION

Some infectious diseases are transmitted to humans through contact with a contaminated animal, called a carrier. Thus, Lyme disease is transmitted by the bite of a tick. Yellow fever, dengue, and malaria are transmitted by the bite of different species of mosquitoes. Typhus is passed on by lice; the plague, by fleas.

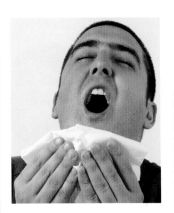

Sneezing
Sneezing is the reflex expulsion of air through the mouth and the nose, in response to an irritation of the nasal mucous membrane (foreign body, infection). The droplets projected by a sneeze can transmit infectious agents.

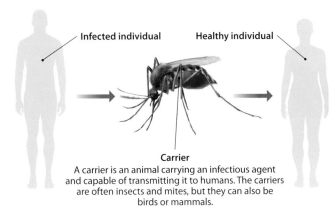

Infected individual · Healthy individual

Carrier
A carrier is an animal carrying an infectious agent and capable of transmitting it to humans. The carriers are often insects and mites, but they can also be birds or mammals.

INCUBATION

Incubation is the period between the infection of an individual by a pathogenic microorganism and the appearance of the first symptoms of the infectious disease it causes. Each disease is characterized by its own incubation period, which lasts from several days to several months or, in some cases, several years. Some diseases, such as measles or chickenpox, are contagious from the incubation period.

SEROPOSITIVITY

Seropositivity is the presence in the blood of antibodies specific to an infectious agent, indicating that the patient has been contaminated by this agent. Seropositivity applies to all infectious diseases, but the term is often used to describe the condition of an individual contaminated by the AIDS virus. Seronegativity characterizes the absence in the blood of the antibodies against an infectious agent.

PUS

Pus is an opaque fluid of varying thickness produced by the body during a bacterial infection. It consists of debris from dead cells, white blood cells and bacteria. Pus may be yellow, green, or brown in color, according to the nature of the infectious agent in question. When a wound or a lesion is infected, the pus tends to concentrate and form an abscess. The latter must be tapped or lanced in order to eliminate the pus. Left untreated, large abscesses tend to become chronic. The bacteria contained in the pus may then infect the blood and spread throughout the body (septicemia).

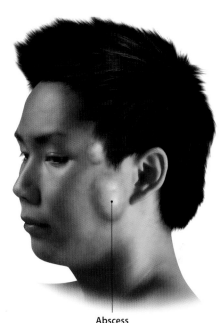

Abscess
An abscess is an accumulation of pus in a tissue infected by a bacterium.

SEPTICEMIA

Septicemia is a generalized infection. It is caused by the release into the blood of large and regular quantities of pathogenic microorganisms from an initial site of infection. Septicemia is manifested by a high fever and a change in overall condition. This is a serious disease that requires emergency hospitalization and prolonged antibiotic treatment.

BACTERIAL CULTURE

A bacterial culture is a laboratory technique that consists of multiplying bacteria in order to identify them. The bacteria, obtained by biopsy or by sampling (blood, wound, pus, secretion), are placed in a solid or liquid medium that promotes their development. They multiply by forming colonies of particular shapes and colors, which makes it possible to recognize them under the microscope. The bacteria may then be put in the presence of different antibiotics (antibiogram) in order to determine which is the most effective for a treatment.

Bacterial culture

Antibiotic
Lozenges impregnated with different antibiotics or in different concentrations are deposited on the culture for several hours.

Positive test
The effective antibiotics cause the destruction of bacteria with which they are in contact.

Negative test

Antibiogram
Performed using a bacterial culture, the antibiogram consists of putting a bacterium in the presence of various antibiotics in order to test its resistance or its sensitivity to each of them.

THE **TREATMENT** OF **INFECTIONS**

Several types of drugs inhibit the spread of certain infectious agents or cause their destruction. Antibiotics are the basic treatment for bacterial infections. Antifungals are used to combat infections caused by microscopic fungi, while antiparasitics such as vermifuges make it possible to treat infections due to parasites. Finally, antivirals are used in the treatment of severe viral infections such as hepatitis, flu, or AIDS. Anti-infective drugs may be injected, administered orally, or applied locally (cream, salve, etc.). The treatment duration varies from a few days to several months. Certain drugs, specifically antibiotics and antivirals, may cause side effects: allergies, digestive problems, neurological problems, etc.

SEROTHERAPY

Serotherapy is a treatment based on the intravenous injection of a therapeutic serum, which contains antibodies specific to an infectious agent. It makes it possible to quickly, but temporarily, protect an infected patient or one at high risk, while waiting for him to develop antibodies or when he is unable to produce them. Serum antibodies are obtained from an animal or a donor immunized against the infectious agent. Serotherapy may be used on a preventive or curative basis, in which the serum is administered before or after the infection.

ANTISEPTICS

An antiseptic is a product intended to destroy the infectious agents present on the skin and the mucous membranes, in order to avoid infections. There are numerous antiseptics such as alcohol, hydrogen peroxide, hexamidine, eosin, or thymol. The majority are exclusively reserved for external use. Some, however, may be administered orally, in order to treat urinary and certain intestinal infections.

Wound
Antiseptics are often used to disinfect a superficial wound, which averts the development of an infection.

VACCINE

A vaccine is a substance prepared from a transformed infectious element (virus, parasite, microbe, toxin), rendered inactive but still capable of stimulating the natural immunity of the body. Inoculating an individual with a vaccine, or vaccination, makes it possible to force the production of antibodies against a particular infectious agent. If the individual then contracts this infectious agent, the immune system quickly recognizes it and destroys it before the disease has the time to develop. Each country has a vaccination schedule, including obligatory vaccines and recommended vaccines, according to its own epidemiological conditions. Vaccination may cause side effects such as temporary pain, passing fever, or an inflammatory reaction (redness, swelling) around the inoculation site. It nevertheless remains the most effective way to avoid the spread of serious infectious diseases.

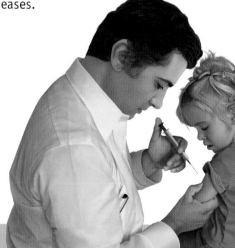

FORTIFYING THE IMMUNE SYSTEM AND PREVENTING INFECTIONS

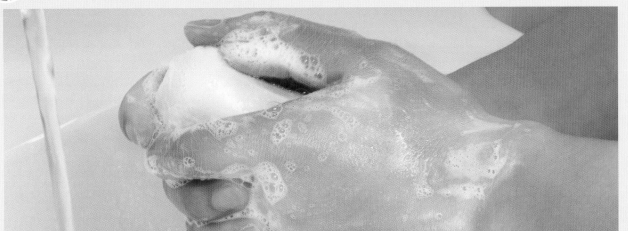

■ **WASH YOUR HANDS AND YOUR BODY REGULARLY**

Regular cleaning of the hands and other parts of the body with soap and water eliminates the potentially infectious agents present.

■ **PROTECT YOURSELF AND OTHERS**

Contagion may be prevented by some simple measures, such as wearing a mask against diseases transmitted by air, the use of condoms against sexually transmitted diseases, and the wearing of gloves against the transmission of pathogenic agents by direct contact. If you are suffering from a contagious disease, avoid direct contact, the exchange of objects, or the sharing of food. Cover your nose and mouth using your elbows or a handkerchief when sneezing or coughing in order to avoid spreading the infectious agent through droplets.

■ **DISINFECT WOUNDS**

The disinfection of a wound using an antiseptic prevents its infection by pathogenic microorganisms.

■ **USE ANTIBIOTICS PROPERLY**

An antibiotic treatment must be undertaken only on a doctor's prescription and must not be interrupted, in order to ensure its effectiveness. The unsuitable use of antibiotics may make some bacteria resistant and compromise the treatment of subsequent infections.

Hygiene and the prevention of infections... page 30

■ **EAT A HEALTHY AND BALANCED DIET**

Excessive consumption of foods rich in sugars, fat, or allergens, as well as the abuse of alcoholic beverages, are capable of weakening the immune system. On the other hand, the regular consumption of foods rich in Vitamins A and C and in minerals, like fruits and vegetables, legumes, nuts, and whole grains, strengthen the immune system. Yogurts based on starter cultures contain beneficial bacteria that make it possible to balance intestinal flora and strengthen immunity. Finally, drinking enough water provides proper hydration for your body and delays the spread of infections.

■ **CONTROL YOUR STRESS**

Prolonged stress weakens the immune system. Control your stress by using various techniques such as meditation or relaxation. In addition, rest, specifically a sufficient number of hours of sleep, makes it possible for the body to regenerate itself and to combat stress. Finally, regular and moderate physical activity makes it possible not only to relieve stress, but also to stimulate circulation and certain elements of the immune system.

■ **AVOID HARMFUL PRODUCTS**

Pesticides as well as certain household cleaning products contain harmful chemical substances that may weaken the immune system. Avoid them as much as possible.

ALLERGIES

Allergy, or hypersensitivity, is an abnormal reaction of the immune system during contact with an allergen, that is a typically harmless substance. Numerous substances can be allergens: pollens, foods, drugs, etc. Hereditary and environmental factors contribute to the development of allergies, without their precise cause being known. Allergic reactions, quick or delayed, may range in severity: redness, eczema, hives, asthma, nasal **inflammation**, swelling of the face and neck, anaphylactic shock. Various treatments make it possible to reduce allergy symptoms or to alleviate an individual's sensitivity to an allergen in a preventive manner.

ALLERGENS

An allergen is a harmless substance that causes an allergic reaction in a sensitive individual. Different types exist in the environment, which may be cutaneous or respiratory (pollens, molds, mites, industrial products, hair, and feathers), ingested (peanuts, shellfish, etc.), or introduced into the body through the blood (insect venom, drugs). A sensitive person is often allergic to several allergens of related chemical composition.

PETS
Certain individuals are allergic to the dead skin, saliva, hair or feathers of certain animals.

DRUGS
Some drugs such as aspirin and certain antibiotics are known to cause serious allergies.

NATURAL OR INDUSTRIAL PRODUCTS
Various substances such as natural latex as well as certain perfumes, cosmetics, cleaning products, or colorants may be allergens.

INSECT BITES
In a sensitized person, the venom of certain insects (bees, wasps, hornets) may trigger an allergic reaction of varying severity.

GRAINS OF POLLEN
According to the country and the season, many plants, such as grasses or the birch tree, release pollen grains that are responsible for hay fever. In autumn, certain molds can also cause allergies.

FOODS
Among the most common food allergens are eggs, peanuts, milk, fish, shellfish, nuts, and strawberries. A food allergy can become very serious if the offending food is not removed from the diet.

MITES
Contact with dust mite feces contained in the dust in homes and in bed linens is one of the main causes of allergic rhinitis, particularly in children.

THE **MECHANISM** OF THE **ALLERGY**

An allergy develops in two stages. An initial contact with the allergen causes a sensitivity in the individual, without appearance of symptoms: the immune system produces specific antibodies, that attach themselves to certain cells present in the tissues and the blood. During the second contact, the antibodies recognize the allergen. The cells to which they are attached then secrete histamine, a chemical substance involved in the inflammation mechanism that causes the symptoms characteristic of the allergic reaction: redness, swelling of tissues, etc. In the case of immediate hypersensitivity, the most frequent of the allergic reactions, the response of the immune system is quick, within a few minutes.

The immune system... page 278

ALLERGIC RHINITIS

Allergic rhinitis is an inflammation of the mucous membranes of the nasal fossae, that affects people who are sensitive to certain airborne allergens. Seasonal rhinitis, or hay fever, is caused by the pollen from certain plants; persistent rhinitis is due to dander (hair, feathers) from pets or dust mites. Allergic rhinitis is manifested during contact with the allergen by sneezing followed by nasal discharge, nasal congestion, itching, watering of the eyes, and, sometimes, conjunctivitis. It may also trigger, in certain cases, an attack of asthma or hives. Treatment is based on eliminating contact with the allergen and the administration of antihistamines. Desensitization may also be undertaken on a case-by-case basis.

ANTIHISTAMINES

An antihistamine is a drug that makes it possible to reduce or block the synthesis of the histamine by the body during an inflammation or an allergy. Antihistamines make it possible to relieve the symptoms of the allergic reaction (edema, nasal discharge, watering of the eyes, etc.) without actually curing the allergy. They exist in the form of tablets, eyedrops, aerosol sprays for the nose, and injectable solutions. Some of these drugs may have side effects: dryness of the mouth, constipation, drowsiness.

ONE OF THE MOST COMMON DISEASES

According to the World Allergy Organization, the number of persons suffering from allergies has considerably increased throughout the world during recent decades. Today, almost 400 million people suffer from allergic rhinitis. Up to 4% of adults and 8% of children are affected by a food allergy. The World Health Organization places allergies 4th among the most common diseases.

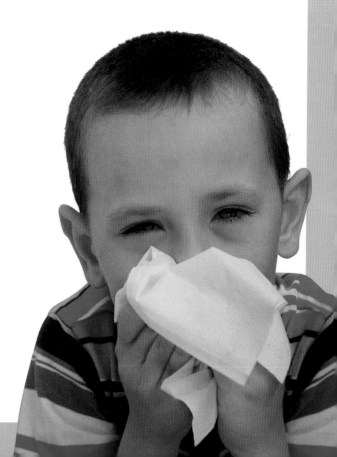

The immune system | Diseases

QUINCKE'S EDEMA

Quincke's edema is a sudden allergic reaction that is manifested by an edema of the deep layers of the skin of the face and the mucous membranes of the throat. It is manifested by a swelling of the lips, tongue, larynx, pharynx, and eyelids, which may be accompanied by fever and muscle and joint pain. A number of allergens can cause Quincke's edema, specifically certain foods (cheeses, eggs, peanuts, shellfish, tomatoes, strawberries, etc.), some drugs (antibiotics, aspirin, etc.), and insect bites. The risk of asphyxia caused by the obstruction of the pharynx is great and Quincke's edema may develop into an anaphylactic shock. Emergency medical treatment, based on the rapid administration of corticosteroids and of adrenaline, is therefore necessary.

ANAPHYLACTIC SHOCK

Anaphylactic shock is a serious allergic reaction that is manifested by severe circulatory insufficiency, accompanied by acute respiratory distress. Left untreated, it can cause death. Several types of allergens (foods, drugs, venoms) are capable of causing an anaphylactic shock in the minutes following the contact. The state of shock is manifested by a drop in blood pressure, breathing difficulties, and various symptoms: shivering, sweating, vomiting, blood diarrhea, hives, Quincke's edema. The risk of asphyxia and of cardiac arrest is significant and emergency hospitalization in an intensive care unit is necessary.

THE POSSIBLE CAUSES OF THE INCREASE IN ALLERGIES

A constant increase in the number of allergies is observed in the populations of several industrialized countries. According to certain researchers, our more sterilized way of life makes the immune system more sensitive to allergies. Thus, contact with certain bacteria, parasites or viruses, specifically during early childhood, makes it possible to stimulate the maturation of the immune system and thus to reduce the risk of developing allergies. Other hypotheses establish a link between the increase in allergies and air pollution, smoking, or diet rich in fat and poor in fruits and vegetables.

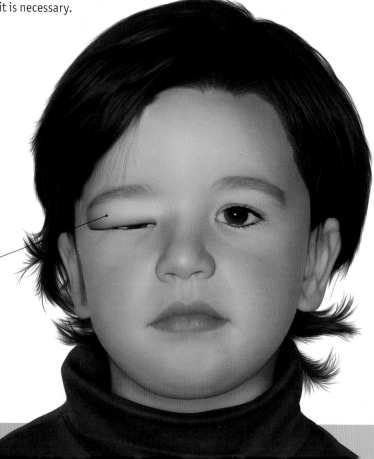

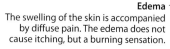
Edema
The swelling of the skin is accompanied by diffuse pain. The edema does not cause itching, but a burning sensation.

THE **SELF-INJECTION** OF **ADRENALINE**

Self-injection of adrenaline is practiced as first aid (Quincke's edema, anaphylactic shock), using a medically prescribed single-use syringe. With the appearance of the first symptoms (redness, heat, itching), the injection must be made in the thigh, while maintaining the position for 10 seconds. Side effects such as nausea, dizziness, hot flashes, or cardiac rhythm problems may occur following the injection. The possession of an adrenaline self-injector at all times is recommended for people suffering from serious allergies, specifically food allergies.

First aid: Respiratory problems... page 548

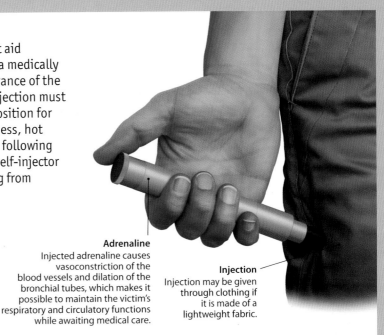

Adrenaline
Injected adrenaline causes vasoconstriction of the blood vessels and dilation of the bronchial tubes, which makes it possible to maintain the victim's respiratory and circulatory functions while awaiting medical care.

Injection
Injection may be given through clothing if it is made of a lightweight fabric.

DESENSITIZATION

Desensitization, or specific immunotherapy, is a treatment that seeks to reduce the sensitivity of an allergic person to a specific allergen. A skin test is first performed on the skin in order to determine to which allergen the patient is sensitive. The treatment then consists in giving regular low-dose injections of this allergen, which are increased progressively, in order to make it possible for the body to develop a tolerance to the substance. The treatment must be followed for several months, even several years, in order to obtain a significant reduction of allergic symptoms. For certain allergies, particularly those related to insect bites, this treatment shows good results. In addition, children demonstrate better receptivity to the treatment than adults.

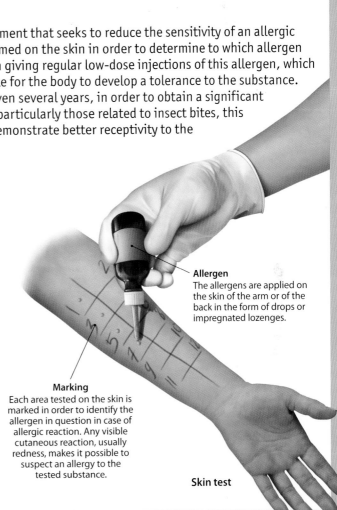

Allergen
The allergens are applied on the skin of the arm or of the back in the form of drops or impregnated lozenges.

Marking
Each area tested on the skin is marked in order to identify the allergen in question in case of allergic reaction. Any visible cutaneous reaction, usually redness, makes it possible to suspect an allergy to the tested substance.

Skin test

ALLERGIES

SYMPTOMS:
Skin reactions (redness, swelling, hives, etc.), eye irritation, digestive problems, inflammation of the upper airways (nose, throat). Breathing difficulties (asthma attack) and cardiovascular problems in the most severe cases.

TREATMENTS:
Antihistamines, corticosteroids, adrenaline, desensitization.

PREVENTION:
Elimination of contact with the allergen.

AIDS

Acquired immunodeficiency syndrome (AIDS) is a serious **infectious** disease caused by the human immunodeficiency virus (HIV). It causes the progressive destruction of certain immune system cells, which results in a major weakening of the entire immune system. The disease, transmitted during unprotected sex or contact with contaminated blood (occurring, for example, when users of injectable drugs share syringes), can remain asymptomatic for several years. The advanced stage of AIDS is characterized by the development of multiple infections that may result in death. Since the 1980s, the AIDS pandemic has been a major public health problem and affects tens of millions of people throughout the world. Despite medical progress, the disease remains incurable and no **vaccine** has yet been found.

THE **HUMAN IMMUNODEFICIENCY VIRUS**

HIV primarily infects the T lymphocytes, on which it depends in order to multiply. The virus spreads primarily in the lymphoid organs, specifically in the lymph nodes. Individuals carrying the virus who do not yet present symptoms of the disease are said to be seropositive for HIV.

Lymphocytes and antibodies... page 280

THE **TRANSMISSION** OF **HIV**

HIV is present in the blood and genital secretions. In 75% of cases, transmission takes place during sex. It may also occur by blood contact, through a dirty syringe, or during a transfusion of contaminated blood. A contaminated mother also has a 25% risk of transmitting the virus to her child during pregnancy, childbirth, or nursing if she does not follow antiviral treatment. Preventive measures, such as the systematic use of a condom during sex, the analysis of transfused blood, the use of sterile injection equipment, and the administration of antivirals to pregnant seropositive women, make it possible to considerably reduce the risks of contagion.

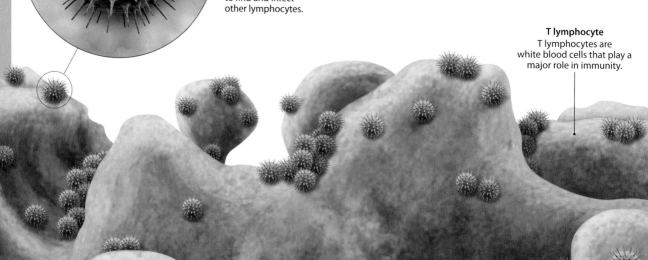

HIV
The virus attaches itself to the surface of the lymphocyte, into which it injects its **genetic** material. It multiplies within the cell before causing its death. Then, the new virus disperses to find and infect other lymphocytes.

T lymphocyte
T lymphocytes are white blood cells that play a major role in immunity.

THE **EVOLUTION** OF **AIDS**

AIDS evolves in several successive phases, at a rhythm that varies from one individual to another. Left untreated, non-specific symptoms (fever, skin eruption, aches, angina) generally appear one to six weeks after the infection, but occasionally it remains asymptomatic for months, even years. In all cases, the anti-HIV antibodies can be detected in the blood (seropositivity) approximately one month after the contamination, which makes it possible to diagnose the disease. The latter evolves, on average at the end of 5 to 10 years, towards a weakening of the patient's immune system. Different symptoms of increasing severity appear next. In the first stage, the individual experiences weight loss, repeated infections of the airways, appearance of skin lesions. The second stage presents with high fever, persistent diarrhea, swelling of the lymph nodes, severe bacterial infections, tuberculosis, and acute inflammation destroying the tissues of the mouth. The final stage is reached (the illness is then called AIDS) when the body becomes the center for opportunistic infections and cancers connected with HIV, such as Kaposi's sarcoma or lymphoma. Recourse to anti-AIDS tritherapy now makes it possible to significantly slow the progress of the disease in a majority of patients.

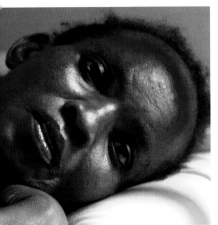

OPPORTUNISTIC INFECTIONS

Opportunistic infections are infections that occur in patients whose immunity is weakened by treatment with immunosuppressants, chemotherapy, or by a disease, such as AIDS. They are caused by different types of infectious agents, often harmless to an individual in good health, but which can cause serious complications, even death, in individuals whose immune system is compromised. Numerous opportunistic infections affect AIDS patients in the skin, the mucous membranes, the internal organs, or the nervous system. Others alter the senses (blindness caused by the cytomegalovirus) or can cause a generalized infection.

KAPOSI'S SARCOMA

The cause of Kaposi's sarcoma, a form of cancer, is not known, but its appearance is associated with a weakening of the immune system, such as in the case of AIDS, or exposure to the human herpes virus type 8 (HHV-8). It develops at the expense of the blood vessel walls and of certain skin cells. This is a rare disease, but one that is frequently encountered in AIDS patients. It is manifested by purplish spots on the mucous membranes and the skin, which are transformed into plaques and nodules. These lesions often reach the digestive tract and the lungs, causing internal hemorrhaging and respiratory insufficiency, which reduce the patient's life expectancy. The treatment is based on chemotherapy, radiation therapy, and surgery. However, when Kaposi's sarcoma is AIDS-related, the use of antivirals (tritherapy) is the best treatment.

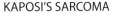

Skin lesions
Kaposi's sarcoma skin lesions can affect all parts of the body. They generally disappear after several weeks of treatment.

THE **PREVALENCE** OF **AIDS** THROUGHOUT THE **WORLD**

Approximately 35 million adults and children throughout the world are now infected by HIV. Africa is the continent most affected by AIDS, with more than one person out of three affected by the disease in certain countries such as Botswana or Swaziland. Eastern Europe, Southeast Asia, Latin America, and the United States are also particularly affected by the pandemic. Since 1981, when the first cases were diagnosed, AIDS has caused the death of more than 25 million people throughout the world. This illness reduces life expectancy in developing countries, where the large majority of new cases of infection are occurring. Access to preventive methods and medical treatments remain a major challenge in these countries.

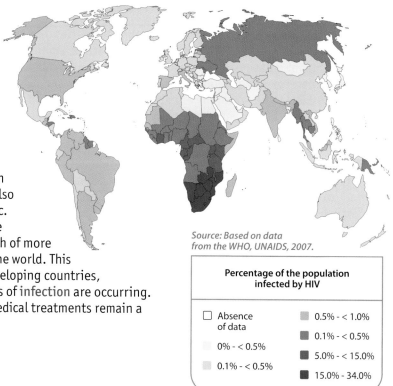

Source: Based on data from the WHO, UNAIDS, 2007.

Percentage of the population infected by HIV

☐ Absence of data

0% - < 0.5%

0.1% - < 0.5%

0.5% - < 1.0%

0.1% - < 0.5%

5.0% - < 15.0%

15.0% - 34.0%

TRITHERAPY

Anti-AIDS tritherapy is based on the administration of three antiviral drugs, whose combined action limits the multiplication of the virus and relieves the symptoms, without actually enabling a cure. First introduced in 1996, it constitutes an advance in the treatment of AIDS. Thanks to tritherapy, a large majority of seropositive individuals do not develop the disease for many years. In addition, tritherapy considerably reduces the appearance of opportunistic infections in patients, which prolongs their life expectancy. However, it is a treatment that can have serious side effects (diabetes, hypercholesterolemia) and which proves ineffective in some patients. Medical advances have made administration of the therapy easier, among other things, by combining the main active ingredients in a single tablet.

AIDS

SYMPTOMS:

Primary infection: fever, rash, aches, angina. Chronic infection: onset is asymptomatic, sometimes lasting for several years, ending with a phase of rapid weight loss, swelling of the lymph nodes, fever, persistent diarrhea, respiratory and skin infections. Final phase: opportunistic infections, cancers.

TREATMENTS:

Tritherapy makes it possible to prevent the disease from evolving. Opportunistic infections are the subject of a curative and sometimes preventive treatment.

PREVENTION:

Use of condoms during sex, antiviral treatment of infected pregnant women, use of sterile single-use syringes, analysis of transfused blood. Avoid direct contact with contaminated blood.

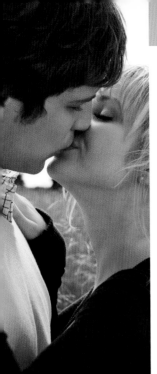

INFECTIOUS MONONUCLEOSIS

Infectious mononucleosis is a harmless disease caused by the Epstein-Barr virus. Contagious, it is basically transmitted by saliva, particularly through kissing. Contamination, which generally occurs during childhood or adolescence, is often asymptomatic. When the symptoms manifest themselves, it generally affects the lymphoid organs (lymph nodes, tonsils, spleen). Treatments make it possible to relieve symptoms but not to eliminate the virus, which remains dormant in the lymph nodes throughout life, without causing recurrence. It is estimated that 80% of adults are carriers of the virus. Between 20% and 30% of them secrete it in their saliva and are therefore capable of contaminating others.

THE **SYMPTOMS** OF **MONONUCLEOSIS**

Although it is most often asymptomatic, mononucleosis may also be manifested by various symptoms, which appear after an incubation that lasts from two to eight weeks. A fever then occurs suddenly, accompanied by headaches and muscular pains. These symptoms are accompanied by a generalized weakened condition and an angina that can make swallowing painful and cause respiratory difficulties. The tonsils are covered by a characteristic gray deposit. An increase in spleen volume and certain lymph nodes (neck, armpit, groin) is also characteristic. More rarely, the skin and the mucous membranes take on a yellowish coloration and a rash appears on the trunk and the base of the limbs. The symptoms generally diminish spontaneously in one to two weeks, but the weakened conditions may continue for several months.

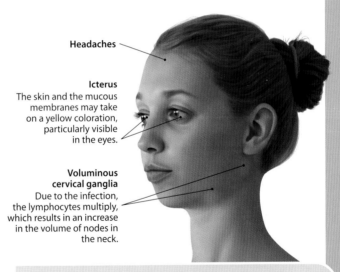

Headaches

Icterus
The skin and the mucous membranes may take on a yellow coloration, particularly visible in the eyes.

Voluminous cervical ganglia
Due to the infection, the lymphocytes multiply, which results in an increase in the volume of nodes in the neck.

INFECTIOUS MONONUCLEOSIS

SYMPTOMS:
Often asymptomatic. Fever, headaches, muscle pain, generalized weakened condition, angina with presence of a gray deposit on the tonsils. Increase in volume of the spleen and of certain lymph nodes (especially those in the neck), yellowing of the skin and mucous membranes, rash.

TREATMENTS:
Treatment of symptoms: rest, antipyretics, antalgics.

LYMPHOCYTOSIS

Lymphocytosis is the increase in the number of lymphocytes in the blood. Frequent in children, it is often the sign of a viral (mononucleosis, chickenpox, mumps, measles, hepatitis) or, more rarely, bacterial (whooping cough) infection.

Lymphocytes and antibodies... page 280

YELLOW FEVER

Yellow fever is an **infectious** viral disease transmitted by the bite of infected mosquitoes. It is endemic in Africa and in South America, where it is sometimes responsible for major epidemics. After an incubation period that lasts from three to six days, the first symptoms appear. This **acute** phase, characterized by congestion of the face, is called the red phase. In 85% of cases, the patient's condition improves and the symptoms quickly disappear. For others, the disease enters the yellow phase, characterized by an attack on the liver and kidneys that can lead to death.

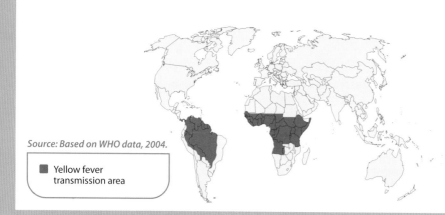

Source: Based on WHO data, 2004.

■ Yellow fever transmission area

YELLOW FEVER

SYMPTOMS:
Red phase: fever, headaches, agitation, nausea, abdominal and muscle pain, congestion and redness of the face, tongue and eyes, intense thirst.
Yellow phase: yellowing of the skin, vomiting and blackish stools, decrease or absence of urine, hemorrhage of the gums, nose and skin, mental confusion.

TREATMENTS:
No curative treatment. Palliative treatment that seeks to support vital functions: hydration, dialysis, transfusion.

PREVENTION:
Protection against mosquitoes. Vaccination, effective for 10 years, must be done at least 10 days prior to a travel to an endemic country.

DENGUE

Dengue is an infectious viral disease generally transmitted by the *Aedes aegypti* mosquito. It manifests itself four to eight days after contamination in a flu-like syndrome, which finally disappears in approximately 10 days. However, in 1% to 2% of cases, the disease can evolve into a more severe and potentially fatal form, hemorrhagic dengue. Endemic in more than 100 tropical and subtropical countries, dengue is spreading and affects more than 50 million people per year.

Flu-like syndrome… page 320

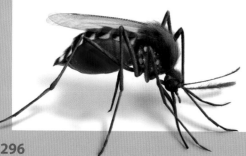

Aedes aegypti
Aedes aegypti is a diurnal mosquito in urban areas in tropical and subtropical countries. It is the main carrier of dengue and yellow fever. The virus is spread by the bite of an infected female.

DENGUE

SYMPTOMS:
Flu-like syndrome with vomiting and rash, disappearing after 10 days or developing into hemorrhagic dengue (hemorrhages of the skin, gums, genital organs and digestive tract).

TREATMENTS:
Antipyretics, rehydration. Hemorrhagic dengue: blood transfusion.

PREVENTION:
Action and protection against the carrier mosquitoes (insect repellant, long clothing).

MALARIA

Paludism, or malaria, is an **infectious** disease caused by parasitic microorganisms, plasmodia, that are transmitted by the bite of the anopheles mosquito. The parasite multiplies in the liver and the blood causing periodic attacks of fever. Left untreated, malaria can quickly evolve into a serious attack on the organs and result in death. Formerly present in temperate countries, today the disease is confined to the tropical regions of the planet.

THE PREVENTION OF MALARIA

When traveling in a country at risk, prevent malaria by using protection against mosquitoes and against plasmodia. In order to protect yourself from mosquito bites, wear long clothing, use insect repellant, avoid outside activities at twilight, and use mosquito screening impregnated with insecticides during the night. Against the plasmodium, there are different drugs (antimalarial) that considerably limit the risks of infection, but not completely. Their use varies according to country and the resistance of plasmodia to their action.

MALARIA

SYMPTOMS:

Approximately 15 days after the infection: fever, shivering, headaches, nausea, vomiting, diarrhea, yellowing of the skin, trembling. Attack (every two or three days according to the type of plasmodium): high fever, shivering, anemia. The attacks may recur months, even years, after the infection.

TREATMENTS:

Differing antimalarial drugs according to the resistance of the plasmodia.

PREVENTION:

Action against mosquitoes, protection against bites, preventive treatment with antimalarials during and after a stay in an endemic area.

ATTACKS OF MALARIA

Malaria is characterized by periodic attacks of fever accompanied by chills, sweats, and weakening. The first outbreak occurs from 8 to 30 days after infection and is then repeated every 2 or 3 days. Neuropaludism is a frequent and often fatal complication of malaria specifically caused by an infection from the parasite *Plasmodium falciparum*. It may cause convulsions, hypoglycemia, respiratory difficulty, and coma.

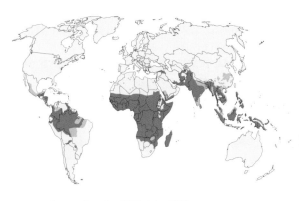

Source: Based on WHO data, 2007.

- ■ Areas with high risk of infection
- ■ Areas with weak risk
- □ Areas without malaria

Worldwide distribution of malaria
Malaria is the most widespread parasitic infection in the world. Each year, approximately 500 million people are infected and 2 million die from it, primarily children. Africa has 90% of all malaria cases, but tropical Asia and America are likewise affected. Plasmodium's resistance to treatments and global warming make the spread of the disease a growing concern.

LEISHMANIASIS

Leishmaniasis is an **infectious** disease caused by microscopic parasites, leishmania, transmitted by a small fly, the sandfly. There are various types of leishmaniasis, of varying degrees of severity. The most serious form, visceral leishmaniasis, affects the liver and the spleen. If untreated, it results in death. Less serious, the cutaneous forms affect the skin and the mucous membranes in the form of ulcerations. Leishmaniasis is rampant in Central and South America, India, the Middle East, and in all of the countries on the Mediterranean perimeter.

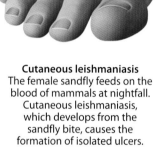

Cutaneous leishmaniasis
The female sandfly feeds on the blood of mammals at nightfall. Cutaneous leishmaniasis, which develops from the sandfly bite, causes the formation of isolated ulcers.

THE FIGHT AGAINST INSECT CARRIERS

Infectious diseases transmitted by insects are responsible for major epidemics, especially in tropical and subtropical countries, where each year they affect hundreds of millions of individuals. Since the end of the Second World War, the fight against carrier insects has been mainly through the use of chemical insecticides. Specifically, dichlorodiphenyltrichlorethane, or DDT, has made it possible to combat the spread of malaria and typhus. However, in the 1970s, it was prohibited in most industrialized countries. The use of DDT and other chemical insecticides remains very controversial. First, insecticides contaminate the air, water, and soil. Furthermore, their residues may cause serious health issues in humans. Biological methods involving the use of natural enemies of insect carriers are increasingly preferred. The latter, however, include risks to be considered for maintaining the ecological balance in an area where new predator species are introduced. Personal protection against insect bites, specifically through the use of mosquito nets, as well as the improvement of sanitary conditions, are also preferred.

LEISHMANIASIS

SYMPTOMS:
Incubation period: one to several months. Visceral form: fluctuating fever, severe anemia, increase in spleen and liver volume. Cutaneous form: ulcers, mutilating lesions of the skin and mucous membranes.

TREATMENTS:
Antimony derivatives or antiparasitics, injected into the lesion or by intramuscular or intravenous administration.

PREVENTION:
Use insect netting and insect repellents. Wear long clothing. Provide dogs with insecticide collars.

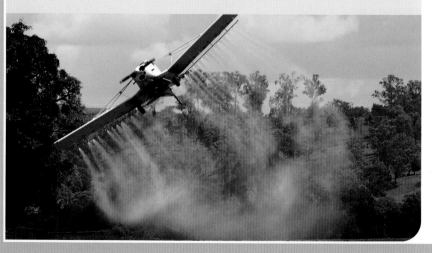

TYPHUS

A serious and contagious **infectious** disease, typhus is caused by a type of bacteria, the rickettsiae. These bacteria live and multiply in the cells of their host, body lice (not head lice) or, more rarely, rat fleas. Present on all continents, typhus especially spreads in environments where hygiene is deficient and crowding significant, such as barracks, prisons, or refugee camps. The disease is often fatal within two or three weeks if no **antibiotic** treatment is started.

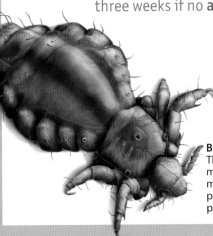

Body louse
The bite of the louse causes itching, which may lead the host to scratch. The resulting skin microlesions make it possible for the bacteria, present in the feces of the infected louse, to penetrate the human body.

TYPHUS

SYMPTOMS:
After an incubation period of approximately 10 days: skin eruption, high fever, diffuse pain, headaches, state of stupor, mental confusion, delirium. Cardiovascular and neurological complications and serious hemorrhages if untreated.

TREATMENTS:
Antibiotics. Hospitalization in an intensive care unit in the most serious cases.

PREVENTION:
Body hygiene. Delousing or rat extermination. Isolation of reported cases in order to avoid contagion.

PLAGUE

Plague is a serious infectious disease caused by the bacterium *Yersinia pestis*. Bubonic plague, the most frequent form of the disease, is caused by the bite of a flea living as a parasite on a rat carrying the bacterium. Pulmonary plague, which is very contagious, occurs when the bacterium invades the lungs and is transmitted through the air from one individual to another. Septicemic plague is a serious complication of bubonic plague, which quickly results in death when untreated. Once the cause of fatal epidemics, today the plague is not widespread. However, it still persists in locations in Africa, Asia, and America.

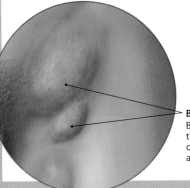

Bubos
Bubonic plague is characterized by the **inflammation** and the swelling of the lymph nodes located in the perimeter of the flea bite. These bubos most often form in the groin and tend to produce pus.

PLAGUE

SYMPTOMS:
High fever, headaches, digestive problems, intense fatigue. Bubonic plague: diffuse pain, painful bubos. Pulmonary plague: respiratory difficulty, coughing, abundant and bloody expectoration, thoracic pains. Septicemic plague: delirium, severe exhaustion, cardiovascular problems, gangrene in the limbs.

TREATMENTS:
Early administration of antibiotics, incision and drainage of bubos.

PREVENTION:
Rat and insect extermination. Reporting and isolation of patients.

BILHARZIASIS

Bilharziasis, or schistosomiasis, is an **infectious** disease caused by a parasitic worm, the schistosome. Contamination occurs by skin contact with water infested with the schistosome larva. The disease, which affects the digestive and urinary tracts, is endemic in the majority of tropical countries. It affects several million people and causes a great number of deaths each year, despite the existence of effective medical treatments.

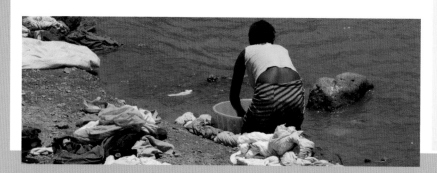

BILHARZIASIS

SYMPTOMS:
Contamination: redness, itching. A few weeks later: fever, headaches, abdominal and joint pain. Several months later: diarrhea, vomiting, swelling of the liver and spleen, presence of blood in the urine, painful urination, abdominal pain.

TREATMENTS:
Antiparasitic treatment by oral means.

PREVENTION:
Avoid contact with fresh water in natural environment in the countries at risk.

TYPHOID FEVER

Typhoid fever is an infectious and contagious disease, caused by the bacterium *Salmonella typhi*. It is most often transmitted by the ingestion of water or food contaminated by the excrement of infected individuals. Once in the body, the bacterium multiplies in the lymph nodes before reaching the circulatory system and causing a generalized infection. It releases toxins into the blood that cause serious complications: intestinal hemorrhages, heart problems, encephalitis. The treatment of typhoid fever is based on **vaccination**, improving hygiene conditions, and the rapid administration of antibiotics.

TYPHOID FEVER

SYMPTOMS:
After a two-week incubation period: fever, weakened state, anorexia, nausea, abdominal pain, headaches, dizziness, insomnia, extreme exhaustion, red spots on the body, diarrhea of a yellow-ocher color.

TREATMENTS:
Antibiotics, rehydration, rest.

PREVENTION:
Vaccination of people residing or traveling in the countries at risk, improvement of hygiene conditions.

Spread of typhoid fever
Endemic in Africa, Asia, and Latin America, typhoid fever is found primarily in regions where hygiene is deficient.

DIPHTHERIA

A contagious, potentially fatal **infectious** disease, diphtheria is caused by the bacterium *Corynebacterium diphteriae*. It is transmitted by saliva (droplets, coughing) and particularly affects children. The bacterium multiplies in the throat, where it causes an **inflammation**, and secretes a toxin in the body that affects the nervous system and the heart. Thanks to systematic **vaccination**, diphtheria has almost disappeared in Western countries. It is, however, on the rise in Eastern European countries and remains a significant cause of infant mortality in developing countries.

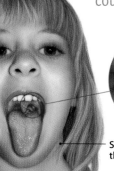

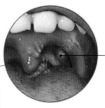

Tonsil
The tonsils are covered with false membranes.

Significant swelling of the lymph nodes

The immune system | Diseases

DIPHTHERIA

SYMPTOMS:
Fever, headaches, intense fatigue, swelling of the lymph nodes in the neck. Sore throat with false membranes on the tonsils, which spread quickly (palate, uvula, larynx), causing the obstruction of the respiratory tract.

TREATMENTS:
Administration of antidiphtheria serum and **antibiotics** once an infection is suspected.

PREVENTION:
Systematic vaccination of persons living or traveling in the countries at risk.

LEPROSY

Leprosy is an infectious disease caused by a bacterium, the Hansen bacillus. It causes **chronic** lesions of the skin and neurological problems causing paralysis, loss of feeling, and disfigurement. The disease is transmitted by direct inhalation of contaminated saliva droplets or by direct contact with the skin lesions of a contagious patient. After an incubation period lasting five years on average, the disease evolves into tuberculoid leprosy (not contagious) or lepromatous leprosy (more severe and contagious), depending on the condition of the patient's immune system. Almost nonexistent in Western countries, leprosy remains endemic in a number of African, Asian, and Latin American countries.

Tuberculoid leprosy
Tuberculoid leprosy, non-contagious, is the most frequent form of leprosy. Its appearance is marked by the formation of large insensitive patches on the skin.

LEPROSY

SYMPTOMS:
Primary stage: depigmented skin patches several millimeters in diameter. Tuberculoid leprosy: large skin patches, swelling of nerves forming palpable cords under the skin, sensitivity and motor problems, disfigurement of extremities. Lepromatous leprosy: lepromes (skin nodules), rhinitis, inflammation and hypertrophy of the nerves, fever, intense fatigue.

TREATMENTS:
Early antibiotic therapy (tritherapy) of long duration.

PREVENTION:
Good personal hygiene, good diet, reporting and rapid treatment of patients in order to prevent complications.

LISTERIOSIS

Listeriosis is an **infectious** bacterial disease caused by *Listeria monocytogenes*. Frequent in animals, it more rarely affects human beings. Transmitted by contaminated food, listeriosis generally appears as a flu-like syndrome (fever, muscle and joint pain) or by gastroenteritis. In pregnant women, newborns, elderly, or **immunodeficient** individuals, it may cause serious complications: miscarriage, generalized infection, meningitis, encephalitis. The disease is treated effectively by **antibiotics**.

Flu-like syndrome... page 320

LISTERIOSIS IN **PREGNANT WOMEN**

Contracted during pregnancy, listeriosis can cause premature childbirth, miscarriage, or an infection of the fetus. In the days following birth, a child infected during pregnancy may develop a lung or blood infection and then, in the following weeks, meningitis. Pregnant women must therefore pay particular attention to the foods they eat, specifically by washing fresh fruits and vegetables, avoiding raw milk cheeses, and cooking meat properly.

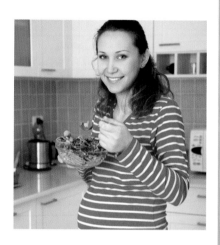

LISTERIOSIS AND **RAW FOODS**

Widespread in the environment, the bacterium *Listeria monocytogenes* frequently contaminates raw foods (sausages, chopped meat, eggs, raw milk cheeses, certain vegetables, certain smoked fish), but in quantities generally insufficient to cause the illness. However, it can multiply easily, even at low temperature. That is why slightly contaminated foods may become dangerous if they are kept for a long time in the refrigerator.

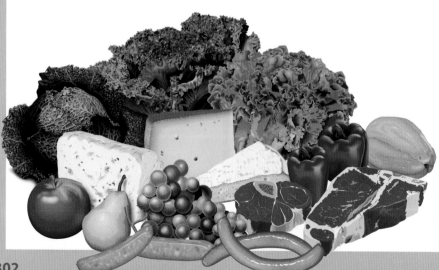

LISTERIOSIS

SYMPTOMS:
Flu-like syndrome, gastroenteritis (diarrhea).

TREATMENTS:
Combination of two antibiotics, one of which is penicillin, administered intravenously.

PREVENTION:
Cook meat adequately, avoid long storage of raw food in the refrigerator, clean the latter regularly with a disinfectant product, and store cooked foods separately from raw foods.

LYME DISEASE

Lyme disease, or Lyme borreliosis, is an **infectious** bacterial disease that is transmitted from an infected animal to a human by a contaminated tick. It is a widespread disease in the temperate and cold regions of the northern hemisphere. It evolves over several months, even several years, and may cause disabling joint and neurological complications. An **antibiotic** treatment beginning with the appearance of the first symptoms (rash) allows rapid recovery and prevents any complications.

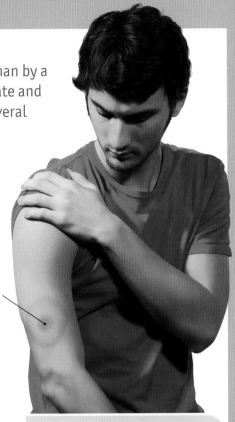

Chronic migrating rash
Chronic migrating rash is a skin lesion characteristic of Lyme disease.

THE **EVOLUTION** OF **LYME DISEASE**

Lyme disease evolves in two phases. After several days incubation, the primary phase appears as a characteristic redness of the skin around the bite, sometimes accompanied by fever. This rash spreads progressively and takes on the appearance of a ring (chronic migrating rash) and ends by disappearing. The second phase, occurring several weeks or several months later, is characterized by various neurological (headaches, neuralgias, facial paralysis), **inflammatory** (arthritis, meningitis, pericarditis, conjunctivitis) or cardiac (arrhythmia, heart failure) manifestations.

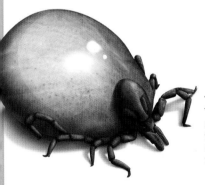

Tick
The tick is a mite parasite of numerous forest animal species. It feeds on the blood of its host, to which it remains attached for four to five days. The risk of contamination by an infected tick increases with the duration of the bite.

LYME DISEASE

SYMPTOMS:
Primary phase: circular rash appearing at the site of the bite and then spreading forming a ring. Second phase: neurological, inflammatory, or cardiac problems that worsen with time.

TREATMENTS:
Orally administered antibiotics, if the treatment is early, or intravenous, if the treatment is late.

PREVENTION:
Use insect repellents, wear long clothing that covers the skin, walk in the center of trails, and avoid contact with tall grasses. Verify the presence of ticks on the skin and on domestic animals, remove them with tweezers without crushing them.

IN CASE OF TICK BITE

Remove the tick as quickly as possible: grab the head using a fine, flat tweezer, as close as possible to the skin, and pull, but without crushing it. Do not use ether or alcohol to put it to sleep because this causes a regurgitation of saliva and increases the risks of infection. Once the tick is pulled off, disinfect the wound with an **antiseptic**. Monitor the bite for three weeks and consult a doctor if a circular rash appears.

LUPUS

Lupus is an **autoimmune** disease characterized by the **chronic inflammation** of one or several organs. The disease, which affects women 15 to 50 years of age in 85% of cases, is connected with **genetic**, hormonal, and environmental factors. It may be triggered by prolonged stress or exposure to ultraviolet rays, certain chemical substances, or certain viruses. Its unpredictable evolution is characterized by outbreaks interspersed with remissions.

THE **FORMS** OF **LUPUS**

Lupus appears in different forms of varying severity. Discoid lupus, less severe, affects only the skin and is manifested by a rash following exposure to the sun. In approximately 15% of cases, discoid lupus evolves into disseminated lupus erythematosus. The latter is a severe form of lupus characterized by sometimes fatal visceral attacks. The symptoms, numerous and non-specific, vary from one patient to another, which makes the initial diagnosis difficult. The illness may affect the skin, joints (pain, arthritis), kidneys, lungs, cardiovascular system, or nervous system.

AUTOIMMUNE DISEASES

Autoimmune diseases, such as lupus, multiple sclerosis, or insulin-dependent diabetes, are caused by a malfunction of the immune system. The latter produces cells (lymphocytes) and antibodies directed against certain elements of the body itself, which results in tissue damage and organ malfunctions: skin, kidneys, nerve fibers, pancreas, etc. The causes of autoimmune diseases are not understood, but they are promoted by genetic and hereditary factors, associated with a triggering event. Their treatment is based on immunosuppressive drugs, which inhibit the activity of the immune system.

Lymphocytes and antibodies... page 280

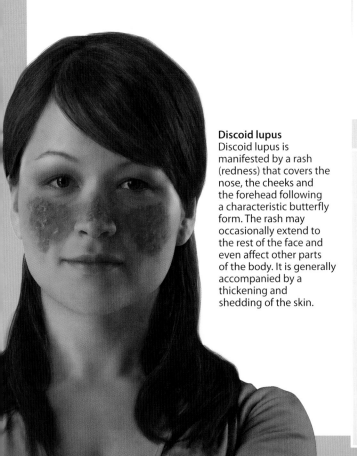

Discoid lupus
Discoid lupus is manifested by a rash (redness) that covers the nose, the cheeks and the forehead following a characteristic butterfly form. The rash may occasionally extend to the rest of the face and even affect other parts of the body. It is generally accompanied by a thickening and shedding of the skin.

LUPUS

SYMPTOMS:
Discoid lupus: rash (redness) particularly affecting the portions of the skin exposed to the sun, specifically the face. Disseminated lupus erythematosus: variable according to the organs affected by the inflammation.

TREATMENTS:
No curative treatment. Treatments designed to reduce the inflammatory reaction and immune response: corticosteroids, non-steroidal anti-inflammatories, immunosuppressants, antimalarials.

PREVENTION:
Prevention of outbreaks: do not expose yourself to ultraviolet rays (sunlight and halogen light), avoid prolonged stress.

INFLAMMATIONS OF
THE LYMPHATIC SYSTEM

Inflammations of the lymphatic system may affect the lymphatic vessels, lymph nodes, or tonsils. They are generally caused by **infections** and affect the adjacent lymphoid organ at the entry point of the infectious agent. Untreated, the inflammation presents complications in the form of an abscess (mass of pus), or reaches the adjacent tissues. The infection may also spread in the lymphatic system, pass into the circulatory system, and cause **septicemia**, a generalized infection.

The lymphatic system... page 281

LYMPHANGITIS

Lymphangitis is an inflammation of the lymphatic vessels, generally caused by a bacterial infection, more rarely by metastases of bronchopulmonary cancers. Lymphangitis appears as a painful and hot rash located around the center of the infection. This rash forms lines that follow the path of the lymphatic vessels to the nearest lymph node, which may become infected in turn (adenitis).

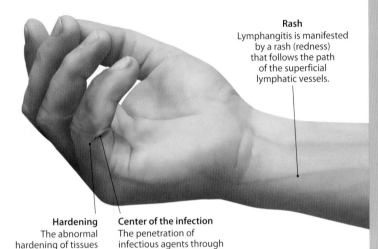

Rash
Lymphangitis is manifested by a rash (redness) that follows the path of the superficial lymphatic vessels.

Hardening
The abnormal hardening of tissues around a wound is often the sign of an infection.

Center of the infection
The penetration of infectious agents through a wound causes an inflammatory reaction around the center of the infection.

ADENITIS

Adenitis is an inflammation of the lymph nodes caused by an infection. It often affects the nodes in the groin, the neck, and the armpits, more rarely those of the abdominal region or the lungs. Adenitis is sometimes expressed by an increase in the volume of lymph nodes, which become hot and painful.

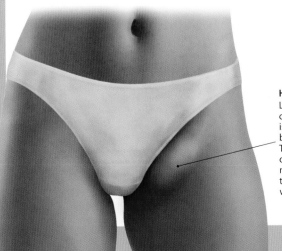

Hypertrophic lymph nodes
Lymph node hypertrophy caused by inflammation is not always visible. It may be diagnosed by palpation. The increase in volume of the nodes is due to the multiplication of lymphocytes that are activated by contact with the virus antigens.

INFLAMMATIONS OF THE LYMPHATIC SYSTEM

SYMPTOMS:
Fever, fatigue. Lymphangitis: painful and hot rash forming an irregular tracing on the skin. Adenitis: swelling of the lymph nodes.

TREATMENTS:
Antibiotics in case of bacterial infection, antipyretics, analgesics.

PREVENTION:
Disinfection of wounds.

LYMPHEDEMA

Lymphedema is an accumulation of lymph in the tissues caused by an obstruction in, or the destruction of, lymph nodes or vessels. This disabling disease is manifested by the sometimes severe swelling of one or several limbs. Lymphedema affects approximately 250 million people throughout the world. There are no curative treatments, but exercise and massage make it possible to reduce its symptoms.

The lymphatic system... page 281

THE **CAUSES** OF **LYMPHEDEMA**
The two main causes are associated with the surgical treatment of breast cancer in industrialized countries and with a parasitic infection, lymphatic filariasis, in many developing countries. More rarely, lymphedema is due to a congenital malformation, a tumor (lymphoma), radiation treatment, or lymphangitis.

Mastectomy
Lymphedema affects approximately 25% of women who undergo a mastectomy (removal of the breast), because this operation is generally accompanied by the removal of ancillary lymph nodes, which drain the lymph from the upper arm.

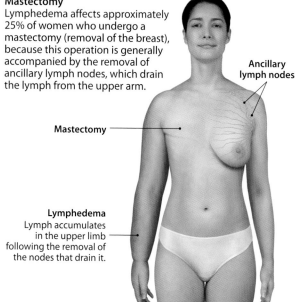

Mastectomy

Ancillary lymph nodes

Lymphedema
Lymph accumulates in the upper limb following the removal of the nodes that drain it.

LYMPHATIC FILARIASIS
Lymphatic filariasis is an infectious disease caused by worms, filaria. These are passed on in larval form by a mosquito bite. They install themselves in the lymphatic system, where they develop, obstructing the vessels, which causes the progressive swelling of one or several limbs, genital organs, and sometimes the breasts in women. Untreated, the disease may evolve into an extreme form of lymphedema called elephantiasis. The excessive swelling of tissues then disrupts the patient's movements.

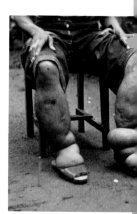

Elephantiasis

LYMPHATIC DRAINAGE
Lymphatic drainage is a type of massage performed on a limb affected by lymphedema. Its effect is to evacuate the accumulated lymph by moving it towards an area of the body where the lymphatic vessels are functional.

LYMPHEDEMA

SYMPTOMS:
Feeling of pressure in a limb, stretching of the skin or heaviness, tingling, pain, sometimes considerable increase in volume of the limb accompanied by a thickening and cracking of the skin in the case of elephantiasis.

TREATMENTS:
Compression, lymphatic drainage and elevation of the affected limb, in extreme cases removal of affected tissues. Lymphatic filariasis: antiparasitic treatment.

PREVENTION:
In women having undergone breast cancer surgery: avoid the heat, skin infections and abrupt movements of the arm, do not wear tight clothing or jewelry.

LYMPHOMAS

Lymphomas are malignant tumors that develop in the lymphoid organs such as the lymph nodes, thymus, tonsils, spleen, or bone marrow. Among them is Hodgkin's disease, an infrequent form of lymphoma of the lymph nodes, and non-Hodgkin's lymphomas, which include numerous forms of malignant tumors of the lymphatic system. Lymphomas are treated with **chemotherapy**, combined with **radiation therapy** or **immunotherapy**, with an effectiveness that depends on the form and the stage of the disease. In the case of Hodgkin's disease, the recovery rate is approximately 80%.

The lymphatic system... page 281

HODGKIN'S DISEASE

Hodgkin's disease, or Hodgkin's lymphoma, is a cancer of the lymph nodes characterized by the typical presence of Reed-Sternberg cells, abnormally large cells containing several nuclei. This infrequent disease most often affects men between 15 and 30 years of age and older than 60. Lymphoma starts in a lymph node, causing its volume to increase, then spreads to adjacent nodes and to other organs. Applied during the first stages of the disease, chemotherapy and radiation therapy, combined with a bone marrow autotransplant in case of recurrence, make it possible to cure the majority of patients.

NON-HODGKIN'S LYMPHOMAS

Non-Hodgkin's lymphomas are cancers of the lymphatic system, other than Hodgkin's disease. They result from the uncontrolled division of lymphocytes in a lymphoid organ. Three to five more times frequent than Hodgkin's disease, non-Hodgkin's lymphomas more frequently affect men over 60 years of age and are promoted by the use of immunosuppressive treatments and by exposure to pesticides or certain pathogenic agents (Epstein-Barr virus and HIV, *Helicobacter pylori* bacterium). Treatments are primarily based on chemotherapy and their effectiveness depends on the type and extent of the lymphoma.

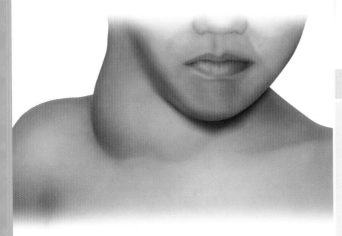

Hodgkin's lymphoma
The proliferation of cancerous cells causes increase in the volume of the affected lymph node.

LYMPHOMAS

SYMPTOMS:
Increase in volume of one or several lymph nodes (visible in the neck, armpits, groin), increase in volume of the spleen, itching, fever, weight loss, general weakness, night sweats, abdominal pain.

TREATMENTS:
Chemotherapy that combines several anticancer agents, radiation therapy, immunotherapy, bone marrow autotransplant.

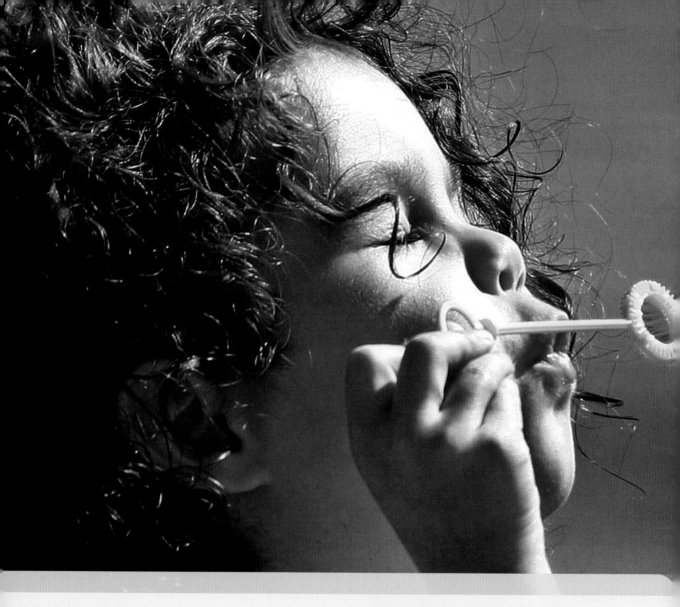

THE BODY

THE **RESPIRATORY SYSTEM**

Respiration is a vital process that enables our body to receive the oxygen necessary for its functioning and to expel carbon dioxide, the waste that is the result of cellular activity. Several organs make up the respiratory system, and it is their combined action that allows for respiration process to be completed. The inhaling movement of the rib cage permits the air loaded with oxygen to reach the alveoli of the lungs, where the exchange of gases takes place. The air loaded with carbon dioxide is then expelled to the outside through the movement of expiration.

The respiratory system organs are heavily exposed to microorganisms and polluting particles from the air. They are therefore subject to **infections** such as colds or the flu as well as diseases related to smoking and atmospheric pollution. Any obstruction to the passage of air in the airways or the distribution of oxygen in the blood causes breathing problems, which, when significant, can lead to respiratory insufficiency and asphyxia.

DISEASES

THE **RESPIRATORY SYSTEM**

The respiratory system is comprised of all of the organs that contribute to the constant exchange between the air and the blood, providing the oxygen needed by the body while eliminating the carbon dioxide it produces. Aside from respiration, the respiratory system plays a fundamental role in speech and smell.

THE **FUNCTIONING** OF THE **RESPIRATORY SYSTEM**

The rhythmic alternation of inhalations and exhalations, thanks to movements of the rib cage, ensures the oxygenation of the blood and the constant renewal of the air contained in the lungs. The inhaled air follows the upper respiratory tract, the trachea, and the bronchial tubes, then reaches the lungs, where the gaseous exchanges take place. Partially reflexive, the respiratory movements are governed by the body's needs for oxygen and the need to expel carbon dioxide, a toxic waste of the metabolism. However, they may also be voluntary, during forced inhalation and exhalation or during deliberate apnea.

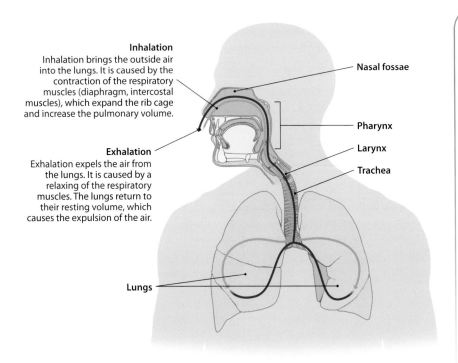

Inhalation
Inhalation brings the outside air into the lungs. It is caused by the contraction of the respiratory muscles (diaphragm, intercostal muscles), which expand the rib cage and increase the pulmonary volume.

Exhalation
Exhalation expels the air from the lungs. It is caused by a relaxing of the respiratory muscles. The lungs return to their resting volume, which causes the expulsion of the air.

Nasal fossae

Pharynx

Larynx

Trachea

Lungs

OXYGEN, A **GAS INDISPENSABLE** TO **LIFE**

Oxygen is naturally present in the air and is assimilated by the body during respiration. It attaches itself to the hemoglobin of the red blood cells, then is transported to each cell of the body through the circulatory system. Oxygen specifically acts by transforming the nutrients provided by the diet into energy that can be used by the cells. A decrease in the contribution of oxygen to the cells can be expressed by the bluish coloration of the skin and mucous membranes and risks causing death by asphyxia.

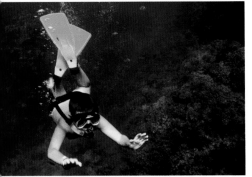

APNEA

Apnea is a temporary stoppage, voluntary or involuntary, of respiratory movements, without cardiac arrest. The maximum duration of an apnea does not generally exceed three minutes, but it can be prolonged up to eight minutes in well-trained individuals, particularly in high-level athletes such as free divers. If it does not stop, the asphyxia that it causes leads to death. Involuntary apnea may be caused by the penetration of liquid into the larynx or by a drug, but its main cause is the obstruction of airways by a foreign body or by tissue from the pharynx (sleep apnea).

THE UPPER RESPIRATORY TRACTS

The nose, sinuses, mouth, and throat, which consists of the pharynx and the larynx, constitute the upper respiratory tracts. They allow the passage of air through the trachea and to the lungs, and play an important role in sound production and immune defense.

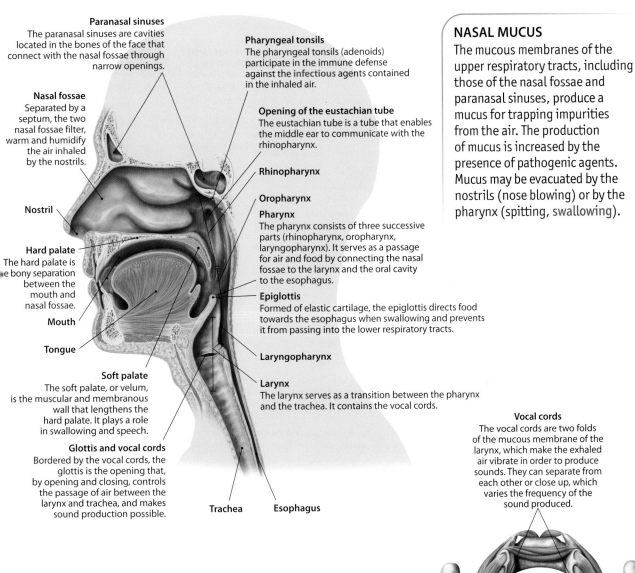

Paranasal sinuses
The paranasal sinuses are cavities located in the bones of the face that connect with the nasal fossae through narrow openings.

Nasal fossae
Separated by a septum, the two nasal fossae filter, warm and humidify the air inhaled by the nostrils.

Nostril

Hard palate
The hard palate is the bony separation between the mouth and nasal fossae.

Mouth

Tongue

Soft palate
The soft palate, or velum, is the muscular and membranous wall that lengthens the hard palate. It plays a role in swallowing and speech.

Glottis and vocal cords
Bordered by the vocal cords, the glottis is the opening that, by opening and closing, controls the passage of air between the larynx and trachea, and makes sound production possible.

Trachea   **Esophagus**

Pharyngeal tonsils
The pharyngeal tonsils (adenoids) participate in the immune defense against the infectious agents contained in the inhaled air.

Opening of the eustachian tube
The eustachian tube is a tube that enables the middle ear to communicate with the rhinopharynx.

Rhinopharynx

Oropharynx

Pharynx
The pharynx consists of three successive parts (rhinopharynx, oropharynx, laryngopharynx). It serves as a passage for air and food by connecting the nasal fossae to the larynx and the oral cavity to the esophagus.

Epiglottis
Formed of elastic cartilage, the epiglottis directs food towards the esophagus when swallowing and prevents it from passing into the lower respiratory tracts.

Laryngopharynx

Larynx
The larynx serves as a transition between the pharynx and the trachea. It contains the vocal cords.

NASAL MUCUS

The mucous membranes of the upper respiratory tracts, including those of the nasal fossae and paranasal sinuses, produce a mucus for trapping impurities from the air. The production of mucus is increased by the presence of pathogenic agents. Mucus may be evacuated by the nostrils (nose blowing) or by the pharynx (spitting, swallowing).

Vocal cords
The vocal cords are two folds of the mucous membrane of the larynx, which make the exhaled air vibrate in order to produce sounds. They can separate from each other or close up, which varies the frequency of the sound produced.

SPEECH

The production of articulated sounds takes place during exhalation, when the air coming from the lungs is put into vibration by the vocal cords. Exiting the larynx, the sound is amplified by the oral cavity, the nasal fossae, the sinuses, and the pharynx. The articulation of sound is provided by the muscles of the pharynx, the soft palate, the tongue, and the lips. All of the sounds produced make up the voice, which varies in amplitude (whispering, cry), in frequency (deep or sharp sounds), and according to gender, age, and state of health.

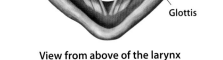

Glottis

View from above of the larynx

THE **LUNGS**

Located inside the rib cage on either side of the heart, the lungs are responsible for gaseous exchanges between the air and the blood. Connected to the upper respiratory tracts by the bronchial tubes and the trachea, these spongy, elastic organs, rich in blood vessels, inflate with air, then deflate, to the rhythm of breathing.

RESPIRATION

Respiration includes ventilation and hematosis. Ventilation is the circulation of air in the lungs, to the rhythm of inhalation and exhalation. Hematosis is the exchange of gases between the air and the blood, which takes place in the area of contact between a pulmonary alveolus and blood capillaries. The rhythm and amplitude of respiration may vary according to the level of carbon monoxide in the blood, age, state of health, physical activity, and environmental factors such as altitude and the quality of the inhaled air. The normal rhythm in an adult in good health and at rest is 12 to 20 respirations per minute.

Trachea
Almost five inches in length, the trachea allows the passage of air between the larynx and the bronchial tubes. Its interior wall is covered with a mucous membrane with cilia, whose movements expel the solid particles and excess mucus towards the upper respiratory tracts.

Bronchus
Stemming from the trachea, the bronchi or bronchial tubes are conduits that allow the air to reach the inside of the lungs. They divide into multiple branches in the pulmonary tissue to form the bronchial tree.

Pulmonary artery
The pulmonary arteries carry the oxygen-poor blood from the heart to the lungs.

Pulmonary vein
The pulmonary veins carry the blood oxygenated by the lungs to the heart.

Bronchioles
The bronchioles are the narrowest subdivisions of the bronchial tree, which end at the pulmonary alveoli.

Arteriole
The pulmonary artery is divided into multiple arterioles that carry the deoxygenated blood to the pulmonary alveoli.

Bronchioles

Venule
The oxygenated blood is transported by venules that meet in the pulmonary veins.

Air heavy with carbon monoxide

Pulmonary alveolus
The pulmonary alveoli are small cavities located at the end of the bronchioles. Arranged in clusters, they are surrounded by a thin wall that permits gaseous exchanges with the adjacent blood capillaries.

Blood capillary
The pulmonary alveoli are surrounded by numerous blood capillaries.

Oxygenated air

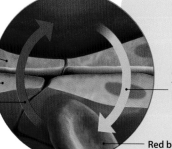

Alveolar cell

Endothelial cell of the blood capillary

Carbon dioxide
Carbon dioxide is carried by the red blood cells towards the lungs, where it is eliminated by respiration.

Oxygen
The oxygen resulting from respiration is carried to the cells by the hemoglobin of the red blood cells.

Red blood cell

THE **PULMONARY LOBES**
The pulmonary lobes are subdivisions of the lungs. More voluminous than the left lung, the right lung consists of three lobes, while the left lung has two due to the space occupied by the heart between the two lungs, in the left center of the thorax.

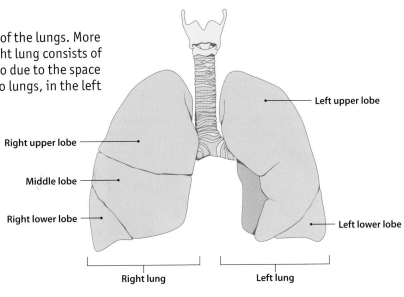

Left upper lobe

Right upper lobe

Middle lobe

Right lower lobe

Left lower lobe

Right lung

Left lung

Pleura
The pleura is a double membrane that envelops the lungs and covers the inside of the ribs. Between its two layers is a small quantity of lubricating liquid that prevents it from being irritated during ventilation.

Rib
The ribs protect the heart and the lungs. During respiration, they expand under the action of the intercostal muscles.

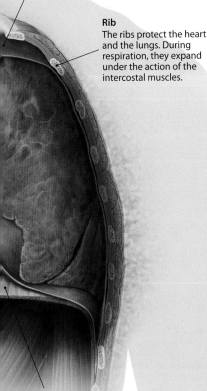

Diaphragm
The diaphragm is a muscle that separates the thorax from the abdomen. During inhalation, it lowers while contracting, which enables the lungs to fill up with air.

THE **HICCUP**
The hiccup is an involuntary spasm of the diaphragm that occurs in episodes whose duration generally does not exceed more than a few minutes. Each spasm is followed by a sound, which results in the sudden closing of the glottis and the vibration of the vocal cords. This is a harmless problem most often related to food ingestion: ingesting food too quickly, in excessive quantity, or that is too hot or too cold, etc. A hiccup attack that persists for several hours can require the use of antispasmodics.

COUGHING
Reflex or voluntary, the cough is an abrupt and noisy exhalation that forces the expulsion of air from the lungs. It allows the elimination of excess mucus or irritating elements (dust, foreign body, chemical agent) present in the larynx, trachea, or bronchial tubes. Normally temporary, it may also indicate a respiratory problem when it becomes chronic. Unlike dry cough, a loose cough is accompanied by expectoration. Persistent dry coughs may be relieved with antitussives, generally in syrup form, while loose coughs are soothed by taking expectorants, which liquefy the mucus and facilitate its expulsion. A spoonful of honey may also soothe slight coughs, because it contains antioxidants and natural antibacterials.

MILLIONS OF ALVEOLI
The lungs contain approximately 300 million alveoli. The total surface of the pulmonary alveoli equals that of a tennis court.

THE HEALTH OF THE RESPIRATORY SYSTEM

The respiratory tract is subject to infections (cold, flu, etc.) and various diseases associated with smoking and atmospheric pollution. In order to preserve its health, the respiratory system should not be exposed to its main irritants.

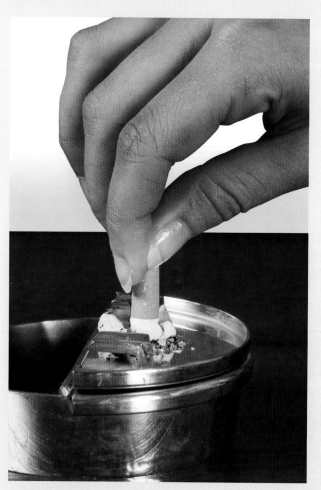

■ DO NOT EXPOSE YOURSELF TO AIR POLLUTION

Prolonged exposure to air pollutants, specifically in major cities where factories are numerous and automobile traffic is very dense, constitutes a risk factor for a number of respiratory diseases such as asthma, emphysema, respiratory insufficiency, and bronchopulmonary cancers. These pollutants may irritate the respiratory tract and make it more sensitive to infections and diseases, particularly in individuals who suffer from asthma, the elderly, and young children. It is therefore recommended that these people abstain from engaging in outdoor physical activity during periods of heavy pollution or smog. According to the World Health Organization, air pollution is responsible for the premature deaths of more than 2 million people worldwide each year.

■ CONTRIBUTE TO IMPROVING AIR QUALITY

You can contribute to reducing air pollution and preserving everyone's pulmonary health by limiting your automobile travel and using, whenever possible, an alternate means of transportation such as walking, bicycling, or public transportation.

■ AVOID SMOKING

Smoking, whether active or passive (secondhand smoke), is one of the main causes of cancer (lungs, bronchial tubes, trachea, throat, mouth, etc.) and pulmonary diseases such as chronic bronchitis, emphysema, or respiratory insufficiency. You can therefore prevent a number of respiratory system problems by avoiding or stopping smoking. Also try to avoid secondhand smoke in public places, at work, and at home.

Nicotine addiction... page 338

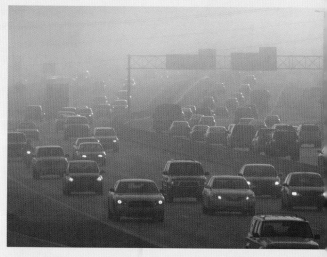

THE HEALTH OF THE RESPIRATORY SYSTEM

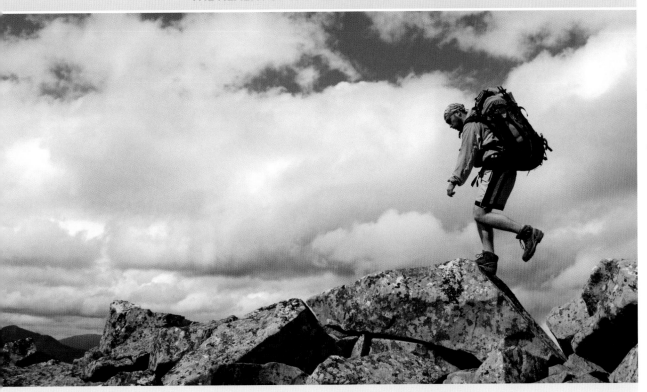

■ EXERCISE REGULARLY

The regular practice of physical exercise such as walking, yoga, or swimming stimulates the supply of oxygen to the lungs and increases their respiratory capacity. In addition to benefiting the entire body by promoting its oxygenation, physical exercise also strengthens immunity against respiratory infections.

■ AVOID HARMFUL PRODUCTS

Chemical products such as certain household cleaners, solvents, paints, and pesticides contain numerous volatile substances that are toxic for the respiratory tract and the lungs. Avoid these products or handle them with care by wearing a protective mask or by airing the premises in order not to inhale their toxic fumes. Pay particular attention to interior air quality both at home and at work. For certain professionals at risk, such as miners or construction workers, the prolonged inhalation of coal dust, asbestos, or cement can cause serious pulmonary diseases. Pulmonary health must therefore be the subject of attentive medical monitoring.

■ PROTECT YOURSELF AND OTHERS FROM INFECTIONS

The transmission of infectious diseases such as the common cold or the flu may be avoided by adopting simple hygiene: wash your hands frequently, and cover your mouth and nose when sneezing or coughing. Proper oral hygiene may also help to prevent respiratory infections or the deterioration of existing respiratory diseases, particularly in the elderly.

■ EAT A HEALTHY AND BALANCED DIET

Eat a sufficient quantity of whole grains, vegetables, and fruits. In addition to helping strengthen the body's natural immunity, these foods rich in antioxidants make your respiratory system more resistant to inflammations and asthma. The abuse of alcoholic beverages may promote or aggravate infections and cancers of the upper respiratory tracts.

Nutrition... page 11

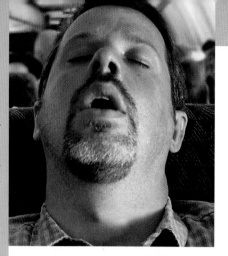

SLEEP APNEA

Sleep apnea is characterized by an intermittent stoppage of respiration that occurs during sleep. It is caused by the obstruction of the upper airways (obstructive apnea) or, more rarely, by the interruption of the contraction of the respiratory muscles.

OBSTRUCTIVE SLEEP APNEA

Obstructive sleep apnea particularly affects obese men over the age of 40. It is due to the combination of two factors: the normal relaxation of muscle tone in the throat during sleep and the reduction in the diameter of the pharynx caused by obesity or anomalies of the palate, the tonsils, the tongue, or the jaw. Obstructive sleep apnea and the lack of rest that accompanies it is manifested by various generally harmless symptoms: snoring, agitated sleep, frequent awakening during the night, sleepiness during the day, general fatigue, memory and attention problems, irritability, depression. Serious forms may cause complications such as respiratory insufficiency, cardiac arrhythmia, or hypertension. The consumption of alcohol or of certain sleeping pills before going to bed is an aggravating factor.

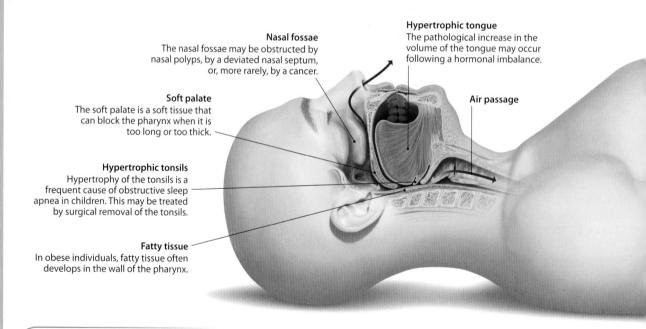

Nasal fossae
The nasal fossae may be obstructed by nasal polyps, by a deviated nasal septum, or, more rarely, by a cancer.

Hypertrophic tongue
The pathological increase in the volume of the tongue may occur following a hormonal imbalance.

Soft palate
The soft palate is a soft tissue that can block the pharynx when it is too long or too thick.

Air passage

Hypertrophic tonsils
Hypertrophy of the tonsils is a frequent cause of obstructive sleep apnea in children. This may be treated by surgical removal of the tonsils.

Fatty tissue
In obese individuals, fatty tissue often develops in the wall of the pharynx.

SNORING

Snoring is the sound generated during sleep by the vibration of the soft tissues of the throat and mouth. It occurs most often during inhalation and is caused by the obstruction of the passage of air through the nose (e.g., during a cold), or by the relaxation of the throat muscles during sleep. In the second case, it may be a symptom of sleep apnea. Snoring particularly affects sedentary men who are overweight. It is aggravated by the consumption of alcohol before going to bed and the taking of sleeping pills.

THE **TREATMENT** OF **SLEEP APNEA**

Sleep apnea treatments are based on surgical techniques (removal of soft tissue of the throat, nasal surgery) or assisted ventilation. The latter consists of blowing in pressurized air at the moment of inhalation and for the duration of the sleep using a pump placed near the bed and connected to a nasal mask. The treatments must be accompanied by a suppression of aggravating factors (obesity, alcohol, tobacco, sleeping pills).

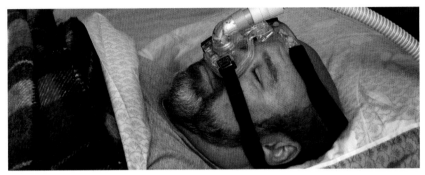

Assisted ventilation

SLEEP APNEA

SYMPTOMS:
Snoring, frequent awakening, daytime drowsiness, fatigue, loss of alertness, irritability, depression.

TREATMENTS:
Assisted ventilation, surgical removal of a portion of the soft tissues of the throat, dieting in the case of excessive weight.

PREVENTION:
Avoiding alcohol and sleeping pills before going to bed, eliminating tobacco, sleeping on the side when the problem habitually occurs when lying on the back.

LESIONS OF THE **NASAL SEPTUM**

The septum that separates the two nasal fossae may be subject to deviations or perforations due to malformations, **traumas**, aging, or the inhalation of chemical substances such as cocaine. These lesions are the cause of numerous respiratory problems: snoring, respiratory discomfort, recurrent **infections** (sinusitis, cold). If these problems are significant or poorly tolerated, a surgical operation, nasal septoplasty, may be performed in order to correct the lesions.

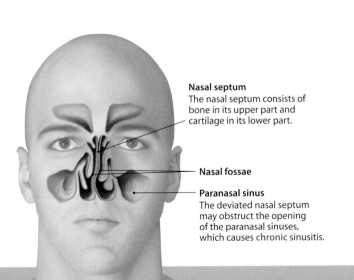

Nasal septum
The nasal septum consists of bone in its upper part and cartilage in its lower part.

Nasal fossae

Paranasal sinus
The deviated nasal septum may obstruct the opening of the paranasal sinuses, which causes chronic sinusitis.

LESIONS OF THE NASAL SEPTUM

SYMPTOMS:
Snoring or wheezing, sleep apnea, nasal congestion, headaches, nosebleeds.

TREATMENTS:
Surgery (septoplasty).

PREVENTION:
Avoiding the inhalation chemical substances such as cocaine, due to risk of perforation of the nasal septum.

RESPIRATORY INFECTIONS

Inhaled air often contains bacteria or viral pathogens capable of causing the **infection** of the respiratory tract. Generally harmless, these infections are resolved spontaneously in a few days, but drugs may relieve their symptoms: local pain, mucus discharge, fever, fatigue, respiratory difficulty. However, sore throat, sinusitis, and laryngitis must be treated and monitored in young children because they may cause serious complications.

Hygiene and the prevention of infections... page 30
Infectious diseases... page 284

THE COMMON COLD

The common cold, or acute rhinitis, is an inflammation of the mucous membranes of the nasal fossae caused by a viral infection. This harmless but very contagious ailment is manifested by nasal congestion, runny nose, irritation of the inside of the nose, sneezing, fatigue, and sometimes fever. The symptoms are relieved by decongestants and antifever drugs.

Warning! If you use a decongestant, be sure to follow the dosage indicated and do not combine it with other drugs without a doctor's approval.

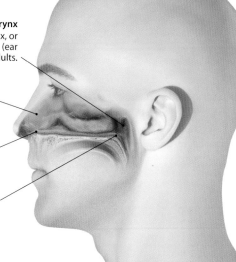

Rhinopharynx
Infection of the rhinopharynx, or rhinopharyngitis, may develop into otitis (ear infection) in children and sinusitis in adults.

Nasal congestion
Nasal congestion is caused by the accumulation of mucus and the increase in the volume of mucous membranes that cover the nasal fossae.

Rhinorrhea
Rhinorrhea (runny nose) is a discharge of abundant and fluid nasal secretions.

Mucus
The discharge of mucus in the throat may spread the infection to the pharynx and larynx.

SNEEZING

Sneezing is a reflux expulsion of air through the nose and mouth, in response to stimulation of the nasal mucous membrane by a foreign body or infection. The air is expelled at a speed of approximately 93 mph (150 km/h)!

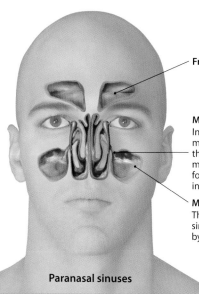

Frontal sinus

Mucous membrane
Inflammation of the mucous membrane closes the discharge path of the mucus towards the nasal fossae and allows the infection to develop.

Maxillary sinus
The maxillary sinus is the sinus most often affected by sinusitis.

Paranasal sinuses

SINUSITIS

Sinusitis is an inflammation of the paranasal sinuses, which is generally caused by the spread of an already existing infection such as a cold or dental infection. It is manifested by nasal congestion, runny nose, fever, pain around the eye sockets, and a feeling of pressure in the head. Sinusitis that persists more than three months may be due to a secondary infection, allergy, deviation of the nasal septum, or an obstruction (due to a polyp, for example) in one of the sinuses. Untreated, sinusitis may develop into meningitis.

SORE THROAT

A sore throat is an infection of the throat. It is often associated with tonsillitis and pharyngitis. Sore throat is normally caused by the common cold or flu virus, but may also be caused by a bacterium, most often a streptococcus. Frequent in children and adolescents, it manifests itself as a sharp pain in the throat, accentuated by swallowing, and the swelling of the lymph nodes in the neck. While a sore throat of viral origin spontaneously resolves, a streptococcal sore throat must be treated by antibiotics due to its possible complications. The viral or bacterial origin of a sore throat is determined by a bacteriological test carried out on a sample.

TONSILLITIS

Tonsillitis is an inflammation of the tonsils. Upon observation, the tonsils may appear red or covered with white spots. A tonsillectomy, or removal of the tonsils, is performed in case of repeated infections or when the tonsils are too large and obstruct the pharynx. The operation requires one day of hospitalization and is performed under general anesthesia.

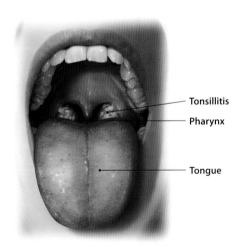

— Tonsillitis
— Pharynx
— Tongue

PHARYNGITIS

Pharyngitis is an inflammation of the pharynx. Acute pharyngitis, of infectious origin, is often associated with tonsillitis. Chronic pharyngitis may be due to chronic rhinitis or sinusitis, gastric reflux, or the irritation of the pharynx by tobacco, alcohol, or chemical products.

LARYNGITIS

Laryngitis is an inflammation of the larynx. Acute laryngitis, most often of viral origin, is frequent in children. It must be monitored because it could cause an obstruction of the larynx and require an emergency intubation. Chronic laryngitis may be caused by the spread of an infection (sore throat, sinusitis, dental infection), by overtaxing the voice, or by smoking. Laryngitis causes a hoarse, dry cough, pain in the throat, as well as an inflammation of the vocal cords, which results in hoarseness of the voice and which can lead to losing the voice altogether.

TRACHEITIS

Tracheitis is an inflammation of the trachea, of viral or bacterial origin, often associated with another respiratory tract infection (cold, bronchitis, etc.). It is manifested by fits of dry coughing, sometimes becoming loose, accompanied by a feeling of discomfort in the chest. Its treatment is based on antitussives.

RESPIRATORY INFECTIONS

SYMPTOMS:
Irritation of the respiratory tract, nasal congestion, respiratory problems, abundant discharge of mucus, sneezing, coughing, localized pain, voice change, fever, fatigue.

TREATMENTS:
Rest, humidification of the air, analgesics, antipyretics, decongestants, anti-inflammatories, antitussives. Bacterial infection: antibiotics. Chronic sinusitis: removal of polyp, if there is one. Repeated sore throats: removal of tonsils.

PREVENTION:
Chronic laryngitis and pharyngitis: reduction of alcohol and tobacco consumption.

THE **FLU**

The flu, or influenza, is a common and generally harmless viral **infection** that primarily affects the respiratory system. Very contagious, each winter the flu affects approximately 10% of the population of industrialized countries and constitutes a significant cause of death in fragile individuals such as the elderly or **immunodeficient**. Although there is no curative treatment against the flu, **vaccination** offers good protection if is renewed each year.

Infectious diseases... page 284

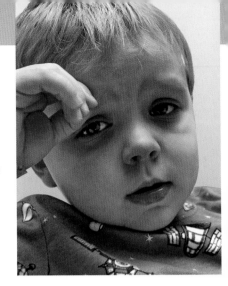

A **COLD** OR THE **FLU?**

Sore throat, nasal congestion, and runny nose are most often the symptoms of a cold. High fever, stiffness and aching, headaches, and intense fatigue are generally associated with the flu.

The common cold... page 318

FLU-LIKE SYNDROME

Flu-like syndrome, or flu-like state, is a combination of symptoms caused by the flu: fever higher than 104°F (40°C), shivering, muscle and joint pain, headaches, and significant fatigue. It is also manifested in connection with other infectious diseases, most often of viral origin. In the case of the flu, flu-like syndrome appears within 48 hours after contamination by the virus and is accompanied by a generalized **inflammation** of the respiratory tract (nose, throat, trachea, bronchial tubes) and a dry cough. In general, the flu spontaneously resolves in one week. In people suffering from **chronic** cardiac or respiratory diseases, a secondary bacterial infection may cause pneumonia.

THE **FLU VIRUS**

The flu is caused by the virus *Myxovirus influenzae*, which has a great ability to mutate. Thus, the flu virus is different each year and the vaccination must be renewed every year in order to be effective. The virus is spread by the microdroplets that come from sneezing and coughing and by direct contact with an infected person. Highly resistant, it is able to survive on objects such as a computer keyboard, a telephone, or a doorknob for at least 24 hours. Frequent washing of the hands in a period of epidemic thus remains one of the effective means of prevention.

RELIEVING FLU SYMPTOMS

Drinking plenty of water or other liquids and getting bed rest usually makes it possible to relieve flu symptoms. Drugs such as **antipyretics** and **analgesics** may also be used to lower the fever and to relieve stiffness, aching, and headaches.

NEW STRAINS OF THE FLU
AND THE RISK OF PANDEMIC

Each year, seasonal flu epidemics cause between 250,000 and 500,000 deaths throughout the world. It is one of the most significant causes of death by an infectious disease. New strains of the flu virus, very different from the seasonal flu virus, appear periodically. They may result from the mutation of an existing virus or the combination of a human flu virus with a porcine or avian flu virus. These flus, against which humans are not immunized, are capable of infecting the population and spreading rapidly, causing a pandemic. For an unknown reason, this phenomenon occurs three or four times per century, as in the 20th century, during which there were pandemics of the Spanish flu (1918–1919), the Asian flu (1957–1958) and the Hong Kong flu (1968–1969). It is difficult to predict the occurrence and the magnitude of a flu pandemic. Its symptoms may be identical to those of the seasonal flu or more severe, presenting a higher risk of death. The virus may also evolve and reappear with greater virulence. Scientists and governments are therefore vigilant when faced with the appearance of these new strains of the flu, as in the case of the avian flu virus of 2003 (H5N1) and the swine flu of 2009 (H1N1).

Faced with the risk of flu pandemic and in order to prepare to fight it, health authorities develop different strategies: implementation by the World Health Organization of a worldwide warning scale consisting of six phases, quarantining infected animals, development of a vaccine (the production of which can take several months). In case of an established flu pandemic and while awaiting a vaccine, it is preferable to limit traveling, particularly by public transportation, to avoid places with large concentrations of people, to wear a protective mask covering the nose and the mouth, and to systematically apply the elementary rules of hygiene such as washing and disinfecting the hands frequently, sneezing into a handkerchief or into one's elbow, etc.

Hygiene and the prevention of infections... page 30

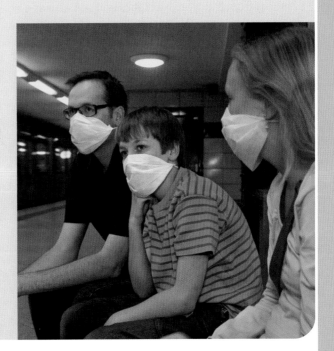

THE FLU

SYMPTOMS:
High fever over 104°F (40°C), shivering, stiffness and aching, joint pain, fatigue, headaches, dry cough, respiratory tract pain.

TREATMENTS:
Analgesics and antipyretics to relieve symptoms. Antibiotics in case of secondary bacterial infection of the respiratory tract.

PREVENTION:
Annual vaccination, antivirals prescribed by a doctor for persons at risk (taken immediately following contact with an infected person). Avoiding contact with sick people.

BRONCHITIS

Bronchitis is an **inflammation** of the bronchial tubes, which is manifested by a loose cough accompanied by expectoration. A distinction is made between **acute** bronchitis, due to an **infection**, and **chronic** bronchitis, caused by smoking, which may evolve into emphysema. The inflammation may extend to the trachea and, in newborns, to the mucous membrane of the bronchial tubes.

Emphysema... 329

ACUTE BRONCHITIS

Most often of viral origin, acute bronchitis is a frequent ailment in autumn and winter. It occurs suddenly and is first manifested by a dry cough, which evolves in three or four days into a loose cough. The latter is accompanied by expectorations of mucus from the bronchial tubes and sometimes a low fever. Acute bronchitis resolves spontaneously in 10 days. However, young children and the elderly or those suffering from respiratory problems are at risk of secondary bacterial infection, which requires **antibiotic** treatment.

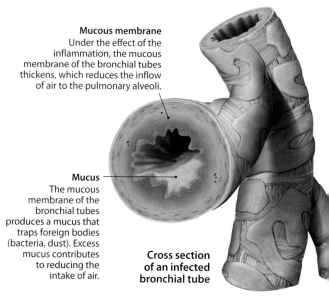

Mucous membrane
Under the effect of the inflammation, the mucous membrane of the bronchial tubes thickens, which reduces the inflow of air to the pulmonary alveoli.

Mucus
The mucous membrane of the bronchial tubes produces a mucus that traps foreign bodies (bacteria, dust). Excess mucus contributes to reducing the intake of air.

Cross section of an infected bronchial tube

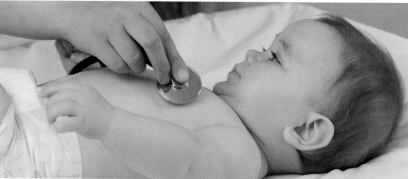

BRONCHIOLITIS

Bronchiolitis is an inflammation of the bronchioles, often caused by a viral infection such as the common cold. Contagious, it particularly affects children younger than 2 years of age. It resolves spontaneously in one week, but it may cause acute respiratory failure by obstruction of the bronchioles, specifically in newborns younger than 6 months old. Treatments are therefore intended to facilitate respiration by aiding in the elimination of mucus obstructing the bronchial tubes (respiratory physical therapy, taking of bronchodilator drugs). Proper hydration and maintaining a level of humidity between 40% and 60% also promotes decongestion of the respiratory tract.

BRONCHITIS

SYMPTOMS:
Dry then loose cough, expectoration of mucus, nasal discharge, low fever. Bronchiolitis: difficult and rapid respiration, wheezing.

TREATMENTS:
Antipyretic, antitussive for dry cough (to be avoided in newborns and children), expectorant for loose cough. Bronchiolitis: respiratory physical therapy, bronchodilators. Antibiotics are prescribed in case of infection or secondary bacterial infection.

PREVENTION:
Bronchiolitis: hygiene, avoiding contact between children in case of epidemic, avoiding contact between adults with a cold and infants.

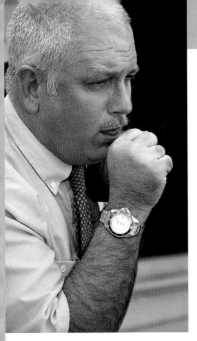

PNEUMONIA

Pneumonia, or pneumopathy, is a lung disease generally caused by a bacterial (pneumococcus, Mycoplasma, staphylococcus) **infection**. It is sometimes caused by a viral infection, particularly in young children. **Acute** lobar pneumonia, caused by the pneumococcus, is the most common, but there are several other forms. The diagnosis is most often made by means of a chest X-ray. **Antibiotic** treatments are effective, but there is a risk of complications in the elderly, young children, and individuals with a weakened immune system or suffering from respiratory failure.

ACUTE LOBAR PNEUMONIA

Acute lobar pneumonia, or pneumococcal pneumonia, is due to a bacterial infection of the lungs by the pneumococcus, most often limited to one or two pulmonary lobes. The symptoms (fever, shivering, chest pain, difficulty breathing, dry cough) appear suddenly and are followed by a loose cough. Recovery occurs within several weeks using an antibiotic treatment. In the elderly or newborns, the disease can develop into meningitis.

Meningitis… page 161

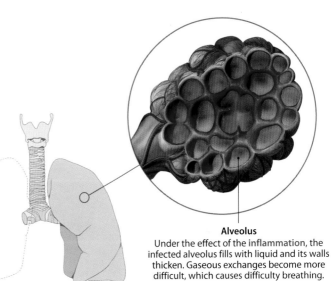

Alveolus
Under the effect of the **inflammation**, the infected alveolus fills with liquid and its walls thicken. Gaseous exchanges become more difficult, which causes difficulty breathing.

LEGIONELLOSIS

Legionellosis, or Legionnaires' disease, is a rare form of pneumonia caused by the bacterium *Legionella pneumophila*. The latter particularly likes tepid water and can contaminate domestic hot water supply pipes, air conditioning systems, or cooling towers. The infection is contracted by inhaling droplets of contaminated water. After 2 to 10 days of incubation, the symptoms are those of a flu-like syndrome then of pneumonia: chest pain, difficulty breathing, dry cough. It can even develop into respiratory failure or death.

Flu-like syndrome… page 320

PNEUMONIA

SYMPTOMS:
High fever, shivering, chest pain, respiratory difficulties, cough becoming loose with greenish or brownish expectoration.

TREATMENTS:
Antibiotics, given intravenously in serious cases.

PREVENTION:
Antipneumococcal vaccination in persons at risk.
Legionellosis: disinfection of air conditioning systems.

TUBERCULOSIS

A very contagious **infectious** disease, tuberculosis is caused by the Koch bacillus, a bacterium that primarily affects the lungs. The disease, in expansion, is responsible for almost 2 million deaths throughout the world each year, especially among young adults. Its progression is promoted by the absence of hygiene measures, malnutrition, poverty, drug abuse, and the expansion of the AIDS epidemic. The diagnosis of tuberculosis is based on a bacteriological examination of expectoration, a chest X-ray, and a skin test using tuberculin (a substance extracted from the Koch bacillus). **Antibiotic** treatment is effective if followed strictly.

PRIMARY TUBERCULAR INFECTION

The primary contact with the Koch bacillus causes a limited infection of the lungs, most often harmless and asymptomatic, called primary tubercular infection or primary tuberculosis. In 90% of cases, the primary tubercular infection is controlled by the immune system.
In the other cases, the latter does not manage to eliminate all of the bacteria, which results in the development of active tuberculosis, after a more or less lengthy latency period, owing to an immunosuppression, for example.

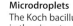

Microdroplets
The Koch bacillus, which can survive several week in the air, enters into the respiratory tract through microdroplets (sputter) from the coughing and sneezing of an infected person.

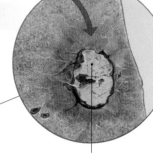

Tuberculous granuloma
A tuberculous granuloma is an **inflammatory** node, consisting primarily of macrophages and lymphocytes, which develops in the pulmonary alveoli following a primary tubercular infection.
The immune system... page 278

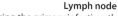
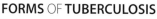

Lymph node
During the primary infection, the bacilli multiply in the pulmonary alveoli and migrate to the lymph nodes that surround the lungs. They then trigger an immune reaction that ends with the formation of a tuberculous granuloma.

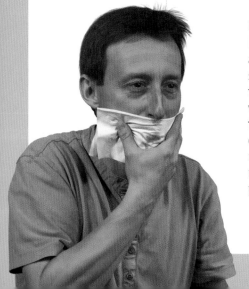

FORMS OF TUBERCULOSIS

Pulmonary tuberculosis is the most common form of tuberculosis. It affects the lungs and is manifested by a loose cough accompanied by sometimes bloody expectoration, chest pains, shortness of breath, fever, and night sweats. It causes general fatigue, loss of appetite, and weight loss. Miliary tuberculosis is a rare and serious form of tuberculosis that primarily affects the elderly or immunodeficient. It is due to the dissemination of the Koch bacillus throughout the body, via the lymph nodes. In addition to the lungs, the organs most frequently affected by miliary tuberculosis are the bones, the pericardium, the meninges, the pleura, the kidneys, and the liver.

DISTRIBUTION OF TUBERCULOSIS BY REGION

The regions most affected by the expansion of the disease are sub-Saharan Africa, Southeast Asia, and, to a lesser degree, Eastern Europe. The spread of tuberculosis, exacerbated by poor living conditions (poor hygiene, poverty, malnutrition, drug addiction, insufficient medical care), is further facilitated by the extension of the AIDS epidemic. The immunodeficiency caused by HIV in fact facilitates the reactivation of the Koch bacillus after a primary infection. The multiplication of cases of Koch bacillus resistance to antibiotic treatments also contributes to the spread of tuberculosis.

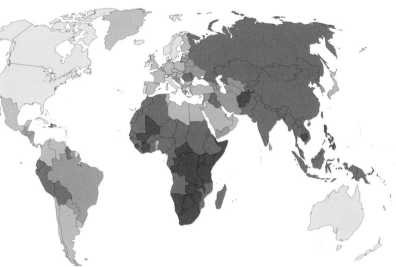

Source: Based on WHO data, 2002.

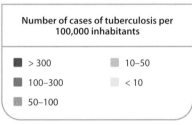

Number of cases of tuberculosis per 100,000 inhabitants

- ■ > 300
- ■ 100–300
- ■ 50–100
- ■ 10–50
- ■ < 10

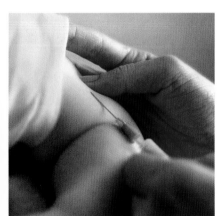

THE BCG VACCINE

The BCG vaccine is a vaccine against tuberculosis. It consists of a weakened live form of *Mycobacterium bovis*, a bacillus very close to the Koch bacillus. The BCG vaccine does not protect against the primary infection, but it enables the immune system to more effectively eliminate the Koch bacillus and to limit the risks of it being spread in the body. It prevents 70% of cases of serious forms (miliary tuberculosis) in children and 50% of cases of pulmonary tuberculosis in adults.

The vaccine... page 286

TUBERCULOSIS

SYMPTOMS:
Coughing, bloody expectoration, chest pains, difficulty breathing, fever, night sweats, fatigue, loss of appetite, weight loss.

TREATMENTS:
Antibiotic therapy based on three or four antibiotics administered orally, for a minimum of six months.

PREVENTION:
The BCG vaccine provides relative protection. Screening to identify contagious patients makes it possible to limit contamination.

ASTHMA

Asthma is a **chronic inflammation** of the bronchial tubes, which is manifested by attacks characterized by significant breathing difficulty. These attacks are caused by triggering factors, variable depending on the patient. Caused by a hereditary factor, asthma is a frequent disease (2% to 5% of the population), particularly in children. Its prevalence has increased regularly over the last 20 years. Early diagnosis, treatment of symptoms, and careful monitoring make it possible to properly control the disease.

ASTHMA ATTACKS

Asthma attacks may occur occasionally or several times in the same day. Attacks often occur at night and generally begin with a dry cough, rapidly followed by other symptoms: shortness of breath, wheezing, feeling of pressure in the chest, expectoration. Not always having the same intensity, asthma attacks may stop spontaneously in a few minutes or worsen and lead to respiratory insufficiency.

TRIGGERING FACTORS OF ASTHMA

An asthma attack is an abnormal reaction of the bronchial tubes to different triggering factors. Asthmatics may be sensitive to one or several factors, with a different sensitivity to each one of them.

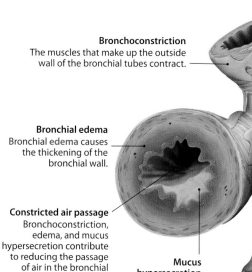

Bronchoconstriction
The muscles that make up the outside wall of the bronchial tubes contract.

Bronchial edema
Bronchial edema causes the thickening of the bronchial wall.

Constricted air passage
Bronchoconstriction, edema, and mucus hypersecretion contribute to reducing the passage of air in the bronchial tubes, which disrupts respiration and causes an asthma attack.

Mucus hypersecretion
The secretion of mucus by the bronchial mucous membrane is increased under the effect of inflammation.

Inflammation of the bronchial tubes

 POLLUTION
Several air pollutants have been recognized as asthma triggers: ozone, sulfur and nitrogen dioxides, cigarette smoke, wood combustion products, aerosols, irritant substances, and strong odors.

 METEOROLOGICAL CONDITIONS
Sudden changes of temperature or high ambient humidity may trigger asthma attacks.

 PHYSICAL EFFORT
A sustained or moderate physical effort may cause an asthma attack, especially when the weather is cold.

 EMOTIONS
Strong emotions, annoyances, and stress are psychological triggering factors.

 INFECTIONS
Infections of the airways (e.g. from a cold) represent 80% of the triggering factors of asthma in children. Asthma does not, however, increase the risk of respiratory infection.

 ALLERGENS
Contact with allergens (dust, dust mites, pollens, animal hair, and saliva) is a frequent cause of asthma.

 DRUGS
Some drugs are known for causing asthma attacks, specifically aspirin, beta blockers, and nonsteroidal anti-inflammatories.

TREATMENTS FOR ASTHMA

Asthma attacks are treated using bronchodilators, drugs that act quickly by relaxing the muscles of the bronchial tubes. The treatments for attacks are generally associated with a basic treatment, based on corticosteroids, whose long-term goal is to eliminate the chronic inflammation of the bronchial tubes. Some drugs are administered directly into the airways, using an inhaler, while others are delivered orally, in tablet form. Some serious attacks may require temporary hospitalization and recourse to artificial oxygenation.

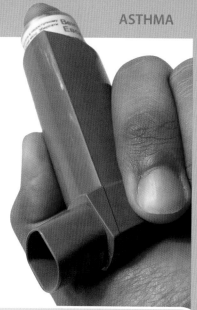

Inhaler
An inhaler, or metered dose inhaler, makes it possible to administer a drug through the airways, by propelling the medicinal substance in the form of droplets or particles (dry powder).

ASTHMATICS AND SPORTS ACTIVITIES

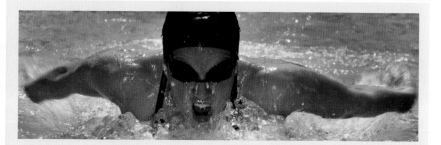

Although physical effort is an asthma-triggering factor, the regular practice of a sport is not contraindicated for an asthmatic. Several minutes of warm-up and the use of a bronchodilator before the effort generally make it possible to avoid the triggering of an attack. While swimming is particularly recommended, it is nevertheless preferable to consult a doctor before practicing certain endurance sports, a high-altitude activity, or scuba diving.

ASTHMA

SYMPTOMS:
Breathing difficulties, shortness of breath, wheezing, feeling of pressure in the chest, expectoration, anxiety.

TREATMENTS:
Attacks: inhaled bronchodilators.
Basic treatment: corticosteroids, inhaled or in tablets.

PREVENTION:
Avoiding triggering factors makes it possible to reduce the frequency of attacks.

SPIROMETRY

Spirometry is a medical examination intended to evaluate the quality of pulmonary ventilation. Seated, the nostrils blocked by a nose clip, the patient performs a series of forced inhalations and exhalations through a tube placed in the mouth and connected to a measuring device. In the case of asthma, the measurement of maximum force of expelled volume during the first second (or FEV1) gives an estimate of the degree of opening of the bronchial tubes. This measurement makes it possible to monitor the evolution of the disease over time.

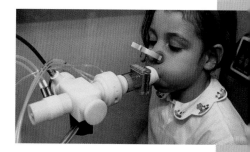

Spirometer
The spirometer measures the speed, volume, and flow of air that passes through the mouth during forced inhalations and exhalations.

CYSTIC FIBROSIS

Cystic fibrosis, or mucoviscidosis, is a recessive hereditary disease that primarily affects the functioning of the mucus glands. It is characterized by the accumulation of viscous secretions of abnormal composition, which causes dilations (cysts), obstructions, and numerous other complications. Cystic fibrosis appears at birth and strongly affects the patient's quality of life and life expectancy, despite the existence of treatments that relieve symptoms.

Heredity... page 50

THE **SYMPTOMS** OF **CYSTIC FIBROSIS**

The symptoms of cystic fibrosis appear early, some of them at birth. Basically, they involve the digestive (pancreas, intestines) and respiratory (bronchial tubes, lungs) systems.

RESPIRATORY PHYSICAL THERAPY

Respiratory physical therapy combines manipulations, postures, and respiratory rehabilitation intended to improve respiration. In the treatment of cystic fibrosis, postural drainage and positive expiratory pressure are intended to unblock the bronchial tubes obstructed by the mucus secretions. Positive expiratory pressure consists of using a mouthpiece or a mask in order to create a resistance to the expiration, which makes it possible to open the bronchial tubes and mobilize the mucus they contain.

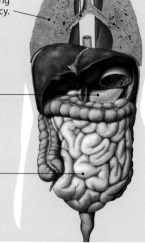

Bronchus
The accumulation of thick mucus obstructs the bronchial tubes and encourages the development of bacterial infections that are very difficult to treat and that are manifested by a constant, loose cough.

Lung
Repeated bacterial infections contribute to a deterioration of the lungs, progressively leading to respiratory insufficiency.

Pancreas
The pancreas does not produce sufficient digestive juices, which makes it difficult for the intestines to assimilate foods, particularly fats. This poor digestion is manifested by oily-looking diarrhea and accompanied by serious nutritional deficiencies and signs of malnutrition.

Intestine
The viscosity of intestinal secretions may cause constipation and intestinal obstructions.

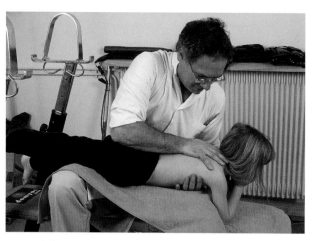

Postural drainage
Postural drainage uses gravity to facilitate the evacuation of mucus from the bronchial tubes.

CYSTIC FIBROSIS

SYMPTOMS:
Persistent loose cough, repeated respiratory infections, breathing difficulty, blue coloration of the extremities, chronic oily-looking diarrhea, intestinal obstruction, signs of malnutrition, male sterility.

TREATMENTS:
Respiratory system: respiratory physical therapy, secretion thinners, bronchodilators, oxygen therapy, antibiotics, corticosteroids. Digestive system: enzyme supplements, adapted diet.

PREVENTION:
Prenatal screening by biopsy of the placenta.

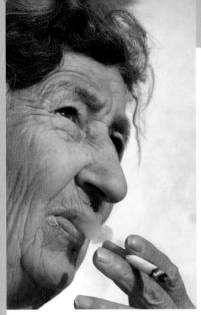

CHRONIC OBSTRUCTIVE BRONCHOPNEUMOPATHY

Smoking and air pollution may cause a progressive deterioration of the bronchial tubes and lungs leading to **chronic** bronchitis and emphysema. Characterized by increasingly difficult respiration, these chronic ailments are combined under the medical terms "chronic obstructive bronchopneumopathy" (COBP), or "chronic obstructive pulmonary disease" (COPD). A disabling disease, COBP is an increasing cause of death in industrialized countries. A spirometer makes it possible to diagnose it.

Spirometry… page 327

EMPHYSEMA

Emphysema is a chronic lung ailment, caused by the enlargement of the pulmonary alveoli by the destruction of their wall. It is often a complication of chronic bronchitis and is primarily caused by smoking. Emphysema is manifested by difficult and noisy breathing (shortness of breath), cough accompanied by expectoration, fatigue, and weight loss. It may progress into chronic respiratory failure or heart failure.

CHRONIC BRONCHITIS

Chronic bronchitis is a permanent or repeated inflammation of the mucous membrane of the bronchial tubes, associated with mucus hypersecretion. Like acute bronchitis, it is manifested by a frequent cough accompanied by fluid or thick expectoration. These symptoms must last at least three months per year for two consecutive years for bronchitis to be declared chronic. Caused primarily by smoking, the disease causes repeated infections. It may develop into emphysema.

Alveolar wall
The destruction of the alveolar wall causes the fusion of the pulmonary alveoli in larger cavities.

Dilated pulmonary alveolus
In growing, the alveoli lose their elasticity, so much so that the air they contain becomes more and more difficult to exhale.

Emphysema

CHRONIC OBSTRUCTIVE BRONCHOPNEUMOPATHY

SYMPTOMS:
Cough, expectoration, breathing difficulty, shortness of breath, noisy breathing, fatigue, weight loss; blue coloration of the skin, lips and nails (advanced stage).

TREATMENTS:
Bronchodilators, corticosteroids, secretion thinners, respiratory physical therapy, antibiotics in case of infection, oxygen therapy.

PREVENTION:
Avoiding tobacco consumption, vaccination against flu and pneumonia.

PNEUMOTHORAX

Pneumothorax is an effusion of air in the pleural cavity, the space located between the two folds of the membrane (pleura) enveloping the lungs. It results in the separation of the two folds and the partial or complete weakening of the affected lung. Pneumothorax is characterized by chest pain, dry cough, faster and more difficult breathing, and an increase in heart rate. The most serious forms are accompanied by **acute** respiratory insufficiency. Pneumothorax often resolves spontaneously. It may also be cured by thoracostomy, which consists in making a small opening in the thorax to withdraw the air from the pleural cavity.

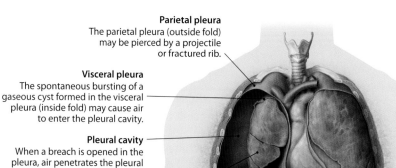

Parietal pleura
The parietal pleura (outside fold) may be pierced by a projectile or fractured rib.

Visceral pleura
The spontaneous bursting of a gaseous cyst formed in the visceral pleura (inside fold) may cause air to enter the pleural cavity.

Pleural cavity
When a breach is opened in the pleura, air penetrates the pleural cavity and the two folds separate.

Lung
The detachment of the two folds causes the lung to weaken.

PNEUMOTHORAX

SYMPTOMS:
Thoracic pain, dry cough that accentuates the pain, breathing difficulties.

TREATMENTS:
Rest, thoracostomy.

PLEURISY

Pleurisy is an acute or **chronic inflammation** of the pleura, which is generally accompanied by an effusion of fluid in the pleural cavity. Its principal causes are cancer, pulmonary **infections**, and heart failure. Pleurisy may manifest itself by a sharp chest pain radiating towards the shoulder, shortness of breath, or a dry cough accentuating the pain. The diagnosis is established from a chest X-ray and a thoracentesis (pleural tap), the analysis of which helps to determine the cause of the pleurisy and choose its treatment.

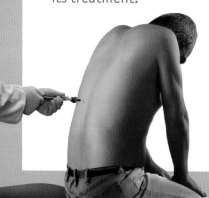

Pleural tap
A pleural tap is a sampling of pleural fluid in order to evacuate excess fluid or for a diagnostic purpose. It is performed under local **anesthesia** by inserting a trocar (puncturing instrument) between the two ribs as far as the pleura.

PLEURISY

SYMPTOMS:
Acute unilateral thoracic pain that irradiates towards the shoulder, respiratory difficulties, fits of dry coughing. The intensity of the symptoms vary with the patient's position.

TREATMENTS:
Antibiotics or anticancer drugs depending on the cause, draining of excessive pleural fluid.

PNEUMOCONIOSIS

Prolonged inhalation of mineral particles is responsible for a pulmonary disease called pneumoconiosis. This is generally an occupational disease whose symptoms manifest themselves after several years of exposure: shortness of breath upon exertion, dry cough, greater sensitivity to **infections**. It is diagnosed following a chest X-ray, sometimes even before the first symptoms appear. The evolution of pneumoconiosis leads more or less rapidly to **chronic** respiratory insufficiency. There are two types of pneumoconiosis: overload pneumoconiosis (anthracosis, siderosis, etc.), which corresponds to the accumulation of particles in the lungs, without toxic effect on the tissues; and fibrogenic pneumoconiosis (silicosis, asbestosis, etc.), which is more serious and is characterized by the irreversible development of pulmonary fibrosis.

ASBESTOSIS

Asbestosis is a pneumoconiosis caused by the inhalation of asbestos fibers. It primarily affects miners or construction workers who are exposed to asbestos. The risks of developing the disease are that much greater when the exposure to the asbestos was extensive and started at a young age. The symptoms (shortness of breath upon exertion, dry cough) are aggravated as the disease progresses, which may lead to respiratory insufficiency or lung cancer.

SILICOSIS

Silicosis is a pneumoconiosis caused by the inhalation of silica particles. It is characterized by the progressive development of hard, rounded pulmonary lesions. Silicosis particularly affects people who work in mines and quarries, or on construction sites.

ANTHRACOSIS

Anthracosis is a pneumoconiosis caused by the accumulation of carbon particles in the lungs. It primarily affects miners, sometimes in association with silicosis.

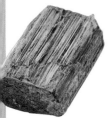

Asbestos
Asbestos is a fibrous mineral that is used industrially, specifically for its insulating properties. Prolonged inhalation of asbestos dust causes a number of diseases of the pleura and the lungs.

Carbon

PULMONARY FIBROSIS

Pulmonary fibrosis is the development of fibrous tissues in the lungs, or the thickening of pulmonary tissues, which is manifested by breathing difficulties during exertion, dry cough, and sometimes a deformation of the nails. Although the exact cause often remains unknown, it may be due to an **inflammation** caused by a drug, radiation, or inhalation of particles. Its evolution leads to respiratory insufficiency.

PNEUMOCONIOSIS

SYMPTOMS:
Shortness of breath after exertion, dry cough, greater sensitivity to pulmonary infections.

TREATMENTS:
No treatment. Oxygen therapy in the case of respiratory insufficiency.

PREVENTION:
Wearing a mask and medical monitoring by chest X-ray for people in occupations at risk.

RESPIRATORY INSUFFICIENCY

Respiratory insufficiency is an **acute** or **chronic** deficiency of the respiratory system, which results in poor oxygenation of the blood, sometimes accompanied by an inability to eliminate the accumulated carbon dioxide. It is caused by an obstruction of the airways, a reduction of respiratory movements, a disruption in gaseous exchanges, or poor circulation of blood in the lungs. Potentially fatal, respiratory insufficiency may be manifested by rapid and difficult breathing, accompanied by significant sweating, cardiac arrhythmia, and bluish coloration of the skin and mucous membranes. Its treatment is intended to reestablish blood oxygenation by different means that may be used according to the severity and origin of the insufficiency.

ACUTE RESPIRATORY INSUFFICIENCY

Acute respiratory insufficiency is the sudden inability of the respiratory system to complete the oxygenation of the blood or eliminate carbon dioxide. It may be caused by various factors: obstruction of the airways (foreign body, tumor, asthma attack, epiglottitis, sleep apnea, etc.), reduction of respiratory movements (neuromuscular ailment, pulmonary lesion), disruption of gaseous exchanges (severe pneumonia, pulmonary edema, acute respiratory distress syndrome), poor circulation of blood in the lungs (heart failure, pulmonary embolism), and complication of a chronic respiratory insufficiency. Whatever its origin, acute respiratory insufficiency may result in death by asphyxia and requires urgent medical attention.

ACUTE RESPIRATORY DISTRESS SYNDROME

Acute respiratory distress syndrome (or ARDS) is an acute respiratory insufficiency caused by a lesion of the alveolocapillary membrane, which corresponds to the location of gaseous exchanges in the pulmonary alveoli. It results in a generalized inflammatory reaction and the formation of a pulmonary edema. The lesion may have diverse origins: pneumonia, contusion, drowning, inhalation of chemical substances, extensive burns, generalized infection, etc. ARDS results in the rapid failure of other vital organs (heart, kidneys) and causes death in 40% to 60% of cases.

Pulmonary edema... page 335

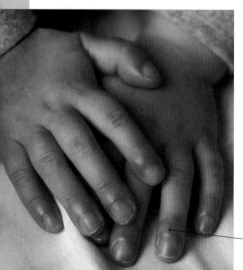

CHRONIC RESPIRATORY INSUFFICIENCY

Chronic respiratory insufficiency is the permanent inability of the respiratory system to ensure proper oxygenation of the blood. It occurs following an obstructive pulmonary disease (chronic bronchitis, asthma, cystic fibrosis, emphysema) or a restriction in volume of inhaled air (tuberculosis, pulmonary fibrosis, pneumectomy, poliomyelitis, amyotrophic lateral sclerosis, severe scoliosis). Chronic respiratory insufficiency is manifested by shortness of breath upon exertion and cyanosis. In the long term, it weakens the body and may develop into an acute form.

Cyanosis
A sign of poor oxygenation of the blood, cyanosis is the bluish coloration of the mucous membranes and skin. It is particularly marked at the extremities of the limbs and in the lips.

OXYGEN THERAPY

Poor oxygenation of the blood may be compensated for by different oxygen therapy treatments that increase the content of oxygen in the inhaled air. Methods of administration vary based on the quantity of oxygen needed. A simple oxygen enrichment may be obtained using oxygen glasses. More precise control of oxygen quantity is obtained using a facial mask, a probe introduced in the trachea, or a catheter connected to a cannula following a tracheotomy. In some cases, oxygen may also be administered at a pressure greater than the barometric pressure (hyperbaric oxygen therapy). Oxygen therapy treatments may be dispensed in a temporary or permanent manner, in a hospital setting or at home.

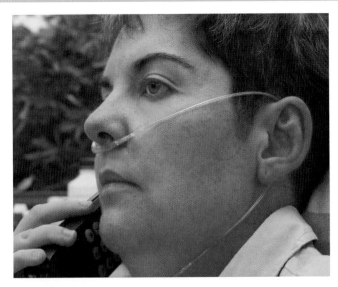

Oxygen glasses
Oxygen glasses consist of a flexible tube, one end of which is placed at the entry to the nostrils and the other connected to a portable oxygen tank.

TRACHEOTOMY

The tracheotomy is a surgical procedure that consists of incising the trachea in the neck area to insert a cannula that connects with the exterior. This technique is used in oxygen therapy in order to facilitate pulmonary ventilation by eliminating the resistance to the passage of air through the upper airways. It also makes it possible to control the quantity of oxygen supplied to the lungs.

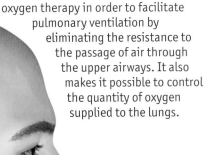

Trachea

Cannula
A cannula is a hollow tube inserted into the body to allow the passage of gas or liquids. In the case of an oxygen therapy treatment, its outside end is connected to an oxygen source.

HYPERBARIC OXYGEN THERAPY

Hyperbaric oxygen therapy is an oxygen therapy technique that consists in administering oxygen at a pressure greater than the barometric pressure. It takes place in an airtight chamber by progressively increasing the air pressure, which increases the quantity of oxygen dissolved in the blood. Hyperbaric oxygen therapy is specifically used in cases of carbon monoxide poisoning, decompression accident (scuba diving), and altitude sickness. It also has a positive effect on certain bacterial infections and accelerates healing of the skin. In addition, it is used by some athletes to increase their physical performance.

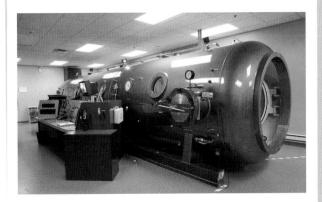

Hyperbaric chamber
A hyperbaric chamber may accommodate one or several persons.

The respiratory system | Diseases

ARTIFICIAL RESPIRATION

Artificial respiration, or artificial ventilation, is a combination of techniques that allow a patient whose respiratory movements are absent or insufficient (paralysis, coma, drowning) to breathe. It consists of forcing in air, which may or may not be enriched with oxygen, at a pressure sufficient to fill the lungs. In the context of emergency cardiopulmonary resuscitation, it is done via the mouth. In other cases, an artificial respirator is used.

First aid: Cardiopulmonary arrest… page 544

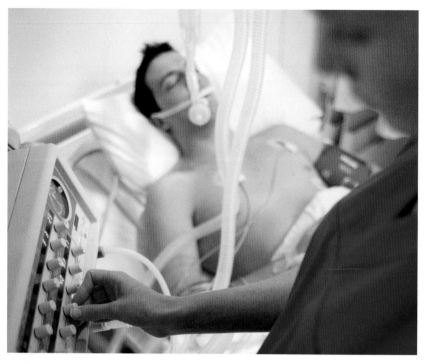

Artificial respiration
An artificial respirator is a device consisting of a pump and system of measurement that allows the regulation of certain respiration parameters (air pressure, volume, frequency, and duration of inhalation). It is often connected to an airtight mask applied to the nose or the entire face.

ENDOTRACHEAL TUBE

An endotracheal tube is a flexible tube introduced through the nose that allows air to be guided into the trachea from an artificial respirator. In comparison with the use of a mask, techniques such as the use of an endotracheal tube or tracheotomy have disadvantages: they are not tolerated as well by the patient, they present a higher risk of infection, and they hamper speech and feeding.

LUNG TRANSPLANT

A lung transplant is a surgical procedure that consists of replacing a deficient lung with a healthy one. It is indicated in cases of pulmonary arterial hypertension or a serious lung ailment endangering the life of the patient. A lung transplant is a delicate operation that is rarely practiced due to the lack of donors and the fragility of the lungs. The transplantation lasts from six to eight hours and then requires several weeks of hospital convalescence. The transplantee must follow lifelong treatment to prevent the risk of rejection.

RESPIRATORY INSUFFICIENCY

SYMPTOMS:
Respiratory rhythm problems, bluish coloration of the skin and mucous membranes, cardiac arrhythmia, sweating, loss of consciousness, feeling of suffocation.

TREATMENTS:
First aid: Heimlich maneuver, mouth-to-mouth. For the longer term: respiratory physical therapy, oxygen therapy, artificial respiration, lung transplant.

PREVENTION:
Avoiding tobacco consumption. Treatment of asthma and obstructive pulmonary diseases.

PULMONARY EDEMA

Pulmonary **edema** is a potentially fatal seepage of blood plasma into the pulmonary alveoli, which results in poor oxygenation of the blood. Its most frequent cause is the increase of blood pressure in the capillaries of the lungs, generally caused by cardiac insufficiency. More rarely, the seepage of plasma is due to a severe **trauma** or an increase in the permeability of the joint surfaces of the capillaries and the pulmonary alveoli. The latter type of edema has various causes (pneumonia, inhalation of toxic gases, altitude sickness, etc.) and is often associated with **acute** respiratory distress syndrome.

Acute respiratory distress syndrome... page 332

SYMPTOMS OF PULMONARY EDEMA

Depending on its origin, the symptoms of pulmonary edema may occur suddenly or take hold more progressively. The first sign is difficult, rapid, and noisy breathing, and a feeling of suffocation, particularly when lying down. It is often accompanied by coughing and expectoration of a pinkish color and frothy appearance. These symptoms are evidence of the obstruction of the airways by the seepage of plasma into the pulmonary alveoli. When the pulmonary edema is large, it is manifested by a bluish coloration of the skin and mucous membranes (cyanosis).

PULMONARY EDEMA

SYMPTOMS:
Shortness of breath, cough, pinkish and frothy expectoration, blue coloration of the skin and mucous membranes. Serious pulmonary edema: consciousness problems, sweats, chilling of the fingers and toes, marble appearance of skin.

TREATMENTS:
Oxygenation of the blood, reduction in pulmonary blood pressure using vasodilators and diuretics.

PREVENTION:
Prevention of cardiovascular diseases. Altitude sickness: progressive ascent.

Expectoration
Pink and frothy expectoration is evidence of the presence of blood plasma in the pulmonary alveoli.

Blood capillary
The alveolus fills with plasma from the blood capillaries.

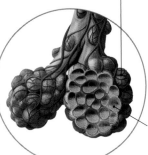

Pulmonary alveolus
The filling of the pulmonary alveoli prevents the exchange of gases. The oxygenation of the blood decreases.

ALTITUDE SICKNESS

In persons who stay in high altitudes (above 8200 feet [2500 meters]) without preparation, the decrease in atmospheric pressure and lack of oxygen may cause altitude sickness. The latter is manifested by nausea, headaches, and sleep problems, and may cause the formation of a pulmonary or cerebral edema. Several days of rest after acclimating to high altitudes and progressive ascent when hiking suffice in preventing altitude sickness.

335

TUMORS OF THE RESPIRATORY SYSTEM

Tumors of the respiratory system may be benign, such as nasal polyps and polyps of the vocal cords, or malignant, such as cancers of the larynx, lungs, or pleura. Benign tumors may be spontaneously cured, but are often surgically removed. Malignant tumors may be treated depending on their stage by surgical removal, **radiation therapy**, or **chemotherapy**, or by a combination of these treatments. Nevertheless, they are a significant cause of death: lung cancer causes approximately 1 million deaths per year worldwide.

Cancer... page 55

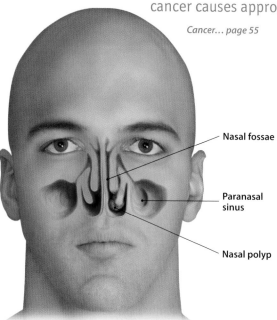

Nasal fossae

Paranasal sinus

Nasal polyp

NASAL POLYPS

Nasal polyps develop in the mucous membrane of the nasal fossae and the paranasal sinuses and may be caused by the chronic inflammation of the mucous membrane (allergic or smoker's rhinitis). The largest polyps cause persistent nasal congestion, discharges, or snoring. In the most serious cases, the polyps cause chronic sinusitis, a loss of sense of smell, or an aggravation of obstructive sleep apnea.

POLYPS OF THE VOCAL CORDS

Polyps may develop on the vocal cords following overuse of the voice or a chronic inflammation caused by an allergy or exposure to irritating substances. They cause a change in the voice (dysphonia). Their treatment consists of surgical removal performed through the natural orifices of the airways. The polyps must not be confused with nodules of the vocal cords, harmless lesions that appear following an overuse of the voice and that most often heal spontaneously.

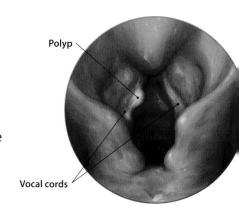

Polyp

Vocal cords

DYSPHONIA

Dysphonia is a voice anomaly signaling a problem with the larynx or the nerves that control it: voice is sharper, lower, hoarse, husky, or throaty, or disappears. It is frequently caused by nodules or polyps appearing on the vocal cords but may also be the symptom of other respiratory system ailments: laryngitis, cancer of the larynx, cancer of the bronchial tubes, etc.

Laryngitis... page 319

TUMORS OF THE PHARYNX

Tumors of the pharynx are sometimes benign, but more often they are cancers that originate in the mucous membrane of the pharynx. These cancers are primarily caused by smoking, alcoholism, and exposure to carcinogenic substances. In certain ethnic groups at risk (Southeast Asia, Mediterranean basin), cancer of the pharynx may be caused by the Epstein-Barr virus, also responsible for mononucleosis.

CANCER OF THE LARYNX

Cancer of the larynx develops in the vocal cords or in the wall of the larynx. Smoking and alcoholism are the main causes of this disease, which primarily affects men 40 to 60 years of age. Cancer of the larynx is manifested by voice, breathing, and swallowing problems, accompanied by ear pain. Treatment is based on radiation therapy (often combined with chemotherapy) and on a laryngectomy. The latter consists of removing part or all of the larynx, according to the extent of the tumor. A partial laryngectomy enables the patient to continue to breathe and speak by normal means, but voice rehabilitation may be necessary. A total laryngectomy results in the loss of the voice and is accompanied by a complete reshaping of the throat involving a tracheostomy.

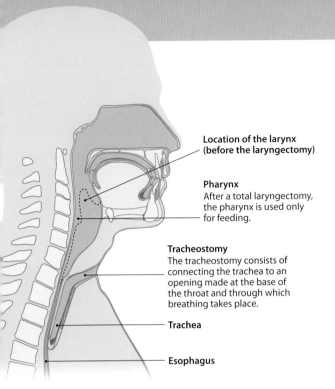

Location of the larynx (before the laryngectomy)

Pharynx
After a total laryngectomy, the pharynx is used only for feeding.

Tracheostomy
The tracheostomy consists of connecting the trachea to an opening made at the base of the throat and through which breathing takes place.

Trachea

Esophagus

Total laryngectomy

BRONCHOPULMONARY CANCER

Bronchopulmonary cancer, or cancer of the lungs, are malignant tumors that develop in the bronchial tubes or, less frequently, in the pulmonary alveoli. The main cause is smoking. Prolonged exposure to air pollutants is also a significant risk factor. Bronchopulmonary cancer is manifested by coughing, expectoration of blood, shortness of breath, or chest pains. These symptoms may be accompanied by fatigue, loss of appetite, and weight loss. Lung cancer treatments depend on the type of tumor and their extent. If they are diagnosed at an early stage, most bronchopulmonary cancers may be treated with some effectiveness by surgical removal of a portion or all of a lung, sometimes followed by radiation therapy or chemotherapy.

TUMORS OF THE RESPIRATORY SYSTEM

SYMPTOMS:
Malignant tumors: voice, breathing and swallowing problems, coughing, expectoration of blood, chest pain, pneumonia, pleurisy.

TREATMENTS:
Benign tumors: rest for the vocal cords, anti-inflammatories, removal. Malignant tumors: removal, chemotherapy, radiation therapy.

PREVENTION:
Quitting smoking makes it possible to reduce the risk of cancer. Avoiding prolonged exposure to carcinogenic substances such as asbestos.

PRIMITIVE CANCER OF THE PLEURA

Primitive cancer of the pleura is a rare form of cancer that primarily affects people who have been exposed to asbestos (miners, construction workers, etc.). It appears 30 to 50 years after the asbestos exposure and is manifested by chest pain and breathing difficulties, combined with an inflammation of the pleura.

Pleurisy... page 330
Pneumoconiosis... page 331

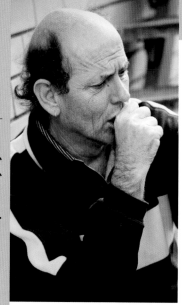

NICOTINE ADDICTION

Consuming tobacco or inhaling secondhand smoke leads to a **chronic** intoxication of the substances that it contains. Consumed for its stimulating effects, particularly due to nicotine, tobacco creates a dependence within a few months of regular consumption. Several substances contained in tobacco or resulting from its burning (tar, carbon monoxide, benzene, etc.) are responsible for cancer and cardiovascular diseases, and also present a risk factor for numerous other diseases. Smoking causes more than 5 million deaths per year worldwide.

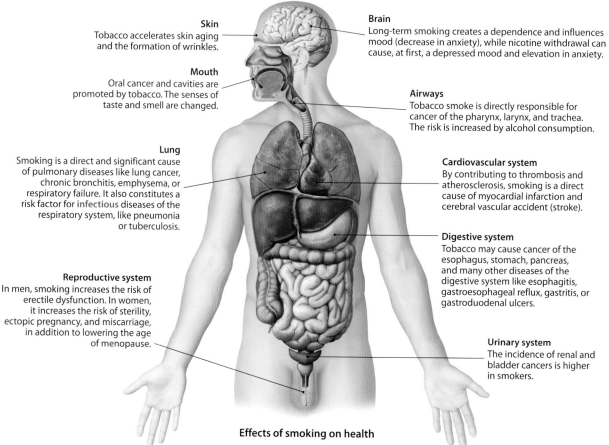

Skin
Tobacco accelerates skin aging and the formation of wrinkles.

Brain
Long-term smoking creates a dependence and influences mood (decrease in anxiety), while nicotine withdrawal can cause, at first, a depressed mood and elevation in anxiety.

Mouth
Oral cancer and cavities are promoted by tobacco. The senses of taste and smell are changed.

Airways
Tobacco smoke is directly responsible for cancer of the pharynx, larynx, and trachea. The risk is increased by alcohol consumption.

Lung
Smoking is a direct and significant cause of pulmonary diseases like lung cancer, chronic bronchitis, emphysema, or respiratory failure. It also constitutes a risk factor for **infectious** diseases of the respiratory system, like pneumonia or tuberculosis.

Cardiovascular system
By contributing to thrombosis and atherosclerosis, smoking is a direct cause of myocardial infarction and cerebral vascular accident (stroke).

Digestive system
Tobacco may cause cancer of the esophagus, stomach, pancreas, and many other diseases of the digestive system like esophagitis, gastroesophageal reflux, gastritis, or gastroduodenal ulcers.

Reproductive system
In men, smoking increases the risk of erectile dysfunction. In women, it increases the risk of sterility, ectopic pregnancy, and miscarriage, in addition to lowering the age of menopause.

Urinary system
The incidence of renal and bladder cancers is higher in smokers.

Effects of smoking on health

SMOKING EPIDEMIC

According to the World Health Organization, the number of smokers is constantly increasing, particularly in developing countries. Nicotine addiction is a real epidemic that affects more than 1.2 billion people around the globe and kills approximately 5.4 million people per year. This number could reach 8 million by 2030.

NICOTINE

Present in a large quantity in tobacco, nicotine is a natural vegetal substance that interacts with the nervous system. Released through burning tobacco, it is absorbed by the lungs and dispersed through the blood. A few seconds after inhalation, it reaches the brain, where it brings slight psychotropic effects such as a calming down, decrease in anxiety, or euphoria. Nicotine stimulates the release of several neurotransmitters, particularly dopamine, responsible for the dependence. Nicotine has several effects: heart rate acceleration, blood vessel constriction, change in breathing rate, stimulation of activity in the digestive system, decrease in appetite, nausea, increase of fat levels in the blood, etc. It is reduced within a few hours, which explains the frequent need to smoke.

NICOTINE ADDICTION

SYMPTOMS:
Craving in the case of abstinence: irritability, difficulty concentrating, insomnia, irrepressible desire to smoke.

TREATMENT:
Complete withdrawal.

PREVENTION:
Refraining from smoking, avoiding secondhand smoke.

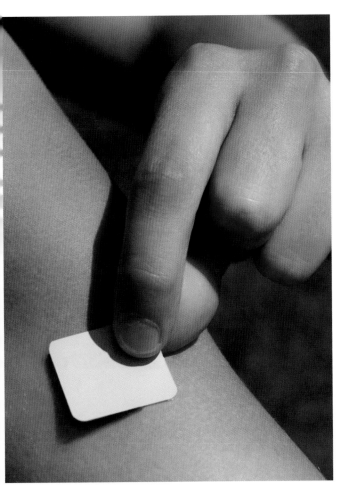

TOBACCO WITHDRAWAL

When there is a dependence on tobacco, tobacco withdrawal appears quickly following the discontinuation of its consumption. It is often associated with sleep problems, irritability, anxiety, and an increase in appetite, which can last several days to several weeks. In most cases, smokers can overcome these symptoms without medical or psychological assistance. More dependent smokers can benefit from different methods to help overcome a nicotine dependence. The most frequently used methods replace the nicotine from tobacco with a skin patch, chewing gum, pills, or aerosols to inhale. These methods allow the elimination of the behavioral dependence associated with the act of smoking, then limit the withdrawal symptoms with a progressive decrease of nicotine doses.

Tobacco, alcohol, and drugs... page 26

Skin patch
In the event of tobacco withdrawal, a skin patch is used to administer decreasing doses of nicotine in the blood by progressive diffusion through the skin.

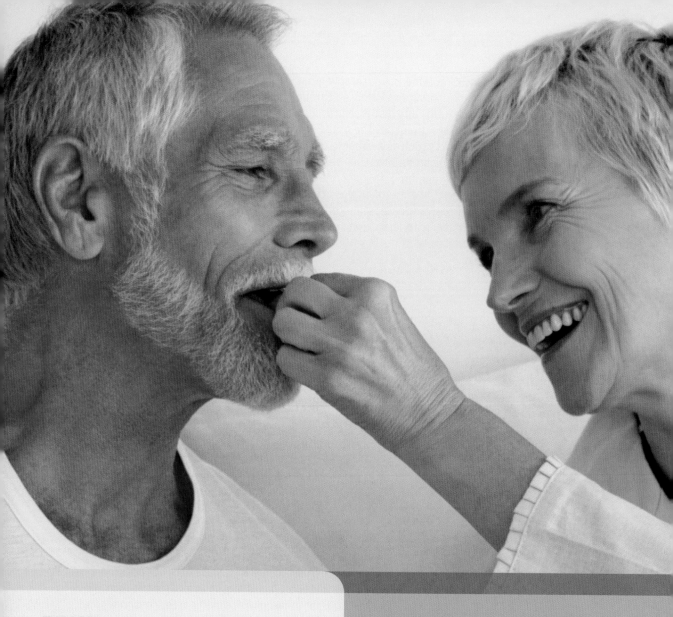

THE **DIGESTIVE SYSTEM**

A balanced diet is necessary for the good health of the human body. Food provides the fuel and raw materials necessary for its proper functioning. The role of the digestive system is to transform this food into particles small enough to be absorbed by the blood and lymphatic circulation. This is digestion. Elements that are not assimilated are eliminated in the form of fecal matter.

An excessive or insufficient diet can have serious consequences on a person's general state of health, and so can the various digestive system diseases that can limit food ingestion, prevent its mechanical or chemical transformation, and harm its transit through the digestive tract or its assimilation. An **infection**, an **inflammation** of the digestive mucous membrane, or a tumor can also interfere with the functioning of digestive organs.

THE **DIGESTIVE SYSTEM**

The digestive system transforms food into nutrients, elements that can be assimilated by the body. It thus provides the energy and raw materials that are essential to the development and functioning of the human body. Close to 95% of food is assimilated during digestion; the rest is eliminated outside the body in the form of fecal matter. Therefore, an unbalanced diet or a digestive tract disease has significant repercussions on the general state of health.

THE **ORGANS** OF THE **DIGESTIVE SYSTEM**

The digestive system is made up of three parts: the mouth, the digestive tract (esophagus, stomach, intestines), and the adjoining organs (salivary glands, liver, biliary vesicle, pancreas). Ingested through the mouth, food is chewed, altered by saliva, and swallowed, which makes it pass through the digestive tract, where it is progressively broken down by mechanical and chemical means. The nutrients are absorbed and the elements that are not used are eliminated through defecation.

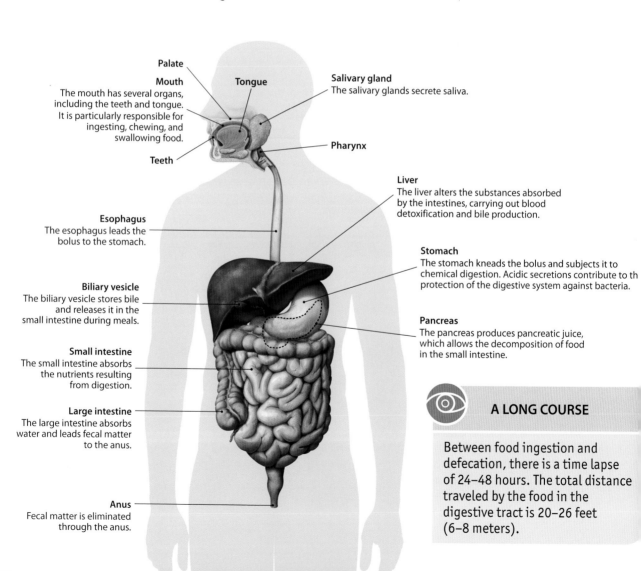

Palate

Mouth
The mouth has several organs, including the teeth and tongue. It is particularly responsible for ingesting, chewing, and swallowing food.

Teeth

Tongue

Salivary gland
The salivary glands secrete saliva.

Pharynx

Liver
The liver alters the substances absorbed by the intestines, carrying out blood detoxification and bile production.

Esophagus
The esophagus leads the bolus to the stomach.

Stomach
The stomach kneads the bolus and subjects it to chemical digestion. Acidic secretions contribute to th protection of the digestive system against bacteria.

Biliary vesicle
The biliary vesicle stores bile and releases it in the small intestine during meals.

Pancreas
The pancreas produces pancreatic juice, which allows the decomposition of food in the small intestine.

Small intestine
The small intestine absorbs the nutrients resulting from digestion.

Large intestine
The large intestine absorbs water and leads fecal matter to the anus.

Anus
Fecal matter is eliminated through the anus.

A LONG COURSE

Between food ingestion and defecation, there is a time lapse of 24–48 hours. The total distance traveled by the food in the digestive tract is 20–26 feet (6–8 meters).

THE **MOUTH**

A means of entry for food into the digestive tract, the mouth (or buccal cavity) completes its first transformation. During mastication, or chewing, food is broken down by the teeth and mixed with saliva to form a paste, the bolus. The bolus is led to the esophagus by **swallowing.** The mouth plays an essential role in taste and also plays a part in breathing and speech production.

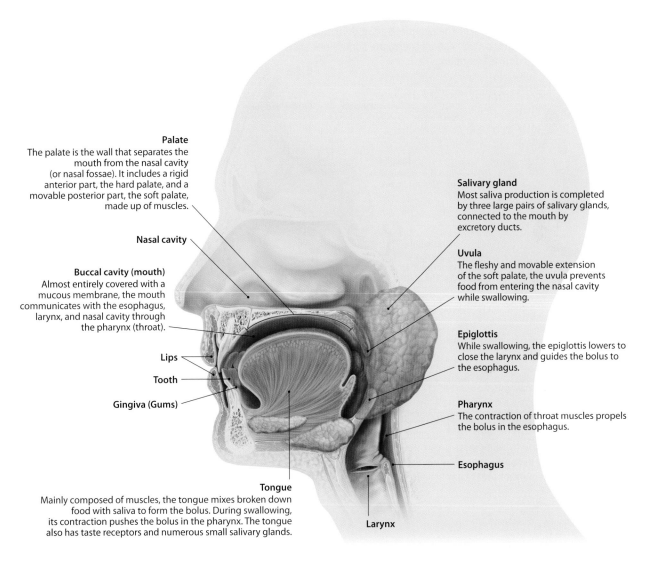

Palate
The palate is the wall that separates the mouth from the nasal cavity (or nasal fossae). It includes a rigid anterior part, the hard palate, and a movable posterior part, the soft palate, made up of muscles.

Nasal cavity

Buccal cavity (mouth)
Almost entirely covered with a mucous membrane, the mouth communicates with the esophagus, larynx, and nasal cavity through the pharynx (throat).

Lips

Tooth

Gingiva (Gums)

Salivary gland
Most saliva production is completed by three large pairs of salivary glands, connected to the mouth by excretory ducts.

Uvula
The fleshy and movable extension of the soft palate, the uvula prevents food from entering the nasal cavity while swallowing.

Epiglottis
While swallowing, the epiglottis lowers to close the larynx and guides the bolus to the esophagus.

Pharynx
The contraction of throat muscles propels the bolus in the esophagus.

Esophagus

Tongue
Mainly composed of muscles, the tongue mixes broken down food with saliva to form the bolus. During swallowing, its contraction pushes the bolus in the pharynx. The tongue also has taste receptors and numerous small salivary glands.

Larynx

SALIVA

Saliva is a viscous liquid secreted by the salivary glands. It is mostly made up of water (97%–99%), mucus, mineral salts, and proteins: enzymes, antibodies, antibacterials, etc. Saliva plays an important role in forming a bolus, in taste, and in the chemical digestion of food because it starts the decomposition of certain carbohydrates. In addition, saliva lubricates the tongue, lips, and cheeks and acts as an antiseptic by destroying microorganisms. Approximately one liter of saliva is produced each day, mainly during meals. The smell, sight, and presence of food in the mouth stimulates salivation.

THE **TEETH**

Anchored in the jawbone, the teeth are hard organs emerging from the gums. They are made up of living tissues and have nerves and blood vessels. All of the teeth together make up the dentition, which has chewing as its primary function, meaning the cutting and grinding of food.

DENTITION

The teeth are distributed symmetrically to form the lower and upper dentition. Until approximately the age of 6, the dentition has 20 temporary teeth. The complete adult dentition has 32 teeth: 8 incisors, 4 canines, 8 premolars, and 12 molars. The last molars, called wisdom teeth, are sometimes absent or poorly positioned. Poor tooth alignment can be corrected by orthodontic treatment.

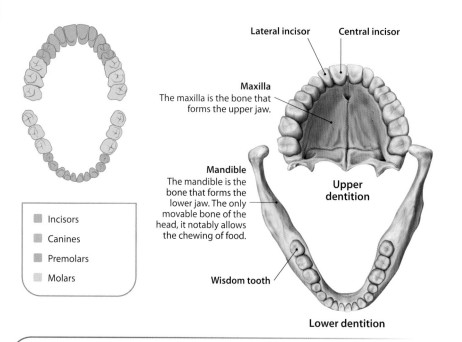

Incisors

Canines

Premolars

Molars

Lateral incisor

Central incisor

Maxilla
The maxilla is the bone that forms the upper jaw.

Mandible
The mandible is the bone that forms the lower jaw. The only movable bone of the head, it notably allows the chewing of food.

Wisdom tooth

Upper dentition

Lower dentition

Ridge

Incisor
Located at the front of the jaw, the eight incisors have a sharp ridge that cuts food.

Crown

Canine
Located between the incisors and premolars, the four canine teeth have a pointed crown capable of piercing and tearing food.

WISDOM TEETH

Wisdom teeth are the third molars. They rarely appear before 18 years of age and may even only partially appear or never appear at all. Their growth can cause the displacement of teeth that are already in place and cause a dental malocclusion.

Dental malocclusion... page 371

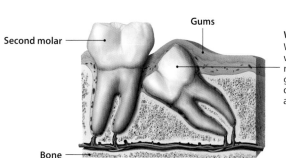

Second molar

Gums

Wisdom tooth
While growing, the wisdom teeth can remain under the gums or in the bone, or even pop up in an abnormal position.

Bone

Cross section of an adult jaw

Premolar
Located between the canines and the molars, the eight premolars have the same role as the molars, but they are smaller.

Crown

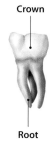

Molar
The molars are the 12 teeth located at the back of the jaw. Large and with two or three roots, they have a flat crown, with points and grooves that allow them to grind food.

Root

DENTAL ANATOMY

The tooth is made up of two parts: the crown, which emerges from the gum and carries out chewing, and the root, which is embedded in the bone. The tooth is primarily made up of a living calcified tissue, dentin. In its center, it houses a cavity filled with dental pulp, which is made of connective tissue, vessels, and nerves. At the crown, the tooth is covered with enamel, a very resistant mineral substance.

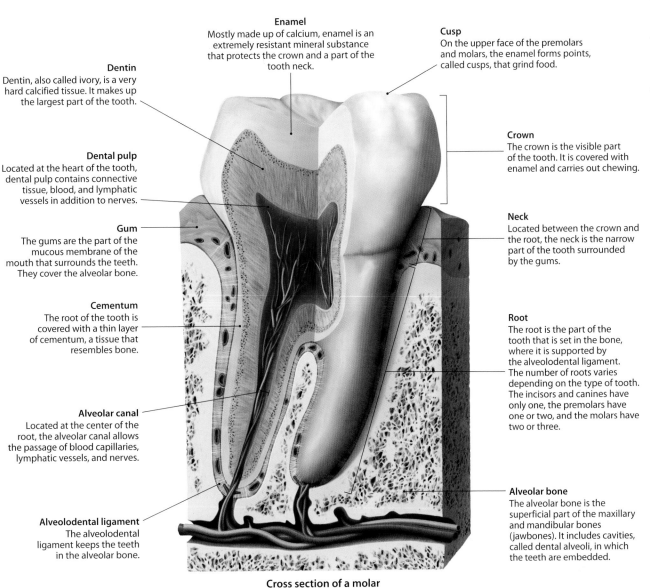

Enamel
Mostly made up of calcium, enamel is an extremely resistant mineral substance that protects the crown and a part of the tooth neck.

Cusp
On the upper face of the premolars and molars, the enamel forms points, called cusps, that grind food.

Dentin
Dentin, also called ivory, is a very hard calcified tissue. It makes up the largest part of the tooth.

Crown
The crown is the visible part of the tooth. It is covered with enamel and carries out chewing.

Dental pulp
Located at the heart of the tooth, dental pulp contains connective tissue, blood, and lymphatic vessels in addition to nerves.

Neck
Located between the crown and the root, the neck is the narrow part of the tooth surrounded by the gums.

Gum
The gums are the part of the mucous membrane of the mouth that surrounds the teeth. They cover the alveolar bone.

Cementum
The root of the tooth is covered with a thin layer of cementum, a tissue that resembles bone.

Root
The root is the part of the tooth that is set in the bone, where it is supported by the alveolodental ligament. The number of roots varies depending on the type of tooth. The incisors and canines have only one, the premolars have one or two, and the molars have two or three.

Alveolar canal
Located at the center of the root, the alveolar canal allows the passage of blood capillaries, lymphatic vessels, and nerves.

Alveolodental ligament
The alveolodental ligament keeps the teeth in the alveolar bone.

Alveolar bone
The alveolar bone is the superficial part of the maxillary and mandibular bones (jawbones). It includes cavities, called dental alveoli, in which the teeth are embedded.

Cross section of a molar

EXTREME RIGIDITY

The layer of enamel that covers the teeth is the hardest structure of the human body. Dentin is less so, but it is almost as hard as a bone.

THE **DIGESTIVE TRACT**

Made up of the esophagus, stomach, and intestines, the digestive tract is responsible for food transit and digestion. These hollow organs succeed one another and form a conduit of approximately 26 feet (8 meters) in length that links the pharynx to the anus. The mucous membrane that covers the internal wall of the digestive tract produces digestive juice and mucus, and absorbs nutrients. It rests on a muscular layer, the involuntary contractions of which allow the progression of food. Residual matter is eliminated through the anus.

ESOPHAGUS

The esophagus is a conduit that is approximately 10 inches (25 cm) long and 1 inch (2.5 cm) in diameter. It propels the bolus to the stomach in four to eight seconds, through involuntary contractions of its wall (peristalsis). The esophagus is closed at its two ends by two ring-shaped muscles, the esophageal sphincters.

ERUCTATION

A meal that is consumed too quickly, the consumption of carbonated soft drinks, or repeated swallowing may be accompanied by a significant ingestion of air. The excessive presence of gas in the stomach leads to a sensation of bloating and may be expelled through the mouth. This is eructation, or burping. The sound emitted from the burp is caused by the vibration of the cardia when the gas passes from the stomach to the esophagus.

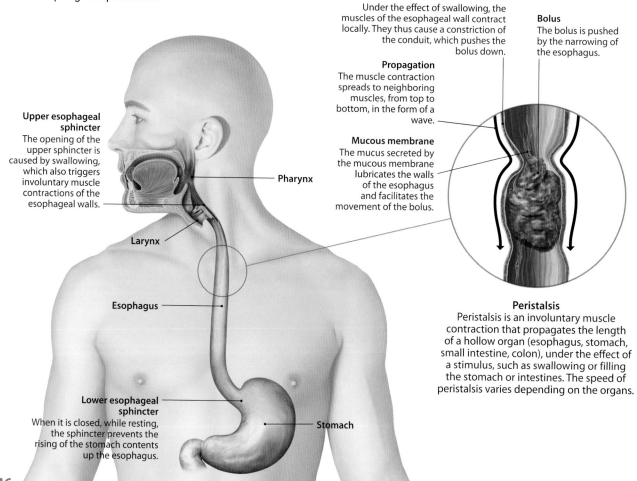

Muscle
Under the effect of swallowing, the muscles of the esophageal wall contract locally. They thus cause a constriction of the conduit, which pushes the bolus down.

Bolus
The bolus is pushed by the narrowing of the esophagus.

Propagation
The muscle contraction spreads to neighboring muscles, from top to bottom, in the form of a wave.

Mucous membrane
The mucus secreted by the mucous membrane lubricates the walls of the esophagus and facilitates the movement of the bolus.

Upper esophageal sphincter
The opening of the upper sphincter is caused by swallowing, which also triggers involuntary muscle contractions of the esophageal walls.

Pharynx

Larynx

Esophagus

Peristalsis
Peristalsis is an involuntary muscle contraction that propagates the length of a hollow organ (esophagus, stomach, small intestine, colon), under the effect of a stimulus, such as swallowing or filling the stomach or intestines. The speed of peristalsis varies depending on the organs.

Lower esophageal sphincter
When it is closed, while resting, the sphincter prevents the rising of the stomach contents up the esophagus.

Stomach

STOMACH

The stomach forms an expandable pocket that transforms food, once it has passed through the esophagus, into a thick fluid mass, called chyme. This transformation, which lasts three to four hours, is completed by abundant secretions of gastric juice (chemical digestion) and the continuous kneading of food by the involuntary contractions of the stomach walls (mechanical digestion). While it is forming, the chyme is expelled into the duodenum, where it is mixed with bile and pancreatic juice to complete chemical digestion.

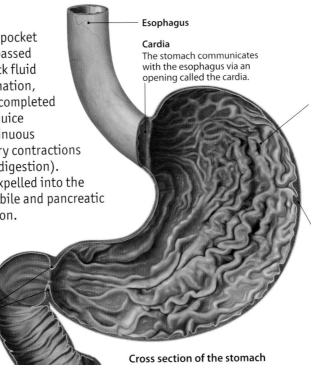

Esophagus

Cardia
The stomach communicates with the esophagus via an opening called the cardia.

Gastric mucous membrane
Heavily folded, the gastric mucous membrane covers the internal surface of the stomach. The thick mucus that it secretes forms a protective barrier against the gastric juice. Extremely acidic, this can in fact cause an inflammation or lesion to the mucous membrane.

Stomach wall
The regular muscle contractions of the stomach wall spread downward and vigorously mix the food with the gastric juice, which contributes to transforming it into chyme.

Pyloric sphincter
The pyloric sphincter closes the lower opening of the stomach. Its repetitive relaxation, under the effect of stomach contractions, lets small quantities of chyme pass into the duodenum.

Duodenum
The duodenum is the first section of the small intestine.

Cross section of the stomach

GASTRIC JUICE

Gastric juice is an acidic liquid produced by the gastric mucous membrane. It particularly contributes to the digestion of food in the stomach by breaking down proteins and carbohydrates. In some conditions, gastric juice can damage the mucous membrane of the stomach or duodenum (gastroduodenal ulcer) or climb the esophagus (gastroesophageal reflux).

Crypt
Numerous creases in the gastric mucous membrane form deep cavities, or crypts.

Surface of the gastric mucous membrane

Gastric mucous membrane

Gastric gland
Located at the bottom of the crypts, small gastric glands produce gastric juice.

AN ELASTIC ORGAN

An empty stomach has an approximate volume of 17 ounces (0.5 liter), but its maximum capacity can reach 135 ounces (4 liters) after a meal.

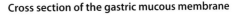

Cross section of the gastric mucous membrane

THE **INTESTINES**

The intestines are made up of the small intestine and the large intestine. The bulk of digestion takes place in this long conduit due to the secretions from the liver, pancreas, and biliary vesicle, and the bacteria of the intestinal flora. The intestines are also responsible for the absorption of nutrients and the elimination of fecal matter. The progression of the intestinal contents lasts on average 24–48 hours, but it may be influenced by different factors: food, stress, sedentary lifestyle, disease, etc.

The liver and pancreas... page 350

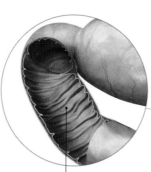

Duodenum
The first segment of the small intestine, the duodenum, accommodates bile and pancreatic juices, which complete the chemical digestion of the chyme. It also produces secretions that neutralize the acidity of the gastric juices.

Large intestine
Made up of the cecum, colon, and rectum, the large intestine connects the small intestine to the anus.

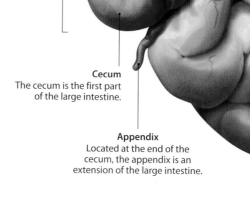

FECAL MATTER

Fecal matter (or stool), the product of elements that are not or cannot be assimilated by the body, is eliminated through the anus during defecation. It is composed of approximately 80% water, 15% dehydrated residues such as vegetal fibers, bacteria from the intestinal flora, and dead cells from the digestive tract. Its brown color comes from bile, while its odor is due to the fermentation gas produced by the intestinal flora. An adult normally excretes ¼–½ pound (100–200 g) of stool per day.

Cecum
The cecum is the first part of the large intestine.

Appendix
Located at the end of the cecum, the appendix is an extension of the large intestine.

CONSTIPATION

Constipation is the difficulty in eliminating fecal matter. It results in dehydrated stools that are hard and less frequent. Constipation is often associated with a slowing of intestinal peristalsis, a diet low in fiber or a lack of physical exercise. It is generally benign and temporary.

Rectum
The rectum is the last section of the large intestine and allows defecation. The arrival of fecal matter in the rectum triggers the defecation reflex.

Anus
The anus is the last opening of the digestive tract, through which fecal matter is eliminated. It is closed by two circular muscles, the anal sphincters. The external sphincter, the relaxation of which is voluntary, allows defecation to be delayed.

Stomach
The stomach begins the digestive process of food and prepares it for its transit in the intestines.

Colon
Approximately 5 feet (1.5 meters) long with a diameter of 2.75 inches (7 cm), the colon is the middle section of the large intestine. It absorbs water and minerals. Due to the intestinal flora, the colon also completes the breakdown of the intestinal contents, which transforms it into fecal matter. Finally, it eliminates the fecal matter by making it progress towards the rectum by involuntary contractions of its wall.

Small intestine
The small intestine, which attaches the stomach to the large intestine, measures approximately 23 feet (7 meters) in length and 1–1½ inches (2–4 cm) in diameter. Due to the numerous creases and folds of its internal mucous membrane, the small intestine absorbs the majority of nutrients, as well as a lot of water and mineral salts. Its mucous membrane also produces intestinal juice, a liquid mostly made up of mucus and water, which facilitates the dissolution and absorption of nutrients.

Fold
The mucous membrane of the small intestine forms large folds covered with villi that increase the surface of absorption.

Intestinal villus
Due to the vessels that irrigate each intestinal villus, the nutrients absorbed pass into the blood circulation, which leads them to the liver, where they are filtered.

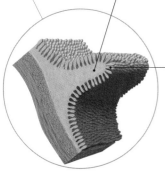

Cross section of the intestinal mucous membrane

INTESTINAL FLORA

Billions of bacteria live in the intestines, particularly in the large intestine, and make up the intestinal flora. These beneficial bacteria break down food that was not digested by the digestive juices and produce certain crucial substances, like Vitamin K. They also prevent the development of pathogenic microorganisms and stimulate natural immunity against infections. Supplied by food, these bacteria colonize the intestines rapidly after birth. Any event that disturbs the balance of the intestinal flora, like taking antibiotics or gastroenteritis, may cause diarrhea or the development of infectious agents.

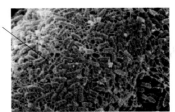

Bacterium

View of intestinal flora through an electronic microscope

INTESTINAL GASES

Mostly made up of hydrogen and methane, intestinal gases (or flatulence) come from the fermentation of food by the intestinal flora. They also contain, in lower quantities, air ingested with food. Intestinal gases escape through the anus (flatulence). The proportion of each gas and the quantity emitted (0.5–1.5 liters per day) varies depending on the individual and diet.

A MASS COLONIZATION

There are approximately 10 times more bacteria in the large intestine than there are cells of the human body! Among these several 100,000 billion bacteria, there are hundreds of different species, the majority of which survive in the absence of oxygen.

THE **LIVER** AND **PANCREAS**

Without the assistance of the liver, pancreas, and biliary vesicle, the digestive tract would not be able to fully carry out the digestion of food. These adjoining organs secrete or store numerous digestive substances, then discharge them in the first segment of the small intestine, the duodenum.

LIVER

A voluminous gland located in the upper right area of the abdomen, the liver plays an important role in digestion and metabolism. It processes the blood filled with nutrients coming from the intestines and uses a part of them to produce bile, cholesterol, and numerous proteins from blood plasma. Other substances are stored there, like vitamins, iron, and glycogen, a type of glucose (sugar) reserve. Additionally, the liver destroys the toxic substances (including alcohol), bacteria and damaged cells circulating in the blood.

Right lobe

Liver
Made up of two lobes, the liver contains a dense network of blood capillaries, which give it its reddish color. Every minute, it receives 50 ounces (1.5 liters) of blood mainly coming from the digestive tract. After having been filtered by the liver, the blood is sent to the heart.

Left lobe

Biliary vesicle
The biliary vesicle is a small pocket lodged under the liver that stores and excretes bile. It collects the bile produced by the liver, concentrates it while reabsorbing part of its water, and excretes it in the duodenum during digestion.

Hepatic portal vein
The hepatic portal vein leads blood to the liver from the intestines, stomach, pancreas, and spleen.

BILE

Bile is a yellow-green fluid produced by the liver and is mainly made up of water and biliary salts. Bile is stored by the biliary vesicle then excreted in the duodenum, where it mixes with the chyme coming from the stomach. It plays an important role in digestion by participating in the breakdown of lipids (fats) and decreasing the acidity of the chyme.

PANCREAS

The pancreas is a long gland, located behind the stomach. It produces pancreatic juice, a digestive fluid released in the duodenum that completes the chemical breakdown of food into nutrients (carbohydrates, lipids, amino acids) that can be absorbed by the small intestine. The pancreas also secretes two hormones (insulin and glucagon) that control glycemia, meaning the level of glucose in the blood.

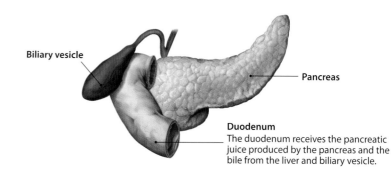

Biliary vesicle

Pancreas

Duodenum
The duodenum receives the pancreatic juice produced by the pancreas and the bile from the liver and biliary vesicle.

METABOLISM

Metabolism is the collection of biochemical reactions that occur in the cells and ensure the functioning of the body. It uses the nutrients provided during digestion and the oxygen supplied by respiration. Depending on the needs of the body, metabolism provides energy or develops living material that makes up the cells, and particularly promotes the growth, renewal, and repair of tissue.

The respiratory system... page 310

BREAKDOWN OF COMPLEX MOLECULES

During digestion, the complex molecules supplied by food are broken down by enzymes contained in the different digestive juices. The resulting simpler molecules, the nutrients, are absorbed by the intestinal mucous membrane and are passed into the blood, which allows them to reach all of the cells of the body. The nutrients provide energy or promote the synthesis of cell constituents. They may also be stored in the adipose tissues (fatty tissues), liver, or muscles.

ENZYMES
Enzymes are protein molecules that accelerate the biochemical reactions of the body. The digestive enzymes, which help break down large molecules of food, are produced by the salivary glands, stomach, pancreas, liver, and small intestine.

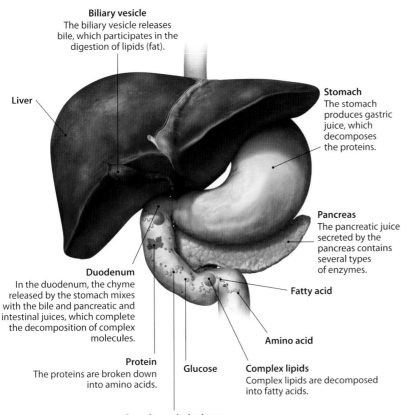

Biliary vesicle
The biliary vesicle releases bile, which participates in the digestion of lipids (fat).

Liver

Stomach
The stomach produces gastric juice, which decomposes the proteins.

Pancreas
The pancreatic juice secreted by the pancreas contains several types of enzymes.

Duodenum
In the duodenum, the chyme released by the stomach mixes with the bile and pancreatic and intestinal juices, which complete the decomposition of complex molecules.

Fatty acid

Amino acid

Protein
The proteins are broken down into amino acids.

Glucose

Complex lipids
Complex lipids are decomposed into fatty acids.

Complex carbohydrates
Complex carbohydrates, such as starch from bread or lactose from milk, are decomposed into glucose molecules (simple carbohydrates) that make up the main source of energy for the body.

ENERGY CONSUMPTION
The body consumes energy in three main ways. The basal metabolic rate, which ensures the vital functions while resting (breathing, blood circulation, basic organ activity), uses approximately 60% of the energy. The maintenance of body temperature consumes approximately 10% of the energy. Physical activity represents 15%–30% of energy consumption, depending on lifestyle. Energy consumption related to basal metabolism is more elevated in men than in women and has the tendency to decrease with age.

HEALTH OF THE DIGESTIVE SYSTEM

Diet and lifestyle have a considerable impact on the health of the digestive system and the body as a whole. Here is some advice that can help prevent certain diseases and bothersome digestive problems like constipation, diarrhea, and bloating.

PREVENTING DIGESTIVE DISORDERS

■ EAT IN A HEALTHY AND BALANCED MANNER

A healthy and balanced diet contributes to preventing obesity, nutritional deficiencies, and numerous diseases of the digestive system. It is particularly important during childhood and adolescence and during pregnancy, because these periods of life require a more significant and complete dietary supply.

Nutrition... page 11

■ OPT FOR FOOD RICH IN FIBER

Dietary fiber is found in abundance in vegetables, fruits, whole grain cereal products, and legumes. Fiber facilitates the displacement and expulsion of fecal matter by increasing its volume and softening it due to the water it retains. Consuming dietary fiber diminishes the risk of certain digestive tract problems such as hemorrhoids, anal fissure, diverticulitis, colorectal cancer, intestinal obstruction, and irritable bowel syndrome.

■ CONSUME PROBIOTICS

Probiotics are the bacteria and yeasts added to foods such as certain yogurts or juices. Consumed in sufficient quantity, they have a beneficial effect on health, particularly on the digestive system. By completing the intestinal flora, they stimulate the immune system, aid digestion, and prevent or cure digestive problems, such as diarrhea caused by antibiotics. The consumption of probiotics may also help to treat irritable bowel syndrome, constipation, ulcerative colitis, and Crohn's disease, but more studies are necessary to confirm these benefits.

■ RECOGNIZE CONSTIPATING OR LAXATIVE FOODS

When constipated, consume dietary fiber (whole grain cereal products, legumes, etc.), but also be sure to drink a lot: to fulfill its laxative function, fiber must be hydrated. Choose water, but also opt for juice, milk, or soybean drinks, which are both hydrating and nutritious. Also consume fruits and vegetables (preferably with the peel), which contain both water and fiber. If you are affected by diarrhea, regardless of the cause (virus, irritation, etc.), let your intestines rest for a day or two by avoiding spicy, fatty, or sugary foods or foods rich in fiber, and by drinking a lot. Stay away from sugary or carbonated drinks. Gradually return to your normal diet.

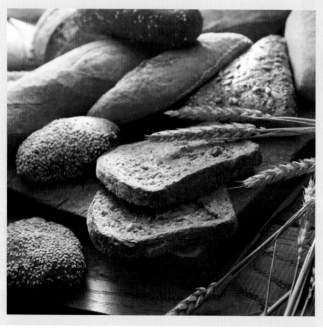

PREVENTING DIGESTIVE PROBLEMS

■ PREVENTING STOMACHACHES AND BLOATING

An excessive presence of gas in the intestine leads to a sense of bloating, heaviness, and discomfort. To prevent such bloating, facilitate the work of your colon by chewing well and slowly, by consuming small meals separated by snacks, and by not chewing gum. You can also diminish your consumption of certain foods that naturally produce (by fermentation) more gas than average: raw or dried fruits and vegetables, legumes, whole cereals, cabbage, broccoli, dairy products, alcohol, and starches. Additionally, you can replace fatty dishes with a lean meat version that is grilled, steamed, or boiled, making it easier to digest. Finally, generally avoid carbonated soft drinks as well as dishes that are high in carbohydrates.

■ FIGHT AGAINST STOMACH BURNING

Several factors can cause a sensation of burning in the stomach: physiological problems, stress, presence of bacterium, overconsumption of certain irritating products (tobacco, alcohol, chocolate, caffeinated or carbonated beverages, citrus, tomatoes, and spices). Reduce the consumption of these products and also avoid those that are rich in fat, since they delay digestion and promote the accumulation of gastric juices. Reduce your meal portions and avoid eating immediately before going to bed. Eat snacks between meals to regularize acid production in your stomach.

■ AVOID SMOKING

Tobacco is harmful to the health of your digestive system. It is recognized as being a risk factor for cancer of the esophagus, stomach, and pancreas. It also promotes other digestive system diseases such as esophagitis, gastroesophageal reflux, gastritis, or gastroduodenal ulcers.

Nicotine addiction... page 338

■ DRINK PLENTY OF WATER

Drink at least 50 ounces (1.5 liters) of water per day to promote your intestinal transit and avoid constipation.

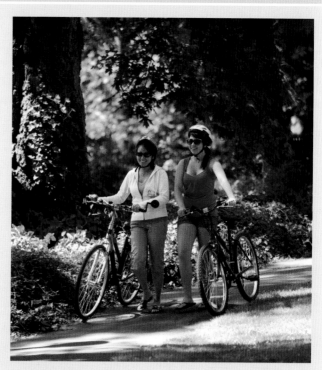

■ EXERCISE

A sedentary lifestyle promotes hemorrhoids, obesity, and numerous intestinal problems (bloating, flatulence, constipation). Exercising regularly can help you avoid these inconveniences, notably by stimulating your intestinal transit.

Exercise... page 22

■ LIMIT YOUR ALCOHOL CONSUMPTION

Alcohol is a toxic and irritating substance for the body. Its abusive and uncontrolled consumption has numerous effects on the metabolism and digestive system. An occasional high consumption will generally lead to intoxication and can be accompanied by digestive problems such as nausea and vomiting. In the long term, frequent and regular alcohol consumption can lead to serious diseases in the digestive tract (cancer of the mouth, esophagus, or stomach, gastritis, colon polyps) and liver (hepatitis, cirrhosis, liver cancer).

Alcoholism... page 358

PREVENTING DIGESTIVE PROBLEMS

■ RELAX

Stress promotes several digestive system problems such as constipation, gastroduodenal ulcers, irritable bowel syndrome, and intestinal obstruction. Relax and eat slowly, taking your time to chew food to facilitate digestion.

Stress control... page 28

■ PROTECT YOUR DIGESTIVE SYSTEM AGAINST INFECTIONS

An infection of your intestines by parasites, bacteria, or viruses can be avoided by observing some basic rules:

- Wash your hands before handling food and clean cooking utensils completely.

- Thoroughly cook meats and wash fruits and vegetables with drinking water.

- Avoid contact between food and utensils (or surfaces) that were used to prepare meat.

- When you vacation in an at-risk country, drink bottled or treated water.

- Pay attention to conserving your food and correctly sterilize your homemade preserves.

- You can be vaccinated against hepatitis B and C.

Hygiene and the prevention of infections... page 30

■ GO TO THE BATHROOM REGULARLY

Try to be regular and avoid delaying defecation. These precautions promote the proper functioning of the digestive system and help to prevent certain diseases, such as hemorrhoids.

■ GET REGULAR MEDICAL CHECKUPS

The incidence of some diseases of the digestive system, such as colon polyps and colorectal cancer, increases with age. People over 50 years of age should get regular medical checkups to detect these diseases early.

■ AVOID OVERMEDICATION

Taken intensively, some medications cause intestinal problems. This is the case with nonsteroidal anti-inflammatories, analgesics, antibiotics, and immunosuppressants, which can promote gastroduodenal ulcers, liver cirrhosis, gastroenteritis, and colitis.

■ PROTECT YOURSELF DURING SEXUAL RELATIONS

Some forms of hepatitis, particularly hepatitis B, are transmitted sexually. Use a condom during sexual relations.

Sexually transmitted diseases... page 444

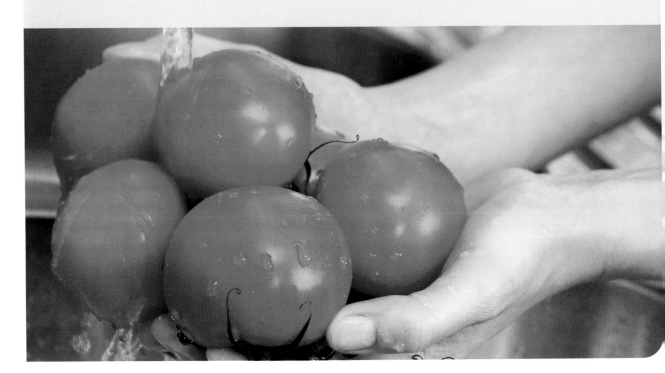

OBESITY

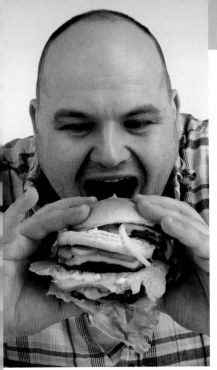

Obesity is the excessive development of adipose tissues, which results in significant weight gain. There are multiple causes: eating disorders, poor nutritional balance, hormonal problems, **genetic** predisposition, stress, and a sedentary lifestyle. This health problem mainly affects industrialized countries, but it progresses in all countries, affecting all age groups. The World Health Organization estimates that, in 2015, the global population will have 400 million obese adults. Obesity presents several degrees of severity and different aspects, depending on the distribution of fat in the body. It is often defined by the value of the body mass index (BMI).

ADIPOSE TISSUES

Adipose tissues comprise 18%–25% of the female body, compared to only 10%–15% in the male body. This difference resides in the fact that in women, adipose tissues constitute an essential reserve of energy during pregnancy and breast-feeding. Crucial to the functioning of the body, the adipose tissues are an important source of energy and heat. They are made up of specialized cells, called fat cells, that store fat. Before birth and during childhood, the number of fat cells increases to reach 20 billion. From the age of 15, the volume of existing fat cells may be multiplied up to 50 times due to an excess in caloric supply. The fats are often located under the skin, but there are deeper fats that encircle the organs, particularly those of the abdominal cavity.

BODY MASS INDEX

The body mass index (BMI) estimates the quantity of adipose tissues in the body and assesses the associated health risks for excess weight in people between the ages of 18 and 65 (with some exceptions). It is calculated by dividing the weight in kilograms (1 kg = 2.2 lbs), by the squared height in meters (1 m = 3.28 ft). A BMI between 18.5 and 25 indicates that the individual's weight has no effect on his health. This is therefore a "healthy weight." As the BMI distances from this interval, weight becomes a health risk factor of increasing importance.

Healthy weight... page 20

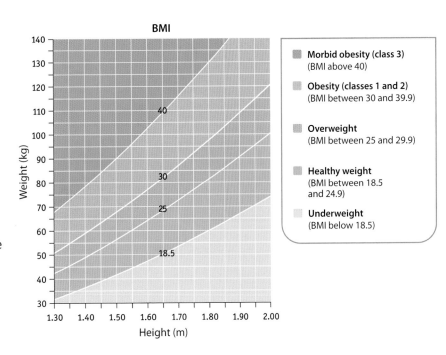

BMI

- Morbid obesity (class 3) (BMI above 40)
- Obesity (classes 1 and 2) (BMI between 30 and 39.9)
- Overweight (BMI between 25 and 29.9)
- Healthy weight (BMI between 18.5 and 24.9)
- Underweight (BMI below 18.5)

STEATOMERY

Steatomery is the formation of localized adipose tissues deep under the skin and in certain regions of the body. On the hips and thighs, this accumulation of fat is better known as saddlebags. Accumulations of adipose tissues may also be located behind the arms, on the neck, on the stomach and on the inside of the knees. Of genetic origin, steatometry generally affects women over 40 years of age and, more rarely, young women. It manifests itself by a change in the figure and weight gain. In an overweight person, it can lead to arthrosis of the knees and can increase the risk of cardiovascular disease.

CELLULITE

Cellulite is the development of adipose tissues in certain regions of the body, most often in the thighs, buttocks, stomach, and arms, which results in the alteration of the skin known as "cottage cheese." It affects, in varying degrees, 90% of women and approximately 2% of men. Cellulite is due in large part to the female hormone estrogen, which stimulates the formation of piles of adipose tissues in the connective tissues located under the skin. It begins during puberty and its development can be accelerated by pregnancy, menopause, and certain estrogen-based medications. Several other factors, such as heredity, poor blood circulation in the legs, an overly rich diet, or a sedentary lifestyle, influence the formation of cellulite.

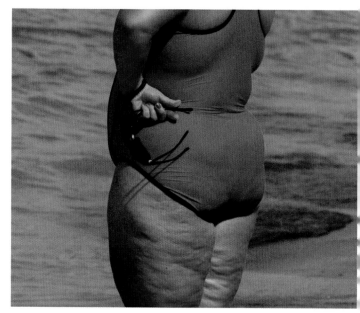

Cottage cheese
The irregular aspect given to the skin by cellulite is due to the growth of piles of adipose tissues.

TYPES OF OBESITY

Depending on the distribution of fat in the body, there are two main types of obesity, often linked to gender and hereditary factors. Gynoid obesity mainly affects women, while android obesity is most common in men.

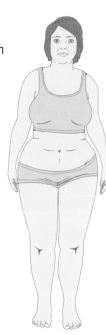

Gynoid obesity
Gynoid obesity is characterized by an accumulation of fat in the lower part of the body, particularly the hips, thighs, and buttocks.

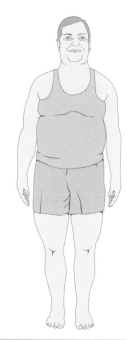

Android obesity
Android obesity, or abdominal obesity, is a excess of adipose tissue in the upper parts of the body, mainly in the stomach, trunk, and neck. This form of obesity is more subject to complications.

COMPLICATIONS OF OBESITY

The health repercussions of obesity are numerous and increase as the body mass index (BMI) rises. Obesity, particularly android obesity, increases the risk of cardiovascular diseases such as heart failure, coronary disease, arterial hypertension, and cerebral vascular accidents. Other diseases, such as type 2 diabetes and hypercholesterolemia, can also be caused by excess weight. It may also cause breathing problems such as sleep apnea or nocturnal snoring. Obesity promotes arthrosis, cholelithiasis, and some cancers such as endometrial, ovarian, colon, and prostate cancer. It may also cause sterility. In its most severe form, obesity has a huge effect on the quality of life, which is affected by respiratory difficulties, sleep problems, excessive sweating, urinary incontinence, and a reduction in mobility and autonomy. Generally, obesity reduces life expectancy.

TREATMENT OF OBESITY

Treatment of obesity varies depending on the cause. The most common approach is to follow a diet that limits caloric intake. This rests on a profound change in dietary habits and must be coupled with regular physical exercise that increases the energy consumption of the body. There are several types of diets. Adapted to each individual, the diet must be balanced and realistic in order not to lead to malnutrition or relapses. It must be monitored by a doctor and may, in certain cases, be accompanied by psychotherapy. In the most severe cases or following the failure of all other treatments, the implementation of a gastric band may be considered. This is a reversible procedure that reduces the volume of the stomach, currently more common than stomach stapling, which is permanent and more invasive.

Nutrition... page 11

OBESITY

SYMPTOMS:
Excess weight, accumulation of fat.

TREATMENT:
Diet, physical exercise, psychotherapy, liposuction, gastric band.

PREVENTION:
Balanced diet, regular physical exercise. Limiting and controling stress.

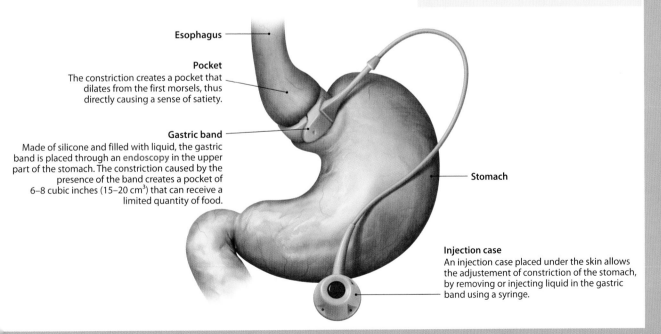

Esophagus

Pocket
The constriction creates a pocket that dilates from the first morsels, thus directly causing a sense of satiety.

Gastric band
Made of silicone and filled with liquid, the gastric band is placed through an **endoscopy** in the upper part of the stomach. The constriction caused by the presence of the band creates a pocket of 6–8 cubic inches (15–20 cm³) that can receive a limited quantity of food.

Stomach

Injection case
An injection case placed under the skin allows the adjustement of constriction of the stomach, by removing or injecting liquid in the gastric band using a syringe.

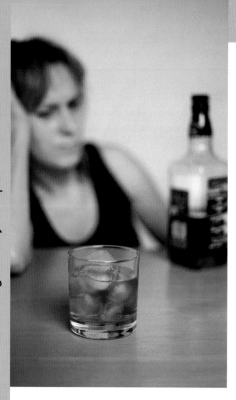

ALCOHOLISM

Alcoholism affects approximately 4% of the global population and more particularly the European population. It is characterized by a dependence (or addiction) to alcohol, which gives rise to the uncontrolled consumption of alcoholic beverages leading to **chronic** intoxication. The quantity necessary to develop an alcoholic dependence varies depending on the individual and depends on **genetic**, psychological, and social factors. Alcoholism is a significant cause of death by diseases, car accidents, suicides, and homicides. In pregnant women, chronic and excessive consumption of alcohol may lead to dangerous fetal alcoholization for the child.

Tobacco, alcohol and drugs... page 26
Fetal alcohol syndrome... page 479

ALCOHOL IN THE BLOOD

After having been completely absorbed by the stomach and small intestine, the ingested alcohol is transported by the blood to the liver, where it is partially transformed into a toxic chemical component. Alcohol being soluble in water and in fats, the portion that cannot be immediately filtered by the liver is spread throughout the body, including breast milk and adipose tissues. The continuous passage of blood in the liver allows for the gradual elimination of alcohol still present in the blood circulation after a first filtering. The blood alcohol level increases proportionally to the quantity of alcohol consumed and does not start to decrease until after consumption stops. The speed of alcohol elimination is 0.1–0.3 grams per hour.

ETHYLOMETER

The ethylometer, also called the alcotest, assesses the blood alcohol level by the quantity of alcohol contained in the exhaled air. Very volatile, alcohol spreads easily in the blood towards the alveoli of the lungs. The quantity of alcohol in the exhaled air is therefore proportional to that in the blood. It can be measured by different types of ethylometers. Some contain a chemical component that intensely changes color on contact with alcohol. A breathalyzer, more precise than the ethylometer, provides a measure of the blood alcohol content in milligrams per liter of exhaled air and in grams per liter of blood.

The lungs... page 312

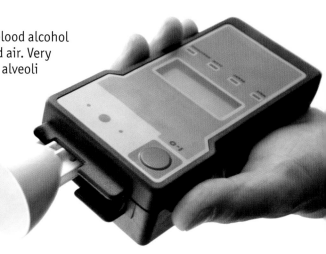

Ethylometer

THE **EFFECTS** OF **ALCOHOL**

Excessive alcohol consumption can lead to acute alcohol intoxication, characterized by a state of drunkenness. Starting around 30 minutes after the ingestion of alcoholic beverages, it generally manifests itself starting at a blood alcohol level of 0.5 grams per liter (g/L). Its effects increase with the blood alcohol level and may be accompanied by nausea and vomiting. A blood alcohol level higher than 3 g/L generally leads to a coma, and to death beyond 6 g/L. The drunk individual presents psychomotor problems such as slowing of the reflexes or difficulty speaking. The effects of alcohol can also lead to the narrowing of the visual field, a slowing of the heart rate, stomach burning, a loss of heat through the skin, and dehydration. Regular, frequent, and abundant alcohol consumption leads to chronic alcohol intoxication, characterized by the development of a dependence on alcohol (alcoholism) and a higher tolerance to its effects. On average and in the long term, alcohol has numerous effects on the metabolism and causes different damage, sometimes irreversible, to various organs.

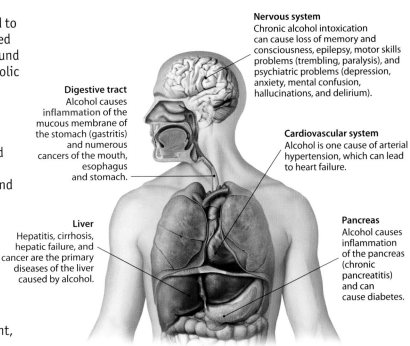

Nervous system
Chronic alcohol intoxication can cause loss of memory and consciousness, epilepsy, motor skills problems (trembling, paralysis), and psychiatric problems (depression, anxiety, mental confusion, hallucinations, and delirium).

Digestive tract
Alcohol causes inflammation of the mucous membrane of the stomach (gastritis) and numerous cancers of the mouth, esophagus and stomach.

Cardiovascular system
Alcohol is one cause of arterial hypertension, which can lead to heart failure.

Liver
Hepatitis, cirrhosis, hepatic failure, and cancer are the primary diseases of the liver caused by alcohol.

Pancreas
Alcohol causes inflammation of the pancreas (chronic pancreatitis) and can cause diabetes.

Effects of chronic alcohol intoxication

TREATMENT OF ALCOHOLISM

The treatment of alcoholism requires, on the part of the patient, a good understanding of the disease, a recognition of his dependence on alcohol, and the desire to overcome it. It consists in following a detoxification cure, generally completed by psychotherapy and medical support. After withdrawal, the risk of recurrence is significant. It can, however, be minimized by psychotherapy and by administering certain medications that cause discomfort during the ingestion of alcohol or prevent the sensation of pleasure that accompanies alcohol consumption.

ALCOHOLISM

SYMPTOMS:
Acute intoxication: slowing of reflexes, reduction of inhibitions, change of mood, difficulty speaking, decrease in motor coordination, loss of balance, nausea, vomiting, dehydration, hypothermia. Chronic intoxication: epilepsy, trembling, paralysis, mental confusion, hallucinations, delirium.

TREATMENT:
Detoxification cure (withdrawal, psychotherapy, medical support, medication).

PREVENTION:
In the absence of dependence: limiting alcohol consumption. In the case of dependence: early diagnosis must be made to treat the disease quickly.

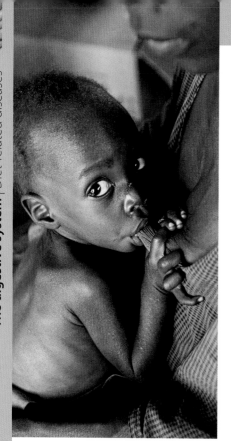

NUTRITIONAL DEFICIENCIES

Nutritional deficiencies are conditions characterized by the lack or absence of one or several substances supplied by food and necessary for the proper functioning of the body. Lack of food, in the case of famine, for example and, more rarely, diseases (**anorexia**, dietary intolerances, etc.), lead to an insufficient supply of food and can lead to a general nutritional deficiency (undernourishment or undernutrition). Malnutrition is a pathological condition caused by the lack of one or several nutrients, whether it is minerals, trace elements, or vitamins. Regardless of origin, nutritional deficiencies have serious and sometimes irreversible consequences on the development of children and can lead to a number of health problems for all ages.

Nutrition… page 11

CONSEQUENCES OF UNDERNOURISHMENT

Undernourishment is accompanied by a permanent sensation of hunger and thirst, muscle weakness, and fatigue. It leads to hypoglycemia, dehydration, weight loss, loss of muscle mass, and death if it is prolonged. Even if temporary, undernourishment is particularly serious for a fetus, newborns, and children because it harms their development and can lead to physical and mental deficiencies.

DISEASES RELATED TO MALNUTRITION

Malnutrition leads to diseases depending on each deficiency: scurvy (Vitamin C), hyperthyroidism (iodine), rachitis and osteomalacia (Vitamin D), xerophtalmia (Vitamin A), beriberi (Vitamin B1), pellagra (Vitamin B3), kwashiorkor (proteins), etc. In most cases, the reintroduction of the missing substances in the diet reverses its effects. But, in the absence of treatment, malnutrition can lead to death.

Thyroid gland diseases… page 225
Skeletal deformities… page 525

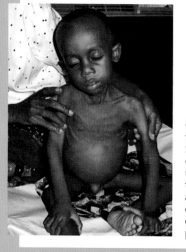

Child suffering from undernourishment
Swelling of the abdomen is characteristic of a state of advanced undernourishment. It is due to two phenomena: weakening of abdominal muscles and the leakage of blood plasma in the abdominal cavity due to the decrease in protein levels in the blood.

A PLAGUE

More than 800 million people in the world, particularly in developing countries, are undernourished, and more than 25,000 die of it every day. Malnutrition affects more than half of the global population.

SCURVY

Scurvy is a disease resulting from a Vitamin C deficiency. It manifests itself after one to three months of the deficiency, through an inflammation of the gums, bleeding (gums, skin, nose), anemia, and weakness. The appearance of these symptoms is accompanied by an elevated risk of heart failure. In children, a Vitamin C deficiency also causes pain in the limbs and increases the risk of sudden death.

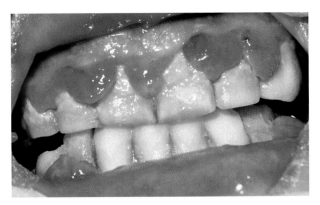

Scurvy

KWASHIORKOR

Kwashiorkor occurs in children after a sudden withdrawal of breast-feeding, necessitated by, for example, the birth of a newborn. It affects children in developing countries, mainly in tropical Africa. Kwashiorkor results from a diet that is very low in proteins. It leads to black skin lesions and a characteristic swelling of the abdomen. It can also cause diarrhea, weight loss, anemia, growth delay, and psychological and mental problems.

XEROPHTALMIA

Xerophtalmia is a disease caused by a Vitamin A deficiency that especially affects children in developing countries. It is characterized by eye dryness, which persists by the appearance of opaque spots on the cornea. These lesions can spread and lead to the destruction or perforation of the cornea. In the absence of treatment, xerophtalmia leads to blindness.

BERIBERI

Beriberi is caused by a Vitamin B1 deficiency. In developing countries, it is promoted by a refined rice-based diet in which the pericarp, or external covering, rich in Vitamin B1 is extracted. It manifests itself by different symptoms: weakness, weight loss, anorexia, constipation, sensitivity problems, muscular atrophy, etc. The disease can then cause impairments on the nerves, heart, or brain.

PELLAGRA

Pellagra is a rare disease caused by a Vitamin B3 (or niacin) deficiency, characteristic of a diet that is low in animal proteins. It is most common in developing countries with undernourishment problems and those where the base food is corn (Central America, South America). Pellagra results in the formation of darker or red defined spots on the areas of skin exposed to the sun. It also causes diarrhea, abdominal pain, and neurological problems such as anxiety, insomnia, or memory loss, which can develop into dementia.

NUTRITIONAL DEFICIENCIES

SYMPTOMS:
Variable depending on deficiency. Symptoms are often reversible when they are treated in a timely manner.

TREATMENT:
Introduction of the missing element into the diet, first in a significant quantity (oral or intravenously), then through a balanced diet.

PREVENTION:
Diversified, sufficient, regular diet.

DIETARY INTOLERANCES

A dietary intolerance is the digestive tract's inability to digest certain foods. Lactose and gluten intolerances are among the most common, even though their significance varies greatly depending on the population and ethnic groups.

LACTOSE INTOLERANCE

Lactose is the main carbohydrate in milk and is only present in dairy products. Lactose intolerance is a common disease that affects approximately three-quarters of adults in the world. It is caused by the absence or deficiency of an enzyme of the small intestine, lactase, which allows the digestion of lactose. Naturally present in all children, lactase decreases or disappears at the adult age in certain people and populations, particularly in Asia, Africa, and South America. When lactase is absent or insufficient, undigested lactose stimulates contractions of the intestine, which causes various digestion and intestinal transit problems. Treatment for lactose intolerance consists of avoiding the consumption of milk and favoring fermented dairy products such as yogurts and cheeses. There are also enzyme supplements in the form of tablets or drops to add to food containing milk or cream.

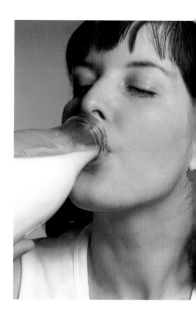

CELIAC DISEASE

Celiac disease, or gluten intolerance, is a chronic disease of the small intestine caused by a protein contained in some cereals. It is relatively common in Northern European populations. In people who are genetically predisposed, gluten causes an immune reaction that results in the inflammation, edema, and destruction of the surface of the intestinal mucous membrane, which reduces its absorption capacity. In addition to digestive problems, poor absorption of nutrients can lead to weight loss, various nutritional deficiencies, and growth and puberty delays in children.

The immune system... page 278

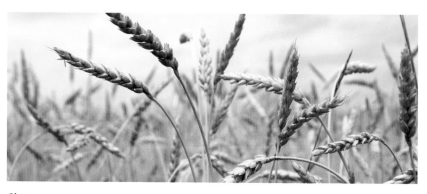

Gluten
Gluten is a protein present in the grains of some cereals containing wheat, rye, and barley. It also is included in many processed foods such as soups, bread crumbs, pasta, or sauces. Several cereals, like corn, amaranth, millet and buckwheat, do not contain gluten. The toxic character of oat for people with celiac disease is being questioned today.

DIETARY INTOLERANCES

SYMPTOMS:
Diarrhea, abdominal cramps and pain, intestinal gas, weight loss, fatigue. Celiac disease is also accompanied by problems linked to malnutrition.

TREATMENT:
Suppression of food responsible for the disease, substitution with a nutritional equivalent, if possible. Lactose intolerance: enzyme supplements.

INDIGESTION

Bloating, nausea, vomiting, and abdominal pain make up a collection of symptoms caused by difficult digestion, or indigestion. While it is most often caused by a meal that is too heavy in food or alcohol, indigestion can be the sign of a more serious problem of the digestive system or other organs, such as gastroenteritis, food poisoning, myocardial infarction, or a brain tumor.

VOMITING

Vomiting is the reflex expulsion of the stomach contents through the mouth. It is produced by the sudden contraction of the diaphragm and abdominal muscles, which constrict the stomach. The circular muscle that closes the upper opening of the esophagus, the upper esophageal sphincter, then relaxes, which lets the gastric contents flow back into the esophagus. Repeated vomiting leads to a risk of dehydration and undernutrition. In some cases, it can also lead to asphyxia. Vomiting can be eased by antispasmodic or antiemetic medications (which prevent vomiting), but the cause must be found and treated.

NAUSEA

Nausea is a disagreeable sensation that generally precedes vomiting. It can be the symptom of a disease of the digestive system, central nervous system, or inner ear. It can also occur during pregnancy or as a result of motion sickness (or travel sickness), stress, or taking medications (notably during chemotherapy), or even be caused by a disagreeable taste or odor. Once its origin is determined, it can be treated by antiemetic medications.

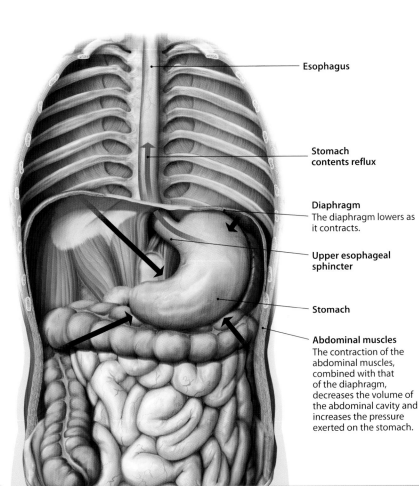

Esophagus

Stomach contents reflux

Diaphragm
The diaphragm lowers as it contracts.

Upper esophageal sphincter

Stomach

Abdominal muscles
The contraction of the abdominal muscles, combined with that of the diaphragm, decreases the volume of the abdominal cavity and increases the pressure exerted on the stomach.

INDIGESTION

SYMPTOMS:
Nausea, vomiting, abdominal pain, bloating, headaches.

TREATMENT:
Diet. Vomiting: treatment of the cause, antiemetics, antispasmodics.

PREVENTION:
Balanced diet. Avoiding excessive alcohol consumption.

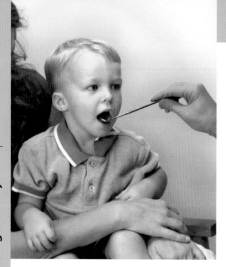

ORAL DISEASES

Diseases that affect the mouth can be caused by poor buccodental (oral) hygiene (cavities, gingivitis, periodontitis), by **infections** or lesions of the buccal mucous membrane (aphtha, thrush, glossitis), or by smoking (oral cancer). They are most often benign, but some, more severe, can limit the functioning of the mouth and interfere with nourishment, speech, and respiration.

Cavities... page 367

GINGIVITIS

The accumulation of dental plaque or tartar on the surface of the teeth can lead to an inflammation of the gums called gingivitis. Gingivitis manifests itself through the redness and swelling of the gums, and by frequent bleeding, particularly during tooth brushing. Some more rare forms of gingivitis can be caused by medication use or immunodeficiency.

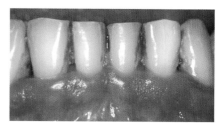

Gingivitis
The inflamed gums present a red and puffy aspect. They may cover a part of the tooth.

PERIODONTITIS

In the absence of treatment, gingivitis can spread to all of the tissues that support the teeth: gums, alveolar bone, cementum, and alveolodental ligaments. It then develops into periodontitis. The gums retract and progressively reveal the base of the teeth, leading to a pronounced mobility of the teeth, which can detach in the most serious cases. Good oral hygiene and a regular periodontal scaling treat gingivitis and prevent or stop the development of periodontitis.

Oral health... page 369

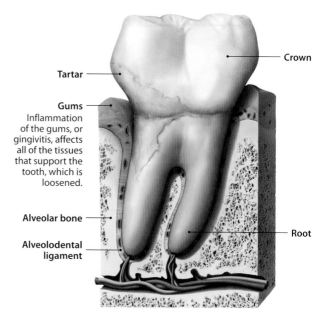

Crown

Tartar

Gums
Inflammation of the gums, or gingivitis, affects all of the tissues that support the tooth, which is loosened.

Alveolar bone

Alveolodental ligament

Root

Periodontitis

DENTAL PLAQUE

A soft and white substance, dental plaque is mainly made up of bacteria from the buccal flora, which settles continuously on the surface of the teeth and gums. In the absence of tooth brushing, it transforms into dental tartar, a hard coating that is the source of caries and gingivitis. Resistant to tooth brushing, tartar must be removed by a dentist using ultrasound or a curette (small scraping tool). The frequency of periodontal scaling varies depending on the person, but semiannual or annual exams limit its formation.

GLOSSITIS

Glossitis is an inflammation of the tongue caused most often by a burn, friction, contact with irritating substances, an infection, allergies, or even iron or vitamin deficiencies. This disease changes the aspect of part of or the entire tongue. Glossitis is generally benign, particularly migratory glossitis (or geographic tongue), especially common in children. Glossitis may be accompanied by pain and discomfort when chewing, swallowing, or speaking. Hospitalization may be necessary when it leads to a swelling of the tongue and obstruction of the pharynx (throat).

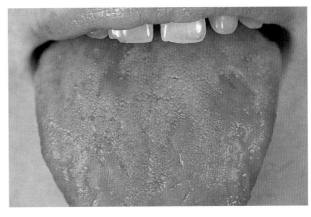

Glossitis
In glossitis, the tongue can increase in volume, its surface may become smooth, and its red coloring can soften or intensify.

THRUSH

Thrush, or buccal mycosis, is an infection in the mouth by the microscopic fungus *Candida albicans*. It causes the appearance of a white coating on the mucous membranes of the mouth, the throat, and sometimes the esophagus and may be accompanied by itching, burning, difficulty swallowing, and loss of appetite. Common and generally benign in very young children, thrush can also develop following a weakening of the immune system caused by a disease such as AIDS or diabetes, or by corticosteroids, antibiotics, or chemotherapy treatments.

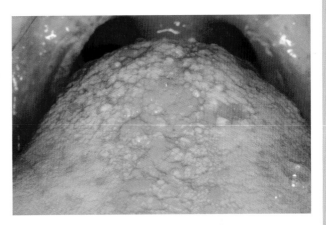

Thrush
The tongue infected with *Candida albicans* is covered with a characteristic whitish pellicle, which can also cover the internal surface of the cheeks and palate, and spread to the pharynx, larynx, and esophagus.

THRUSH IN NEWBORNS

During pregnancy, hormonal variations sometimes cause the proliferation of *Candida albicans* in the maternal vagina. The fungus can be transmitted to the child during birth. The newborn is at risk of developing thrush, which can interfere with nourishment. The fungus can also be transferred to the mother during breast-feeding, which generally causes pain in the nipples.

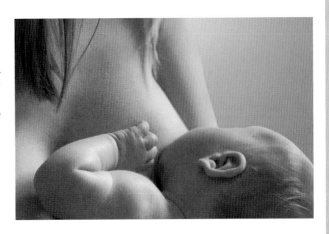

APHTHA

Aphtha is a small painful ulcer located on the mucous membrane of the mouth. It is characterized by a small yellowish spot that is round or oval, surrounded by a red halo showing an inflammation. Aphthas are most often benign and isolated lesions. They have multiple causes: trauma (rubbing from a device or dental ridge), dietary intolerance, infection, stress, fatigue, etc. They do not require any treatment and disappear spontaneously after 8–10 days. However, the eruption of multiple aphthas may be the sign of a chronic infection.

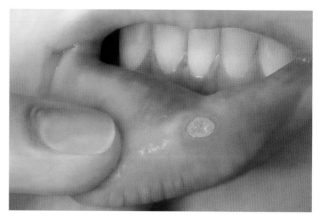

Aphtha of the mouth
Aphthas appear on the internal surface of the cheeks and lips, on the gums, or on the tongue.

MOUTH CANCER

Mouth cancer, or oral cancer, is a malignant tumor affecting one or several organs of the mouth (lips, tongue, gums, cheeks, palate, salivary glands). Often painless at onset, it can take different forms: a small wound, red or white plaque, an ulceration, or a nodule on the lip or in the neck. These lesions are aggravated over time and are accompanied by other symptoms: bleeding, persistent pain in the mouth and throat, difficulty chewing, swallowing, or moving the tongue, numbness. The alcohol-tobacco association and poor oral hygiene are significant risk factors for mouth cancer, which particularly affects men over 50 years of age. The success of its treatment depends on how early it is diagnosed.

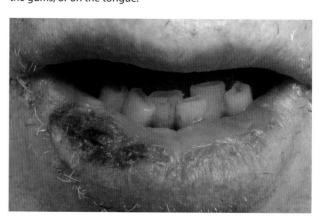

Lip cancer
The risk of developing lip cancer increases with smoking and prolonged exposure to the sun.

ORAL DISEASES

SYMPTOMS:
Inflammation, lesion, or change in aspect of the affected organ, may be accompanied by pain and change in certain functions: chewing, swallowing, phonation, breathing.

TREATMENT:
Gingivitis, periodontitis: periodontal scaling. Glossitis: corticosteroids in mouthwash and antibiotics or antifungals in the case of infectious origin. Thrush: antifungals in mouthwash. Oral cancer: surgical ablation, radiation therapy, chemotherapy when the tumors are very extended.

PREVENTION:
Oral hygiene, regular exam by a dentist (at least once a year).

Oral health… page 369

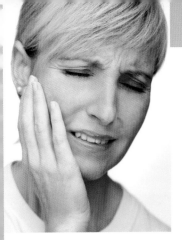

CAVITIES

Bacteria present in the dental plaque can proliferate, nourished by the sugars coming from food. While developing, they progressively destroy the different hard tissues of the tooth, forming a cavity. The significant or frequent consumption of sugar, poor oral hygiene, and the insufficient production of saliva promotes the formation of cavities. In the absence of treatment, a cavity can develop into an abscess.

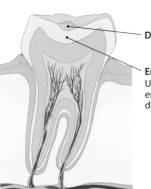

Dental plaque

Enamel
Under the effect of acids, enamel progressively disappears.

1. Breakdown of enamel
The bacteria in the dental plaque transform the sugars from food into acids, which dissolve the enamel layer of the tooth.

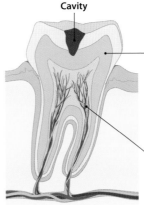

Cavity

Dentin
When the infection attacks the dentin, the progression of the cavity causes irreversible destruction of the dentin. The dentist can stop the cavity at this stage.

Nerve
With the absence of enamel to protect the dentin, the nerves of the tooth receive stimulations from the buccal cavity. The tooth thus becomes sensitive to cold, heat, pressure, and certain foods.

2. Destruction of dentin
The breakdown of the enamel creates a breach by which bacteria penetrate the tooth. The infection spreads to the dentin and destroys it.

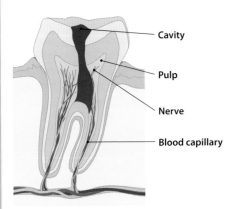

Cavity

Pulp

Nerve

Blood capillary

3. Inflammation of the pulp
The infection attacks the heavily innervated pulp and causes its inflammation. The pain is therefore intense and continuous.

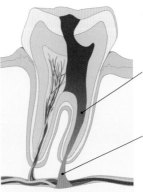

Alveolar canal

Abscess
The accumulation of pus beyond the root of the tooth creates an abscess. It manifests itself by redness and painful swelling of the gums, sometimes associated with a fever and headaches.

4. Creation of an abscess
In the absence of treatment, the infection spreads to the alveolar canal. It can lead to necrosis of the tooth and form an abscess. The infection can spread to the entire body and cause serious complications, like meningitis, endocarditis, and joint infections.

DENTAL X-RAYS
Rapid and painless, dental X-rays make visible the hard tissues of the tooth as well as any prior treatment to establish the diagnosis of a tooth or gum affliction.

TREATMENT OF A CAVITY

Drilling is the first step in treating a cavity. It consists of eliminating all of the infected tissues of the tooth with a metal drill. The cavity created is then filled with a resistant and nontoxic material, which may be an amalgam filling or composite resin. The dentist molds the filling material while respecting the shape of the tooth and then polishes it, which restores the aspect of the tooth and its function of chewing food. A treated tooth is more fragile and must be monitored carefully because new cavities can form under an old filling. When the cavity is deep, a root canal and placement of an artificial crown may be necessary.

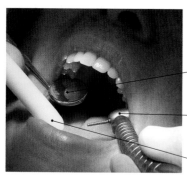

Mirror
A mirror allows the dentist to see less accessible areas of the mouth. It is also used to push aside the cheeks, lips, and tongue.

Dental drill
A drill is a small rod, the end of which is covered with diamond dust or has cutting blades. It is animated by a rapid rotating movement that allows it to dig into the tooth.

Suction tube
A suction tube eliminates saliva, rinsing liquids and debris produced during drilling that accumulate in the mouth.

Drilling

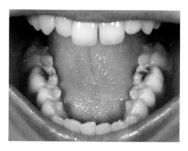

Amalgam filling
An amalgam filling, also called sealing, is a very resistant gray material made up of a mix of metals. The composite resin is a mix of organic and mineral materials.

ROOT CANAL

In the case of deep cavities, dental abscesses, or even a broken tooth, a root canal (devitalization or pulp removal) may be completed under local anesthesia. After having removed all of the pulp from the tooth, the alveolar canals are cleaned, widened, disinfected, and filled with a filling material. The upper part of the tooth is filled with an amalgam filling or composite resin. Deprived of pulp, the tooth is no longer irrigated by blood vessels and becomes more fragile. When the natural crown is very damaged, a root canal is often followed by the placement of an artificial crown. The entire treatment is painless, but it is a long and meticulous process that may be divided into multiple sessions.

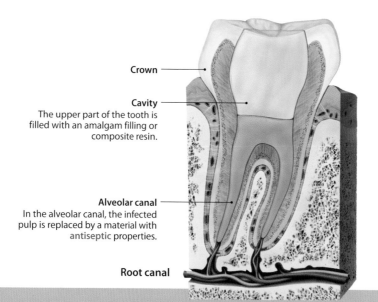

Crown

Cavity
The upper part of the tooth is filled with an amalgam filling or composite resin.

Alveolar canal
In the alveolar canal, the infected pulp is replaced by a material with antiseptic properties.

Root canal

CAVITIES

SYMPTOMS:
Localized, sometimes intense pain triggered by the cold, heat, pressure on the tooth or certain foods.
Abscess: permanent pain, swelling and redness of the gums, which may spread to the cheek.

TREATMENT:
Removal of the decayed tissues through drilling, dental filling. Significant cavity: root canal and placement of an artificial crown, if needed.
Abscess: antibiotics to control infection, analgesics to relieve pain.

PREVENTION:
Good oral hygiene. Regular tooth examination by a dentist. Limited consumption of sweets.

ORAL HEALTH

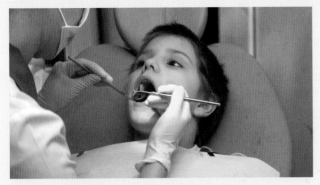

■ ADOPT PROPER ORAL HYGIENE PRACTICES

Oral hygiene consists of regularly eliminating dental plaque, which continuously forms on the teeth, by brushing and flossing. When properly practiced, this preserves the health of the teeth, gums, and mucous membranes of the mouth by preventing the appearance of cavities and infections of tissues that support the teeth (gingivitis, periodontitis). Tooth brushing must be done at least twice a day for three minutes after each meal. Dental floss must be passed daily between each tooth before brushing. Poor oral hygiene promotes the proliferation of bacteria of the buccal flora, which causes bad breath. This problem, called halitosis, can also be caused by a lack of saliva, a cold, sinusitis, or the ingestion of substances such as garlic, onion, coffee, cauliflower, tobacco, or alcohol.

■ LIMIT YOUR CONSUMPTION OF SUGARY OR ACIDIC FOOD AND BEVERAGES

Certain processed foods and certain drinks (soda, fruit juice) contain large quantities of simple carbohydrates such as sucrose, glucose, and fructose, which promote the formation of cavities. Choose food and drinks without added refined sugars. Food that is high in acid (sports drinks, carbonated drinks, coffee, wine, etc.) causes erosion of the dental enamel, which can lead to the appearance of cavities, discoloration, and tooth pain. Therefore, avoid sipping acidic drinks for long periods of time and limit the time the acid is in contact with your teeth. Do not brush your teeth immediately after having consumed acidic drinks; instead, rinse your mouth by drinking water, milk, or a soybean beverage in order to avoid damaging the weakened enamel.

Nutrition... page 11

■ HAVE YOUR TEETH EXAMINED REGULARLY BY A DENTIST

Depending on the individual, annual or semiannual cleanings and exams at a dental clinic prevent the development of cavities and tartar accumulation.

■ AVOID SMOKING

The active consumption of tobacco promotes the development of cavities, periodontitis, and mouth cancer.

Nicotine addiction... page 338

■ TAKE CARE OF YOUR CHILDREN'S HEALTH

• To avoid the appearance of cavities, limit your children's consumption of sugary foods, particularly before bed. Also avoid giving them a bottle of milk or fruit juice just before they fall asleep.

• Your child's first teeth can be wiped with a damp cloth. Later on, use a small soft children's toothbrush and toothpaste to clean your child's teeth twice a day. Progressively teach your child to do it himself.

• Take your child to the dentist after the eruption of his first tooth and regularly thereafter.

• To prevent misalignment of the teeth, discourage prolonged thumb sucking.

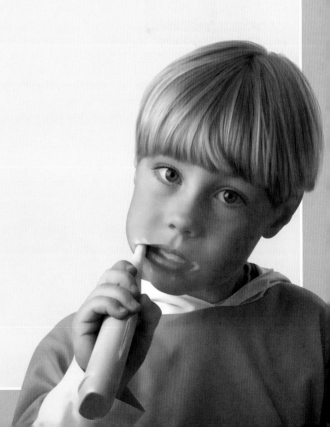

DENTAL PROSTHESES

A dental **prosthesis** is a fixed or removable device, designed to replace one or several teeth. It improves chewing and particularly prevents periodontitis of the teeth and problems affecting jaw articulation. A dental prosthesis also plays an aesthetic and psychological role by restoring the aspect of normal teeth.

ARTIFICIAL CROWN

When a natural crown is very damaged or following a root canal, an artificial crown is normally implanted to protect the rest of the tooth against further damage. Artificial crowns can be composed of a metal alloy, ceramic or ceramic-covered metal.

BRIDGE

A bridge (or fixed bridgework) replaces one or several missing teeth by resting on the neighboring teeth. It is made of only one piece including the artificial tooth or teeth and their fastening device.

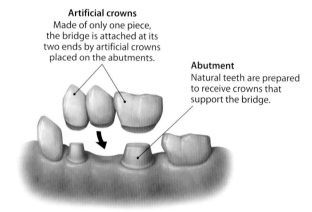

Artificial crowns
Made of only one piece, the bridge is attached at its two ends by artificial crowns placed on the abutments.

Abutment
Natural teeth are prepared to receive crowns that support the bridge.

Bridge

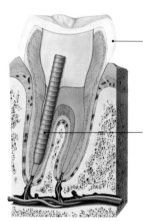

Artificial crown
The color of the ceramic crown is adjusted to the natural color of the tooth.

Dental pivot
Some artificial crowns are supported by a rod implanted in the root of the tooth.

DENTURES

A denture is a removable dental prosthesis that serves to replace several or all of the teeth. Wearing dentures requires adaptation time during which pain and difficulty speaking and eating may be experienced.

DENTAL IMPLANT

When the natural root of a tooth has been extracted, a dental implant made of a metal rod is integrated in the jawbone to support the artificial crown, a bridge (fixed bridgework), or dentures. Its installation is completed in multiple stages under local anesthesia, after incision of the gums. Several months are needed for the integration of the implant to the bone. A prosthesis can then be attached to the implant.

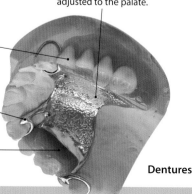

Prosthetic tooth
Prosthetic teeth are made of a metal armature covered with a composite resin whose color corresponds to that of the natural teeth.

Fake palate
The two sides of the dentures are attached by a piece adjusted to the palate.

Hook
Partial prostheses are supported by the remaining teeth by means of metal hooks.

Fake gums
Molded on the gums, the base of the dentures naturally adheres to the gum due to saliva.

Dentures

DENTAL MALOCCLUSION

Poor tooth alignment leads to an imperfect superimposition of the upper denture and lower denture, called malocclusion. Tooth alignment anomalies are generally due to a **congenital** malformation, too many or too few teeth, or thumb sucking. Malocclusions can lead to problems chewing or **swallowing**. They can also make tooth brushing difficult and be the source of cavities and oral diseases. Malocclusions can be corrected with orthodontic treatments. Orthodontics exert mild and continued pressure on the teeth for a period of six months to three years using fixed or removable devices (braces).

BRACES
Braces are temporary devices attached to the teeth that correct the dental alignment. They are made up of several brackets attached to the teeth with cement or glue and attached to each other with an archwire. The force exerted by the wire is regulated to slowly and progressively reposition the teeth.

THE END OF ORTHODONTIC TREATMENT
Orthodontic treatment ends with a period of contention, which consists in immobilizing the teeth to maintain the obtained result. For a variable duration, contention is realized using grooves molded in transparent resin or metal wires glued on the interior surface of the teeth.

Archwire
The archwire is a metal or elastic wire that connects each bracket and applies force on the teeth. It must be readjusted every four to seven weeks. A readjustment may be accompanied by pain for several days.

Bracket
A bracket, or ring, is a metal, composite or ceramic piece glued or sealed to a tooth. It transmits the force exerted by the archwire.

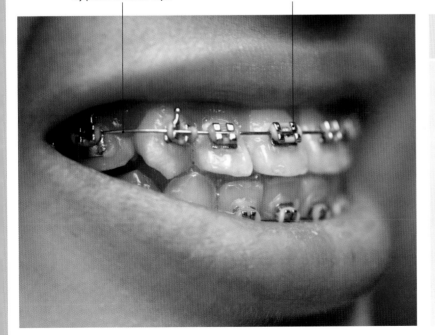

Braces

DENTAL MALOCCLUSION

SYMPTOMS:
Problems chewing, swallowing, speaking or breathing, pain or muscle spasms in the jaw, headaches.

TREATMENT:
Slight grinding of the teeth, orthodontics. Orthodontic treatments are more effective before adult age.

PREVENTION:
Discourage thumb sucking.

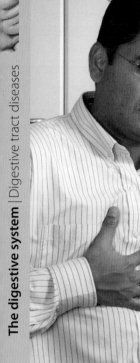

GASTROESOPHAGEAL REFLUX

Affecting 10% to 20% of the population, gastroesophageal reflux is a digestive problem that is relatively benign, characterized by the return of some of the stomach contents in the esophagus. It is accompanied by acidic regurgitations and burns along the esophagus. These symptoms occur generally one to three hours after meals and are aggravated when lying down. Gastroesophageal reflux occasionally occurs in adults, particularly after a large meal, and more regularly in newborn babies until the age of three months. Its complications are exceptional but serious (stenosis, ulcer, cancer).

CAUSES OF GASTROESOPHAGEAL REFLUX

Gastroesophageal reflux is mainly caused by the weakening of the esophageal sphincter, the muscle located between the stomach and the esophagus. In predisposed individuals with family histories, the relaxation of this muscle can be triggered or aggravated by certain food substances (fat, chocolate, coffee, alcohol), smoking, or some medications. Other factors can also promote gastroesophageal reflux: decrease in saliva production, peristalsis failure of the esophagus, hiatal hernia, asthma, obesity, diabetes, pregnancy, etc.

PREVENTING GASTROESOPHAGEAL REFLUX

If you are subject to gastroesophageal reflux, follow these tips to avoid or limit its aggravation:

- Stop your consumption of tobacco, alcohol, coffee, and fatty or spicy food.
- Lose excess weight.
- Eat small meals.
- Avoid physical effort after meals.
- Sleep with the head of the bed raised.
- Avoid wearing tight clothing.

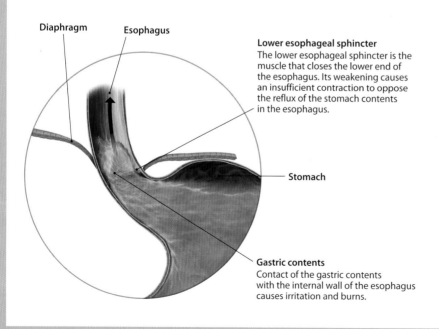

Diaphragm

Esophagus

Lower esophageal sphincter
The lower esophageal sphincter is the muscle that closes the lower end of the esophagus. Its weakening causes an insufficient contraction to oppose the reflux of the stomach contents in the esophagus.

Stomach

Gastric contents
Contact of the gastric contents with the internal wall of the esophagus causes irritation and burns.

TREATMENTS FOR GASTROESOPHAGEAL REFLUX

The treatment of gastroesophageal reflux depends on its severity. In most cases, medication is taken to neutralize the acidic secretions of the stomach or inhibit their production. Other medications act by promoting the transit of bolus to the stomach and by strengthening the lower esophageal sphincter. These treatments must be accompanied by measures aiming to limit aggravating factors. In the case of severe lesions of the esophagus or intolerance to medications, a surgical operation may be performed. Completed under general anesthesia, fundoplication consists of folding the upper part of the stomach to form a sleeve around the lower end of the esophagus. The operation may cause temporary difficulty swallowing and a feeling of distension in the stomach. In 85% of cases, it completely eliminates gastroesophageal reflux.

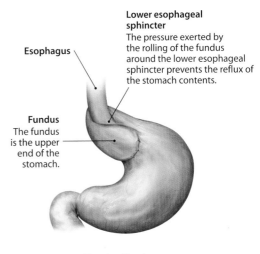

Esophagus

Lower esophageal sphincter
The pressure exerted by the rolling of the fundus around the lower esophageal sphincter prevents the reflux of the stomach contents.

Fundus
The fundus is the upper end of the stomach.

Fundoplication

HIATAL HERNIA

A hiatal hernia is an anatomic anomaly characterized by the protrusion of a part of the stomach in the thorax through the diaphragm. This disorder, still poorly explained, can be caused by a congenital malformation of the diaphragm, a trauma, or increase in abdominal pressure, particularly caused by obesity, pregnancy, or chronic constipation. Generally asymptomatic, a hiatal hernia can sometimes aggravate gastroesophageal reflux and result in inflammation of the esophagus (esophagitis).

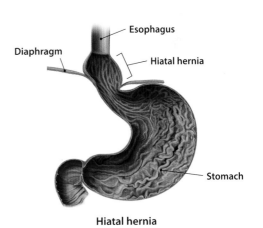

Esophagus

Diaphragm

Hiatal hernia

Stomach

Hiatal hernia

ESOPHAGEAL STENOSIS

Esophageal stenosis is the constriction of the lumen (interior diameter) of the esophagus. It can be caused by an inflammation, a benign or malignant tumor that causes the thickening of the wall or by the presence of a scar following radiation therapy, gastroesophageal reflux, or the ingestion of corrosive substances. Esophageal stenosis is characterized by a difficulty swallowing and sometimes by regurgitations. Depending on its cause and severity, treatment consists in mechanically dilating the lumen of the esophagus or surgically removing the constricted segment.

GASTROESOPHAGEAL REFLUX

SYMPTOMS:
Acidic regurgitations, burns at the top of the stomach climbing the length of the esophagus, difficulty swallowing, nocturnal cough. These symptoms appear or are accentuated after meals and while lying down.

TREATMENT:
Medications neutralizing the acidic secretions or their production, or promoting the transit towards the stomach, surgical operation (fundoplication).

PREVENTION:
Limiting of aggravating factors.

GASTRODUODENAL ULCER

The gastroduodenal ulcer is a lesion of the wall of the stomach or duodenum that results in pains and cramps in the upper and center abdomen, radiating sometimes to the middle of the back. These symptoms are experienced regularly between meals and are eased by eating food. An ulcer is characterized by the progressive erosion of the wall of the stomach or duodenum. It occurs when the acidic secretions of the stomach are too abundant or when the production of protective mucus is insufficient. The main cause of this deregulation is **infection** by *Helicobacter pylori*, a bacterium that may contaminate the stomach. The repeated use of **nonsteroidal anti-inflammatories**, an excess of alcohol, an **inflammatory** disease (like Crohn's disease), and cancer are among the risk factors. Slightly declining in industrialized countries, gastroduodenal ulcer particularly affects people over 50 years of age.

GASTRITIS

Gastritis is an inflammation of the mucous membrane of the stomach. It can be due to the same factors that are at the origin of gastroduodenal ulcer (infection by *Heliobacter pylori*, repeated use of nonsteroidal anti-inflammatories, excess alcohol, Crohn's disease, cancer). It manifests in stomachaches (pyrosis or heartburn, burns), bloating, gastroesophageal reflux, and difficult digestion, sometimes accompanied by nausea.

GASTROSCOPY

Gastroscopy is an endoscopy of the stomach, esophagus, and duodenum that allows the diagnosis of digestive tract diseases such as gastritis, gastroduodenal ulcer, esophageal cancer, and stomach cancer. The exam, uncomfortable but painless, is completed following a six-hour fast. The flexible tube of the endoscope is introduced through the mouth or nose, under local anesthesia, during which the patient is lying on his back or side. The progression of the endoscope along the digestive tract is facilitated by the insufflation of air, which slightly dilates the organs. The exam lasts less than 10 minutes, during which samples are collected.

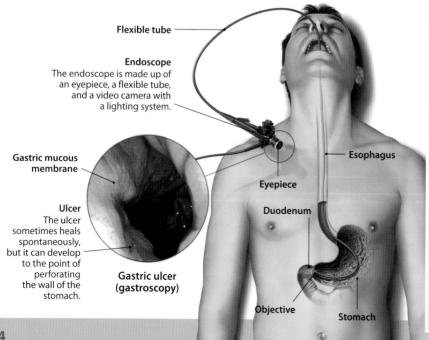

Flexible tube

Endoscope
The endoscope is made up of an eyepiece, a flexible tube, and a video camera with a lighting system.

Gastric mucous membrane

Ulcer
The ulcer sometimes heals spontaneously, but it can develop to the point of perforating the wall of the stomach.

Gastric ulcer (gastroscopy)

Eyepiece

Duodenum

Objective

Esophagus

Stomach

GASTRODUODENAL ULCER

SYMPTOMS:
Pain, cramps from the abdomen to the top of the stomach, may extend to the middle of the back. Serious ulcer: vomiting that may contain blood, dark stool.

TREATMENT:
Medications neutralizing acidic secretions or their production, antibiotics in the case of infection due to *Heliobacter pylori*.

PREVENTION:
Abstinence from alcohol and nonsteroidal anti-inflammatories.

DIGESTIVE TRACT CANCERS

Any portion of the digestive tract can be the location of a malignant tumor, particularly the large intestine, stomach, and esophagus. Cancer of the digestive tract especially affects people over 45 years of age, more frequently men. Cancer is promoted by smoking and alcoholism (esophageal cancer), gastritis and gastric ulcer (stomach cancer), family histories, certain types of colon polyps, a diet low in fiber, a sedentary lifestyle and obesity (colorectal cancer). Cancer is a serious disease that may have an unfavorable prognosis. The treatment of digestive tract cancers often consists in surgical removal of the affected area. Its success depends on the extent of the tumor and it is often completed by **chemotherapy** or **radiation therapy**.

ESOPHAGEAL CANCER

Esophageal cancer is a malignant tumor that develops in the wall of the esophagus. It manifests first through a difficulty swallowing (dysphagia), followed by weight loss, rib pain, and, sometimes, vomit containing blood. Generally diagnosed at an advanced stage, this cancer is treated by the surgical removal of the esophagus (partial or total esophagectomy), associated with chemotherapy and radiation therapy treatments. The stomach is then stretched or a segment of the colon is transplanted in place of the esophagus. If the state of the patient and the size of the tumor make operation impossible, only chemotherapy and radiation therapy treatments are administered. While surgical removal is the most effective curative treatment of esophageal cancer, its long-term success rate is limited.

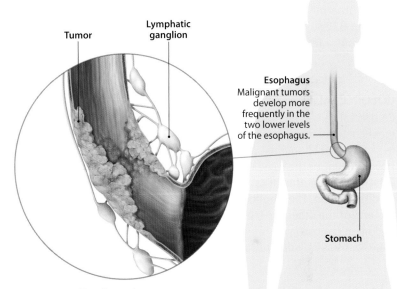

Tumor

Lymphatic ganglion

Esophagus
Malignant tumors develop more frequently in the two lower levels of the esophagus.

Stomach

Esophageal cancer
The tumor spreads rapidly to all of the tissues of the esophageal wall (mucous membrane, smooth muscles). It can also invade the neighboring organs: lymphatic ganglions, trachea, aorta. During the esophagectomy, the tumor, lymphatic ganglions, and the portion of the esophagus and the stomach that surround it are removed.

DYSPHAGIA

Dysphagia is a difficulty swallowing. It may be mechanical (obstruction by a foreign body, constriction of the esophagus, gastroesophageal reflux) or be due to an infection (laryngitis, pharyngitis, amygdalitis), a tumor (cancer of the pharynx, larynx, or esophagus), or a neurological disease (achalasia, muscular dystrophy, Parkinson's disease). Dysphagia can also be caused by a saliva deficiency, stress or intense emotion.

STOMACH CANCER

Stomach cancer is a malignant tumor that develops in the wall of the stomach. It first manifests in vague signs: stomach pains, difficult and sometimes painful digestion, and vomiting. These symptoms are often followed by anorexia, weight loss, and general fatigue. A diagnosis is established by the internal examination of the stomach (gastroscopy) and by analyzing samples of the mucous membrane. Stomach cancer is the second greatest cause of death by cancer in the world. Its treatment consists of surgically extracting a part or all of the stomach (gastrectomy), a part of the esophagus or duodenum, as well as neighboring lymph nodes. The esophagus or the remaining portion of the stomach is then reattached to the small intestine. In some cases, the operation must be followed by chemotherapy treatments and sometimes radiation therapy. The absence or reduction in volume of the stomach has several negative consequences: difficult or impossible digestion of raw vegetable fiber, decrease in quantity of absorbable foods, bloating, diarrhea. The patient must also regularly receive Vitamin B12 supplements to avoid the development of pernicious anemia.

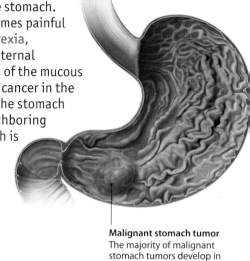

Malignant stomach tumor
The majority of malignant stomach tumors develop in the mucous membrane.

COLORECTAL CANCER

Colorectal cancer is a malignant tumor that develops in the wall of the colon or rectum. It is one of the most common forms of cancer. It manifests itself by intestinal transit problems, the presence of red blood in stools, and abdominal pains. These symptoms can also be accompanied by frailty and weight loss. Development of the tumor can lead to intestinal obstruction or perforation of the large intestinal wall. Treatment of colorectal cancer consists in ablation of the tumor (colectomy). After having removed a part or all of the colon, the surgeon reattaches the two ends of the digestive tract that remain in place. In some cases, the end of the digestive tract can be connected, temporarily or permanently, to an opening pierced in the abdomen (colostomy).

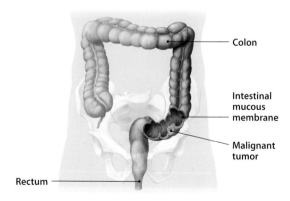

Colorectal cancer
Colorectal cancer develops first in the mucous membrane, then progressively invades other tissues of the intestinal wall. It can spread to neighboring organs (small intestine, bladder, vagina, prostate, sacrum), invade the lymphatic system, and form metastases in the liver, lungs, bones, peritoneum, and brain.

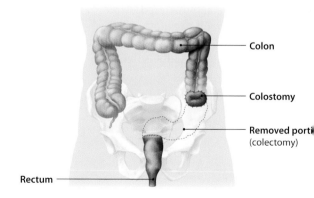

Colostomy
Colostomy, or artificial anus, allows for the evacuation of fecal matter in a plastic pocket attached to the skin that has a filter to eliminate odors.

SCREENING FOR COLORECTAL CANCER

Regular screening for colorectal cancer is recommended in people over 50 years of age or in those having familial histories. It begins with a stool examination aiming to detect the presence of blood, followed by a colonoscopy. This endoscopic exam of the colon, completed with or without general anesthesia, consists in introducing a flexible tube of approximately ½ inch (1 cm) in diameter in the intestine through the anus. The colonoscopy also allows for the collection of samples for analysis and the ablation of polyps. A barium enema or virtual colonoscopy (coloscanner) may also be completed. These two painless radiological exams lasting approximately 30 minutes make visible the intestines by using an opaque liquid and X-rays. They also allow the detection of noncancerous anomalies of the large intestinal wall, like polyps, diverticula, or an inflammation. The night before the colonoscopy or radiological exam, the patient must drink a laxative substance to eliminate all fecal matter from the intestines. To screen for rectal cancer, a rectal exam must be completed.

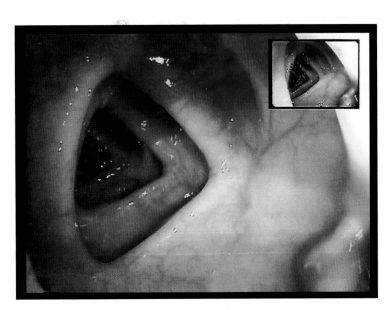

Internal view of the colon taken during a colonoscopy

DIGESTIVE BLEEDING

Digestive bleeding is the bleeding of the internal wall of the digestive tract. Upper bleeding, which affects the esophagus, stomach, or duodenum, results in bloody vomiting or blackish stools, colored by the digested blood. It indicates the existence of a gastroduodenal ulcer, tumor, or inflammation of the esophagus or stomach. Lower bleeding (e.g. in the colon, rectum, or anus) generally results in bright red stools. It may be the sign of lesions in the anus (hemorrhoid, anal fissure, tumor) or intestines (diverticulitis, colorectal cancer).

DIGESTIVE TRACT CANCERS

SYMPTOMS:
Difficulty swallowing, digesting, vomiting (sometimes containing blood), diarrhea, constipation, blood in stools, localized pain, weight loss, frailty.

TREATMENT:
Ablation of the malignant tumor, chemotherapy, radiation therapy.

PREVENTION:
Abstinence from tobacco and alcohol. Diet rich in fruit and fiber. Regular screening for colorectal cancer after 50 years of age.

GASTROENTERITIS

Gastroenteritis is an **inflammation** of the mucous membrane in the stomach and intestines, causing diarrhea and vomiting, among other symptoms. It is most often caused by an **infection** from the ingestion of water or food that has been contaminated by pathogens, such as bacteria, viruses (noroviruses or rotaviruses), or intestinal parasites. Gastroenteritis can also be caused by dietary intolerances or food poisoning. Food poisoning is the result of ingesting foods that contain toxic substances (poisonous mushrooms, ground beef, or mayonnaise contaminated by a toxin, etc.).

Hygiene and the prevention of infections… page 30
Dietary intolerances… page 362

NOROVIRUSES

Noroviruses are highly contagious viruses that are responsible for gastroenteritis (stomach flu). They are usually transmitted by contaminated water or food, especially seafood. They can also be passed from one person to another when standards of hygiene have not been followed. The symptoms of gastroenteritis appear 1–2 days after contamination and then disappear spontaneously 2–3 days later.

SALMONELLAE

Salmonellae are infectious diseases of the intestines, caused by bacteria of the *Salmonella* genus. Contamination comes from the consumption of water or food that has been infected by these bacteria (dairy products, raw eggs, poultry, and seafood). The first symptoms of gastroenteritis appear 12–24 hours after ingestion of the contaminated products. In most cases, people recover spontaneously within 3–5 days. However, in people with a weakened immune system, the infection may be more severe and may require hospitalization and the administration of antibiotics.

TRAVELER'S DIARRHEA

Traveler's diarrhea is a form of infectious gastroenteritis contracted while traveling abroad. Also called "Montezuma's revenge," it is generally caused by the consumption of water or food contaminated with the bacteria *Escherichia coli*, although it can also be caused by a virus or parasite. Symptoms usually disappear after a few days. If they persist, or if they are accompanied by a high fever or blood in the stool, a doctor should consulted.

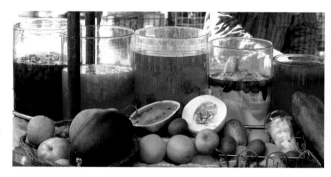

Fruit and vegetables
Fruit and vegetables must be peeled or washed with treated water before being eaten.

DIARRHEA AND ITS RELIEF

Diarrhea resulting from infectious gastroenteritis begins suddenly. In most cases, gastroenteritis disappears spontaneously after a few days of rest and a diet of high-calorie liquids (electrolyte solutions). Taking antidiarrheal medication can temporarily relieve the symptoms, but may delay elimination of the pathogen and the patient's recovery. These medications should only be used when necessary (e.g. if you need to travel).

BOTULISM

Botulism is a rare but serious form of food poisoning caused by a toxic substance produced by the bacterium *Clostridium botulinum*. Contamination comes from eating infected food, most often contaminated meat or poorly sterilized preserves. The first symptoms of gastroenteritis (abdominal pain, vomiting, and diarrhea) are followed by disruptions of the nervous system: difficulties in terms of swallowing, speaking, and vision. The more severe forms of botulism lead to paralysis and cardiac and respiratory problems, which can sometimes be fatal.

FOOD POISONING
FROM **POISONOUS MUSHROOMS**

A number of mushrooms are poisonous, meaning they contain substances that are toxic to human beings when ingested. Some examples are the death cap, the fly agaric, and the red-brown parasol. The consumption of poisonous mushrooms leads to gastroenteritis or a variety of more serious ailments. Symptoms may appear anywhere between 15 minutes and more than 10 hours after consumption of the poisonous mushroom. Treatment depends on the toxin that was ingested and on the severity of the symptoms. Medical assistance over several days may be necessary in some cases. To prevent poisoning, have a specialist identify any mushrooms you gather and do not place different species in the same container.

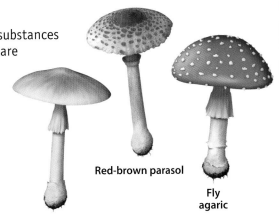

Red-brown parasol

Fly agaric

Death cap

GASTROENTERITIS

SYMPTOMS:
Diarrhea, vomiting, stomach cramps and pains, sometimes fever.

TREATMENT:
Bacterial infection: antibiotics, if needed. Antidiarrheals only in exceptional cases. Electrolyte solutions (for rehydration) must be administered until the symptoms have disappeared.

PREVENTION:
Washing your hands and food, using adequate methods for the conservation, and cooking food. Traveler's diarrhea: consuming only cooked food, treated or bottled water, and fruit and vegetables that have been peeled or washed with treated water.

HAMBURGER DISEASE

Hamburger disease got its name from its primary cause: undercooked ground beef. This is a form of food poisoning caused by a toxin produced by the bacterium *Escherichia coli* 0157:H7, which is present in cow intestines and which can contaminate meat prepared at the time of slaughter. The symptoms of the resulting gastroenteritis are usually limited to strong abdominal pain and diarrhea (sometimes with blood). There may also be a moderate fever. In children under the age of 15, this illness may be more severe and may lead to acute kidney failure, requiring dialysis.

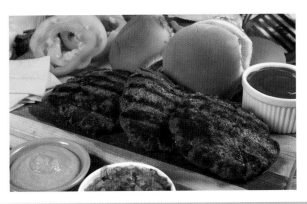

Ground meat
Ground meat must be cooked until it has lost its pinkish color before being eaten.

INTESTINAL PARASITES

The intestines can be infected by parasites, primarily worms. Contamination occurs through the ingestion of larvae or eggs, carried via the hands, objects, water, or food. Parasites grow in the intestines by feeding off the food that they contain, and cause a number of digestive disorders, some of which can be severe.

Infectious diseases... page 284

OXYURIASIS

Widespread in countries with temperate climates and especially prone to infecting children under the age of 2 and the elderly, oxyuriasis is a parasitic disease of the large intestine caused by a small, round worm a few millimeters long: the pinworm. The adult worm travels through the colon and lays several thousand eggs around the anus, which causes severe itching.

TAENIASIS

Taeniasis is caused by flatworms called taenia (or tapeworms). Ingested via undercooked pork (pork tapeworm) or beef (beef tapeworm), the tapeworm larvae attach to the walls of the small intestine and develop into adult tapeworms. Weight loss and the presence of rings in the stool or underwear are signs of taeniasis. Less frequently, tapeworm larvae can affect the muscles, the brain, the spinal cord, and the eyes, by forming cysts.

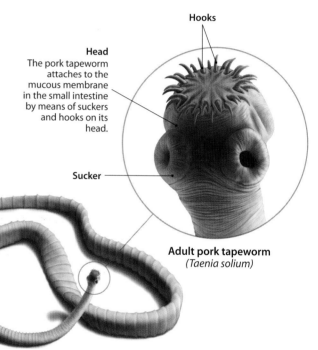

Hooks

Head
The pork tapeworm attaches to the mucous membrane in the small intestine by means of suckers and hooks on its head.

Sucker

Adult pork tapeworm
(Taenia solium)

Rings
A whitish ribbon measuring several yards in length, the tapeworm is formed of many rings, the last of which detach easily, which allows for the dissemination of the eggs that they contain, via the stool.

ASCARIASIS

Caused by the ascaris, a roundworm 2–14 inches (5–35 cm) long, ascariasis affects one-quarter of the world's population, particularly children in tropical countries. This parasite in transmitted in tiny eggs, carried by unclean water and food. Once hatched, the larvae cross through the wall of the small intestine and travel through the bloodstream. They then move into the lungs, often leading to difficulty breathing. They travel up to the larynx, are swallowed, and return to the small intestine, where, after their metamorphosis, they can continue this cycle as adults. Without treatment, ascariasis can lead to serious complications, such as intestinal obstruction, pancreatitis, and peritonitis.

INTESTINAL PARASITES

SYMPTOMS:
Digestive problems: nausea, vomiting, diarrhea, abdominal pain, weight loss.

TREATMENT:
Special antiparasitics (vermicides), in topical form or taken orally or intravenously.

PREVENTION:
Maintaining hygiene. Washing and cooking food.

DYSENTERY

Dysentery primarily affects children under the age of 5 in developing countries, where it is responsible for approximately 1 million deaths each year. This type of **infectious** disease, very common in tropical regions, is transmitted by contaminated water and food. It attacks the mucous membrane of the colon, causing abundant, bloody, viscous diarrhea. The different forms include amoebiasis, caused by an amoeba, and shigellosis, from bacteria of the *Shigella* genus. Without treatment, dysentery leads to serious complications.

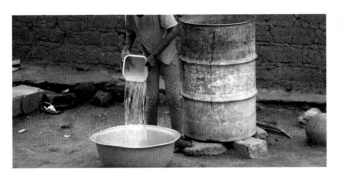

Epidemics
In countries at war or plagued by natural disasters, overpopulation (particularly in refugee camps) and a lack of access to clean drinking water can cause serious epidemics of cholera and dysentery. Quickly restoring a network of clean drinking water and a sanitation and sewage system can help prevent the spread of these diseases.

DYSENTERY

SYMPTOMS:
Bloody, viscous diarrhea, abdominal cramps and pain, vomiting, painful anal spasms.

TREATMENT:
Rehydration (oral or intravenous). Antiparasitics or antibiotics, depending on the cause.

PREVENTION:
In at-risk countries: drinking treated water or sealed bottled water, washing fruit using this same water or peeling it, washing your hands before eating.

CHOLERA

Cholera is an infectious disease caused by the bacterium *Vibrio cholerae*. Once ingested through water or food contaminated by the stool of infected people, the bacterium multiples in the small intestine. It causes frequent, abundant diarrhea, vomiting, and strong abdominal cramps. Cholera is widespread in many developing countries, across all continents. *Vibrio cholerae* can survive for several months in warm, stagnant water, and for several days in fish and shellfish. Without treatment, the disease and its complications can lead to death by dehydration.

CHOLERA

SYMPTOMS:
Sudden, frequent, abundant liquid diarrhea, abdominal cramps, vomiting, rapid dehydration and weight loss. Convulsions in children.

TREATMENT:
Rehydration by IV drip containing mineral salts and glucose. Antibiotics.

PREVENTION:
In at-risk countries: drinking bottled, treated water, following basic hygiene measures. Vaccination provides temporary protection for people with a high risk of exposure or with a weakened immune system.

COLITIS

Inflammation of the colon, or colitis, may arise following the use of **laxative** or **antibiotic** medications, but it is most often caused by an **infection** from the bacterium *Clostridium difficile*. In this case, it is accompanied by diarrhea, fever, nausea, and abdominal cramps, and may lead to dehydration and more serious complications, such as dilation or perforation of the colon. The more rare **chronic** forms of colitis, including Crohn's disease and ulcerative colitis, affect young people ages 15–30 in particular, and do not have any clearly defined cause. These are incapacitating diseases that develop in bursts.

CHRONIC COLITIS

Ulcerative colitis is a chronic ailment affecting the mucous membrane of the rectum, usually extending to the colon. It causes bloody diarrhea and stomach pains and may lead to a number of complications (dilation of the colon, perforation of the intestine, etc.). Crohn's disease is a chronic inflammation of the digestive tract, affecting, in particular, the ileum (the final segment of the small intestine), the colon, and the anus. It can have any of a number of digestive symptoms: intermittent diarrhea (possibly containing blood and pus), constipation, obstruction, abdominal cramps, vomiting, and anal lesions. Chronic colitis also has nondigestive symptoms: chronic inflammation of the spinal joints, inflammation of the eye, aphthas, cholelithiasis, and urolithiasis.

CLOSTRIDIUM DIFFICILE

Clostridium difficile (or *C. difficile*) is a bacterium responsible for infections of the intestinal mucous membrane. It is naturally present in the ground and in excrement, and is a part of the intestinal flora. It becomes pathogenic when its proliferation is favored by antibiotic treatments or by immunosuppressants, which destroy a portion of the intestinal flora. The toxins that it secretes then attack the intestinal wall, causing abundant diarrhea. *Clostridium difficile* is resistant to most antibiotics.

COLITIS TREATMENTS

Infectious forms of colitis disappear after the end of an antibiotic treatment that has disturbed the intestinal flora. Chronic colitis can be controlled by anti-inflammatory or immunosuppressant treatments. If these treatments are not effective, surgical removal (ablation) of the rectum and, sometimes, the anus (proctectomy) are considered. Proctectomy may be combined with partial or complete ablation of the colon (coloproctectomy).

COLITIS

SYMPTOMS:
Diarrhea, abdominal cramps and pain, vomiting, loss of appetite, weight loss, fever. Crohn's disease and ulcerative colitis: bloody stool, constipation, arthritis, aphthas, uveitis, urolithiasis, and cholelithiasis.

TREATMENT:
Infectious colitis: interruption of antibiotics or switching to different antibiotics. Chronic colitis: anti-inflammatories, immunosuppressants, surgical ablation of the colon, rectum, or anus.

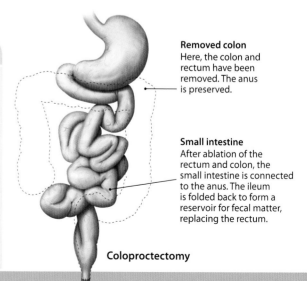

Removed colon
Here, the colon and rectum have been removed. The anus is preserved.

Small intestine
After ablation of the rectum and colon, the small intestine is connected to the anus. The ileum is folded back to form a reservoir for fecal matter, replacing the rectum.

Coloproctectomy

COLON POLYPS

Colon polyps are benign tumors that form in the mucous membrane of the colon, projecting inward from its surface. They appear in all age ranges, but increase with age. The causes of their development are relatively unknown, except in the case of **genetic** forms. Their onset is favored by **inflammations** of the colon (colitis), by alcohol consumption, a sedentary lifestyle, and obesity. In general, colon polyps have no symptoms when they are small. However, larger polyps may be indicated by digestive problems (diarrhea, constipation, etc.) and by the occasional presence of red blood in the stool. Colon polyps are usually diagnosed during **colonoscopy** and are removed during the examination, by polypectomy, because they present a risk of developing into colorectal cancer.

Benign tumors… page 54

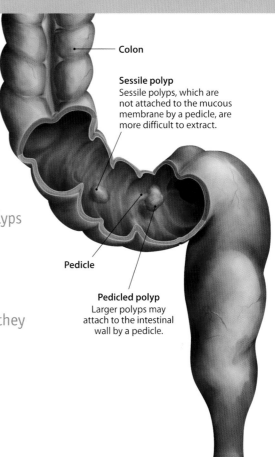

Colon

Sessile polyp
Sessile polyps, which are not attached to the mucous membrane by a pedicle, are more difficult to extract.

Pedicle

Pedicled polyp
Larger polyps may attach to the intestinal wall by a pedicle.

TYPES OF COLON POLYPS

Most colon polyps are the result of an increase in the number of cells in the mucous membrane of the digestive tract (colon, rectum, etc.) and remain benign. They generally appear in the form of smooth, round outgrowths, 3/16 inch (5 mm) in diameter, that may or may not be attached to the mucous membrane by a connecting stalk (pedicle). Certain large, pedicled polyps are adenomas. These less frequent, but more dangerous, polyps can form in any segment of the large intestine. After 5–10 years, on average, some adenomas may develop into cancer of the colon and rectum.

POLYPECTOMY

Surgical ablation of a polyp (polypectomy) is performed by colonoscopy, with or without general anesthesia. The surgical instruments are inserted into the flexible tube of the endoscope via the anus. The polyps are severed, then analyzed at the laboratory to determine whether they are benign or malignant tumors.

COLON POLYPS

SYMPTOMS:
Small polyps have no symptoms. Larger polyps may be indicated by blood in the stool, diarrhea, or constipation.

TREATMENT:
Surgical ablation of the tumors (polypectomy, colectomy).

PREVENTION:
Regular testing starting at the age of 50, diet rich in fiber and fruit, avoiding tobacco and excessive alcohol intake.

IRRITABLE BOWEL SYNDROME

Contractions of the intestinal muscles are normally coordinated to move fecal matter towards the anus. In irritable bowel syndrome, strong, uncoordinated contractions disrupt intestinal transit and lead to irregular defecation. Multiple factors have been identified as triggering these spasms: stress (family problems, new job, etc.), anxiety, depression, certain foods (dairy products, coffee, chocolate, and alcohol), and gastroenteritis. However, the precise causes of irritable bowel syndrome are unknown and no anomaly in the intestinal wall has been shown. Usually occurring in young adults, this **chronic** disorder affects some 20% of the population and affects twice as many women as men. Symptomatic treatment aims to return intestinal transit to normal and to relieve abdominal pain.

SYMPTOMS OF IRRITABLE BOWEL SYNDROME

Irritable bowel syndrome is indicated by episodes of diarrhea or constipation. These intestinal transit problems are often combined with abdominal pain and cramps and, in some cases, bloating caused by the production of intestinal gas. In addition, a clear, transparent mucus may be excreted with the stool. These symptoms vary in severity, depending on the person, and may occur intermittently. In severe cases, they will diminish the quality of life of the patient.

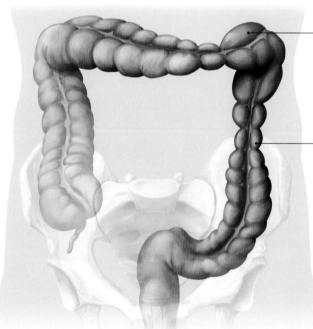

Dilation
Intestinal gas can accumulate in a segment of the intestine, causing painful distension of its wall.

Spasms
Spasms in smooth (nonstriated) muscles can accelerate the movement of fecal matter (diarrhea) or slow it down (constipation).

Irritable bowel

IRRITABLE BOWEL SYNDROME

SYMPTOMS:
Diarrhea and constipation (possibly alternating), abdominal pain and cramps, bloating, mucus in the stool.

TREATMENT:
Symptomatic treatments to return intestinal transit to normal (**anticonvulsants**, antidiarrheals, laxatives) and treatment of abdominal pain.

DIVERTICULOSIS

Diverticulosis is the formation of multiple small pouches (diverticula) on the wall of the digestive tract. It most often affects the large intestine, particularly the sigmoid colon (just before the rectum). The cause of diverticulosis is unknown, although it is more common in diets lacking in fiber: such a diet itself can cause constipation and an increase in the pressure exerted by fecal matter on the walls of the large intestine. This benign, often asymptomatic disease may cause abdominal cramps. Diverticulosis is often diagnosed by chance, during an examination of the digestive tract. It is a common ailment that affects nearly one in two people over 65 years of age. Its main complication, which arises in 10%–25% of cases, is **infection** of the diverticula (diverticulitis).

DIVERTICULOSIS

SYMPTOMS:
Abdominal cramps. Diverticulitis: pain in the lower left of the abdomen, constipation, nausea, fever, in some cases bleeding from the anus.

TREATMENT:
Diverticulitis: antibiotics and analgesics. In the event of complications (abscess, perforation, intestinal obstruction, fistula, etc.): ablation of the affected area (colectomy).

PREVENTION:
Diet rich in fiber, fruit, and liquids.

Cross section of the colon

Diverticulum

Fecal matter
The fecal matter trapped in a diverticulum creates conditions that favor the local proliferation of the bacteria of the intestinal flora and the formation of a focus of infection.

Infected diverticulum
In the case of diverticulitis, an infected diverticulum may burst and the infection can spread to the abdominal cavity.

INTESTINAL OBSTRUCTION

An intestinal obstruction is a blockage of intestinal transit. It can have a number of causes: stoppage of the peristaltic reflex due to an abscess or peritonitis; obstruction of the intestine by a tumor or gallstone; or strangulation by an inguinal hernia, torsion, or scar tissue. It results in intense abdominal pain, vomiting, and swelling of the abdomen. Intestinal obstruction is a serious ailment that can quickly lead to dehydration and a state of shock. It may cause **necrosis** (death) of the tissues in the intestine and, in some cases, their perforation.

INTESTINAL OBSTRUCTION

SYMPTOMS:
Intense abdominal pain (colic), vomiting, abdominal swelling.

TREATMENT:
Emergency treatment consists in emptying the contents of the intestine using a stomach tube and, if necessary, treatment of the cause of the obstruction, usually by surgery.

PREVENTION:
Identifying the triggers, avoiding stress, avoiding gas-inducing foods, increasing fiber in the diet.

Distended intestine
The accumulation of fecal matter, intestinal gases, and digestive secretions causes the intestine to distend and the abdomen to swell.

Strangulation

HERNIAS

Hernias are anatomic anomalies characterized by the displacement of an organ, or part of an organ, outside its natural cavity. The organ may be displaced through a natural orifice (hiatus hernias) or through the membrane surrounding the organ, either via a lesion (herniated disc) or a weak point (inguinal and umbilical hernias). Inguinal and umbilical hernias are usually benign and painless, although they can choke off a portion of the intestines, blocking the movement of fecal matter and causing an intestinal obstruction. The only effective treatment is surgery.

INGUINAL HERNIAS

An inguinal hernia is the outward protrusion of a part of the peritoneum or the intestines at the groin or scrotum. These account for 90% of abdominal hernias and most often affect men over 50 years of age. Inguinal hernias are usually caused by the weakening of the abdominal muscles and may be induced by repeated efforts. They cause swelling of varying degrees, depending on the pressure exerted on the abdomen through effort, position, transit of fecal matter, and coughing.

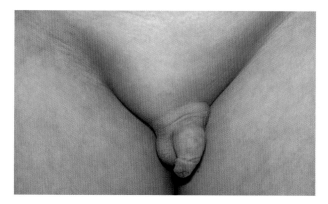

Inguinal hernias
The swelling of the groin is painless and may be temporarily reduced by pressure from the hand.

UMBILICAL HERNIAS

An umbilical hernia is the are outward protrusion of a portion of the intestines at the naval. This fairly rare type accounts for just 5% of abdominal hernias and mainly affects infants under the age of 2 (primarily premature newborns), women over 50 having had multiple pregnancies, and the obese. In children, umbilical hernias spontaneously resolve before the age of 4 in 90% of cases.

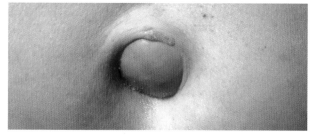

Umbilical hernias
In children, the gradual development of the abdominal muscles around the naval can spontaneously reduce umbilical hernias.

HERNIAS

SYMPTOMS:
Localized (naval, groin, or scrotum), painless swelling of the abdomen, which can be temporarily reduced by applying pressure with the fingers. If the hernia turns red or blue, hardens, or causes pain or vomiting, this may be a sign of a complication and will require emergency surgery.

TREATMENT:
Surgery to put the intestines back in place and close off the point of passage, possibly using a synthetic lattice.

APPENDICITIS

Appendicitis is the **acute inflammation** of the appendix, an outgrowth of the large intestine, typically caused by its **infection**. It is a common illness, affecting 7% of the population of industrialized countries, primarily people ages 15–30. Once diagnosed, the only curative treatment is the surgical ablation (removal) of the appendix, which must be performed rapidly due to the high risk of complications (peritonitis, **septicemia**, etc.). It takes place under general **anesthesia**, via an incision in the wall of the abdomen or by **celiosurgery**.

SYMPTOMS OF APPENDICITIS

The onset of appendicitis is sudden, indicated by intense pain. This pain starts above or around the naval, then rapidly localizes in the lower right of the abdomen, which may contract when touched. The pain may be combined with loss of appetite, nausea, vomiting, and moderate fever (100°F–101°F [38°C]). Appendicitis may be difficult to diagnose if the symptoms are limited or if the appendix is in an abnormal position.

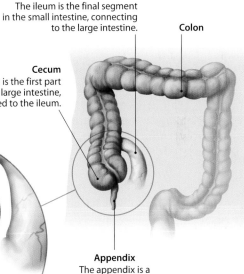

Ileum
The ileum is the final segment in the small intestine, connecting to the large intestine.

Colon

Cecum
The cecum is the first part of the large intestine, connected to the ileum.

Appendix
The appendix is a narrow outgrowth, about 4 inches (10 cm) long, extending from the cecum.

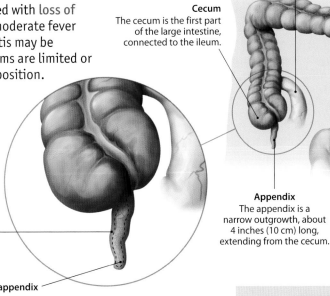

Infected appendix
As an effect of inflammation, the appendix increases in size, which can cause it to burst, leading to peritonitis.

Normal appendix

PERITONITIS

Peritonitis is the inflammation of the peritoneum, caused by the spread of an infection or the perforation of a digestive organ. It appears as an intense, continuous pain in the abdomen, which becomes extremely hard. Peritonitis is accompanied by vomiting, stoppage of intestinal transit, high fever, and several other general symptoms: rapid breathing and heartbeat, low blood pressure, weakness, and pallor. It is a serious ailment that requires emergency medical attention. Once the source of the infection has been treated, medical care consists in surgically washing the peritoneum and administering antibiotics to fight off the infection.

APPENDICITIS

SYMPTOMS:
Intense, continuous pain in the lower right of the abdomen, nausea, vomiting, loss of appetite, constipation, moderate fever, abdominal wall hard to the touch. When lying on the left side of the body, the pain increases when the right leg is raised and extended.

TREATMENT:
Ablation of the appendix, antibiotics if needed.

HEMORRHOIDS

Hemorrhoids are the dilation of a blood vessel in the anus or the lower part of the rectum. There are two different types: external hemorrhoids and internal hemorrhoids, which differ in terms of their location, their symptoms, and their associated complications. Hemorrhoids are usually benign and are a common disorder in people over 45 years of age. In some cases, the discomfort, pain, or complications that they produce may require surgical treatment.

RISK **FACTORS** FOR **HEMORRHOIDS**

The formation of hemorrhoids is affected by multiple factors, particularly heredity and chronic irritation of the anus, especially due to a spicy diet or the use of laxatives. It is also favored by a slowing of the venous return, caused by a sedentary lifestyle or by a prolonged seated position, and by increased pressure in the abdomen, caused by a variety of factors: constipation, obesity, pregnancy, and certain sports activities.

PREGNANCY

Approximately one in three pregnant women suffers from hemorrhoids, usually during the second trimester of pregnancy. This may be triggered by constipation or by the pressure exerted by the uterus on the blood vessels in the abdomen.

HEREDITY

In some families, hemorrhoids are common, due to a congenital weakness of the walls of the blood vessels. This hereditary characteristic can also appear in the form of venous incompetence and varicose veins in the lower limbs.

Varicose veins... page 272

DIET

Diet has a major impact on the formation of hemorrhoids. Consuming spicy foods, alcohol, coffee, and tea may foster their development. Conversely, a diet rich in fiber and water encourages the production of softer stool and reduces the risk of hemorrhoids.

INTERNAL HEMORRHOIDS

Internal hemorrhoids are located in the mucous membrane of the lower part of the rectum or the anal canal. They cause mild bleeding (bright red), during and shortly after defecation. Internal hemorrhoids are usually painless and invisible. When they increase in size, they may drop outside the anus, leading to itching, sharp pain, and spasms in the anus. If they do not rise back up spontaneously or if they cannot be pushed back manually, the extruding hemorrhoids are surgically removed.

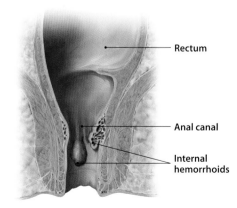

Rectum

Anal canal

Internal hemorrhoids

EXTERNAL HEMORRHOIDS

Located around the anus, external hemorrhoids are usually painful, owing to the many sensitive nerves running through the skin in that area. They may involve the formation of blood clots, which cause substantial, continuous pain in the area around the anus. The resulting edema may regress spontaneously after around two weeks, leaving behind just a fold in the skin.

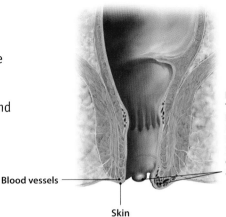

External hemorrhoids
The accumulation of blood in an external hemorrhoid may cause blood clots to form. In turn, these lead to edema, appearing as a bluish swelling.

Blood vessels

Skin

ANAL FISSURES

An anal fissure is a superficial wound in the folds of the anus, accompanied by the constant contraction of the internal muscle of the anus. Its causes are relatively unknown and, although sometimes combined with hemorrhoids, the two are separate pathologies. An anal fissure appears as a very painful burning and tearing sensation during defecation. Its treatment is based on good hygiene, appropriate diet, and local application of anesthetics, medicated creams, and muscle relaxants. Healing may, however, take some time. If the medical treatment is not effective, surgery may be recommended to remove the fissure and relax the sphincter.

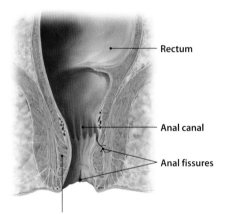

Rectum

Anal canal

Anal fissures

Internal anal sphincter
The pain experienced is partially due to the continuous contraction of the internal anal sphincter.

HEMORRHOID TREATMENT

Hemorrhoid treatment depends on the severity of the symptoms experienced. To reduce the inflammation, alleviate the pain, and reabsorb the dilated segments of the blood vessels, a medical treatment may be administered orally or applied locally in the form of a cream or suppository. Another type of treatment may be considered in the case of failure of the initial treatment or recurrence of hemorrhoids. Several nonsurgical techniques can be used to burn the hemorrhoids (photocoagulation, electrocoagulation, and cryotherapy) or to cause their necrosis (ligation of the hemorrhoids and sclerotherapy). In the case of infection or when a hemorrhoid drops too far outside the anus or forms a blood clot, it is surgically removed. This operation, performed under anesthesia, requires a short hospital stay. During recovery, the patient must temporarily follow a diet to soften the stool.

HEMORRHOIDS

SYMPTOMS:
Slight bleeding caused by defecation, itching and irritation, spasms, and strong, constant pain in some cases. External hemorrhoids are visible; internal hemorrhoids may or may not be.

TREATMENT:
Anti-inflammatories, vein tonics, analgesics (painkillers). Photocoagulation, cryotherapy, sclerotherapy, ligation or removal of the hemorrhoids.

PREVENTION:
Diet rich in fiber and liquids, physical activity. Prompt defecation.

HEPATITIS

Hepatitis is the **acute** or **chronic inflammation** of the liver, which causes the destruction of its cells. Acute hepatitis is usually caused by a viral **infection** or, more rarely, by alcohol poisoning or drug intoxication. Some of the viruses that cause acute hepatitis can infect the liver on a lasting basis and may lead to cirrhosis. Chronic hepatitis is a serious illness that brings about the gradual destruction of the liver and, in some cases, the onset of liver cancer. It may necessitate a liver transplant.

Cirrhosis of the liver... page 392

VIRAL HEPATITIS

The viral forms of hepatitis are classified from A to G, depending on the type of virus. The viruses that cause hepatitis may be communicated by the digestive pathway (hepatitis A, E, and F) after ingesting contaminated water or food (seafood, poorly washed fruit and vegetables, etc.), by the blood (hepatitis B, C, D, and G) via a contaminated syringe or transfusion, or by sex or pregnancy (hepatitis B, D, and G). After a variable period of incubation, acute viral hepatitis causes faintness, nausea, vomiting, fever, and fatigue. After a few days, icterus (jaundice) may develop, accompanied by discomfort in the area of the liver and loss of appetite. The urine darkens and the stool may become light in color. In most cases, acute hepatitis is cured on its own after a few weeks. However, some types (hepatitis B, C, and D) may develop into a chronic form, lasting over six months. In exceptional cases, acute hepatitis can lead to the rapid deterioration of the liver and the patient's condition, often requiring an emergency liver transplant. Hepatitis A and B, which may pose a threat to the immunodeficient and to young children, can be prevented by vaccination.

HEPATITIS: KEY FIGURES

The most frequently occurring types are hepatitis A, B, and C. Hepatitis A, the most common and most benign, affects approximately 90% of the population of developing countries due to insufficient sanitary conditions. Hepatitis B affects some 350 million people around the world and hepatitis C, around 170 million.

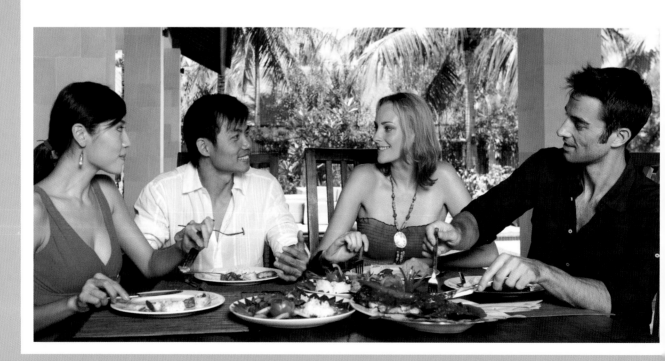

ACUTE ALCOHOLIC HEPATITIS

The regular consumption of large quantities of alcoholic beverages can lead to the destruction of the cells in the liver, causing acute alcoholic hepatitis. This disease is usually indicated by the appearance of specific symptoms (loss of appetite, nausea, fatigue, icterus, pains, and mild fever), possibly accompanied, in the most severe cases, by swelling of the abdomen (ascites), digestive hemorrhage, and impairment of consciousness and of the heart rhythm. Patients may also develop cirrhosis in the long term. The severe forms have a poor prognosis, with a mortality rate around 50%. In the less serious forms, a cure requires completely stopping all alcohol consumption and may take up to six months.

ICTERUS

Icterus, or jaundice, is a yellow coloration of the skin and of the mucous membrane owing to the excessive presence of bilirubin (a pigment derived from hemoglobin) in the blood. It may be caused by a disease of the liver, bile duct, pancreas, or blood. Icterus is accompanied by the production of dark urine and, in some cases, light-colored stool. It disappears after treatment of its cause. There is a common form of physiologic icterus in newborns, due to the immaturity of the liver, which normally dissipates after a few days.

Icterus of the newborn... page 515

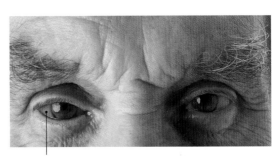

Eye
Yellow coloration of the eye
is a sign of icterus.

LIVER TRANSPLANTS

An irreparably damaged liver (due to hepatitis, cirrhosis, cancer, etc.) can no longer fulfill its functions; this is referred to as "hepatic failure." A liver transplant is then planned to replace the diseased liver with a healthy liver. This is the most common type of transplant after kidney transplants. During the four- to six-hour operation, the patient's liver is completely removed and replaced by either a whole liver taken from a brain-dead patient or a portion of a liver taken from a voluntary donor. After the operation, at least 20 days of hospitalization is required in order to verify that the new liver is functioning properly. The risk of rejection, which is highest in the first months, is kept in check by an immunosuppressant treatment, which must be taken for life. The patient can gradually return to a normal life, but must refrain from consuming alcohol and must undergo regular medical follow-ups.

HEPATITIS

SYMPTOMS:
May be asymptomatic. Icterus (jaundice), dark urine, light-colored stool, loss of appetite, weakness, nausea, weight loss, fever, painful discomfort around the liver. Severe cases may be accompanied by confusion.

TREATMENT:
Chronic nonviral hepatitis: corticosteroids. Chronic viral hepatitis: antivirals, interferon. Severe hepatic failure: liver transplant.

PREVENTION:
Moderate alcohol consumption, safe sex (condoms), use of sterile syringes, strict hygiene in developing countries and at-risk environments (hospitals, housing centers, and laboratories), vaccination against hepatitis A and B, compliance with prescribed dosages in acetaminophen treatments.

CIRRHOSIS OF THE LIVER

The hepatitis virus, long-term excessive consumption of alcohol or medications, cystic fibrosis, and some **autoimmune** diseases attack the liver and may cause a gradual disruption of the structure of its tissues. The result is a **chronic** disease, cirrhosis of the liver. Initially asymptomatic, cirrhosis of the liver appears as a swelling of the spleen, yellow coloring of the skin and mucous membrane (icterus), characteristic rashes (arterial spiders), reddening of the palms of the hands, **edema** (swelling) of the lower limbs, significant weakness, and weight loss. It is a serious, irreversible disease that can lead to numerous complications: liver cancer, hepatic failure, digestive hemorrhage, swelling of the abdomen, osteoporosis, and confusion. Cirrhosis treatments are limited to slowing its development and alleviating its symptoms. In the most serious cases, a liver transplant may be necessary.

THE **CIRRHOTIC LIVER**

Cirrhosis changes the structure of the liver. Its tissues are destroyed by repeated attacks and regenerate, forming small clusters called "regenerative nodules." Although these nodules are composed of functioning cells, they are disorganized and separated by scarring of the fibrous conjunctive tissue, which disrupts the circulation of blood in the liver. The liver gradually becomes incapable of efficiently filtering the blood.

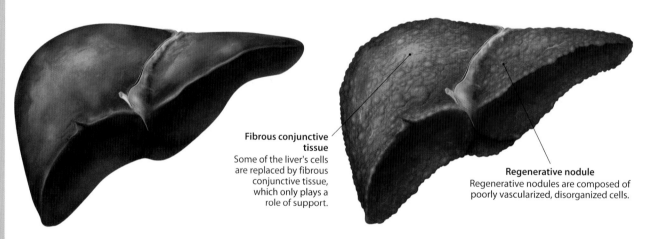

Fibrous conjunctive tissue
Some of the liver's cells are replaced by fibrous conjunctive tissue, which only plays a role of support.

Regenerative nodule
Regenerative nodules are composed of poorly vascularized, disorganized cells.

Healthy liver
A healthy liver is reddish-brown in color, with a smooth, even surface.

Cirrhotic liver
A cirrhotic liver is smaller or larger than a normal liver. Its mottled appearance is caused by the presence of cords of conjunctive tissue separating the regenerative nodules.

LIVER BIOPSY

To diagnose illnesses like cirrhosis and hepatitis, a small piece of the liver may be sampled by means of a liver biopsy. Performed under local anesthesia, this procedure consists in inserting a hollow needle between two ribs and into the liver. It takes only about 10 minutes, but the patient must then remain in bed for several hours in order to reduce the risk of bleeding.

HEPATIC FAILURE

The liver's inability to perform its functions is called "hepatic failure." Its onset is indicated by a variety of disorders, depending on its severity: significant weakness, icterus (jaundice), dermatological problems (arterial spiders, redness of the palms of the hands), impaired coagulation (hemorrhage), repeated infections, and neurological disorders (apathy, sleepiness, confusion, and coma). Hepatic failure is the result of the destruction of the liver's cells by various agents: alcohol, viruses, medications, inflammation, malignant tumors, etc. It is often a complication of cirrhosis. It is a serious ailment for which there are only fairly ineffective, symptomatic treatments. In the most severe cases, a liver transplant may be the only possible recourse.

ASCITES

Ascites is excess liquid accumulated between the two layers of the peritoneal cavity, caused by cirrhosis of the liver, heart failure, cancer of the digestive system, or ovarian cancer. It appears as the generally rapid, often painless, swelling of the abdomen, possibly accompanied by nausea. The main complications are infection of the liquid contained in the peritoneum, the formation of an umbilical hernia, and difficulty breathing due to the pressure exerted on the diaphragm. Treatment of ascites is based on a low-sodium diet and the use of diuretics. In the case of treatment failure, the liquid may be drained.

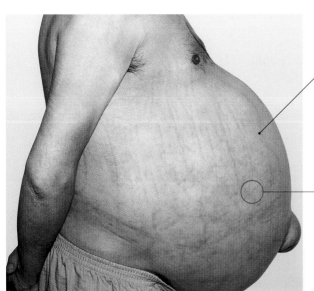

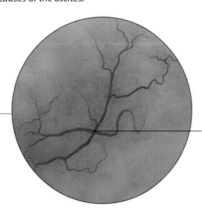

Abdomen
Ascites can be detected when the amount of liquid in the abdomen exceeds 2.5 quarts (2.4 liters). Drainage of the liquid relieves the patient and helps to identify the causes of the ascites.

Arterial spiders
An arterial spider is a spider-shaped lesion of the blood vessels in the skin. Arterial spiders are a characteristic of cirrhosis of the liver, in particular.

CIRRHOSIS OF THE LIVER

SYMPTOMS:
Weakness, weight loss, swelling of the spleen, icterus (jaundice), arterial spiders, redness of the palms of the hands, edema of the lower limbs, steatosis (presence of fat in the liver).

TREATMENT:
Treatment aims to alleviate the symptoms. A liver transplant is planned in the case of severe hepatic failure.

PREVENTION:
Avoiding excessive alcohol intake. Vaccination against hepatitis B.

LIVER CANCER

Liver cancer is most often due to the presence of metastases, meaning that it develops from a cancer of another organ (organs of the digestive tract, pancreas, lungs, breast, kidney, or prostate). When it is a primary cancer (originating in the liver), its main form is hepatocellular carcinoma. Although increasingly frequent in Western countries, it is most common in Asia and Africa, where it is the 5th leading cause of cancer in men. Liver cancer is a serious disease, with a generally negative prognosis. In the case of primary cancer of the liver, and in the absence of metastases, surgical treatment may be required, ranging from partial ablation of the liver (hepatectomy) to a liver transplant.

Cancer... page 55

HEPATOCELLULAR CARCINOMA

Hepatocellular carcinoma is a primary cancer of the liver that, in most cases (90%), develops in cirrhotic livers. Asymptomatic at onset, it is often discovered during cirrhosis complications, such as icterus (jaundice), ascites, or digestive hemorrhage, or during a screening test performed on patients with cirrhosis. Other symptoms appear once the malignant tumor has become very developed: loss of appetite, weight loss, weakness, fever, pains, enlargement of the liver. The diagnosis is established using an imaging technology (ultrasound, scanner, or magnetic resonance) and, in some cases, via a needle biopsy. The treatment selected will depend on the spread of the tumor: partial removal of the liver, chemotherapy, localized destruction of the tumor, or liver transplant.

ABLATION OF THE LIVER

Partial or total ablation (removal) of the liver, or hepatectomy, is chiefly performed as part of the treatment of a hepatocellular carcinoma. Partial ablation of the liver (up to 75% of its volume) is followed by regeneration of the missing section via the tissues left in place. As a result, its success depends primarily on the quality of the remaining tissues. Total hepatectomy must immediately be followed by a liver transplant.

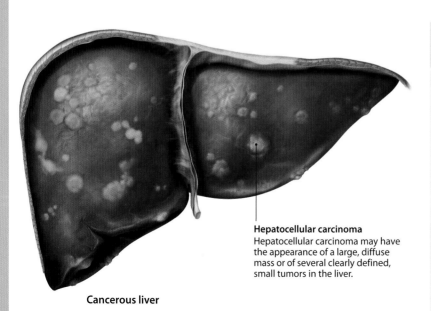

Hepatocellular carcinoma
Hepatocellular carcinoma may have the appearance of a large, diffuse mass or of several clearly defined, small tumors in the liver.

Cancerous liver

CANCER OF THE LIVER

SYMPTOMS:
Asymptomatic at onset. Loss of appetite, weight loss, significant weakness, fever, liver pain with an increase in the size of the liver.

TREATMENT:
Partial ablation of the liver, chemotherapy, localized destruction of the tumor or liver transplant.

PREVENTION:
Vaccination against hepatitis B, prevention of alcoholism.

CHOLELITHIASIS

Cholelithiasis is a disease characterized by the formation of small stones (gallstones) in the gallbladder. Common in industrialized countries—particularly among women—its onset is favored by age, obesity, fasting, some hormonal treatments, pregnancy, and diseases such as Crohn's disease and cystic fibrosis. The main symptom, which only appears in 20% of cases, is a sharp pain (hepatic colic) arising suddenly under the sternum or under the ribs on the right side. If it persists for several hours, it may be a sign of a complication requiring medical care. Surgical extraction of the gallbladder, or cholecystectomy, may become necessary. This operation is usually performed by **celiosurgery**, under general **anesthesia**.

GALLSTONES

A gallstone is a solid mass measuring $1/32$–1 inch (1 mm–3 cm) in length, formed in the gallbladder. Chiefly composed of cholesterol and bile pigment, gallstones appear when the amount of cholesterol produced by the liver is greater than the quantity that can be dissolved in the bile. In most cases, gallstones remain in the gallbladder and have no symptoms. However, when a stone moves along the bile ducts, it blocks the excretion of bile, causing the walls of the ducts to distend. This situation causes a sharp pain called hepatic colic. If the obstruction continues, it can lead to inflammation and, potentially, infection of the gallbladder. This is referred to as cholecystitis. Conversely, if the stone is ejected into the duodenum or if it returns to the gallbladder, the symptoms disappear.

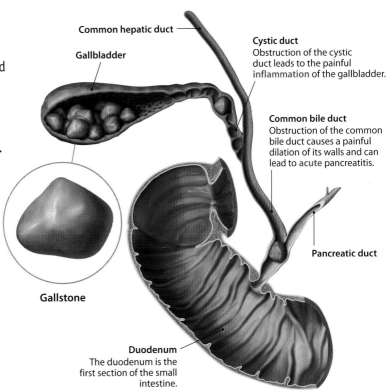

Common hepatic duct

Gallbladder

Cystic duct
Obstruction of the cystic duct leads to the painful **inflammation** of the gallbladder.

Common bile duct
Obstruction of the common bile duct causes a painful dilation of its walls and can lead to **acute** pancreatitis.

Pancreatic duct

Gallstone

Duodenum
The duodenum is the first section of the small intestine.

HEPATIC COLIC

Obstruction of the bile ducts by a gallstone causes a severe pain called hepatic colic. Located under the sternum, on the right side of the abdomen, it often extends to the back, to the tip of the shoulder blade. Hepatic colic can last between 15 minutes and a few hours. More intense during inhalation, it can lead to respiratory discomfort and is sometimes accompanied by vomiting. It may stop as suddenly as it started.

CHOLELITHIASIS

SYMPTOMS:
Often asymptomatic. In some cases, sharp pain under the sternum.

TREATMENT:
Analgesics, antibiotics, removal of the gallbladder.

PREVENTION:
Avoiding overindulging and drastic weight-loss diets.

PANCREATITIS

Pancreatitis is the **acute** or **chronic inflammation** of the pancreas. It is marked by intense pain in the mid and upper abdomen, radiating out to the sides and the back, in some cases accompanied by vomiting and bloating. In chronic pancreatitis, the symptoms may be less pronounced and appear some time after onset.

ACUTE PANCREATITIS

The leading causes of acute pancreatitis are cholelithiasis and alcoholism. Less frequently, it may be a complication arising after a surgical operation of the digestive system. In most cases, pancreatitis is restricted to the occurrence of an edema. More rarely, it can lead to the gradual destruction of the pancreas, which may, depending on its severity, give rise to localized complications (digestive hemorrhage, cysts, or abscesses) or general complications (respiratory failure, kidney failure, or state of shock). Treatment of acute pancreatitis consists in relieving the pain and feeding the patient intravenously. The cause of the pancreatitis must be treated: withdrawal of alcohol from the diet, cholecystectomy (removal of the gallbladder), etc.

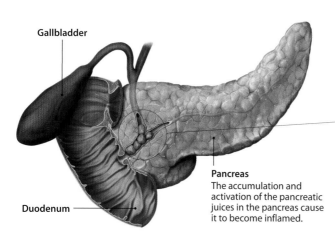

Gallbladder

Common bile duct

Pancreatic duct
Obstruction of the pancreatic duct prevents the ejection of pancreatic juices into the duodenum.

Pancreas
The accumulation and activation of the pancreatic juices in the pancreas cause it to become inflamed.

Duodenum

Gallstone
Gallstones from the gallbladder can obstruct the common bile duct and the pancreatic duct.

Acute pancreatitis caused by cholelithiasis

CHRONIC PANCREATITIS

Chronic pancreatitis, most often caused by alcoholism, is characterized by the gradual, irreversible destruction of the pancreas. Dysfunction of the pancreas results in poor assimilation of food, due to lack of pancreatic juices, physically expressed as weight loss and soft, foul-smelling, oily stool. The endocrine function of the pancreas is also affected, usually leading to diabetes. Treatment of chronic pancreatitis aims to relieve pain and to counterbalance the dysfunction of the pancreas via supplements in digestive enzymes and in insulin (in the case of diabetes). Chronic pancreatitis in children is usually caused by cystic fibrosis.

PANCREATITIS

SYMPTOMS:
Acute form: intense pain in the mid and upper abdomen, radiating out to the sides and the back, more pronounced after meals, accompanied by bloating and vomiting. Chronic form: weight loss; soft, foul-smelling, oily stool; abdominal and back pain.

TREATMENT:
Acute form: strict fasting, hydration, treatment of the cause, stomach tube to relieve the patient. Chronic form: enzyme supplements, insulin (in the case of diabetes). Surgical treatment is possible.

PREVENTION:
Avoiding excessive alcohol intake.

PANCREATIC CANCER

Pancreatic cancer is a rare, malignant tumor caused by a **chronic inflammation** of the pancreas (chronic pancreatitis) and by smoking. It primarily affects men over 45 years of age. The disease, whose symptoms do not appear immediately, can be indicated by a pain in the upper abdomen or by yellow coloration of the skin and mucous membranes (icterus) frequently accompanied by itching, or by the emission of dark urine and light-colored stool. These symptoms are often accompanied by other, less specific signs: weight loss, diarrhea, digestive hemorrhage, swelling of the abdomen (ascites), diabetes, and depression. The most effective treatment of pancreatic cancer is the surgical removal of the tumor, but this operation is delicate and may be impossible in some cases. Pancreatic cancer entails a generally negative prognosis.

Cancer... page 55

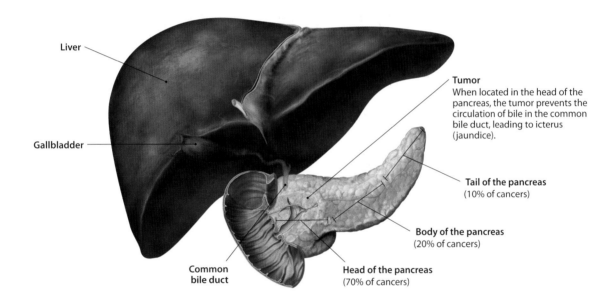

Liver

Gallbladder

Common
bile duct

Tumor
When located in the head of the pancreas, the tumor prevents the circulation of bile in the common bile duct, leading to icterus (jaundice).

Tail of the pancreas
(10% of cancers)

Body of the pancreas
(20% of cancers)

Head of the pancreas
(70% of cancers)

INSULINOMA

Insulinoma is a rare, typically benign tumor of the endocrine tissues of the pancreas. It causes an excessive secretion of insulin, resulting in hypoglycemia, which leads to various disorders: impaired vision, palpitations, perspiration, weakness, dizziness, confusion, shaking, and loss of consciousness. These symptoms occur mainly between meals and disappear rapidly after ingesting sugar. Treatment of insulinoma consists in surgically removing the tumor or, if this is not possible, inhibiting the production of insulin by means of medication.

PANCREATIC CANCER

SYMPTOMS:
Icterus (jaundice), pain in the upper abdomen, deterioration of the general state of health (weight loss, loss of appetite, significant weakness).

TREATMENT:
Surgical removal of the tumor (possible in 20% of cases), radiotherapy, chemotherapy.

PREVENTION:
Abstinence from smoking and avoiding excessive alcohol intake.

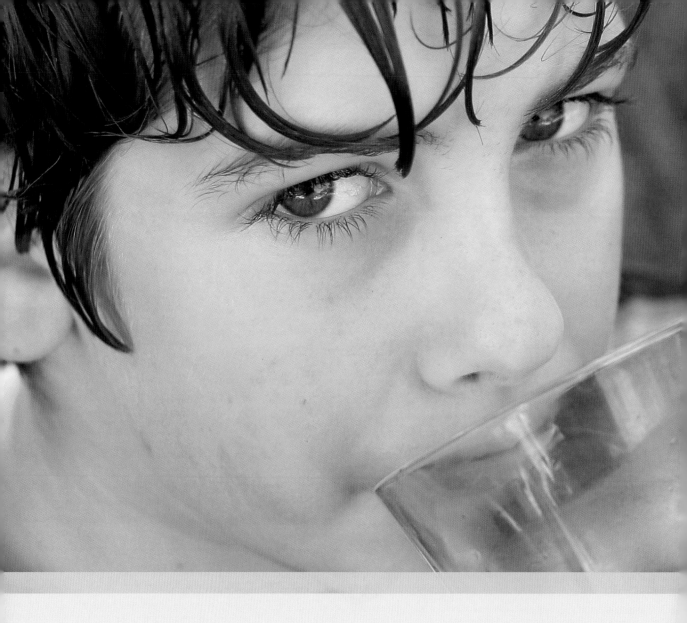

THE **URINARY SYSTEM**

The urinary system includes all of the body's organs that produce, circulate, store, and eliminate urine. It connects to the circulatory system at the kidneys. The kidneys filter the blood to remove the body's waste and any excess water and to balance the mineral salt levels in our bodies. The product of this filtration—urine—is temporarily stored in the bladder before being eliminated during micturition (urination).

The urinary system can be the site of various disorders, such as urinary tract **infection**, kidney stones, and incontinence. Without treatment, some of these ailments can dangerously alter the functioning of the kidneys, which can have serious health consequences. However, the body can function with a single healthy kidney and, today, treatments such as kidney dialysis and kidney transplants allow people suffering from kidney failure to lead virtually normal lives.

HOW THE **URINARY SYSTEM WORKS**

The nutrients obtained from food, and the waste produced by the functioning of the cells, travel through our bodies, mixed with water, which accounts for 60% of our total weight. This water circulates through the body, primarily via the blood, whose composition is regulated by the urinary system, which eliminates certain substances in the form of urine. The main organs of the urinary system are the kidneys, which filter the blood and produce urine, and the bladder, which stores the urine until it is eliminated via the urethra.

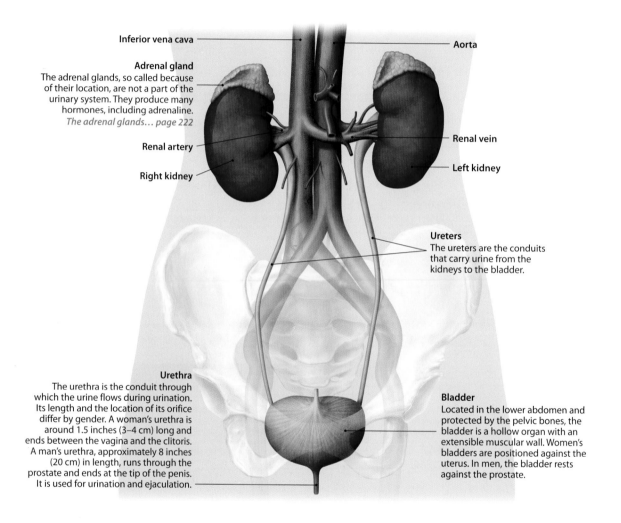

Inferior vena cava

Aorta

Adrenal gland
The adrenal glands, so called because of their location, are not a part of the urinary system. They produce many hormones, including adrenaline.
The adrenal glands... page 222

Renal artery

Renal vein

Right kidney

Left kidney

Ureters
The ureters are the conduits that carry urine from the kidneys to the bladder.

Urethra
The urethra is the conduit through which the urine flows during urination. Its length and the location of its orifice differ by gender. A woman's urethra is around 1.5 inches (3–4 cm) long and ends between the vagina and the clitoris. A man's urethra, approximately 8 inches (20 cm) in length, runs through the prostate and ends at the tip of the penis. It is used for urination and ejaculation.

Bladder
Located in the lower abdomen and protected by the pelvic bones, the bladder is a hollow organ with an extensible muscular wall. Women's bladders are positioned against the uterus. In men, the bladder rests against the prostate.

1. Blood filtration
Contaminated blood enters the kidneys through the renal arteries. It is then filtered in several stages, ending with the production of clean blood and urine. Urine is composed of water, waste, and mineral salts.

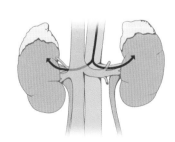

2. Waste elimination
The clean blood returns to the bloodstream via the renal veins, while the urine flows through the ureters to the bladder, where it is temporarily stored before being eliminated during micturition (urination).

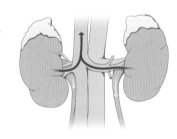

THE **KIDNEYS**

Located at the back of the abdomen, level with the first lumbar vertebra, the two kidneys are shaped like beans. They are dark red and roughly 4.5 inches (12 cm) long. Their primary function is to produce urine by filtering the blood. All of the body's blood is filtered every 45 minutes, but just 1 to 4 pints (0.5 to 2 liters) of urine are eliminated daily, because most of the filtrate is reabsorbed into the bloodstream. The kidneys are vital organs, but one kidney alone can meet the body's needs.

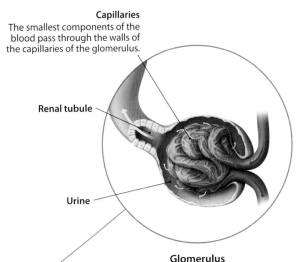

Capillaries
The smallest components of the blood pass through the walls of the capillaries of the glomerulus.

Renal tubule

Urine

Glomerulus
The glomerulus filters the blood, allowing the smaller molecules (water, mineral salts, glucose, etc.) to pass into the renal tubule. The larger molecules, like proteins, remain in the blood.

Arteriole
The blood is carried into the glomerulus by an arteriole stemming from the renal artery.

Renal tubule
The renal tubule carries the urine to the collecting tubule. During this transit, part of the substances contained in the urine is reabsorbed by the capillaries.

Collecting tubule
The collecting tubule gathers the urine produced by multiple nephrons.

Glomerulus

Capillaries

Urine

Renal cortex
The renal cortex is the outer part of the kidney, where the blood is filtered by the nephrons.

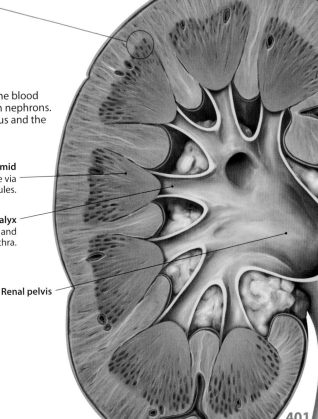

Nephron
Nephrons are the functional units of the kidneys, filtering the blood and producing urine. Each kidney contains around one million nephrons. A nephron is composed of two main elements: the glomerulus and the renal tubule.

Renal pyramid
The renal pyramid collects urine via several thousand collecting tubules.

Calyx
Each calyx gathers urine from the collecting tubules and directs it towards the renal pelvis of the urethra.

Renal pelvis

URINE PRODUCTION

The urinary system produces an average of 12,000 gallons (approx. 45,000 liters) of urine over a lifetime, enough to fill a swimming pool 16 feet (5 meters) in diameter and 6 feet (1.8 meters) deep.

401

URINATION

Urination, or micturition, is the elimination of the urine stored in the bladder. The bladder can contain up to 1 pint of urine (0.5 liter), but the need to urinate is a reflex that is triggered as soon as the bladder is half full. Urination may be voluntarily deferred for a certain amount of time, but the reflex will continue to assert itself, becoming more and more difficult to control.

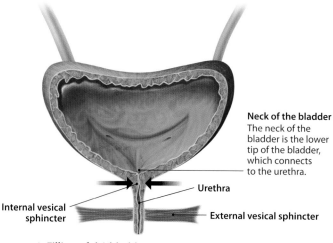

Neck of the bladder
The neck of the bladder is the lower tip of the bladder, which connects to the urethra.

Urethra

Internal vesical sphincter

External vesical sphincter

1. Filling of the bladder

The vesical sphincters are muscles running around the neck of the bladder and the urethra. Between urinations, these sphincters contract to prevent the leakage of urine.

Bladder

Detrusor muscle
The detrusor is the muscle that forms the wall of the bladder.

Internal vesical sphincter

External vesical sphincter

Urethra

2. Retention of urine

When the bladder fills, the stretching of its walls triggers the reflexive contraction of the detrusor urinal muscle and the involuntary relaxation of the internal vesical sphincter. Urination is delayed by intentionally contracting the external vesical sphincter. The contractions will then stop temporarily.

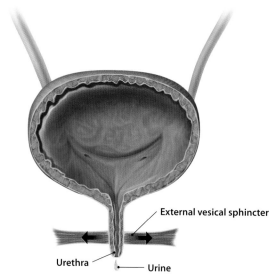

External vesical sphincter

Urethra

Urine

3. Urine emission

Filling of the bladder continues and the reflex to urinate is triggered again. Voluntary relaxation of the external vesical sphincter leads to the elimination of urine via the urethra at the desired time.

URINE

Usually pale yellow, clear, and with a slight odor, urine is 95% water, containing various dissolved organic substances (urea, creatinine, uric acid, vitamins, hormones, etc.) and minerals (sodium, potassium, calcium, etc.). In a healthy person, it has no or little content in proteins, glucose, blood cells, and hemoglobin. It is usually germ-free, and the presence of bacteria is a sign of a urinary tract infection. Any change in the appearance of the urine (color, odor, or clarity) may be an indication of a urinary tract illness. However, some medications and certain foods, such as beets and asparagus, can color or change the odor of urine without any repercussions on the person's health.

EXAMINATIONS OF THE URINARY SYSTEM

In the case of disorders of the urinary system, different methods, such as medical imagery and **biopsy**, are used to establish a diagnosis. However, the basic examination to evaluate the urinary function remains the urine test, which can also provide information on other diseases, such as diabetes.

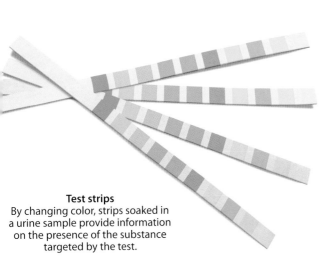

Test strips
By changing color, strips soaked in a urine sample provide information on the presence of the substance targeted by the test.

URINE TESTS

Urine tests can detect a number of diseases, particularly those of the urinary system, by recognizing and measuring each of the components of the urine. They are also performed in contexts other than the diagnosis of an illness (e.g. to confirm a pregnancy or to check for the absorption of illicit substances). The level of analysis may vary from a simple qualitative test using colored strips (pregnancy tests) to precise measurements performed in a laboratory. This second group of tests includes the urine culture, which is used to count the blood cells present in the urine and to identify the germs responsible for an infection. The presence of red blood cells in the urine may be a sign of certain diseases: cystitis, urolithiasis, glomerulonephritis, polycystic kidney, or bladder cancer.

CYSTOSCOPY

The inside of the bladder can be examined to search for a tumor or other lesion. This visual examination is called a cystoscopy. It consists in introducing a thin, supple, or rigid tube containing an optical system and lighting via the urethra. This uncomfortable but painless examination is quick and performed under local anesthesia. The bladder is engorged with sterile water so as to open out its walls for observation. After cystoscopy, the patient may feel a frequent need to urinate and/or a burning sensation for two to three days. These disturbances disappear more quickly when the person drinks and urinates frequently.

Urinary system tumors… page 411

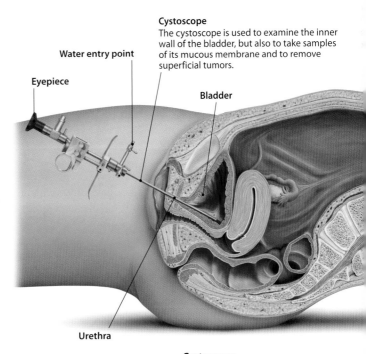

Cystoscope
The cystoscope is used to examine the inner wall of the bladder, but also to take samples of its mucous membrane and to remove superficial tumors.

Water entry point

Eyepiece

Bladder

Urethra

Cystoscopy

URINARY INCONTINENCE

Urinary incontinence is the involuntary leakage of urine. There are several types of urinary incontinence, of which the two most common are effort incontinence and hyperactive bladder. These may have different causes, such as weakening of the muscles that control the bladder, genital prolapse, neurological disorders, or physical **trauma**. Incontinence is not to be confused with nocturnal urination, or enuresis, in children, which is a passing disorder.

Enuresis... page 178
Genital prolapse... page 433

EFFORT INCONTINENCE

Effort incontinence is the most common form of incontinence. It is caused by the contraction of the abdominal muscles, which is caused by sneezing, coughing, bursts of laughter, or muscular effort. This is due to a weakening of the perineum (pelvic floor, which extends from the anus to the genitals), particularly the external vesical sphincter. Promoted by numerous pregnancies or difficult deliveries, effort incontinence is most common in older women.

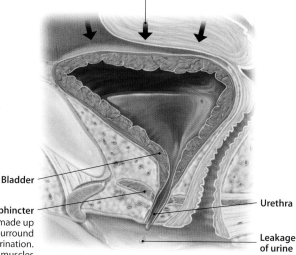

Abdominal contraction
Abdominal muscle contraction (sneezing, cough, etc.) leads to compression of the bladder.

Bladder

External vesical sphincter
The external vesical sphincter is made up of the muscles of the perineum that surround the urethra and allow the voluntary delay of urination. When they are weakened, these muscles let a small quantity of urine escape.

Urethra

Leakage of urine

Effort incontinence

HYPERACTIVE BLADDER

Hyperactive bladder causes uncontrollable, sometimes copious, urination. It is caused by involuntary contractions—often of unknown origin—of the bladder muscle, which can be the result of a lesion of the nervous system, a fracture of the pelvis or an infection of the bladder or urethra.

Urinary tract infections... page 406

URINARY INCONTINENCE

SYMPTOMS:
Effort incontinence: limited leakage of urine during abdominal muscle contractions.
Hyperactive bladder: sudden and uncontrollable need to urinate.

TREATMENT:
Effort incontinence: retraining of the perineum muscles often yields good results.
Hyperactive bladder: treatment of the cause is essential.

PREVENTION:
Limit diuretic drinks (coffee, tea), sugar, and alcohol, which irritate the bladder; drink plenty of water; fight constipation; do not hold in urine. Muscle exercises of the external vesical sphincter and the perineum.

PREVENTING URINARY INCONTINENCE

■ **AVOID EXTREME EFFORT**

Favor light sports and activity, particularly during and after pregnancy.

■ **STRENGTHEN THE MUSCLES OF THE PELVIC FLOOR**

The strengthening of the perineum and the external vesical sphincter with specific exercises makes it possible to better support the bladder and reduce the urgency and frequency of urinations. Kegel exercises consist of contracting these muscles for 10 seconds and relaxing them for a few seconds, for 10–20 repetitions, at least 6 times a day. To learn which muscles to contract, stop the urination several times in a row, without contracting the muscles of the abdomen, buttocks, or thighs.

■ **AVOID IRRITATING AND DIURETIC FOODS AND BEVERAGES**

Avoid diuretic foods and beverages, particularly those that contain caffeine, such as tea, coffee, chocolate, and carbonated soft drinks. Also limit the consumption of foods that are irritating to the bladder, such as alcohol, citrus, sugar, and sweeteners (artificial sugars).

■ **MAINTAIN A HEALTHY WEIGHT**

Excess weight increases pressure on the bladder and contributes to leakages of urine.

■ **PREVENT AND TREAT CONSTIPATION,**
URINARY TRACT INFECTIONS AND PROSTATE DISORDERS

Constipation promotes urine leakage by putting pressure on the bladder. To prevent this, consume foods that are rich in fiber, such as legumes, green vegetables, fruits, or whole grains. Treat urinary tract and prostate infections, which cause urgent needs to urinate.

Health of the digestive system... page 352

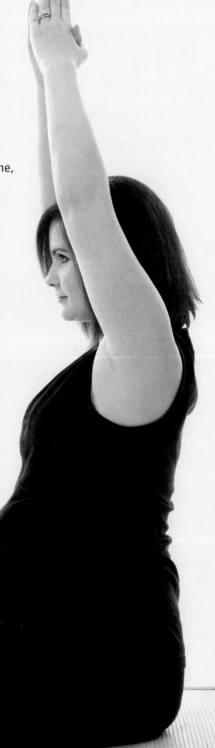

URINARY TRACT INFECTIONS

Bacteria may be introduced in the urinary tract and multiply, causing a urinary tract **infection**. The germ responsible is often *Escherichia coli*, a bacterium that is part of the normal intestinal flora. Contamination of the urinary tract may occur upon sexual relations, but may also be due to hygienic negligence, malformations of the urinary tract, or obstruction of urine flow (urinary stone, prostate adenoma, etc.). Urinary tract infections may also result from physiological changes that occur during pregnancy or may arise spontaneously in girls under 2 years of age.

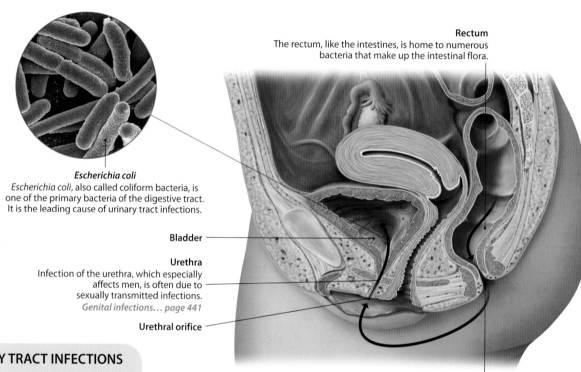

Rectum
The rectum, like the intestines, is home to numerous bacteria that make up the intestinal flora.

Escherichia coli
Escherichia coli, also called coliform bacteria, is one of the primary bacteria of the digestive tract. It is the leading cause of urinary tract infections.

Bladder

Urethra
Infection of the urethra, which especially affects men, is often due to sexually transmitted infections.
Genital infections... page 441

Urethral orifice

Anus

Cross section of lower urinary tracts in women
In women, urinary tract infections are often caused by the passing of bacteria from the rectum to the urethral orifice, then to the bladder.

URINARY TRACT INFECTIONS

SYMPTOMS:
Painful, urgent, and frequent urination; cloudy and smelly urine, containing blood. Pyelonephritis: back and abdominal pains near the affected kidney, high fever with chills.

TREATMENT:
Antibiotics and elimination of risk factors.

PREVENTION:
Proper hydration, frequent urination, good personal hygiene.

CYSTITIS

Bladder infection, or cystitis, is generally benign and relatively common. A woman's anatomy, characterized by the short length of the urethra and the proximity of the anus and the urethral orifice, makes her more susceptible to this type of infection. Cystitis notably entails painful, urgent, and frequent urination. A cytobacteriological analysis of the urine will recognize an infectious agent and antibiotic treatment will begin if a bacterium is detected. Cystitis can reoccur and, in the absence of treatment, the infection can spread to the kidneys.

Urine analysis... page 403

PYELONEPHRITIS

Pyelonephritis is a kidney infection. In its acute form, it often follows cystitis when the bacteria present in the bladder ascend the ureters to reach the kidneys. The slowing down of the urinary flow, caused by the presence of a urinary stone or malformation, also promotes the multiplication of bacteria in the bladder and their ascent to the kidneys. Chronic pyelonephritis, which is more rare and develops slowly, may lead to kidney atrophy and kidney failure.

Kidney failure... page 412

PREVENTING URINARY TRACT INFECTIONS

Here is some advice for preventing urinary tract infections and their recurrence.

■ DRINK SUFFICIENTLY

Drink 1½ to 2 quarts (1.4 to 1.9 liters) of water every day. Berry-based juices, such as cranberry juice, are also recommended to prevent the recurrence of urinary tract infections.

■ URINATE AS SOON AS YOU FEEL THE URGE

Retaining urine promotes the proliferation of germs.

■ MAINTAIN PROPER PERSONAL HYGIENE

Regularly wash the anal and vulvar regions, but not excessively. Avoid vaginal douching as well as irritating soaps and cosmetic products (deodorants, bath products, etc.). After defecation, wipe from front to back and wash your hands with soap and water.

■ WEAR PROPER CLOTHING

Avoid overly tight clothing and synthetic undergarments, which promote perspiration and the proliferation of germs. Change undergarments regularly.

■ URINATE AFTER SEXUAL RELATIONS

Urinate after each sexual encounter to eliminate certain germs.

■ FIGHT CONSTIPATION

Treat or prevent constipation to avoid the proliferation and propagation of bacteria towards the urethra. Fibers contained in foods such as legumes, green vegetables, fruits, or whole grains encourage proper functioning of the intestines.

■ DO NOT HESITATE TO CONSULT A DOCTOR

Avoid self-medication that may mask symptoms of more serious illnesses and consult a doctor, particularly in the event of recurrence of the infection.

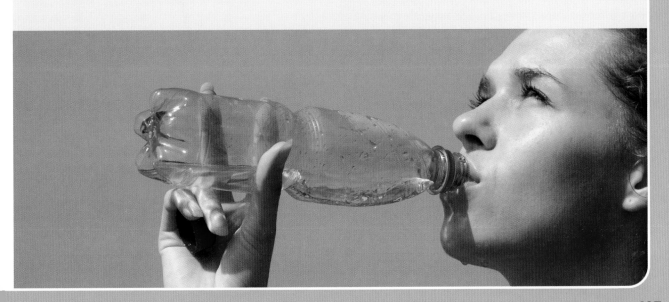

UROLITHIASIS

Small stones, or calculi, may form in the organs or urinary tract and cause urolithiasis. Most often, the stones measure less than ¼ inch (5 mm) in diameter and are eliminated spontaneously by natural means. Sometimes, a larger stone may obstruct a ureter and cause intense pain in the lumbar region, called nephritic colic. The stone must therefore be removed immediately to alleviate the pain and avoid complications. The presence of these stones in the ureter or kidneys may promote the development of pyelonephritis (kidney **infection**).

Urinary tract infections... page 406

RENAL CALCULI

Certain substances contained in urine may form crystals that gather together to form renal calculi. Most often it is calcium, phosphate, or uric acid. Their crystallization is promoted by a lack of hydration or a diet rich in dairy products. The formation of stones is also promoted by repeated urinary tract infections, metabolism disorders (hypercalciuria), and, in men, the slowing of urine flow due to a malformation or prostate adenoma.

Prostate adenoma... page 429

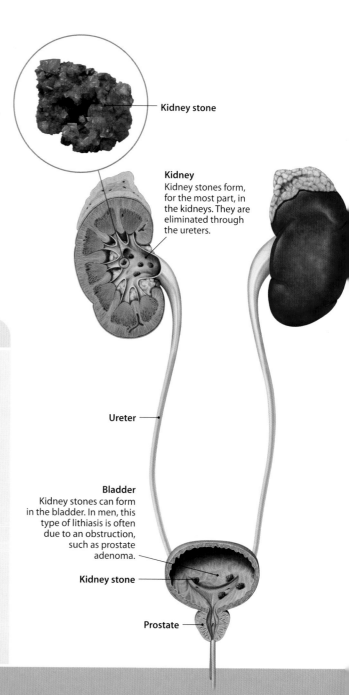

Kidney stone

Kidney
Kidney stones form, for the most part, in the kidneys. They are eliminated through the ureters.

Ureter

Bladder
Kidney stones can form in the bladder. In men, this type of lithiasis is often due to an obstruction, such as prostate adenoma.

Kidney stone

Prostate

UROLITHIASIS

SYMPTOMS:
Presence of blood in urine, pain and burning sensation when urinating, false desire to urinate, nephritic colic (intense pain in the lumbar region) in the event of stone blockage in the ureter. Small stones often do not present any symptoms.

TREATMENT:
Analgesics, anti-inflammatories, medications capable of dissolving certain types of stones, lithotripsy, surgical endoscopy, open surgery. Absorption of alkaline mineral water promotes the dissolution of uric acid stones.

PREVENTION:
Treatment of the cause helps to prevent recurrences. Proper hydration, adapted diet.

LITHOTRIPSY

Lithotripsy is a treatment for kidney stones that consists of fragmenting or pulverizing the stones with forceps, ultrasounds, shock waves, or laser ray. Extracorporeal lithotripsy is the most common and least traumatizing treatment. It consists of emitting shock waves in the direction of the stone, without surgical intervention, to reduce them into fragments that are then eliminated naturally with urine.

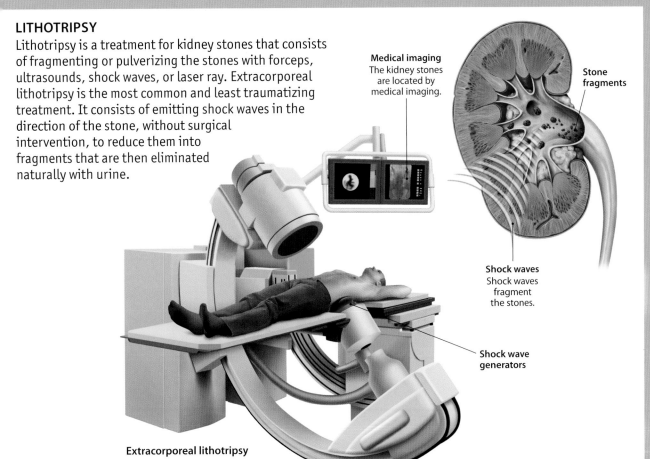

Medical imaging
The kidney stones are located by medical imaging.

Stone fragments

Shock waves
Shock waves fragment the stones.

Shock wave generators

Extracorporeal lithotripsy

PREVENTING KIDNEY STONES

Kidney stones have the tendency to recur. Here is some preventative advice, particularly for people who have already suffered from this problem.

■ STAY HYDRATED

Proper hydration is the primary recommendation to follow to avoid the formation of kidney stones. Drink more than 2 quarts (1.9 liters) of liquid (at least 10 glasses) every day, spread out throughout the day and night, and increase the amount in the event of significant perspiration due to heat or physical exercise. Drink water and limit alcoholic and sugary drinks.

■ ADAPT YOUR DIET

If you have already suffered from calcium oxalate stones, do not surpass the daily recommendation of 800 to 1000 mg of calcium and avoid food rich in oxalate, like chocolate, tea, and leeks. Also abstain from consuming large quantities of Vitamin C (4 g and more per day). Fruits and vegetables rich in potassium, such as unpeeled potatoes, cantaloupes, avocados, lima beans, and bananas are beneficial in preventing stones.

■ CONSULT A DOCTOR

After having analyzed the type of stone that you are predisposed to, a doctor can prescribe the appropriate medical treatment.

GLOMERULONEPHRITIS

Glomerulonephritis is an **inflammation** of the renal glomeruli. The **acute** form is often a complication of a streptococcus **infection**. It especially affects children, but is easily cured in most cases. **Chronic** glomerulonephritis, which may be primary (limited to the kidneys) or secondary (consecutive to another disease such as diabetes or lupus), may lead to kidney failure. It is shown by an elevated level of proteins in the urine, a low level of albumin in the blood, and edema.

Sore throat... page 319
Kidneys... page 401

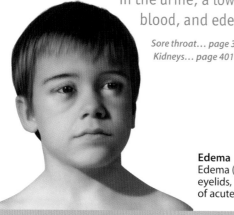

Edema
Edema (swelling) of the face, particularly the eyelids, is one of the more visible symptoms of acute glomerulonephritis.

GLOMERULONEPHRITIS

SYMPTOMS:
Edema, dark urine that is foamy and not copious, lumbar pains, headaches, vomiting.

TREATMENT:
Antibiotics (to eliminate the streptococcus that triggered the inflammation), salt-free diet, diuretics, corticosteroids, immunosuppressants, anticoagulants (to prevent complications).

KIDNEY CYSTS

Often associated with aging, isolated cysts on a kidney are generally benign and asymptomatic. On the other hand, multiple cysts that are present on both kidneys are the sign of a more serious condition: polycystic kidney disease. This hereditary disease affects 1 in 1000 people in Western countries. The recessive form of the disease, transmitted by both parents, appears from childhood, even before birth, and interferes with the development of the kidneys and liver. The dominant form, transmitted by only one parent, appears habitually after 40 years of age. The cysts develop progressively and, little by little, affect the functioning of the kidneys, which can lead to kidney failure. They can also affect other organs, such as the liver or brain.

Heredity... page 50
Cysts... page 52

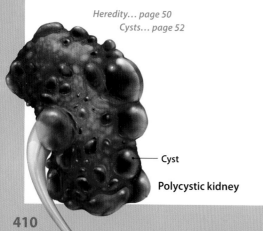

Cyst

Polycystic kidney

KIDNEY CYSTS

SYMPTOMS:
Simple cyst: mostly asymptomatic. Polycystic kidney disease: arterial hypertension, sometimes abdominal pain, and presence of blood in urine.

TREATMENT:
Simple cyst: generally none. Monitoring in the event of abnormal aspect (possibility of tumor).
Polycystic kidney disease: decrease in arterial pressure, puncture of cysts, dialysis, kidney graft.

PREVENTION:
Polycystic kidney disease: screening of family members of the afflicted person.

URINARY SYSTEM TUMORS

Tumors of the urinary system often affect the bladder and, less often, the kidneys. Smoking is recognized as being one of the main causes of these diseases. Obesity, exposure to certain chemical substances, and **chronic** cystitis are also significant risk factors.

Cancer... page 55

KIDNEY CANCER

Kidney cancer is a rare disease that develops slowly before producing metastases in the bones, lungs and liver. Asymptomatic at first, the tumor is often discovered by accident, during an ultrasound or abdominal scan. As long as it does not produce metastases, it can be treated effectively by total or partial ablation of the affected kidney. When the metastases appear, anticancerous treatments are necessary but their efficiency is limited.

BLADDER TUMORS

Bladder tumors originate in the mucous membrane that covers the inside of the bladder. They are often distinguished by the presence of blood in the urine. Malignant bladder tumors must be surgically treated by bladder ablation and the implantation of a replacement bladder. Superficial tumors are generally benign and can be removed by cystoscopy.

Examinations of the urinary system... page 403

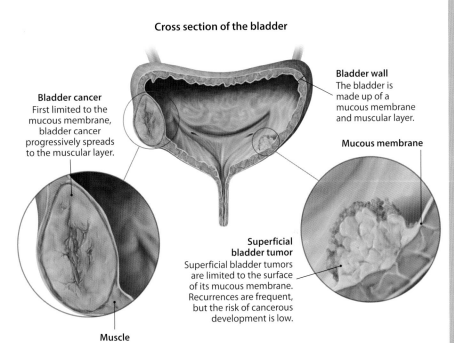

Cross section of the bladder

Bladder wall
The bladder is made up of a mucous membrane and muscular layer.

Bladder cancer
First limited to the mucous membrane, bladder cancer progressively spreads to the muscular layer.

Mucous membrane

Superficial bladder tumor
Superficial bladder tumors are limited to the surface of its mucous membrane. Recurrences are frequent, but the risk of cancerous development is low.

Muscle

URINARY SYSTEM TUMORS

SYMPTOMS:
Presence of blood in the urine, sometimes pain.

TREATMENT:
Surgery, radiation therapy, chemotherapy, medications preventing the formation and dissemination of cancerous cells (antiangiogenics), immunotherapy in the event of metastases.

PREVENTION:
Limiting risk factors: smoking (which multiplies the risk fourfold), prolonged exposure to toxic products (ink, paint), chronic cystitis.

KIDNEY FAILURE

Kidney failure is the decrease or loss of the kidneys' capacity to fulfill their function of filtering and eliminating waste from the blood. It is a serious issue that may lead to death if it is not treated quickly. In its **acute** form, the failure appears suddenly, when the kidneys stop working following a fall in arterial pressure, poisoning, **infection**, presence of an obstruction (urinary stone, tumor), or even glomerulonephritis. Recovery generally does not leave sequelae. **Chronic** kidney failure begins progressively and irreversibly. It can be the result of acute kidney failure or any other form of kidney disease. Kidney failure must be treated quickly by dialysis (**hemodialysis**, peritoneal dialysis) or a kidney graft.

HEMODIALYSIS

Hemodialysis consists of diverting the blood outside of the cardiovascular network, purifying it through an artificial membrane located outside the body, then reintroducing it into the blood system. Blood purification is completed by a dialyzer, or artificial kidney, that absorbs waste from the blood. Hemodialysis can be prescribed for the short term in the event of acute kidney failure or for the long term in the event of chronic kidney failure. A hemodialysis session is completed in the hospital, in a specialized center, or at home. It lasts from four to five hours and, in the event of chronic kidney failure, it must be carried out at least three times per week.

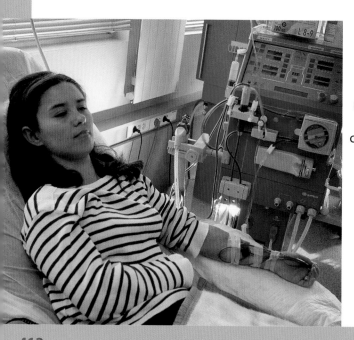

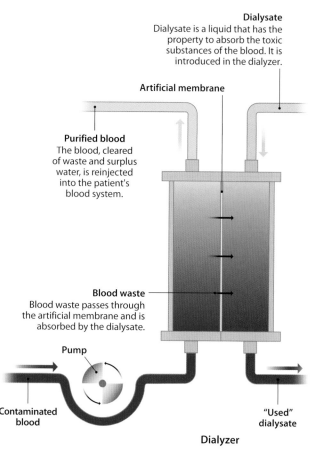

Dialysate
Dialysate is a liquid that has the property to absorb the toxic substances of the blood. It is introduced in the dialyzer.

Artificial membrane

Purified blood
The blood, cleared of waste and surplus water, is reinjected into the patient's blood system.

Blood waste
Blood waste passes through the artificial membrane and is absorbed by the dialysate.

Pump

Contaminated blood

"Used" dialysate

Dialyzer

PERITONEAL DIALYSIS

Peritoneal dialysis consists in filtering the blood through a membrane naturally present inside the abdomen, the peritoneum. The dialysate, identical to the one used for hemodialysis, is introduced in the abdominal cavity by a small tube implanted through the skin. During the hours that follow, the dialysate absorbs the blood waste issued from numerous small blood vessels of the peritoneum. Four times per day, the patient must eliminate the "used" dialysate and reintroduce a new dialysate, which may be completed manually during the day or automatically during the night. Peritoneal dialysis is less aggressive for the body than hemodialysis and it does not immobilize the patient, who may attend to their daily routines.

KIDNEY GRAFT

When both kidneys stop functioning, a kidney graft may provide an alternative to dialysis to treat kidney failure. The healthy kidney, removed from a deceased or living donor, is implanted below the sick kidney to facilitate the operation. After the operation, performed under general anesthesia, the patient must remain in the hospital for about two weeks. Taking immunosuppressants, which must be taken for life, helps to prevent rejection of the new organ by the immune system.

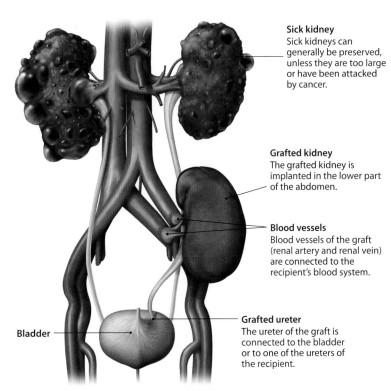

Sick kidney
Sick kidneys can generally be preserved, unless they are too large or have been attacked by cancer.

Grafted kidney
The grafted kidney is implanted in the lower part of the abdomen.

Blood vessels
Blood vessels of the graft (renal artery and renal vein) are connected to the recipient's blood system.

Grafted ureter
The ureter of the graft is connected to the bladder or to one of the ureters of the recipient.

Bladder

KIDNEY FAILURE

SYMPTOMS:
Nausea, vomiting, significant fatigue, lumbar pains, thirst in chronic cases, frequent or rare urination (depending on the cause of the failure).

TREATMENT:
Acute kidney failure: treatment of the cause, temporary dialysis. Chronic kidney failure: low protein and low salt diet, medication to lower arterial pressure (antihypertensors). Advanced stage: dialysis and kidney graft.

PREVENTION:
Treatment of kidney diseases.

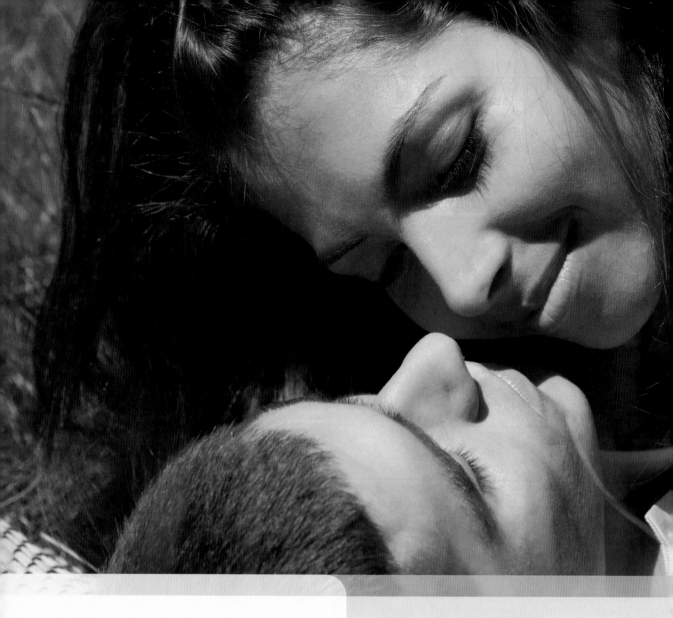

THE **REPRODUCTIVE SYSTEM**

Conceiving a child is the result of an elaborate process undertaken by the genital organs, which make up the reproductive system. Different in men and women, these organs that are both internal and external are present from birth, but they do not become able to fulfill their functions until puberty, when they reach maturity. In women, the fertility period, regulated by ovarian and menstrual cycles, ends with menopause. Men remain fertile their entire lives.

The genital organs are subject to numerous **infections**. Several may be transmitted sexually (sexually transmitted diseases). They can cause **inflammation** of the affected organs and may result in sterility. Genital organs may be affected with other illnesses, like malformations or tumors.

THE **GENITAL ORGANS**

The reproductive system is made up of organs that ensure reproductive functions. Differing between the sexes, the genital organs comprise the gonads (testicles, ovaries), other sexual glands (prostate, seminal vesicles, Cowper's glands, Bartholin glands), genital canals (vasa deferentia, uterus, fallopian tubes, vagina), and the external organs (penis, vulva). The genital organs must reach maturity during puberty to fulfill their reproductive functions. This is possible due to, notably, the production of sex cells (sperm cells and ova), whose unique character guarantees the diversity of human beings.

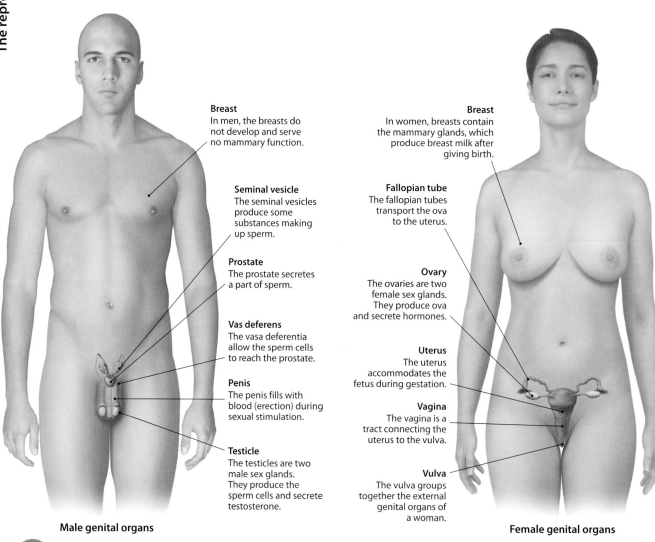

Breast
In men, the breasts do not develop and serve no mammary function.

Seminal vesicle
The seminal vesicles produce some substances making up sperm.

Prostate
The prostate secretes a part of sperm.

Vas deferens
The vasa deferentia allow the sperm cells to reach the prostate.

Penis
The penis fills with blood (erection) during sexual stimulation.

Testicle
The testicles are two male sex glands. They produce the sperm cells and secrete testosterone.

Male genital organs

Breast
In women, breasts contain the mammary glands, which produce breast milk after giving birth.

Fallopian tube
The fallopian tubes transport the ova to the uterus.

Ovary
The ovaries are two female sex glands. They produce ova and secrete hormones.

Uterus
The uterus accommodates the fetus during gestation.

Vagina
The vagina is a tract connecting the uterus to the vulva.

Vulva
The vulva groups together the external genital organs of a woman.

Female genital organs

MILLIONS OF SPERM CELLS AND SEVERAL HUNDRED OVA

Starting from puberty, the testicles of a man produce from 100 to 400 million sperm cells per day. In contrast, of the hundreds of thousands of oocytes contained in the ovaries at birth, only approximately 400 will transform into ova during a woman's adult life.

MALE GENITAL ORGANS

The genital organs that make up the male reproductive system ensure the sexual and endocrine functions. Some are located outside of the body, like the testicles. They are contained in the scrotum (or bursa), whose dense skin supports and protects them. Also external, the penis is traversed by the urethra and ends with the glans. It is made up of three cylindrical parts: the urethra, the cavernous body, and the spongy body. When not sexually stimulated, it is soft and hangs in front of the scrotum. Sexual stimulation provokes blood flow into the penis, leading to an erection, and then to ejaculation, the expulsion of sperm through the urethra. The male internal glands (prostate, seminal vesicles, and Cowper's glands) secrete the seminal liquid that contains sperm cells and makes up sperm.

Endocrine glands and hormones... page 220

CONCEPTION REQUIRES COOLNESS

The testicles are located outside the body because the production of sperm cells can only be completed at a temperature approximately 3.5°F (2°C) below that of the body.

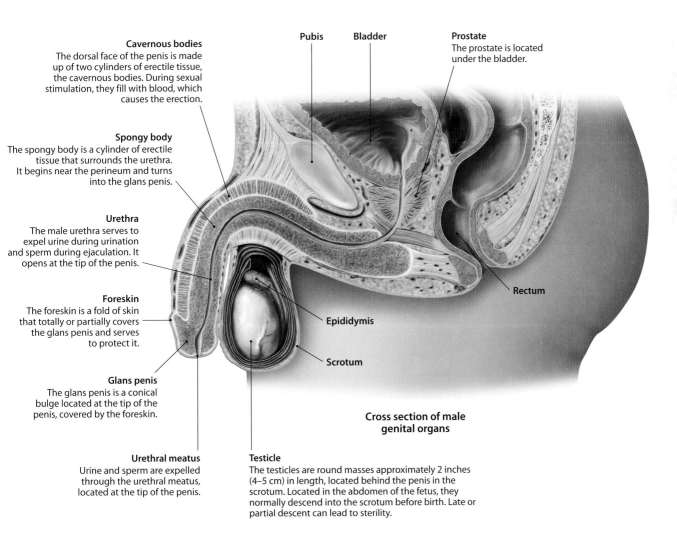

Cavernous bodies
The dorsal face of the penis is made up of two cylinders of erectile tissue, the cavernous bodies. During sexual stimulation, they fill with blood, which causes the erection.

Spongy body
The spongy body is a cylinder of erectile tissue that surrounds the urethra. It begins near the perineum and turns into the glans penis.

Urethra
The male urethra serves to expel urine during urination and sperm during ejaculation. It opens at the tip of the penis.

Foreskin
The foreskin is a fold of skin that totally or partially covers the glans penis and serves to protect it.

Glans penis
The glans penis is a conical bulge located at the tip of the penis, covered by the foreskin.

Urethral meatus
Urine and sperm are expelled through the urethral meatus, located at the tip of the penis.

Pubis

Bladder

Prostate
The prostate is located under the bladder.

Rectum

Epididymis

Scrotum

Cross section of male genital organs

Testicle
The testicles are round masses approximately 2 inches (4–5 cm) in length, located behind the penis in the scrotum. Located in the abdomen of the fetus, they normally descend into the scrotum before birth. Late or partial descent can lead to sterility.

TESTICLES

The testicle is both an exocrine and endocrine gland. Its exocrine activity consists of producing sperm cells, which are led from the testicle by a complex network of ducts (seminal tubes, epididymis, vas deferens). Testicular endocrine secretions (testosterone and other male hormones) come from the tissue located between the seminal tubes.

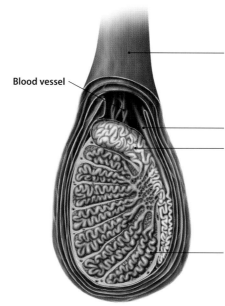

Blood vessel

Spermatic cord
The spermatic cord is a cylindrical envelope that connects the testicles to the abdominal cavity and contains the vas deferens, blood vessels, lymphatic vessels, and nerves.

Vas deferens

Epididymis
The epididymis is a long duct wound around itself, located above and behind the testicles. Sperm cells produced by the seminal tubes are stored there and reach maturity there, until ejaculation.

Seminal tube
The seminal tubes are small ducts located in the testicles. They produce sperm cells. These are then led to the epididymis.

Testicular cross section

SPERM

A white and slightly sticky liquid, sperm is composed of sperm cells (approximately 60 million per milliliter) and secretions, the seminal liquid. The latter contains chemical substances like mineral salts, sugars and proteins that, notably, protect the sperm cells and promote their movement.

Ejaculation… page 453

TESTOSTERONE

Testosterone is the primary male hormone. Primarily secreted by the testicles, it is notably responsible for the development of the genital organs, for the formation of sperm cells, and for secondary sexual characters. The adrenal glands, ovaries and placenta also secrete testosterone.

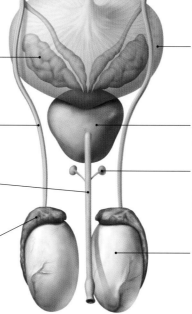

Seminal vesicle
Located above the prostate, behind the bladder, seminal vesicles are two male genital glands, the secretions of which form approximately 60% of sperm.

Vas deferens

Urethra
The male urethra serves to expel urine (miction) and sperm (ejaculation). It opens at the end of the penis.

Epididymis
The sperm cells stored in the epididymis are led to the prostate by the vas deferens during ejaculation.

Bladder

Prostate
The prostate surrounds the urethra and releases its secretions there, which compose about 30% of sperm.

Cowper's gland
The Cowper's glands are two male glands located under the prostate. They secrete part of the sperm into the urethra.

Testicle
The testicles are sexual glands that notably secrete testosterone and produce sperm cells. Once formed, the sperm cells are led to the epididymis.

Anterior view of male secreting ducts

FEMALE GENITAL ORGANS

The female genital system essentially comprises the internal organs (ovaries, fallopian tubes, uterus, vagina) located in the pelvic cavity, which is defined by the pelvic bones. The vulva represents all of the external female genital organs. Made up of the two labia majora partially covering the two labia minora, it protects the clitoris as well as the vaginal opening. Breasts are not genital organs, but they participate in reproduction by allowing breast-feeding and in sexuality by constituting an erogenous area.

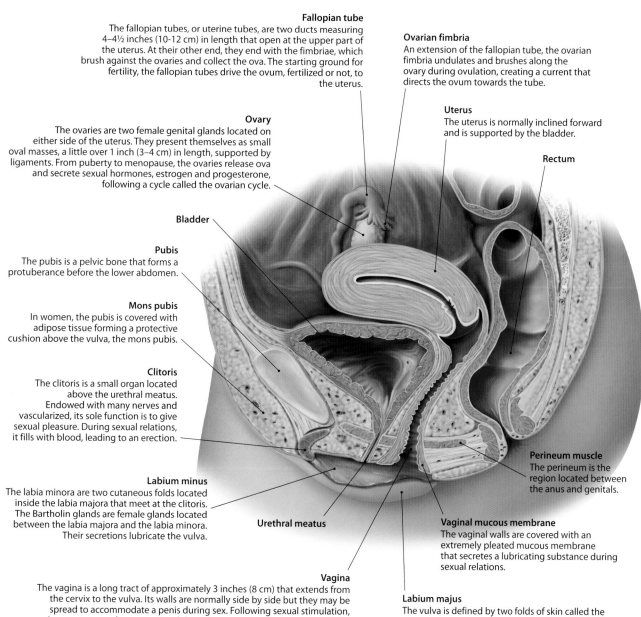

Fallopian tube
The fallopian tubes, or uterine tubes, are two ducts measuring 4–4½ inches (10-12 cm) in length that open at the upper part of the uterus. At their other end, they end with the fimbriae, which brush against the ovaries and collect the ova. The starting ground for fertility, the fallopian tubes drive the ovum, fertilized or not, to the uterus.

Ovarian fimbria
An extension of the fallopian tube, the ovarian fimbria undulates and brushes along the ovary during ovulation, creating a current that directs the ovum towards the tube.

Ovary
The ovaries are two female genital glands located on either side of the uterus. They present themselves as small oval masses, a little over 1 inch (3–4 cm) in length, supported by ligaments. From puberty to menopause, the ovaries release ova and secrete sexual hormones, estrogen and progesterone, following a cycle called the ovarian cycle.

Uterus
The uterus is normally inclined forward and is supported by the bladder.

Rectum

Bladder

Pubis
The pubis is a pelvic bone that forms a protuberance before the lower abdomen.

Mons pubis
In women, the pubis is covered with adipose tissue forming a protective cushion above the vulva, the mons pubis.

Clitoris
The clitoris is a small organ located above the urethral meatus. Endowed with many nerves and vascularized, its sole function is to give sexual pleasure. During sexual relations, it fills with blood, leading to an erection.

Perineum muscle
The perineum is the region located between the anus and genitals.

Labium minus
The labia minora are two cutaneous folds located inside the labia majora that meet at the clitoris. The Bartholin glands are female glands located between the labia majora and the labia minora. Their secretions lubricate the vulva.

Urethral meatus

Vaginal mucous membrane
The vaginal walls are covered with an extremely pleated mucous membrane that secretes a lubricating substance during sexual relations.

Vagina
The vagina is a long tract of approximately 3 inches (8 cm) that extends from the cervix to the vulva. Its walls are normally side by side but they may be spread to accommodate a penis during sex. Following sexual stimulation, its mucous membrane secretes lubricating substances and the upper part of the muscular wall dilates. It is through the vagina that blood flows during menstruation and that a baby passes through during delivery.

Labium majus
The vulva is defined by two folds of skin called the labia majora. Their internal face is covered with a mucous membrane and their external face has sweat glands, sebaceous glands, and pubic hair.

Cross section of the female genital system

THE UTERUS

The uterus is a hollow organ located between the bladder and the rectum in which the fetus develops during gestation. It is connected to the fallopian tubes and the vagina. The uterus is made up of a dense wall of smooth tissue, the myometrium, covered with a mucous membrane, the endometrium. Highly expandable, the uterus stretches during pregnancy to reach 30 times its initial size.

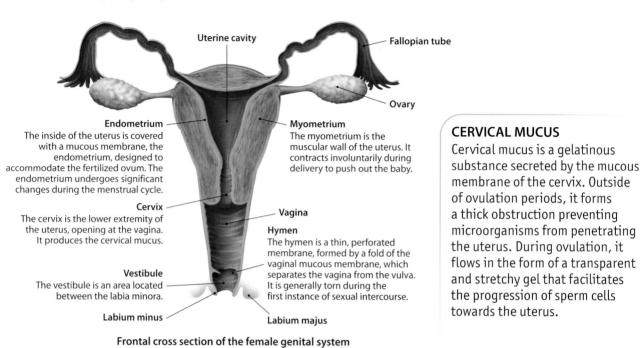

Uterine cavity

Fallopian tube

Ovary

Endometrium
The inside of the uterus is covered with a mucous membrane, the endometrium, designed to accommodate the fertilized ovum. The endometrium undergoes significant changes during the menstrual cycle.

Myometrium
The myometrium is the muscular wall of the uterus. It contracts involuntarily during delivery to push out the baby.

Cervix
The cervix is the lower extremity of the uterus, opening at the vagina. It produces the cervical mucus.

Vagina

Hymen
The hymen is a thin, perforated membrane, formed by a fold of the vaginal mucous membrane, which separates the vagina from the vulva. It is generally torn during the first instance of sexual intercourse.

Vestibule
The vestibule is an area located between the labia minora.

Labium minus

Labium majus

Frontal cross section of the female genital system

CERVICAL MUCUS

Cervical mucus is a gelatinous substance secreted by the mucous membrane of the cervix. Outside of ovulation periods, it forms a thick obstruction preventing microorganisms from penetrating the uterus. During ovulation, it flows in the form of a transparent and stretchy gel that facilitates the progression of sperm cells towards the uterus.

THE BREASTS

The breasts are two glandular organs rich in adipose tissue that cover the pectoral muscles. In women, each breast contains a mammary gland. Under the action of different hormones, these glands slowly increase in volume during the days preceding periods, while during pregnancy they develop considerably to prepare to produce milk for the newborn. They become atrophied at menopause. The nipples and the pigmented area surrounding them, the areola, are made up of muscular tissue that involuntarily contracts when exposed to cold or to sexual stimulation.

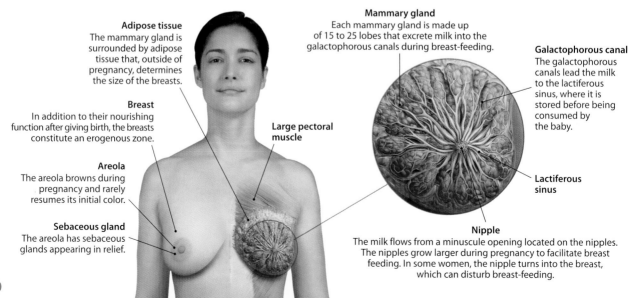

Adipose tissue
The mammary gland is surrounded by adipose tissue that, outside of pregnancy, determines the size of the breasts.

Mammary gland
Each mammary gland is made up of 15 to 25 lobes that excrete milk into the galactophorous canals during breast-feeding.

Galactophorous canal
The galactophorous canals lead the milk to the lactiferous sinus, where it is stored before being consumed by the baby.

Breast
In addition to their nourishing function after giving birth, the breasts constitute an erogenous zone.

Large pectoral muscle

Areola
The areola browns during pregnancy and rarely resumes its initial color.

Lactiferous sinus

Sebaceous gland
The areola has sebaceous glands appearing in relief.

Nipple
The milk flows from a minuscule opening located on the nipples. The nipples grow larger during pregnancy to facilitate breast feeding. In some women, the nipple turns into the breast, which can disturb breast-feeding.

THE **SEX CELLS**

The male sex cells, called sperm cells, and the female sex cells, called ova, are produced by the gonads (testicles and ovaries). They are formed by a specific mechanism of cell division, meiosis. Completely different genetically, the sex cells comprise only 23 chromosomes, that is, one chromosome of each 23 pairs that make up the other cells of the body.

Human cell... page 46

THE **FORMATION** OF **SPERM CELLS**

The production of sperm cells begins during puberty and does not end until death. It takes place via cell division in the seminal tubes of the testicles, through the stem cells, the spermatogones. These give birth to spermatocytes, which produce spermatids, which in turn develop into sperm cells. The process takes approximately 74 days. Once born, the sex cells are led to the epididymis, where they complete their maturation. Some factors can provoke the formation of abnormal sperm cells, like exposure to radiation or overconsumption of alcohol.

Cell division... page 49
Testicles... page 418

Seminal tube
The seminal tubes are located in the testicles. They are the location of formation of the sperm cells.

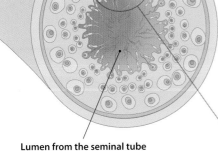

Lumen from the seminal tube
Little by little during their transformation, the sperm cells approach the lumen of the seminal tube, by which they are led towards the epididymis.

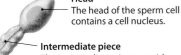

Head
The head of the sperm cell contains a cell nucleus.

Intermediate piece
The intermediate piece provides the energy necessary for the sperm cell to move.

Flagellum
Resembling a long, vibrant cilia, the flagellum allows the sperm cell to move.

Sperm cell
Sperm cells have the role of reaching and penetrating the ovum to fertilize it. They move at the rate of approximately .04 inches (one millimeter) per minute and their life span in the uterus is 72 hours on average.

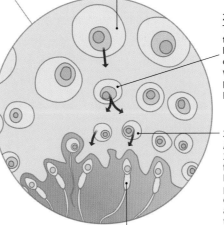

1. Spermatogone
A spermatogone is a seminal tube stem cell, the precursor to sperm cells. The spermatogones reproduce by cell division to assure their renewal, but some transform into spermatocytes.

2. Spermatocyte
The spermatocyte gives birth to spermatids by meiosis. During this specific process of cell division, the mother cell, which has 46 chromosomes, produces daughter cells possessing 23 chromosomes.

3. Spermatid
A spermatid is a 23-chromosome cell formed from spermatocyte division. It undergoes a maturation process (disappearance of a part of its cytoplasm, appearance of a flagellum) that transforms it into a sperm cell.

4. Sperm cells
The sperm cells produced in the seminal tubes possess an imperfect mobility and capacity of fertilization. They reach their maturity in the epididymis.

THE **FORMATION** OF **OVA**

The production of ova occurs in the ovaries. Started during the fetal life and interrupted at birth, it restarts at puberty and continues until menopause. An ovum is produced during a cycle of approximately 28 days that begins at the same time as the menstrual cycle. The expulsion of the ovum outside of the ovary, or ovulation, takes place between the 11th and 14th day of the ovarian cycle. It can cause pain in the lower abdomen. Several ova can be expelled at the same time, which can cause multiple pregnancies.

Multiple pregnancies… page 461

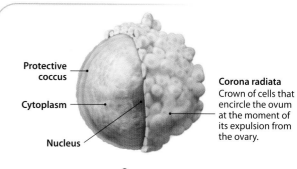

Protective coccus

Cytoplasm

Nucleus

Corona radiata
Crown of cells that encircle the ovum at the moment of its expulsion from the ovary.

Ovum
After ovulation, the ovum travels through the fallopian tubes towards the uterus, where it can be fertilized by a sperm cell. Without fertilization, its life span is approximately 24 hours.

THE **OVARIAN CYCLE**

The ovarian cycle is the series of changes that periodically intervenes in the ovaries allowing them to produce ova and hormones. It occurs parallel to the menstrual cycle. The ovarian cycle begins on the first day of menstruation and lasts for approximately 28 days. It is divided into three successive phases (follicular phase, ovulatory phase, luteal phase), during which a follicle develops, expels an ovum, and then transforms into the corpus luteum.

1. Follicular phase
During the first 10 days of the ovarian cycle, an ovarian follicle pursues its maturation.

Ovarian follicle
An ovarian follicle is a small structure of the ovary inside which an oocyte develops during the ovarian cycle.

Oocyte
The oocyte is a developing sex cell. At birth, an ovary contains hundreds of thousands of oocytes, but only approximately 400 will transform into ova (from puberty to menopause).

Ovary

2. Ovulatory phase
The ovulatory phase occurs in the middle of the ovarian cycle, when the wall of one of the ovaries is torn at the protuberance formed by a graafian follicle. An ovum is expelled from the ovary.

Ovum
An ovum is a sex cell produced from the maturation of an oocyte.

Graafian follicle
The graafian follicle is an ovarian follicle containing a mature oocyte (or ovum) ready to be expelled in the fallopian tube.

Fallopian tube
The ovum, expelled from the ovary, travels in the fallopian tube until it reaches the uterus.

Ovulation
Ovulation is the phenomenon by which an ovum is expelled from an ovary, then captured by a fallopian tube.

3. Luteal phase
The luteal phase is characterized by the transformation of the graafian follicle into the corpus luteum, which secretes progesterone.

Graafian follicle
After having expelled the ovum, the graafian follicle transforms into the corpus luteum.

Corpus luteum
The corpus luteum is a temporary endocrine gland secreting progesterone, a hormone with the primary function of preparing the gestation. It develops in the ovary from the graafian follicle disturbed during ovulation. If the ovum is not fertilized, the corpus luteum degenerates at the end of the ovarian cycle.

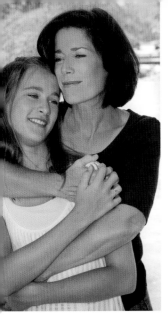

THE **MENSTRUAL CYCLE**

In order for a potential fertilized ovum to attach itself to the mucous membrane of the uterus, the uterus periodically undergoes a series of transformations called the menstrual cycle. This cycle is governed by the hormones produced by the ovaries and the pituitary gland and occurs parallel to the ovarian cycle. The menstrual cycle occurs in all healthy women, from puberty to menopause and outside periods of pregnancy. It may be accompanied by abdominal cramps, particularly during ovulation or periods. Premenstrual syndrome corresponds to various issues that affect some women during the days preceding periods.

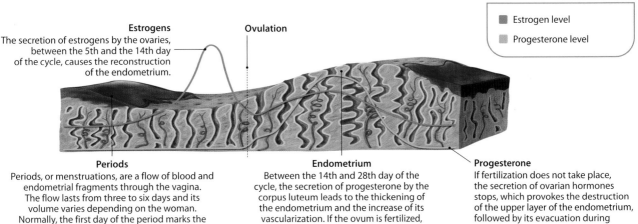

Estrogens
The secretion of estrogens by the ovaries, between the 5th and the 14th day of the cycle, causes the reconstruction of the endometrium.

Ovulation

- ■ Estrogen level
- ■ Progesterone level

Periods
Periods, or menstruations, are a flow of blood and endometrial fragments through the vagina. The flow lasts from three to six days and its volume varies depending on the woman. Normally, the first day of the period marks the beginning of menstrual and ovarian cycles.

Endometrium
Between the 14th and 28th day of the cycle, the secretion of progesterone by the corpus luteum leads to the thickening of the endometrium and the increase of its vascularization. If the ovum is fertilized, it implants itself in the endometrium and begins its development.

Progesterone
If fertilization does not take place, the secretion of ovarian hormones stops, which provokes the destruction of the upper layer of the endometrium, followed by its evacuation during periods.

MENSTRUAL CYCLE PHASES

Like the ovarian cycle, the menstrual cycle lasts an average of 28 days. It is comprised of three phases: the menstrual phase, during which the endometrium sheds and flows through the vagina (periods); the proliferative phase, during which the endometrium is reconstituted, and the secretory phase, during which it thickens to accommodate the fertilized ovum. These phases, which succeed in a cyclical manner, are strictly related to hormones (estrogens and progesterone) secreted by the ovaries during the ovarian cycle.

HEAVY PERIODS

A woman suffers from menorrhagia when her periods last more than seven days and when the overabundance of the flow forces her to frequently change her menstrual protection. This trouble may be accompanied by debilitating abdominal cramps and may cause iron deficiency anemia causing fatigue and breathlessness. Menorrhagia is frequent in the approach to menopause and at the beginning of adolescence, periods marked by significant hormonal fluctuations that cause exaggerated development of the endometrium. More rarely, it results from disorders affecting the uterus, endometrium, ovaries, etc. Ectopic pregnancy and miscarriage also provoke copious vaginal bleeding, but outside the menstrual period.

Iron deficiency anemia... page 242

PREMENSTRUAL SYNDROME

In some women, the hormonal changes of the ovarian cycle may cause several physical and psychological issues a few days before and sometimes at the beginning of periods. Called premenstrual syndrome (PMS), these varying symptoms affect 5% to 10% of women in a severe and highly debilitating manner. Though some PMS-like symptoms can manifest starting from puberty, premenstrual syndrome appears generally around age 30, particularly in women having familial antecedents and in those who suffer from stress, anxiety, or depression. In some women, pain in the lower abdomen persists and intensifies during menstruation. This disorder, called dysmenorrhea, is frequent in adolescence. It generally decreases with age and often after pregnancy. Even if it often results from hormonal factors, dysmenorrhea can sometimes reveal an anomaly in reproductive organs: endometriosis, infection, tumor, etc.

ABSENCE OF PERIODS

The absence of periods, or amenorrhea, is said to be primary when a woman has not yet had a period after the age of 16. It generally results from a genetic or anatomical anomaly. Amenorrhea is secondary if a woman who normally has her period has not had a period for three consecutive cycles. It may be caused by pregnancy, chemotherapy, or illness: tuberculosis, kidney failure, hypophyseal adenoma, anorexia, etc. It can also be linked to the intensive practice of sports or have a psychological origin. After 40, amenorrhea associated with other characteristic signs leads to the diagnosis of menopause, which may be confirmed by a test that assesses the level of sex hormones in the blood. In younger women, secondary amenorrhea may also be the sign of premature menopause.

Menopause... page 426

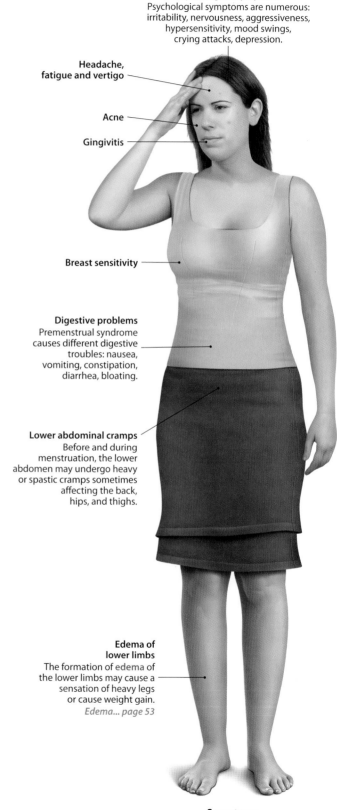

Psychological symptoms
Psychological symptoms are numerous: irritability, nervousness, aggressiveness, hypersensitivity, mood swings, crying attacks, depression.

Headache, fatigue and vertigo

Acne

Gingivitis

Breast sensitivity

Digestive problems
Premenstrual syndrome causes different digestive troubles: nausea, vomiting, constipation, diarrhea, bloating.

Lower abdominal cramps
Before and during menstruation, the lower abdomen may undergo heavy or spastic cramps sometimes affecting the back, hips, and thighs.

Edema of lower limbs
The formation of edema of the lower limbs may cause a sensation of heavy legs or cause weight gain.
Edema... page 53

Symptoms of premenstrual syndrome

ALLEVIATING MENSTRUAL PAINS

Some measures may contribute to the relief the various discomfort that arises before and after periods, notably cramps in the lower abdomen, back pain, and edema in the legs. However, if the symptoms are particularly intense or irregular, a doctor should be consulted.

■ EXERCISE

Exercising regularly (walking, swimming) is beneficial in preventing or relieving symptoms related to periods. To minimize abdominal cramps, you can also adopt yoga stances like the arch or the cobra.

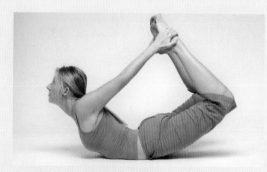

Arch

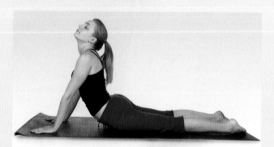

Cobra

Attention! If you have any health problems, consult your doctor before beginning a physical exercise program. Some positions may be contraindicated. If a position or movement causes pain, stop practicing it.

■ MAKE YOURSELF WARM

As heat can minimize lower abdominal cramps, take a hot bath or apply a hot water bottle to your abdomen. If these methods are not effective, you can, alternatively, apply a bag of ice to your abdomen for 15 minutes.

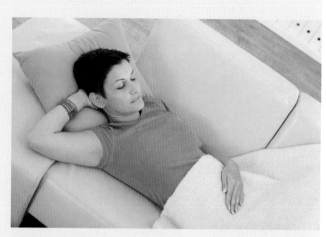

■ REST AND RELAX

Before and during menstruation, do not hesitate to rest and practice relaxing activities: deep and regular breathing through the abdomen, massaging painful areas, etc.

■ ADAPT YOUR DIET

Your diet must be balanced, rich in fruits and vegetables. Also, the consumption of food rich in unsaturated fatty acids, like fatty fish (salmon, mackerel, etc.), vegetable oils, grains, etc., is encouraged. A good calcium source, especially present in dairy products, would also be beneficial. Limit your consumption of salt and stimulants like alcohol, coffee, tea, spices, sugar products, and saturated fats (red meat, whole milk products, etc.).

Nutrition... page 11

■ TAKE MEDICATION WHEN NEEDED

Nonsteroidal anti-inflammatories like ibuprofen can minimize pain and discomfort related to periods. If they are not effective, a doctor can prescribe different treatments to block ovulation and others adapted to different symptoms: diuretic medication, antispasmodics, anxiolytics, etc.

MENOPAUSE

Menopause is a normal stage of life for a woman that corresponds to the stopping of ovarian activity. It signals the end of the hormonal production of progesterone, the end of ovulation, and, thus, fertility, as well as the stopping of periods. Menopause generally occurs between the ages of 45 and 55. Hormonal fluctuations that precede it bring on various physiological changes accompanied by various physical and psychological disorders. They can also cause osteoporosis and cardiovascular diseases. To minimize the negative effects of menopause, it is recommended to practice a healthy lifestyle, particularly by having a balanced diet and exercising regularly. Substitutive hormonal treatments that compensate for hormonal deficiency may also be prescribed. In addition to the natural process of aging, menopause may have **genetic**, **autoimmune**, or medical causes, like ovary ablation or **chemotherapy**.

Osteoporosis... page 106

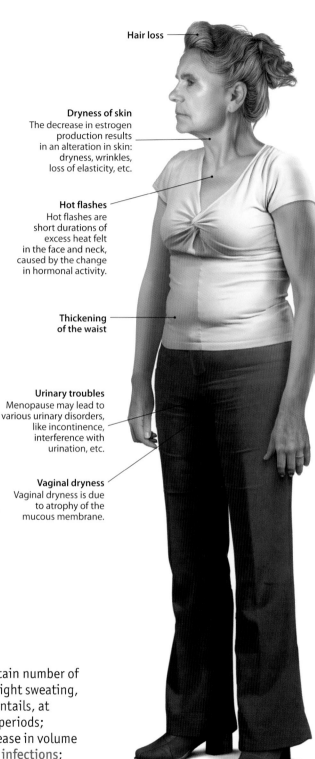

Hair loss

Dryness of skin
The decrease in estrogen production results in an alteration in skin: dryness, wrinkles, loss of elasticity, etc.

Hot flashes
Hot flashes are short durations of excess heat felt in the face and neck, caused by the change in hormonal activity.

Thickening of the waist

Urinary troubles
Menopause may lead to various urinary disorders, like incontinence, interference with urination, etc.

Vaginal dryness
Vaginal dryness is due to atrophy of the mucous membrane.

SIGNS OF MENOPAUSE

Approaching menopause, 80% of women experience a certain number of physical and psychological issues, including hot flashes, night sweating, insomnia, mood swings, and irritability. Menopause also entails, at varying degrees, changes in the female body: stopping of periods; changes in skin, nails, hair, and mucous membranes; decrease in volume of mammary glands; greater susceptibility to urinary tract infections; sometimes incontinence. Before stopping, the menstrual cycle is irregular. Continuing to use a method of contraception during the first 12 months of amenorrhea is recommended.

SUBSTITUTIVE HORMONAL TREATMENT

To minimize or eradicate the functional issues related to menopause, some women may be prescribed substitutive hormonal treatment (SHT). This hormone therapy, designed to replace the hormones that the ovaries cease to produce during menopause, generally combines estrogens and progestin. There are several types that differ in dosage or method of administration (pills, transdermal patches, gels, nasal solutions). Taking an SHT may be contraindicated, particularly in the event of liver disease, unexplained vaginal bleeding, or thrombosis or breast cancer antecedents. As SHT does not prevent ovulation, it cannot be used as a contraceptive.

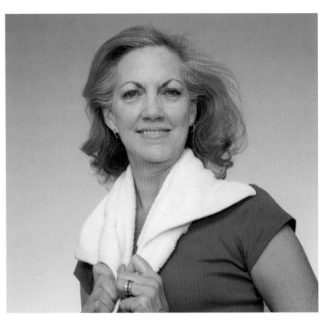

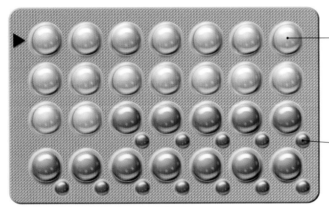

Estrogens
The administration of estrogens combats the disagreeable symptoms of menopause.

Progestin
A progestin is a natural or artificial substance that produces effects similar to those of progesterone. The progestin administered by SHT compensates for the negative effects of estrogens on the endometrium (risk of cancer).

Substitutive hormonal treatment
in pill form

CONTROVERSY SURROUNDING SHT

SHT allows many women to limit the negative effects of menopause, like hot flashes, mood swings, vaginal dryness, and night sweats. This treatment also decreases the risk of colon cancer and osteoporosis. However, numerous studies put the beneficial effects of SHT into question. They claim that some types of SHT, especially those that are taken over the long term, can increase the risk of cardiovascular disorders (vein thrombosis, myocardial infarction, cerebral vascular accidents). They can also increase the risks of developing breast or ovarian cancer. Studies on a larger scale must corroborate these results, but, in the interim, a doctor can determine case by case the necessity of following the treatment and the existing risk factors. An adapted dose and medium-term treatment, supplemented by regular medical monitoring (gynecological exam, mammogram, colonoscopy, etc.), may present lower risks.

TESTICULAR CANCER

Testicular cancer is a malignant tumor that affects testicular tissue and of which various types exist. It is a rare disease, but it constitutes the most common form of cancer in young men, particularly in the case of undescended testicles or testicular atrophy. Treatment requires ablation of the affected testicle. Cancer generally only affects one testicle, but it can cause sterility. As a precaution, a reserve of sperm cells is often stored once the diagnosis is established. A testicle self-exam completed regularly may allow an individual to detect a tumor and treat it as soon as possible, which increases the chances of recovery. The testicles are also the location of benign tumors or cysts.

Cancer... page 55

SELF-EXAM
OF THE **TESTICLES**

To check for testicular cancer, a man should, from puberty, carry out a testicle self-exam every month, preferably after a hot shower or bath, when the skin of the scrotum is softened. The exam consists in delicately palpating each testicle with both hands, while placing the thumbs on top and the other fingers below. The testicles should normally be smooth and firm. If a suspicious lump is detected, a doctor should be consulted.

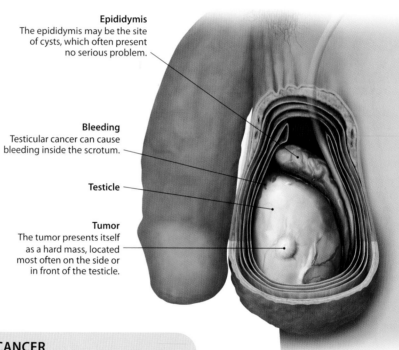

Epididymis
The epididymis may be the site of cysts, which often present no serious problem.

Bleeding
Testicular cancer can cause bleeding inside the scrotum.

Testicle

Tumor
The tumor presents itself as a hard mass, located most often on the side or in front of the testicle.

TESTICULAR CANCER

SYMPTOMS:
Palpable hard mass (nodule), increase in volume of testicle, fertility issues, sometimes increase in volume of one or both breasts. Testicular cancer is generally painless.

TREATMENT:
Ablation of the testicle, followed by radiation therapy or chemotherapy. For aesthetic reasons, the ablated testicle can be replaced by a prosthesis.

A RARE AND CURABLE CANCER

Testicular cancer affects between 3 and 6 men out of 100,000 in industrialized countries and its recovery rate exceeds 95%.

SPERMATIC CORD DISEASES

Spermatic cords connect the abdominal cavity and the testicles. They contain the blood vessels that ensure the irrigation of the testicles. The spermatic cords can be the site of different diseases, such as spontaneous testicular torsion or the permanent dilation of spermatic veins (varicocele), which lead to blood circulation dysfunctions and can cause irreversible damage, like sterility or **necrosis** of the testicle.

SPERMATIC CORD DISEASES

SYMPTOMS:
Testicular torsion: acute pain in the lower abdomen, swelling of the testicle. Varicocele: sensation of heaviness. Varicocele is often asymptomatic.

TREATMENT:
Testicular torsion: emergency surgical intervention. Varicocele: binding or embolization of spermatic veins.

PREVENTION:
Testicular torsion: surgical fixation of the testicle to the scrotum in the event of acute isolated pain indicating a risk of torsion or to avoid recurrences.

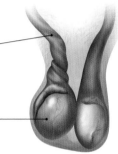

Spermatic cord
The spermatic cord winds around itself, which causes the compression of blood vessels. The torsion of the cord is promoted by abnormal mobility of the testicle or by a cord that is too long.

Testicle
Deprived of blood, the testicle swells, becoming painful and slightly elevated.

Testicular torsion

PROSTATE ADENOMA

Prostate adenoma is a benign tumor that develops in the central part of the prostate, surrounding the urethra. The increase in volume of the prostate, which in turn compresses the urethra, can cause various urinary issues. Prostate adenoma does not cause sexual disorders and cannot develop into prostate cancer. It is a common disease that affects close to 50% of men 60 years of age and approximately 90% of men 80 years of age.

Benign tumors… page 54

PROSTATE ADENOMA

SYMPTOMS:
Frequent and sometimes uncontrollable urge to urinate, interference with urinating, decrease in force of the urine stream, presence of blood in urine. Often, no particular symptoms at first.

TREATMENT:
Treatment with medication, adenoma removal if it is very large, implantation of a prosthesis in the urethra.

PREVENTION:
Certain life habits permit the minimization of interference due to prostate adenoma: avoid spicy dishes, alcoholic beverages, and carbonated soft drinks; exercise regularly.

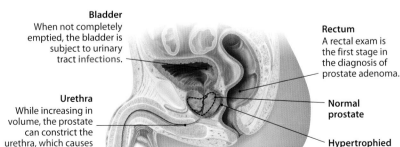

Bladder
When not completely emptied, the bladder is subject to urinary tract infections.

Urethra
While increasing in volume, the prostate can constrict the urethra, which causes difficulties urinating.

Rectum
A rectal exam is the first stage in the diagnosis of prostate adenoma.

Normal prostate

Hypertrophied prostate

PROSTATE CANCER

Prostate cancer is a very common malignant tumor that affects close to three-quarters of men 80 years and older, but one that causes relatively few deaths due to its late appearance and its generally slow development (one-third of men affected will die). It occurs most often in men over 50 years of age and is promoted by a diet rich in animal fat, smoking, alcohol abuse, familial antecedents, and a selenium deficiency. Its treatment depends on the development stage of the tumor and may require the removal of the prostate. The operation requires a five- to 10-day hospitalization and the placement of a catheter in the urethra to evacuate urine. Removal of the prostate causes sterility and may cause erectile dysfunction, and sometimes urinary incontinence.

Cancer... page 55

RECTAL EXAM

To detect colorectal cancer, prostate cancer, or prostate adenoma, the doctor may perform a rectal exam. He introduces a gloved and lubricated finger in the rectum of the patient and palpates the anus, rectum, and prostate to detect any suspicious anomalies. Other exams, like blood analysis or an ultrasound, complete the diagnosis of prostate cancer, but only a biopsy can confirm it. A rectal exam must be completed regularly after 50, or earlier in the event of familial antecedents.

PROSTATE CANCER

SYMPTOMS:
Presence of blood in urine, trouble urinating, fatigue, anemia, weight loss. Prostate cancer is often asymptomatic and discovered by chance.

TREATMENT:
Prostate ablation, radiation therapy, hormone therapy, chemotherapy, cryotherapy, ultrasound treatment. Hormone therapy aims to suppress the production of testosterone, which promotes the development of cancerous cells.

PREVENTION:
A diet low in fat and rich in Vitamin E (vegetable oil, nuts, grains), selenium (seafood), and lycopene (fruits and vegetables, particularly tomatoes) decreases the risk of developing the disease. After prostate ablation, blood analyses provide screening for recurrence.

Bladder **Penis** **Scrotum** **Rectum**

Prostate
The malignant tumor presents itself as a hard excrescence often located on the periphery of the prostate.

Rectal exam
The doctor palpates the prostate through its wall. If it is hard and knotted, it may indicate the presence of cancer.

PHIMOSIS

Phimosis is a narrowness of the foreskin orifice, rendering it difficult or impossible to retract the foreskin behind the glans penis (capping), particularly during sexual relations. In infants, the presence of phimosis is normal and temporary. However, phimosis may persist or even appear following repeated **infections**, disease (diabetes, syphilis, glans penis cancer), or capping maneuvers damaging the tip of the foreskin. Ablation of the foreskin (circumcision) may be necessary.

CONGENITAL PHIMOSIS

Most boys are born with congenital phimosis that almost always disappears spontaneously with the development of the genital organs. In approximately 1% of cases, however, phimosis persists to adulthood, causing infections and pain during erections and sexual relations. Forced capping of the glans penis, once recommended, is strongly discouraged today. In fact, it risks tearing the tip of the foreskin or causing strangulation of the base of the glans penis. In this last case, strangulation leads to painful edema of the foreskin, which requires emergency treatment, because it can cause lesions or necrosis of the glans penis and foreskin.

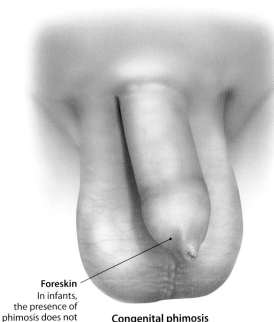

Foreskin
In infants, the presence of phimosis does not interfere with any penal hygiene.

Congenital phimosis

CIRCUMCISION

Surgical ablation of the foreskin, called circumcision, is a ritual practiced by some peoples for religious and cultural reasons. It also constitutes the primary medical treatment of pathological phimosis. However, it is discouraged by the majority of medical organizations for children presenting congenital phimosis. When it is necessary, circumcision can be completed at any age, under general or local anesthesia. Sexual relations and masturbation must be avoided until healing is complete, which occurs in two to four weeks. Once the foreskin is excised, the glans penis always remains visible. With time, permanent rubbing against clothing provokes the thickening and drying of the surface, which can lead to a loss of sensitivity.

PHIMOSIS

SYMPTOMS:
Difficult or impossible capping. If the orifice is very limited, difficulty urinating.

TREATMENT:
Surgical enlargement of the foreskin; with the risk of recurrence, circumcision. When phimosis is not too tight, some doctors recommend the application of a corticosteroid-based salve.

PREVENTION:
Rigorous personal hygiene, avoid forced capping.

ENDOMETRIOSIS

Endometriosis is a gynecological disease characterized by the presence of endometrial cells (mucous membrane of the uterus) outside of the uterus. It affects approximately 10% of women 25 to 45 years of age, and they often have familial antecedents. Generally diagnosed late, endometriosis leads to sterility in approximately one-third of cases and is treated by **hormone therapy** or **coeliosurgery**. It rarely develops into cancer and generally disappears during menopause due to hormonal changes.

DAMAGE CAUSED BY ENDOMETRIOSIS

Endometrial cells are normally destroyed by the immune system if they leave the uterus. In women with endometriosis, these cells implant themselves on other organs of the peritoneal cavity: peritoneum, ovaries, fallopian tubes, ligaments and external wall of the uterus, intestines, and bladder. They form characteristic lesions there, called endometriosis implants. These fragments of the endometrium develop under the influence of hormones produced by the ovaries. Governed by the menstrual cycle, they bleed during periods. This phenomenon causes cramps and local inflammation, and can lead to the formation of nodules, ovarian cysts, and adherences (abnormal joining) between the affected organs. Endometriosis frequently causes adherences between the uterus and the ovaries or fallopian tubes, which can lead to sterility (reversible in some cases).

COELIOSCOPY

Coelioscopy, or laparascopy, is a technique that allows the visualization of the interior of the abdomen through an optical instrument, the coelioscope, introduced through the abdominal wall. It is used for the diagnosis and surgical treatment (coeliosurgery) of several diseases: endometriosis, ovarian cyst, uterine fibroid, prostate cancer, cholecystitis, appendicitis, etc. Its barely invasive character limits the duration of hospitalization and convalescence.

Endometrium
The endometrium is the mucous membrane that covers the interior of the uterus.

Endometrioma
The endometrioma (or endometriosis cyst) is a cyst forming on the ovary in women suffering from endometriosis. Made up of endometrial cells, it is often filled with blood, is a dark red color, and can break and bleed during periods.

Fallopian tube

Ovary

Myometrium
When endometriosis affects the myometrium (muscular wall of the uterus), it is called adenomyosis.

Endometriosis implant
An endometriosis implant is a characteristic nodule of endometriosis, made up of clusters of endometrial cells.

Lower view of the cervix

ENDOMETRIOSIS

SYMPTOMS:
Abdominal pain, particularly during periods and sexual relations. Long and copious or irregular periods. The symptoms disappear at menopause. Sterility.

TREATMENT:
Hormone therapy to inhibit the hormonal secretion of the ovaries, surgical ablation of cysts by coeliosurgery, removal of the uterus.

GENITAL PROLAPSE

Genital prolapse (or descent of an organ) is the progressive sliding down of one or several pelvic organs in a woman, particularly the uterus, but also the bladder, rectum, or urethra. It is caused by the relaxing of ligaments and muscles that support them, most often following repeated births or after menopause. Genital prolapse is a relatively common disorder that affects approximately 40% of woman over 45 years of age. It is treated by the implementation of a pessary (a device inserted into the vagina to support the uterus) or by surgery, depending on the stage of development and the patient's age and level of sexual activity.

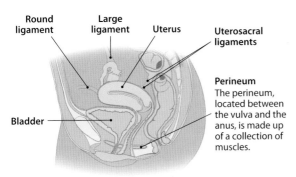

Normal uterus
In a normal state, the uterus is suspended by a series of ligaments and supported by the perineum. Inclined towards the front, it is supported on the bladder.

Round ligament · Large ligament · Uterus · Uterosacral ligaments · Bladder

Perineum
The perineum, located between the vulva and the anus, is made up of a collection of muscles.

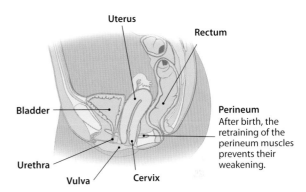

Uterine prolapse
Uterine prolapse is the progressive descent of the uterus into the vagina. In a very pronounced prolapse, the cervix exits through the vaginal orifice. The uterus can even completely exit through the vulva. Surgical intervention is then necessary.

Uterus · Rectum · Bladder · Urethra · Vulva · Cervix

Perineum
After birth, the retraining of the perineum muscles prevents their weakening.

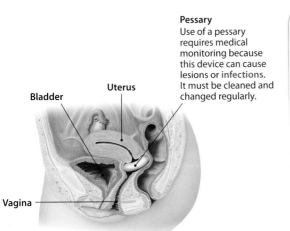

Pessary
Use of a pessary requires medical monitoring because this device can cause lesions or infections. It must be cleaned and changed regularly.

Bladder · Uterus · Vagina

Using a pessary
The pessary is a flexible device that is introduced into the vagina to support the uterus or other organs exiting the vagina, in the event of genital prolapse. Using a pessary constitutes an alternative to surgery in the event of moderate prolapse.

CYSTOCELE
Cystocele, the prolapse of the bladder, generally appears during menopause and particularly affects women who have had multiple childbirths. The bladder exits the vagina, which causes pain and difficulty completely evacuating the bladder.

GENITAL PROLAPSE

SYMPTOMS:
Sensation of heaviness, lumbar pains, effort incontinence, difficulty urinating or defecating, cervix exiting through the vulva.

TREATMENT:
Pessary, surgery (fixation of organs using ligaments or prosthesis), removal of the uterus.

PREVENTION:
Perineal retraining after delivery.
Postpartum... page 474

UTERINE TUMORS

The uterus can be subject to various types of benign tumors, like uterine fibroids and polyps, or malignant tumors, like cervical cancer or endometrial cancer. Regular gynecological and cytological exams make it possible to screen for and treat them as soon as possible. Depending on the disease, treatments call for **hormone therapy**, **chemotherapy**, or surgery.

UTERINE FIBROIDS

The muscle of the uterus, the myometrium, may be the site of benign tumors called uterine fibroids, or uterine myomas. Often asymptomatic and developing slowly, they very rarely turn into cancer and regress during menopause. The causes and factors promoting the appearance of these tumors, which may affect up to 70% of women, are not well known. The size of fibroids is variable. Their presence can cause pain or menstrual hemorrhaging and can even interfere with pregnancy, birth, and the functioning of neighboring organs.

Benign tumors... page 54

UTERINE CANCER

Uterine cancer is a malignant tumor that can develop in the cervix or in the mucous membrane that covers it, the endometrium. Cervical cancer is promoted by certain sexually transmitted viruses from the papillomavirus family. A vaccine or using a condom during sexual relations serve as protection (efficiency of the vaccine has yet to be confirmed). In Western countries, endometrial cancer is more common than cervical cancer. Rare before the age of 40, it develops under the influence of female hormones—estrogen—and is promoted by premature puberty, late menopause, absence of pregnancy, and especially obesity. Early diagnosis of uterine cancer through a cervical smear or biopsy of the endometrium makes it possible to treat it quickly and avoid its spread, thereby considerably increasing the chance of recovery.

Cancer... page 55

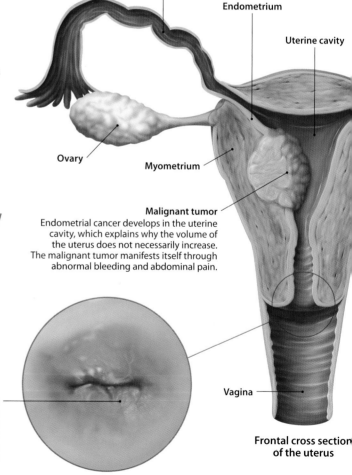

Fallopian tube

Endometrium

Uterine cavity

Ovary

Myometrium

Malignant tumor
Endometrial cancer develops in the uterine cavity, which explains why the volume of the uterus does not necessarily increase. The malignant tumor manifests itself through abnormal bleeding and abdominal pain.

Vagina

Frontal cross section of the uterus

Precancerous lesions
The development of cervical cancer is characterized by the appearance of precancerous lesions, detectable by a cytology and colposcopy. Abnormal bleeding is the first symptom of cervical cancer.

Lower view of the cervix

GYNECOLOGICAL EXAMS AND CYTOLOGIES

Every year, women should undergo a routine gynecological exam that includes a breast palpation and vaginal exam. This allows the detection of potential anomalies like infection, malformation, genital prolapse, or of the endometrium cysts and tissues that surround it. Every year for women under 30 and every three years following that, the exam should be supplemented by a gynecological cytology (Pap smear), that is, a microscopic analysis of cells sampled from the cervix (cervical smear). This test makes it possible to detect abnormal cells that may indicate the onset of cancer. So as to not falsify results, the sample must not be preceded by a vaginal douche, sexual relations, or local treatment and cannot be performed during periods. When the results of the smear are abnormal, a visual exam of the vagina and cervix, a colposcopy, can be completed using an optical magnifying instrument, the colposcope, which makes it possible to locate the lesions for a biopsy. A uterine exam, hysteroscopy, can also be carried out to diagnose or treat diseases such as uterine fibroids or endometrial cancer.

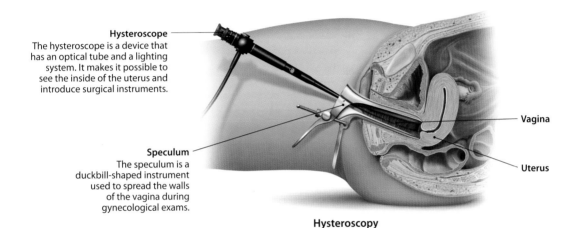

Hysteroscope
The hysteroscope is a device that has an optical tube and a lighting system. It makes it possible to see the inside of the uterus and introduce surgical instruments.

Speculum
The speculum is a duckbill-shaped instrument used to spread the walls of the vagina during gynecological exams.

Vagina

Uterus

Hysteroscopy

ABLATION OF THE UTERUS

The surgical ablation of the uterus, or hysterectomy, is performed to treat different gynecological conditions: endometriosis, uterine fibroids, endometrial cancer, uterine prolapse. A hysterectomy stops periods and leads to irreversible sterility. It is therefore mainly reserved for women who have undergone menopause or those who no longer wish to have children. In women of reproductive age, it is done only after the failure of other treatments. A hysterectomy may be partial if the cervix remains in place, total in the event of complete ablation of the uterus and cervix, or radical when a small part of the upper vagina and certain pelvic lymph nodes are removed as well. A hysterectomy may be accompanied by the ablation of the ovaries and fallopian tubes. It can be performed via the abdomen or the vaginal tract.

UTERINE TUMORS

SYMPTOMS:
Uterine fibroid: copious periods, bleeding between periods, cramps in the lower abdomen, feeling of heaviness, urinary issues, constipation. Cervical cancer: often asymptomatic, sometimes bleeding during sexual relations, white discharge streaked with blood. Endometrial cancer: copious periods, bleeding between periods or after menopause, abdominal pain, white discharge, difficulties urinating.

TREATMENT:
Uterine fibroids: hormone therapy, surgery. Cancer: surgery, radiation therapy, brachytherapy, chemotherapy.

PREVENTION:
Cervical cancer: use of condoms during sexual relations, vaccination, regular gynecological monitoring to screen at early stages.

OVARIAN CYSTS

Poor functioning of the ovaries, particularly from adolescence and at the beginning of pregnancy, can lead to the formation of functional cysts on the ovaries. Most of them are benign and disappear spontaneously. More rarely, an alteration in the structure of the ovaries can cause organic cysts, at risk of developing into ovarian cancer. Some ovarian cysts secrete masculine hormones in excess, which can often cause the abnormal development of hair, acne, and obesity. This is notably the case when the ovaries present numerous cysts (polycystic ovary syndrome). This syndrome also frequently leads to sterility and increases the risk of diabetes and myocardial infarction.

Cysts... page 52

Cysts... page 52

OVARIAN CYSTS

SYMPTOMS:
Sensation of heaviness, pain during sexual relations, amenorrhea, bleeding, difficulty urinating. Ovarian cysts are often asymptomatic. Torsion, rupture or infection of the cyst: violent pain, sometimes fever.

TREATMENT:
Determination of the size and nature of the cysts by ultrasound and X-ray. Functional cyst: no treatment, except in the case of complications. Polycystic ovary: hormonal or antidiabetic treatment, slimming diet. Organic cyst: surgical removal.

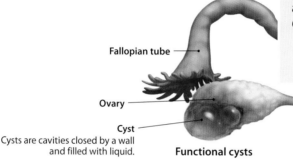

Fallopian tube

Ovary

Cyst
Cysts are cavities closed by a wall and filled with liquid.

Functional cysts

OVARIAN CANCER

Ovarian cancer is a malignant tumor that develops in an ovary. Not very common, it generally occurs after menopause and more often in the event of familial antecedents. Since the symptoms are not very specific, the disease is often detected late, after spreading to other organs and structures in the abdomen, which considerably decreases the chances of recovery. Diagnosis relies on **ultrasound** and surgical exploration by **coelioscopy**. Blood analyses and complementary exams allow monitoring of the development of the disease.

Cancer... page 55

Cancer... page 55

OVARIAN CANCER

SYMPTOMS:
Abdominal pain, swelling of the abdomen (ascites), change of frequency or aspect of stools, fatigue, thinning, anemia.

TREATMENT:
Removal of ovaries and surrounding fatty tissues, fallopian tubes, uterus, a part of the peritoneum, and local lymphatic ganglions. Complementary chemotherapy.

PREVENTION:
Early screening by regular gynecological monitoring. Taking an oral contraceptive and having had multiple childbirths seem to be protective factors.

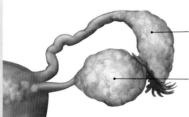

Fallopian tube

Ovary
The malignant tumor can develop inside the ovary or on its surface, and can spread to the fallopian tube and neighboring organs (uterus, bladder). It presents itself as a hard and irregular mass.

BENIGN BREAST TUMORS

Breast tumors form singular or multiple palpable masses that can cause swelling or pain. Discovered during a gynecological exam, mammogram, or breast self-exam, roughly 80% are benign. However, when a suspicious mass is detected, a doctor should be consulted since the distinction between a benign tumor and breast cancer can only be established by examining punction or **biopsy** samples. In addition, some benign breast tumors must be removed because they can become malignant.

Benign tumors… page 54

DIFFERENT BENIGN BREAST TUMORS

Several types of benign tumors can develop in the breasts. The most common are adenofibroma and cysts. Generally not serious, they are often left in place and monitored regularly. Breast adenofibromas primarily affect women under 40 years of age, while breast cysts occur most often in women between 40 and 50 years of age. Cyst can be treated by proceeding to their surgical removal, or by draining them through a small needle (punction). They never develop into cancer and sometimes disappear spontaneously. The intraductal papillomas, which develop inside the galactophorous canal, and phyllodes tumors, voluminous and rapidly developing, are systematically removed because they can develop into cancer.

Cysts… page 52

Breast adenofibroma
Breast adenofibroma develops in the mammary gland and generally presents as a firm, smooth, and mobile ball that is normally painless. It can be left in place if the size is modest and it does not present the risk of cancerous development.

Galactophorous canal
An intraductal papilloma develops inside the galactophorous canal (duct through which milk is excreted). It can cause a blood discharge from the nipple. Multiple papillomas are a risk factor for breast cancer.

BENIGN BREAST TUMORS

SYMPTOMS:
Singular or multiple palpable masses, swelling, pain, blood discharge through the nipple (intraductal papilloma).

TREATMENT:
Cysts: punction or removal. Adenofibroma: simple monitoring or removal. Phyllodes tumor and intraductal papilloma: removal. Samples are systematically analyzed to ensure the benign character of the tumor.

PREVENTION:
The breast self-exam and regular monitoring by a doctor make it possible to quickly detect tumors and ensure their benign character.

437

BREAST CANCER

Breast cancer is a malignant tumor that develops in the mammary glands. These tumors are primarily located in the upper external half of the breast or in the nipple. They affect the left breast more frequently than the right, although in rare cases, they are present in both breasts. Some tumors develop very slowly while others spread quickly to neighboring tissues and create metastases, particularly in young women. Breast cancer constitutes the most common type of cancer and is among the biggest killers of women in the Western world. The regular practice of screening exams, like breast self-exams and mammograms, makes it possible to detect the disease at an early stage, thereby increasing the chances of recovery.

Cancer... page 55

THE **RISK FACTORS** OF **BREAST CANCER**

Some factors contribute to an increased risk of developing breast cancer. The most significant are aging and **genetic** predispositions. In fact, women who have several family members (mother, sister, daughter, etc.) who have suffered from breast cancer, notably before 50 years of age, have a higher risk of developing the disease. This is also the case for women who experience premature puberty, pregnancy later in life, or late menopause, as well as those who have never been pregnant. Taken over the long term, the contraceptive pill slightly promotes the occurrence of breast cancer while some substitutive hormonal treatments for menopause increase the risk in a significant manner. Obesity and a sedentary lifestyle can also increase the risk of cancer.

TYPES OF **BREAST CANCER**

Close to 95% of breast cancer cases develop in the galactophorous canals (canal carcinoma) or in the mammary lobules (lobular carcinoma). Canal carcinoma is the most common form of breast cancer (80% of cases). Most often, it is an invasive cancer that creates metastases in the axillary (of the axilla) lymph nodes and in the surrounding and distant organs. Less common than canal carcinomas, lobular carcinomas are also becoming less often invasive. Sometimes no symptoms occur and it can affect both breasts.

Mammary lobule
The mammary lobule is the smallest subdivision of the mammary gland, grouping together the milk-producing cells.

Lobular carcinoma

Mammary lobe
The mammary lobe is a subdivision of the mammary gland, made up of mammary lobules.

Nipple

Canal carcinoma

Galactophorous canal
The galactophorous canal is the duct through which milk is excreted.

Adipose tissue

MAMMOGRAM

The X-ray of the mammary gland, called a mammogram, aims to screen for breast cancer or to specify the diagnosis of an anomaly detected by a clinical breast exam. However, approximately 20% of cancers escape detection by this technique. A mammogram should be performed every two years, starting at 50 years of age, or, for women who run a higher risk of breast cancer (family history), starting at 40 years of age.

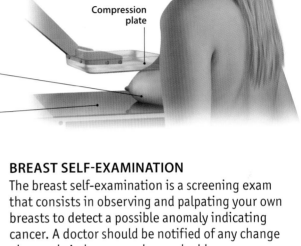

X-ray emitter

Compression plate

Breast
Each breast is X-rayed at different angles. The exam can cause a more or less disagreeable sensation depending on the breast sensitivity of the patient, because they are compressed between two plates.

Compression plate
The breast is kept in place by two plates that compress it. The lower plate contains an X-ray-sensitive film.

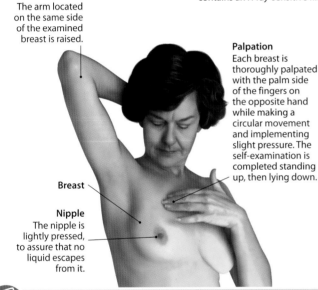

Raised arm
The arm located on the same side of the examined breast is raised.

Palpation
Each breast is thoroughly palpated with the palm side of the fingers on the opposite hand while making a circular movement and implementing slight pressure. The self-examination is completed standing up, then lying down.

Breast

Nipple
The nipple is lightly pressed, to assure that no liquid escapes from it.

BREAST SELF-EXAMINATION

The breast self-examination is a screening exam that consists in observing and palpating your own breasts to detect a possible anomaly indicating cancer. A doctor should be notified of any change observed. A change can be a palpable mass, thickening of skin, change in shape, size or color of skin or nipple, spontaneous bloody discharge, bump on the axilla, retraction of the nipple, or permanent redness. From the age of 25 onwards, it is recommended that women conduct a breast self-examination once a month, five to seven days after the beginning of periods, in addition to regular exams by a physician.

PROMISING PROSPECTS

Between 1980 and 2000, the incidence of breast cancer rose sharply, in part due to the generalization of screening, which led experts to declare the existence of a true epidemic. But since then this number has decreased significantly, notably due to the decrease of substitutive hormone treatments in women who have undergone menopause. According to current statistics, approximately 1 in 9 women will be affected with breast cancer during her lifetime and 1 in 27 with breast cancer will die. However, the mortality rate of breast cancer is steadily decreasing. More frequent and more efficient screenings enable early diagnosis and better prognosis. Treatments for breast cancer have also improved. Today they are more targeted and cause less undesirable side effects. Moreover, numerous researchers are developing new promising paths, like antiangiogenic treatments that aim to block the development of blood vessels that feed cancerous tumors. The genetic screening and MRI of high-risk women or those predisposed to breast cancer are also signs of significant progress.

BREAST CANCER TREATMENT

Surgery is the main treatment for breast cancer. Depending on the size of the tumor, partial or total ablation of the breast, a mastectomy, is performed. The operation is generally associated with the ablation of axillary lymph nodes and sometimes followed by radiation therapy. Mammary reconstruction can then be planned. Anticancerous chemotherapy has achieved significant progress in the treatment of breast cancer, in addition to anticancerous hormone therapy.

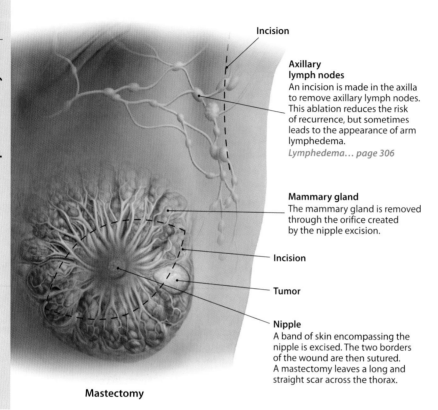

Incision

Axillary lymph nodes
An incision is made in the axilla to remove axillary lymph nodes. This ablation reduces the risk of recurrence, but sometimes leads to the appearance of arm lymphedema.
Lymphedema... page 306

Mammary gland
The mammary gland is removed through the orifice created by the nipple excision.

Incision

Tumor

Nipple
A band of skin encompassing the nipple is excised. The two borders of the wound are then sutured. A mastectomy leaves a long and straight scar across the thorax.

Mastectomy

MAMMARY RECONSTRUCTION

Mammary reconstruction is a reparative surgical technique that allows the reconstitution of the breast and nipple after their removal. The curving contour of the breast may be reconstructed using muscle flap and skin lifted from the back or stomach, sometimes combined with the implantation of a mammary prosthesis. Three months later, the nipple and the areola are reconstructed through tattooing or a sampled skin graft from the inside of the thigh, the vulva, or the areola of the opposite breast. The operative sequelae of mammary reconstruction are quite painful.

BREAST CANCER

SYMPTOMS:
Palpable hard mass, swelling, thickening of skin, fatty clusters of breast tissues, clear or bloody liquid discharge through the nipple, permanent redness, retraction of the nipple, deformation of the curving contour of the breast. Pain is rare. Breast cancer is sometimes asymptomatic.

TREATMENT:
Breast removal (partial or total) with ganglionic curage, radiation therapy, chemotherapy, hormone therapy if the cancer is hormone-dependent.

PREVENTION:
Early screening improves the prognosis: breast self-examination, regular exam by a doctor, mammograms.

BREAST CANCER IN MEN

Approximately 100 times more rare than in women, breast cancer in men is often diagnosed later, which makes it more dangerous. It generally manifests itself in a small, firm, and painless mass and is treated by surgery or hormone therapy. Male breast cancer is associated with hormonal problems or testicular illnesses.

GENITAL INFECTIONS

Bacteria, viruses, fungi, or parasites can cause **infections** in the genital organs. These diseases lead to an **inflammation** characterized by redness, pain, swelling, or heat sensation, as well as discharge, itching, fever, and sometimes the formation of an abscess. Their treatment, most often with **antibiotics**, depends on the affected organ and the cause of the infection. Some genital infections, like orchitis, epididymitis, and salpingitis, can cause sterility.

PROSTATITIS

Prostatitis is the inflammation of the prostate, of infectious origin or not. It is a common affliction, the prevalence of which increases with age. Sometimes associated with a urinary infection, acute bacterial prostatitis manifests itself by fever, chills, and difficulties with urination. Poorly treated, it can develop into chronic bacterial prostatitis, notably causing pain during ejaculation. Nonbacterial prostatitis is the most common form. Its cause is not well known and its treatment consists mostly of dietary measures (avoid spicy food and alcohol) and hygiene.

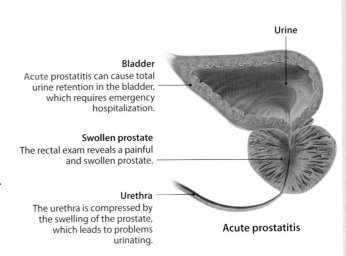

Urine

Bladder
Acute prostatitis can cause total urine retention in the bladder, which requires emergency hospitalization.

Swollen prostate
The rectal exam reveals a painful and swollen prostate.

Urethra
The urethra is compressed by the swelling of the prostate, which leads to problems urinating.

Acute prostatitis

TESTICULAR INFECTIONS

Testicular infections can be caused by urinary infections, sexually transmitted infections (chlamydia, gonorrhea), or the mumps. They cause inflammation of the testicles (orchitis), epididymis (epididymitis), or often of both tissues (orchi-epididymitis). The symptoms are characterized by pain and testicular swelling.

Penis
A discharge of pus may be produced from the penis and problems urinating may be observed.

Epididymitis

Orchitis

Hydrocele
Hydrocele is an accumulation of serous liquid surrounding the testicle, resulting in an increase in volume of the scrotum. It can be caused by the inflammatory reaction in the event of orchi-epididymitis.

Orchi-epididymitis

PENIS INFECTIONS

Penis infections mainly affect the glans penis (balanitis) and the urethra (urethritis). Balanitis may have an infectious origin (candidiasis, chlamydia, genital herpes, syphilis) or be caused by dermatitis. It can also result from a lack of hygiene (for example, in the event of phimosis) or by an irritation caused by certain hygienic products or condoms. Balanitis can cause painful erythema (redness) of the glans penis or intense itching. As for urethritis, it particularly affects young men and is generally caused by sexually transmitted diseases (gonorrhea, chlamydia). It causes discharge, burning accentuated by urination, and sometimes fever.

VAGINITIS

Vaginitis is an inflammation of the vaginal walls that is generally manifested through discharge (leukorrhea), burning, itching, and pain during sexual relations. It is often associated with inflammation of the vulva, or vulvitis. Infectious vaginitis can be caused by an imbalance in the vaginal flora or by the introduction of a pathogenic agent into the vagina (candidiasis, vaginosis, streptococcus). Treatment is often local, but taking oral antibiotics is sometimes necessary. Vaginitis can also be the result of an irritation caused by a forgotten foreign body (notably a tampon) or by an allergy to a hygienic product. It is sometimes caused by the atrophy of the vaginal mucous membrane observed during menopause.

VAGINAL FLORA

The vaginal flora is a collection of bacteria normally present in the surface of the vaginal mucous membrane as a defense against infections. Several factors (antibiotics, diabetes, hormonal disorders, certain hygienic products, some methods of contraception, wearing synthetic undergarments or tight pants) can cause an imbalance in the vaginal flora and cause bacterial vaginosis or vaginal mycosis, both responsible for vaginitis.

UPPER GENITAL TRACT INFECTION

Upper genital tract infection, or pelvic inflammatory syndrome, is an infection of the internal genital organs of a woman. It may cause sterility. The infection progresses from the cervix (cervicitis) to the endometrium (endometritis) before affecting the fallopian tubes (salpingitis) and the ovaries. It can also spread to the peritoneum. Upper genital tract infections are often caused by chlamydia or, more rarely, gonorrhea. Their diagnosis can be difficult because their symptoms are not specific (lower abdominal pain, leukorrhea, pain during periods and sexual relations) and are often barely noticed, if at all.

Salpingitis
Salpingitis is the inflammation of the fallopian tube. It causes the formation of scar tissue capable of obstructing the tubes, which leads to a risk of ectopic pregnancy and sterility.

Ovary

Endometritis

Cervicitis

Vagina

Upper genital tract infection

LEUKORRHEA

Leukorrhea, also called vaginal discharge or white discharge, is vaginal discharge that is more copious than normal vaginal secretions and does not contain blood. Leukorrhea can be a symptom of a genital infection, like vaginitis. It can be more or less copious, watery or thicker, sometimes crumbly, of variable color (white, yellowish, or greenish), sometimes with a foul odor. Its appearance gives an indication of the cause of the infection.

PREVENTING VAGINITIS

Vaginitis is promoted by different factors and has the tendency to recur. Here are some measures to follow to prevent its occurrence.

■ **PRACTICE ADEQUATE HYGIENE**
Your personal hygiene should be regular but not excessive. Clean the genital area from front to back and dry well. Do not use scented products or acids and avoid vaginal douches that damage the vaginal flora. During your periods, change your tampon or sanitary napkin regularly.

■ **AVOID HUMIDITY**
A humid environment promotes the development of infectious vaginitis and fungi (candidiasis). Therefore, wear underwear made of natural materials (white cotton) rather than those made of synthetic fibers, change them every day, and wash them in warm water, possibly with a little bleach. Avoid wearing tight pants. Places like public pools, saunas, and steam baths encourage the development of fungi. Avoid them if you are prone to vaginitis. After a bath or sauna session, rinse yourself right away with clean water and do not wear a wet bathing suit for too long.

■ **ADAPT YOUR DIET**
To avoid recurrences of vaginitis, have a balanced diet. Limit your consumption of sugars because they promote the proliferation of fungi implicated in vaginal mycosis. You can also consume dairy products that are high in beneficial bacteria for intestinal and vaginal flora: yogurt, kefir, probiotic enhanced products, etc.

Nutrition... page 11

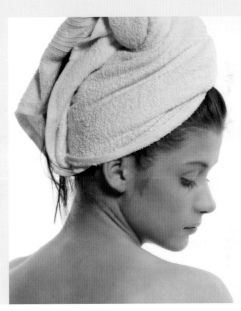

GENITAL INFECTIONS

SYMPTOMS:
Fever; inflammation of the affected organ (pain, swelling, redness, itching); trouble urinating; pain during sexual relations; bloody, purulent, and smelly discharge.

TREATMENT:
Antibiotics, antifungals, analgesics. Sometimes treatment must also be administered to sexual partners.

PREVENTION:
Use condoms during sexual relations. Use appropriate hygienic products. Chronic prostatitis: avoid spicy food and alcohol. Vaginal mycosis: avoid humid environments and oversugary food and drinks, wearing synthetic underwear or tight pants.

Condoms... page 454

SEXUALLY TRANSMITTED INFECTIONS

A sexually transmitted **infection** (STI), or a sexually transmitted disease (STD), is an infectious disease that is generally transmitted by sexual relations. It may be caused by a virus, a bacterium, a microscopic fungus, or a parasite. These infections may manifest in burning or itching sensations, abnormal discharges, urination problems, pains in the lower abdomen, and sometimes by lesions on the skin or the mucous membranes. Some of them may have serious consequences: sterility, **chronic** pain, cancer, premature birth, extrauterine pregnancy, or major problems in a child whose mother transmitted the disease before or during childbirth (**congenital** malformations, cerebral or pulmonary problems, etc.). In addition, many STDs increase the risks of contracting other similar infections, including AIDS. Diagnosing an STD may be done by clinical examination, by microscopic examination of discharges, or by a blood analysis.

AIDS... page 292

PREVENTING STDs

Sexually transmitted diseases are often very contagious. The best way to protect yourself is to know how they are transmitted and to follow the recommendations below.

■ TALK ABOUT STDs

Do not hesitate to ask a new sexual partner if he or she has an STD or inform him or her of your state of health. Also discuss the ways of protecting yourselves from STDs.

■ PROTECT YOURSELF

It is wrong to think that the contraceptive pill, withdrawal before ejaculation, or the absence of penetration prevent you from contracting an STD. Only the systematic use of a condom when having sexual relations, including oral sex, can prevent you from being contaminated by or infecting your partners.

The condom... page 454

■ BE SCREENED

If you have regular or unprotected sexual relations, with one or several partners, periodic screening tests are advised. It is, in fact, possible that you are a carrier without knowing it, some illnesses being asymptomatic.

■ IF YOU HAVE AN STD

Adopt meticulous personal hygiene measures in order not to spread the infection. Follow your treatment scrupulously until the end. It is also important that your partner receive care in order to avoid a recurrence.

■ BE CAREFUL WITH NEEDLES

Make sure that sterile needles are used for any medical treatment, but also for piercing and tattooing.

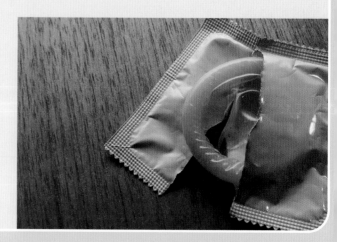

SYPHILIS

Syphilis, or the pox, is a serious and very contagious sexually transmitted **infection** caused by a bacterium, the treponema pallidum. This bacterium usually enters the body through lesions of the skin or the mucous membranes, which can be avoided by using condoms when having sexual relations. Syphilis may be transmitted to the fetus from the fourth month of pregnancy and can cause **congenital** malformations.

THE **EVOLUTION** OF **SYPHILIS**

After an incubation period lasting from two to six weeks, syphilis evolves in three stages characterized by different symptoms and separated by more or less defined periods of latency during which the symptoms disappear. The evolution of the disease may be accelerated in cases of HIV seropositivity or of AIDS.

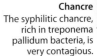

Chancre
The syphilitic chancre, rich in treponema pallidum bacteria, is very contagious.

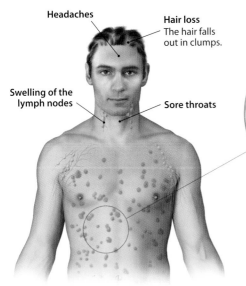

Headaches

Hair loss
The hair falls out in clumps.

Swelling of the lymph nodes

Sore throats

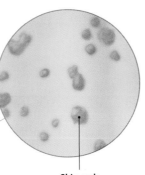

1. Primary stage
The primary stage is characterized by the appearance at the point of infection (genital organs, mouth, tongue) of an ulceration that is hard to the touch and generally painless, called a chancre. It is accompanied by a swelling of the lymph nodes located in the same area.

Skin rash
Skin marks characterizing the secondary stage are pink and not very striking. The syphilides are small lesions located in the folds of the face, the palms of the hands, and the soles of the feet, and around the mouth and the anus.

2. Secondary stage
The secondary stage starts between one and three months after the infection and lasts an average of two years. It corresponds to the spreading of the bacteria in the body. This stage is characterized by skin rashes (red spots, then syphilides), accompanied by a flu-like syndrome and generalized swelling of the lymph nodes.
The flu-like syndrome... page 320

Syphilitic gumma
The syphilitic gumma is a large nodule that progressively softens, ulcerates, and leaves a round scar.

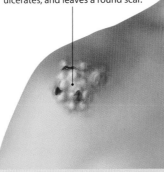

3. Tertiary stage
The tertiary stage occurs after a period of latency capable of lasting several years. It is marked by the appearance of lesions of the skin (syphilitic gumma), of the mucous membranes, and of certain internal organs (bones, liver, pylorus, larynx, kidneys, cardiovascular system, central nervous system), sometimes causing serious problems: blindness, paralysis, dementia, heart disease, etc.

SYPHILIS

SYMPTOMS:
Primary stage: chancre, swelling of lymph nodes. Secondary stage: flu-like syndrome, lesions of the skin and mucous membranes (red spots, syphilides). Tertiary stage: skin lesions, numerous internal lesions (nervous system, bones, liver, stomach, kidneys, etc.).

TREATMENTS:
Treatment with antibiotics (penicillin, in particular), more or less extensive according to the stage. Sexual partners must also be treated.

PREVENTION:
Use a condom when having sexual relations, including oral sex.

CHLAMYDIA

Chlamydias are **infectious** diseases caused by bacteria of the genus Chlamydia. These are primarily sexually transmitted infections such as genital chlamydia and venereal lymphogranuloma. The bacteria may also infect the eyes and cause conjunctivitis or trachoma. They may also affect the lungs and cause pneumonia or psittacosis. Chlamydias may cause serious complications: sterility, extrauterine pregnancy, blindness, etc.

TRACHOMA

Trachoma is an infectious disease caused by the bacterium *Chlamydia trachomatis*, which affects the conjunctiva and the cornea. It causes a deformation of the upper eyelid and an opacification of the cornea. The disease is transmitted by direct or indirect contact with ocular secretions (handkerchiefs, fingers, etc.) and by certain flies. It occurs mainly in the poor areas of the world and constitutes the primary cause of preventable blindness.

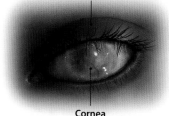

Upper eyelid
The inside of the eyelid thickens, becomes sclerotic and deformed, causing the eyelashes to rub against the cornea and damage it.

Cornea
The opacification of the cornea, caused by the successive damage, progressively masks the pupil, resulting in blindness.

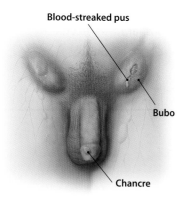

Blood-streaked pus

Bubo

Chancre

VENEREAL LYMPHOGRANULOMA

Also called Nicolas-Favre disease, venereal lymphogranuloma is caused by the bacterium *Chlamydia trachomatis* and primarily affects the lymph system. It may cause the appearance of a chancre on the penis, a painful swelling of the lymph nodes in the groin (bubos), and a discharge of blood-streaked pus.

THE CHLAMYDIAS

SYMPTOMS:
Genital chlamydia: often asymptomatic. Yellowish foul-smelling vaginal discharges, lower abdominal pain, vaginal bleeding, fever; in men, inflammation of the urethra, with discharge, burning sensations during urination. Venereal lymphogranuloma: chancres, bubos in the groin, inflammation of the rectum in case of anal contamination. Trachoma: inflammation of the conjunctiva, opacification of the cornea.

TREATMENTS:
Antibiotics. Sexual partners must be treated. Recontamination possible.

PREVENTION:
Sexual relations, including oral sex, protected by a condom. Screening test recommended for persons at risk who have unprotected sex or multiple partners.

The condom... page 454

GENITAL CHLAMYDIA

Genital chlamydia is a very common and very contagious sexually transmitted infection, caused by the bacterium *Chlamydia trachomatis*. More common in women, it usually affects the cervix of the fallopian tubes and is often asymptomatic. In men, the illness affects the urethra and may spread to the epididymis. Often diagnosed late, genital chlamydia constitutes the world's foremost cause of female sterility.

GENITAL HERPES

Genital herpes is a sexually transmitted **infection** caused by the *Herpes simplex* virus. It is characterized by the eruption of small, transparent blisters, herpetic vesicles, on or near the genital organs. The virus remains latent in the nerve lymph node and causes the periodic reappearance of symptoms (herpes outbreaks). An infected person remains a carrier of the virus for life. Genital herpes is a common disease that is transmitted by direct contact with the lesions, which are very contagious. The treatment is intended to calm the attacks and must be administered with the first signs in order to reduce the duration of the symptoms. The spreading of the disease to the eyes or to the brain involves risks of blindness, encephalitis, or meningitis. The contamination of a newborn during childbirth can cause cerebral damage or even death.

Labial herpes... page 86

THE **SYMPTOMS** OF **GENITAL HERPES**

Outbreaks of genital herpes are manifested by the appearance of herpetic vesicles on the genital organs, accompanied by a burning sensation, itching and sometimes fever, headaches, and stomachaches. After several days, the vesicles burst and cause ulcerations, then form scabs and disappear. The first outbreak of genital herpes is generally very painful and lasts two to three weeks. The pain, which is very sharp, is exacerbated by contact with urine. Shorter and less intense, recurrences are caused by emotional shocks, fatigue, stress, menstruation, pregnancy, and the wearing of tight pants. Certain individuals feel the warning signs of herpes outbreaks (stinging, itching, burning) from a few hours to a few days before the start of an attack. It is possible to be a carrier of the virus and to transmit it without presenting any symptoms. The use of a condom must therefore be systematic.

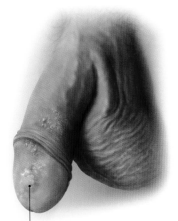

**Genital herpes
in men**

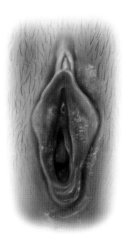

**Genital herpes
in women**

Herpetic vesicle
Herpetic vesicles are small blisters filled with liquid, in clusters. In men, genital herpes vesicles are usually located on the penis and sometimes on the testicles. In women, they are located on the vulva, but also in the vagina or even on the cervix. In both sexes, they may also be present on the anus, the buttocks, and the upper thigh.

GENITAL HERPES

SYMPTOMS:
Painful herpetic vesicles, open wounds, scabs. Burning, stinging, itching.

TREATMENTS:
Antiviral (aciclovir) in cream or in tablet form, sometimes intravenous, making it possible to reduce the duration of the symptoms and to slow down the multiplication of the virus.

PREVENTION:
Have protected sex, even when the illness is not presenting any symptoms. Abstain from sexual relations during herpes outbreaks. Adopt personal hygiene measures in order not to spread the virus.

GENITAL WARTS (CONDYLOMA)

Genital warts are benign, painless growths caused by a papillomavirus and found on the skin and the mucous membranes of the genital organs and the anus. These lesions multiply and their rate of growth varies according to the individual. They sometimes cause irritation, itching, and pain during sexual relations or defecation. Genital warts are among the most frequent STIs and the infected individuals remain carriers for life. Transmission of the virus generally takes place through direct contact during sexual relations. The incubation period may last from three weeks to eight months and the disease is often unobtrusive at the start, which promotes its transmission.

THE **LOCATION** OF **GENITAL WARTS**

In men, genital warts may be found on the penis, the testicles, the urethra, and the anus. In women, they are most often found on the vulva and sometimes in the vagina and on the cervix. Flat or raised, genital warts can be pink, grayish, or whitish in color. They may spread considerably, grow bigger, and take on the appearance of a cauliflower. Lesions may also ooze and, although it is very rare, give off a putrid odor.

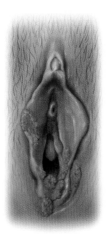

Genital warts
in women

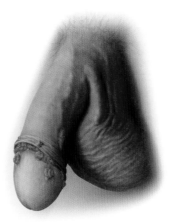

Genital warts
in men

THE **PAPILLOMAVIRUS**

The papillomavirus, or human papilloma virus, is a virus of which certain types cause the appearance of benign tumors on the skin (warts) or on the genital organs (genital warts). It may promote the development of certain malignant tumors, specifically cervical cancer. If either of the partners is infected with genital warts, periodic screening for cervical cancer (Pap test) is recommended. In immunodeficient individuals, specifically those with AIDS, the papillomavirus often causes extensive and persistent lesions.

Warts... page 75

GENITAL WARTS

SYMPTOMS:
Growths on the skin or mucous membranes, capable of reaching a very large size with the appearance of a cauliflower (specifically in immunodeficient subjects). Genital warts may be annoying, but they are rarely painful. Sometimes asymptomatic.

TREATMENTS:
Removal (trichloroacetic acid, podophyllin, cryotherapy, electrocoagulation, laser, surgery). Application of antiviral ointment. Sexual partners must be treated. Genital warts are difficult to treat and recurrences are frequent, especially when the immune system is weak.

PREVENTION:
Protected sex using a condom.
The condom... page 454

GONORRHEA

Gonorrhea, or blennorrhagia, is a sexually transmitted **infection** caused by a bacterium, the gonoccus. Particularly common, its transmission generally occurs through direct contact during sex. It is often associated with a genital chlamydia. Untreated, the infection spreads to the uterus, the fallopian tubes, and the ovaries in women and to the epididymis in men, and may become a cause of extrauterine pregnancy or sterility. Often asymptomatic (especially in women), blennorrhagia may manifest in abnormal discharge from the vagina or urethra (purulent in men), burning sensations during urination, and inflammation of the infected organs (cervix in women, urethra in men). In some cases, the blennorrhagia manifests itself by atypical symptoms: orogenital sex may cause infection of the mouth or the throat.

GONORRHEA

SYMPTOMS:
In men: **inflammation** of the urethra (purulent, yellowish discharge, burning sensation at urination). Blennorrhagia is often asymptomatic, specifically in women.

TREATMENTS:
Antibiotics. Sexual partners must be treated. Recontamination is possible.

PREVENTION:
Sexual relations, including oral sex, protected using a condom. Screening test recommended for persons at risk who have unprotected sex or multiple partners.
The condom… page 454

TRICHOMONIASIS

Trichomoniasis is a sexually transmitted disease caused by the parasite *Trichomonas vaginalis*. Very common, it manifests in women in vaginitis accompanied by strong itching and significant, often foul-smelling, vaginal discharge. In men, it may cause urethritis, but it is often asymptomatic. Transmission is primarily sexual, but it is also possible through contact with contaminated objects: towels, bathing suits, sauna benches. The disease is promoted in women by an imbalance in vaginal flora and a reduction in the natural acidity of the vagina.

TRICHOMONIASIS

SYMPTOMS:
Often asymptomatic, especially in men. Women: vaginitis with abundant, greenish, foul-smelling discharge, strong itching, urination problems. Men: inflammation of the urethra.

TREATMENTS:
Antibiotics. Sexual partners must be treated. Recontamination is possible.

PREVENTION:
Protected sex using a condom.
The condom… page 454

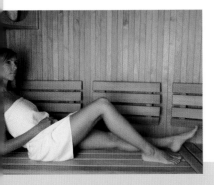

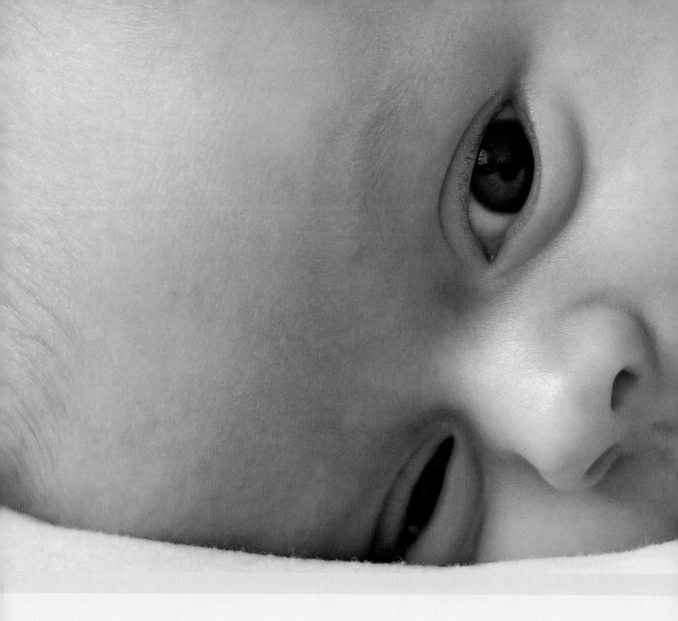

REPRODUCTION

Reproduction refers to all of the processes used by living beings in order to give birth to another generation. In human beings, the fertilization, or meeting of a sperm and an ovum, usually results from a sexual relationship between a man and a woman (coitus). The merger of these two cells creates an embryo, which implants itself in the mother's uterus. The embryo is develops progressively into a fetus, thanks to the placenta, which acts as a filter and permits exchanges of gas, hormones, antibodies, and nutrients between it and the mother. Childbirth normally takes place after nine months of pregnancy, when the development of its organs make it possible for the child to live outside of the uterus.

The development of the embryo or the fetus may be disrupted by various problems. Depending on the individual case, there may be fetal distress, delay in growth, premature birth, malformations, or miscarriage. Some pregnancies must be carefully monitored and may necessitate in a birth by cesarean section. Different factors affecting the man, the woman, or the couple may also prevent fertilization, causing sterility.

SEXUALITY

Sexuality is all of the behaviors, partly instinctive, connected with reproduction and the search for sexual pleasure. It develops primarily with adolescence and simultaneously puts into play both psychological (love, libido) and physical (erection, ejaculation, orgasm) phenomena. These phenomena are given concrete expression through sexual relations. These involve two partners and are generally preceded by a period of excitation, helped by the libido. During sex, the partners feel pleasure, which, excited by the stimulation of erogenous zones, may end with orgasm. The development of sexuality contributes to the development of well-being.

COITUS

Coitus is sex between a man and a woman, with penetration of the erect penis into the vagina. The repetitive movements of the penis and of the vagina generally end in an orgasm and the expulsion of the sperm (ejaculation) into the vagina. Coitus may also lead to the fertilization of an ovum by a sperm cell and the conception of a child.

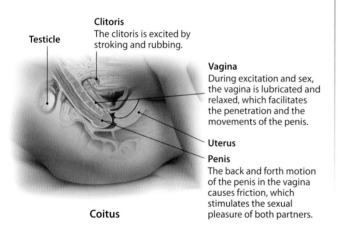

Testicle

Clitoris
The clitoris is excited by stroking and rubbing.

Vagina
During excitation and sex, the vagina is lubricated and relaxed, which facilitates the penetration and the movements of the penis.

Uterus

Penis
The back and forth motion of the penis in the vagina causes friction, which stimulates the sexual pleasure of both partners.

Coitus

LIBIDO

Libido, or sexual desire, is the psychological energy at the origin of sexual impulses. It results from visual, chemical (hormones), and mental (fantasies) stimulation. In men, the libido triggers the secretion of male hormones (testosterone), which, in turn, stimulate desire. In women, the libido is at its maximum at the moment of ovulation, when the female hormones (estrogens) are secreted in large quantity.

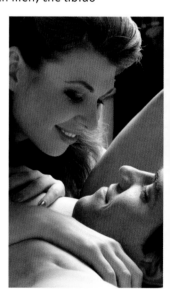

ORGASM

Orgasm is a sensation of intense pleasure that occurs at the end of sexual excitation, during sex or masturbation. It results from the repetitive stimulation of the sexual organs and the erogenous zones. In men, orgasm is associated with ejaculation. In women, it is accompanied by vaginal contractions and an increase in vaginal secretions. Orgasm is followed by muscular and psychological relaxation causing a drop in sexual excitation, which is longer in men than in women.

EROGENOUS ZONES

Erogenous zones are very sensitive parts of the body, whose tactile stimulation may result in sexual excitation and pleasure. The penis, glans, and foreskin in men, and the clitoris and vagina in women, are erogenous zones. There are many others, specifically around the genital organs, on the breasts, the buttocks, the lips, etc.

ERECTION

Erection is the swelling and hardening of certain organs and tissues: penis, clitoris, nipples. Penal erection corresponds to the sudden rush of blood into the penis and its retention in the cavernous body. It is controlled by a nervous reflex and often triggered by sexual stimulation. Erection is necessary for coitus. The inability to obtain an erection and to maintain it long enough to obtain an ejaculation may occur occasionally or in a chronic manner, specifically with age or in the case of diseases such as diabetes. Smoking and alcoholism may also affect the erection.

Sterility… page 486

Vein
The dilation of the spongy and cavernous bodies during erection compresses the veins, which prevents the blood from leaving the penis.

Nerve

Cavernous body
During the erection, the blood flows into the cavernous body.

Artery

Urethra

Spongy body

Cross section of penis in erection
The penis in erection hardens, grows larger, grows longer, and stands up straight.

EJACULATION

Ejaculation is the expulsion of sperm by the urethra at the moment of male orgasm. It occurs during sexual relations or masturbation, after the repetitive stimulation of the penis. A nervous reflex first causes the contraction of the vas deferens and related glands (seminal vesicle, prostate, Cowper's glands), which discharge their secretions (sperm cells and seminal fluid) into the urethra. The 2 to 5 milliliters of sperm thus accumulated are then propelled inside the penis by spasmodic contractions of the muscles of the perineum. Ejaculation is followed by a rapid deflating of the erection.

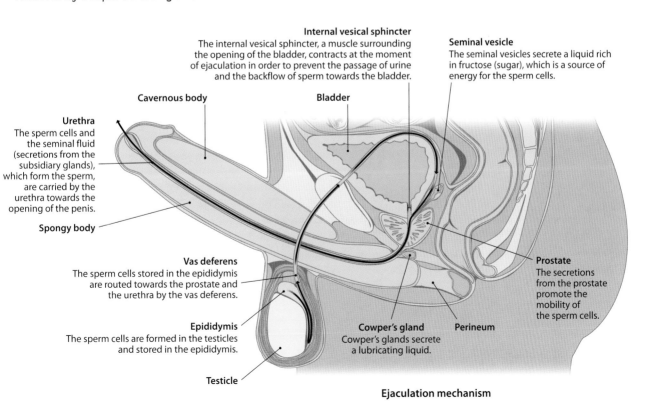

Internal vesical sphincter
The internal vesical sphincter, a muscle surrounding the opening of the bladder, contracts at the moment of ejaculation in order to prevent the passage of urine and the backflow of sperm towards the bladder.

Seminal vesicle
The seminal vesicles secrete a liquid rich in fructose (sugar), which is a source of energy for the sperm cells.

Cavernous body

Bladder

Urethra
The sperm cells and the seminal fluid (secretions from the subsidiary glands), which form the sperm, are carried by the urethra towards the opening of the penis.

Spongy body

Vas deferens
The sperm cells stored in the epididymis are routed towards the prostate and the urethra by the vas deferens.

Epididymis
The sperm cells are formed in the testicles and stored in the epididymis.

Testicle

Cowper's gland
Cowper's glands secrete a lubricating liquid.

Perineum

Prostate
The secretions from the prostate promote the mobility of the sperm cells.

Ejaculation mechanism

453

CONTRACEPTION

Contraception is the use of a method intended to prevent pregnancy, which makes it possible to plan a birth and to reduce the number of unwanted children. Contraceptive methods may be mechanical (condom, intrauterine device, diaphragm), hormonal (contraceptive pill, transdermal patch, vaginal ring, subcutaneous implant), or surgical (tubal ligation, vasectomy). In case of unwanted fertilization, an abortion may be considered in numerous countries.

THE CONDOM

The condom is used as a method of contraception and as protection against sexually transmitted infections. It is a sheath of latex or of impermeable polyurethane used to cover the penis in erection before sex. The condom is very effective when it is carefully handled and when its expiration date is respected. Easy to purchase and to use, it has no side effects, with the exception of rare allergies to latex. Nevertheless, it changes the tactile sensations of both partners and its use requires a brief interruption in the act.

Sexually transmitted infections… page 444

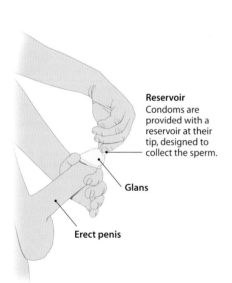

Reservoir
Condoms are provided with a reservoir at their tip, designed to collect the sperm.

Glans

Erect penis

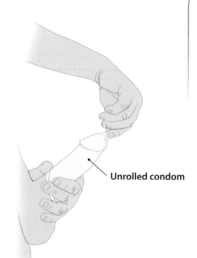

Unrolled condom

FEMALE CONDOM
Since the 1990s, a female condom has been available. Based on the principle of the male condom and adapted to female anatomy, it is placed in the vagina.

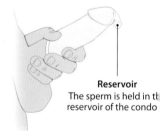

Reservoir
The sperm is held in th[e] reservoir of the condo[m]

1. Application
The packaging must be opened without using cutting instruments, nails, or teeth, so as not to perforate the condom. It is applied on the end of the erect penis (glans) while pinching lightly on the reservoir in order to expel the air.

2. Unrolling
The condom is unrolled up to the base of the penis while taking care not to introduce air.

3. Withdrawal
After ejaculation, the man must withdraw quickly, before the loss of the erection, while securing the condom at the base of the penis.

"NATURAL" CONTRACEPTION METHODS

The withdrawal of the penis prior to ejaculation or periodic abstinence associated with the woman's menstrual cycle and period of fertility (basal body temperature method, Ogino method) are called "natural" contraceptive methods. However, their effectiveness is limited and the failure rate remains high.

THE **CONTRACEPTIVE PILL**

The contraceptive pill makes it possible to control the menstrual cycle using sex hormones administered orally, in the form of pills. The most commonly used and most effective pills contain a mixture of estrogen and a progesterone derivative, progestin. They block ovulation, change the cervical mucus (secreted in the cervix), and prevent the preparation of the endometrium for implantation. In case of contraindication connected with estrogens, pills containing only progestin (micro-pills) may be prescribed, but they are less effective. The contraceptive pill requires a prescription and medical monitoring. Its use may have negative side effects, such as fatigue, weight gain, breast pain, migraines, or nausea. The pill may also have positive effects: reduction of functional ovarian cysts, acne, and ovarian cancer risks.

The menstrual cycle... page 423
Nidation... page 459

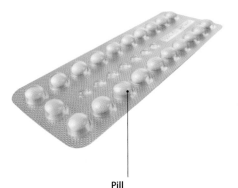

Pill
The contraceptive pill is usually available in the form of a packet of 21 pills. The first pill must be taken on the first day of menstruation. The following pills are taken each day, at the same time. A seven-day break then allows for menstruation to occur. When the packets contain 28 pills, they must be taken without interruption.

THE **INTRAUTERINE DEVICE**

The intrauterine device is a removable device inserted in the uterine cavity for contraceptive purposes. Its contact with the uterine wall creates an inflammation that is slight but sufficient to prevent implantation of the fertilized egg in the endometrium. The intrauterine device is inserted by a doctor in a few minutes, after having verified the absence of contraindications. Its placement must be regularly checked by the woman. At first, the intrauterine device may cause uterine spasms, some bleeding, and heavier and longer periods. It also increases the risk of extrauterine pregnancy and of pelvic infection.

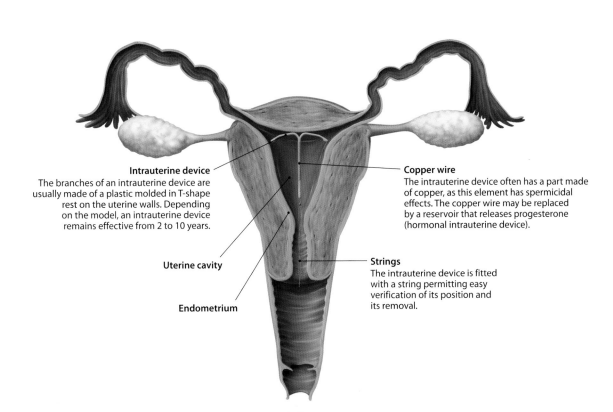

Intrauterine device
The branches of an intrauterine device are usually made of a plastic molded in T-shape rest on the uterine walls. Depending on the model, an intrauterine device remains effective from 2 to 10 years.

Copper wire
The intrauterine device often has a part made of copper, as this element has spermicidal effects. The copper wire may be replaced by a reservoir that releases progesterone (hormonal intrauterine device).

Uterine cavity

Endometrium

Strings
The intrauterine device is fitted with a string permitting easy verification of its position and its removal.

455

STERILIZATION

Sterilization is a permanent method of contraception, most often irreversible, performed surgically. It may be done for medical reasons, specifically when a pregnancy would present a vital risk, or for personal convenience. In this case, it is generally subject to rules and evaluation criteria that vary according to the country: information on the consequences, observance of a waiting period, number of children, age, etc.

VASECTOMY

Men may choose to have a vasectomy, which consists of interrupting the passage of the sperm cells in the vas deferens, most often by severing the latter. After surgery under local anesthesia lasting less than 30 minutes, the patient returns home and engages in normal activity, even though he may feel discomfort for three or four days. The vasectomy does not affect either erection or ejaculation. It is only completely effective after a period of two to three months, during which time the liquid ejaculated still contains sperm cells. The operation is reversible in approximately 25% of cases.

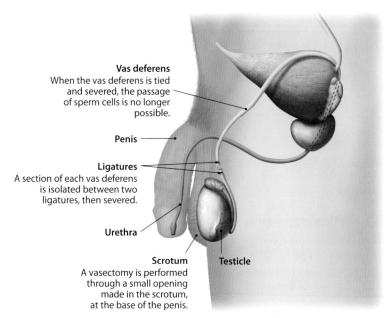

Vas deferens
When the vas deferens is tied and severed, the passage of sperm cells is no longer possible.

Penis

Ligatures
A section of each vas deferens is isolated between two ligatures, then severed.

Urethra

Scrotum
A vasectomy is performed through a small opening made in the scrotum, at the base of the penis.

Testicle

Vasectomy

TUBAL LIGATION

Women may choose to undergo a tubal ligation, which is intended to prevent the passage of ova in the fallopian tubes. It may be done by severing the tubes or by closing them using clips. Surgery, which requires one day of hospitalization at most, is done in the majority of cases under general anesthesia by making a small incision in the wall of the abdomen. The tubal ligation may also be done without incision by placing a device in the tubes that results in their obstruction. The tubal ligation is an effective method of birth control that does not alter the menstrual cycle. It is generally irreversible.

Incision

Ligature

Fallopian tube
A portion of each fallopian tube is isolated between two ligatures then incised, which prevents any meeting between an ovum and a sperm cell.

Ovary

Uterus

Ligation of the fallopian tubes

ABORTION

Voluntary interruption of pregnancy, or abortion, is the stopping of gestation done at the mother's request. It may be done by taking abortion drugs, which stop implantation and cause uterine contractions and natural expulsion, or surgically, which requires one day of hospitalization. The principal surgical method used is endouterine aspiration, which consists of aspirating the contents of the uterus through the vagina. This may also be done following a miscarriage. Endouterine aspiration is done under local, regional, or general **anesthesia,** after the dilation of the cervix. The operation may cause bleeding for several days, but it rarely causes complications. In countries where abortion is legal, its application is subject to strict conditions defined by law: waiting period, age, circumstances, stage of pregnancy, etc.

THERAPEUTIC ABORTION

Gestation stopped for medical reasons is called therapeutic abortion, or medical interruption of pregnancy. In many countries, it may be done at any time during the pregnancy with parental and medical consent. Therapeutic abortion may be specifically considered if the mother has a serious illness: heart, renal or respiratory failure, AIDS, cancer, etc. It may also be done when prenatal tests reveal a serious anomaly in the fetus: Down's syndrome, spina bifida, etc.

THE **MORNING-AFTER PILL**

The morning-after pill is not an abortion drug, but rather an emergency contraceptive method used in case of risk of pregnancy, after sex without contraception or with the tearing of a condom, the dislodging of an intrauterine device, or forgetting a contraceptive pill. The morning-after pill, which prevents fertilization or the implantation of the egg, must be taken as quickly as possible after sexual intercourse. It may cause minor, short-term side effects, such as nausea, headaches, and stomachaches or slight bleeding.

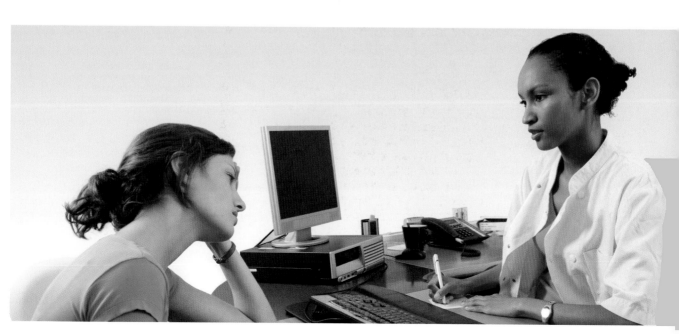

FERTILIZATION

Fertilization is the fusion between an ovum and a sperm cell. It occurs following coitus that ends with the man ejaculating into the woman's vagina during her ovulation period. The meeting of male and female sex cells, if not voluntarily prevented by contraception or involuntarily by sterility, takes place in the fallopian tubes. The fertilized egg then migrates to the uterus, where it implants itself into the endometrium.

THE STAGES OF FERTILIZATION

After having been deposited in the far end of the vagina at ejaculation, millions of sperm cells travel through the uterus towards the fallopian tubes. Only a few hundred of them manage to reach the ovum. The penetration of one of the sperm cells into the ovum, or fertilization, results in the merging of their respective cellular nuclei. The fertilized ovum, called the zygote, descends through the fallopian tube towards the uterus. It divides progressively into a number of cells in order to form an embryo, or blastocyst, which implants itself in the endometrium (nidation).

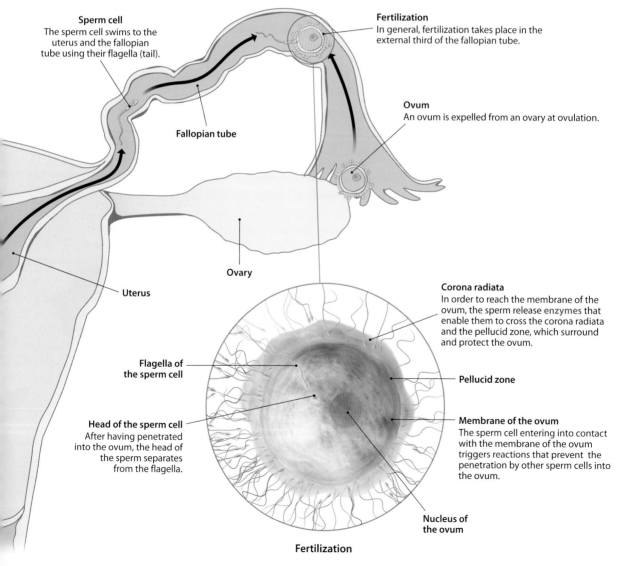

Sperm cell
The sperm cell swims to the uterus and the fallopian tube using their flagella (tail).

Fertilization
In general, fertilization takes place in the external third of the fallopian tube.

Ovum
An ovum is expelled from an ovary at ovulation.

Fallopian tube

Ovary

Uterus

Corona radiata
In order to reach the membrane of the ovum, the sperm release enzymes that enable them to cross the corona radiata and the pellucid zone, which surround and protect the ovum.

Flagella of the sperm cell

Pellucid zone

Head of the sperm cell
After having penetrated into the ovum, the head of the sperm separates from the flagella.

Membrane of the ovum
The sperm cell entering into contact with the membrane of the ovum triggers reactions that prevent the penetration by other sperm cells into the ovum.

Nucleus of the ovum

Fertilization

458

NIDATION

Nidation is the implantation of a fertilized egg in the endometrium, six or seven days after fertilization. The cells of its outer layer (trophoblast) multiply and erode the endometrium, which enables the blastocyst to anchor itself there. The implantation phase lasts approximately one week.

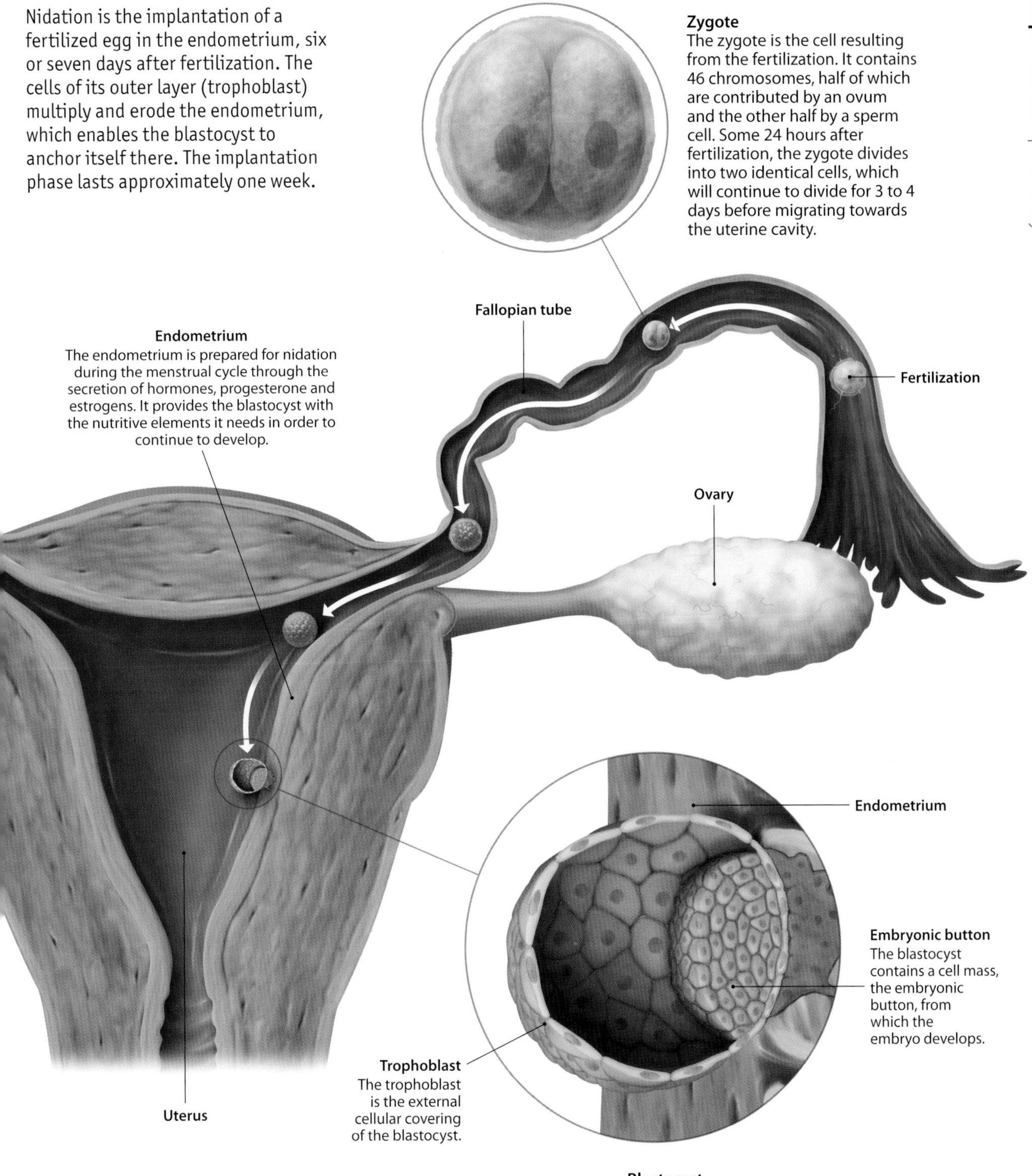

Zygote
The zygote is the cell resulting from the fertilization. It contains 46 chromosomes, half of which are contributed by an ovum and the other half by a sperm cell. Some 24 hours after fertilization, the zygote divides into two identical cells, which will continue to divide for 3 to 4 days before migrating towards the uterine cavity.

Fallopian tube

Endometrium
The endometrium is prepared for nidation during the menstrual cycle through the secretion of hormones, progesterone and estrogens. It provides the blastocyst with the nutritive elements it needs in order to continue to develop.

Fertilization

Ovary

Endometrium

Embryonic button
The blastocyst contains a cell mass, the embryonic button, from which the embryo develops.

Trophoblast
The trophoblast is the external cellular covering of the blastocyst.

Uterus

Blastocyst
A blastocyst is an embryo 5 to 7 days old, following fertilization. It consists of a central cavity and two distinct types of cells, the trophoblast and the embryonic button.

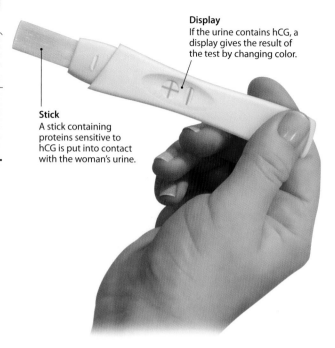

Display
If the urine contains hCG, a display gives the result of the test by changing color.

Stick
A stick containing proteins sensitive to hCG is put into contact with the woman's urine.

THE **PREGNANCY** TEST

A pregnancy test makes it possible to determine whether or not a woman is pregnant. It is based on the detection of a hormone, the human chorionic gonadotropin (hCG) hormone, in the urine or the blood. One week after fertilization, blastocyst cells begin to secrete hCG, which prolongs the production of female hormones (progesterone, estrogens) and which prevents the triggering of menstruation during the time needed for the blastocyst to attach itself in the endometrium. The amount of hCG increases up to the second month of pregnancy before suddenly dropping. Urine tests may be easily done by the woman herself, while blood analyses must be done in the laboratory.

THE **DETERMINATION** OF **GENDER**

The sex cells (ova and sperm cell) are haploids, which means they contain 23 chromosomes, of which only one participates in determining the gender of the unborn child, the sex chromosome. During fertilization, an ovum and a sperm cell merge to form a diploid cell, the zygote. The latter contains 46 chromosomes, of which two are sex chromosomes. Each child of the couple inherits one of two X chromosomes from its mother, together with an X chromosome or a Y chromosome from its father.

DNA and genes... page 48

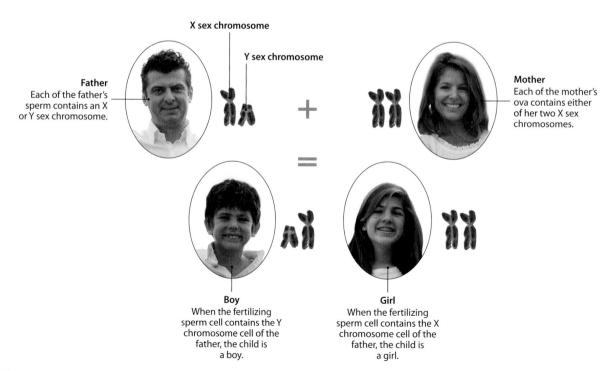

X sex chromosome

Y sex chromosome

Father
Each of the father's sperm contains an X or Y sex chromosome.

Mother
Each of the mother's ova contains either of her two X sex chromosomes.

+

=

Boy
When the fertilizing sperm cell contains the Y chromosome cell of the father, the child is a boy.

Girl
When the fertilizing sperm cell contains the X chromosome cell of the father, the child is a girl.

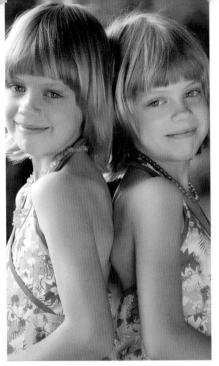

MULTIPLE PREGNANCIES

When several fetuses develop simultaneously in the uterus, it is called multiple pregnancy, or multifetal pregnancy. The most frequent case is the presence of two fetuses, twins, but sometimes the fetuses are more numerous (triplets, quadruplets, etc.). There are two types of multiple pregnancies, due to two very different processes. Monozygote twins come from a single ovum while dizygote twins come from two separate ova. Multiple pregnancies must be closely monitored and often end in premature delivery.

The formation of ova… page 422

MONOZYGOTE TWINS

Monozygote twins, or "identical twins," are two people born from the same fertilized ovum (zygote), which divided into two. This division occurs for reasons as yet unknown, during the first 14 days after fertilization. If it takes place early enough, the embryos have separate placentas, but it often happens that they share the same placenta. Monozygote twins are of the same gender, have the same genetic code, and closely resemble each other.

DIZYGOTE TWINS

Dizygote twins, or "fraternal twins," are two people resulting from the same pregnancy, but who developed from two separate ova. The ova fertilized by the different sperm cells produce two zygotes that evolve separately. Dizygote twins may be of different genders and have their own genetic code. The frequency of this type of pregnancy is increasing due to fertility treatments such as artificial insemination. It is also higher in certain ethnic groups and in women over age 30.

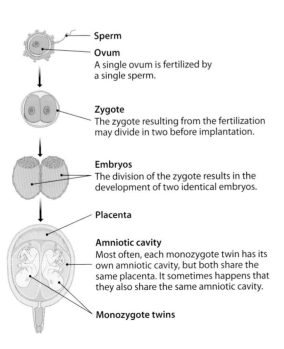

Sperm

Ovum
A single ovum is fertilized by a single sperm.

Zygote
The zygote resulting from the fertilization may divide in two before implantation.

Embryos
The division of the zygote results in the development of two identical embryos.

Placenta

Amniotic cavity
Most often, each monozygote twin has its own amniotic cavity, but both share the same placenta. It sometimes happens that they also share the same amniotic cavity.

Monozygote twins

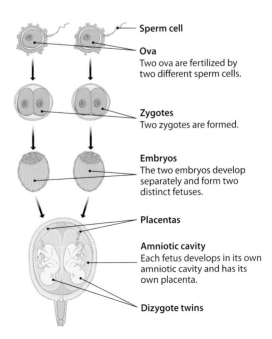

Sperm cell

Ova
Two ova are fertilized by two different sperm cells.

Zygotes
Two zygotes are formed.

Embryos
The two embryos develop separately and form two distinct fetuses.

Placentas

Amniotic cavity
Each fetus develops in its own amniotic cavity and has its own placenta.

Dizygote twins

461

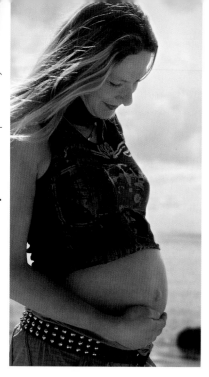

PREGNANCY

Pregnancy is all of the physiological phenomena that occur in a pregnant woman between fertilization and childbirth. It normally lasts between 40 and 42 weeks from the last menstrual period. After fertilization, the egg divides to form an embryo, which implants itself in the uterine wall and progressively develops into a fetus. During pregnancy, the woman experiences a number of physical transformations, which often involve minor problems. In some cases, the pregnancy cannot continue to term and ends with a premature birth or a miscarriage. In industrialized countries, pregnant women benefit from prenatal examinations that make it possible to detect possible complications.

THE **EMBRYO**

From fertilization to the the 8th week of pregnancy, the human being developing in the uterus is called an embryo. It develops from a fertilized egg (blastocyst) implanted in the endometrium. Some blastocyst tissues evolve to create the placenta, the umbilical cord, and the amniotic sac, while others are at the origin of different organs. From the end of the 3rd week, the embryo has an outline of a nervous system. Its heart begins to beat and blood circulation is in place, while an outline of its digestive system and urinary system appear. Subsequently, the organs develop and the skeleton hardens. At the end of eight weeks, the embryo appears human and its limbs are well-defined: it becomes a fetus.

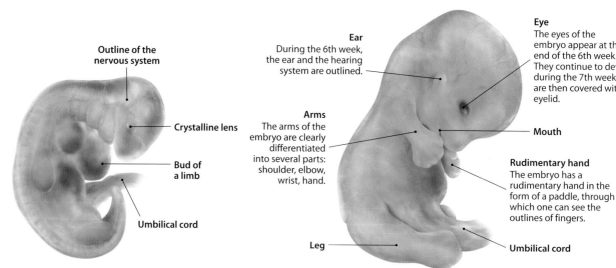

Outline of the nervous system

Crystalline lens

Bud of a limb

Umbilical cord

Ear
During the 6th week, the ear and the hearing system are outlined.

Arms
The arms of the embryo are clearly differentiated into several parts: shoulder, elbow, wrist, hand.

Leg

Eye
The eyes of the embryo appear at the end of the 6th week. They continue to develop during the 7th week and are then covered with an eyelid.

Mouth

Rudimentary hand
The embryo has a rudimentary hand in the form of a paddle, through which one can see the outlines of fingers.

Umbilical cord

Four-week embryo
A four-week embryo is bent over in the form of a C and measures approximately ³/₁₆ inch (5 mm). It has the buds of limbs and its crystalline lenses begin to form.
The eye... page 190

Six-week embryo
A six-week embryo measures almost ½ inch (13 mm) and weighs approximately 1.5 g. Its limbs are already differentiated and its face is beginning to have a human appearance.

THE **FETUS**

Between the 8th week of pregnancy and birth, the human being developing in the uterus is called a fetus. It undergoes significant growth, especially during the second trimester, growing from 3 to nearly 20 inches (from 8 to 50 cm). It straightens out and its features become finer while its weight increases from ¼ ounce to 7 pounds (8 g to 3.2 kg). From the 12th week, its kidneys function and it starts to urinate in the amniotic fluid. Its cardiovascular system develops until the 3rd month and its digestive system until the 7th month. The fetus is aware of tactile stimuli from the 4th month and begins to perceive sounds from the outside world at seven months. At birth, the skeleton is formed, but the bones are still partially cartilaginous. The bones, as well as several other organs such as the brain, the cerebellum, and the genital organs continue their maturation after birth.

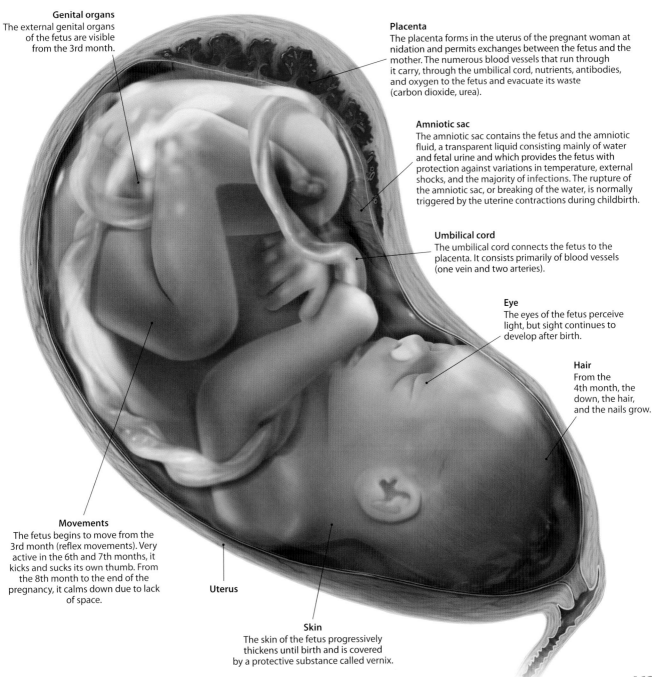

Genital organs
The external genital organs of the fetus are visible from the 3rd month.

Placenta
The placenta forms in the uterus of the pregnant woman at nidation and permits exchanges between the fetus and the mother. The numerous blood vessels that run through it carry, through the umbilical cord, nutrients, antibodies, and oxygen to the fetus and evacuate its waste (carbon dioxide, urea).

Amniotic sac
The amniotic sac contains the fetus and the amniotic fluid, a transparent liquid consisting mainly of water and fetal urine and which provides the fetus with protection against variations in temperature, external shocks, and the majority of infections. The rupture of the amniotic sac, or breaking of the water, is normally triggered by the uterine contractions during childbirth.

Umbilical cord
The umbilical cord connects the fetus to the placenta. It consists primarily of blood vessels (one vein and two arteries).

Eye
The eyes of the fetus perceive light, but sight continues to develop after birth.

Hair
From the 4th month, the down, the hair, and the nails grow.

Movements
The fetus begins to move from the 3rd month (reflex movements). Very active in the 6th and 7th months, it kicks and sucks its own thumb. From the 8th month to the end of the pregnancy, it calms down due to lack of space.

Uterus

Skin
The skin of the fetus progressively thickens until birth and is covered by a protective substance called vernix.

THE **PREGNANT WOMAN**

During pregnancy, the pregnant woman experiences numerous physiological transformations and frequently suffers from minor discomforts. She gains weight (an average of 27.5 pounds, or 12.5 kg, at term), her abdomen and her uterus expand as the fetus grows and her breasts get larger. These morphological changes often involve pain in the breasts, the groin, the pubis, and the back, as well as shortness of breath. Pregnant women frequently suffer from anemia, which causes a general state of weakness (fatigue, sleepiness, general discomfort), particularly marked in the first trimester. She becomes more prone to infections, specifically to urinary tract infections (cystitis), and her digestive system is disturbed: nausea, vomiting, constipation. Circulatory problems such as varicose veins, hemorrhoids, and edema (swelling) are also common, because the blood volume is increasing and the heart rate is accelerating. Vaginal discharge and itching, as well as increased salivation and perspiration, are also common. To these physiological problems are sometimes added psychological problems, at times pronounced: nervousness, irritability, emotionalism, insomnia and food cravings and aversions.

THE FIRST SIGNS OF PREGNANCY

The most convincing sign is the late period, but it is not systematic because many women have an irregular menstrual cycle and slight bleeding can occur during pregnancy. To this may be added the numerous changes associated with pregnancy, specifically changing breasts, psychological and digestive problems, as well as major fatigue. A pregnancy test eliminates all doubt.

Mask of pregnancy
The skin takes on a specific pigmentation, particularly on the face (mask of pregnancy) and the midline of the abdomen.

Nose
The sense of smell is more developed.

Gums
The gums are more sensitive to inflammations (gingivitis).

Breasts
From the start of the pregnancy, the breasts increase in volume and become heavier in preparation for nursing. The nipples swell and become darker.

Stomach
In stretching, the uterus compresses the digestive organs and pushes the stomach up, which causes frequent gastro-esophageal reflux.

Skin
The stretching of the skin sometimes causes an alteration of the elastic fibers, which appears as stretch marks, specifically on the breasts, the buttocks, and the abdomen.

Uterus
Normally 3 inches (8 cm) in length, the uterus reaches almost 14 inches (35 cm) at the end of the pregnancy.

Bladder
The uterus presses on the bladder, which increases the need to urinate.

Leg
Circulatory problems often affect the legs, which are subject to cramps, varicose veins, and edemas.
Edema... page 53

Physiological changes during pregnancy

SUGGESTIONS FOR LIMITING NAUSEA

During the first trimester of pregnancy, nausea is common in pregnant women. Here are some recommendations that will help you alleviate it:

• Eat upon awakening, if possible before getting up, and do not do too much in the morning.

• Eat less and more often: three meals and two snacks per day.

• Avoid drinking during meals.

• Eat what you want, but avoid food with pronounced taste, as well as strong odors.

• Inhale the smell of a cut lemon or eat a piece of one.

• Breathe fresh air.

A healthy pregnancy and a healthy child… page 466

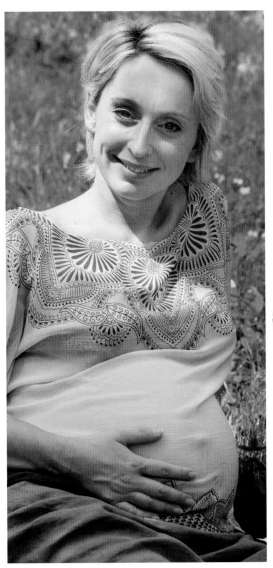

LATE PREGNANCY

A woman's fertility begins to diminish significantly at age 35 and declines progressively until menopause (between ages 45 and 55). Having a child after age 35, or even 40, is entirely possible, but the pregnancy involves more risks: gestational diabetes, pregnancy-induced hypertension, fibroids, preeclampsia, etc. After age 35, a pregnant woman is more tired and also more prone to miscarriages, as well as to premature or cesarean births. With advancing age, the risks of fetal malformation increase slightly, but cases of Down syndrome are multiplied (a prenatal test makes it possible to detect them). Despite this, late pregnancies have a good chance of progressing properly if the mother is in good health and is the subject of regular medical monitoring.

Gestational diabetes… page 229
Menopause… page 426

THE DURATION OF THE PREGNANCY

From fertilization, the date of which is determined at the first ultrasound, the average length of a pregnancy is 38 to 40 weeks. The starting date of the last period is also often used as a baseline date, the average then being 40 to 42 weeks from amenorrhea. These two calculation methods are valid; it is important to know which one is used in a document or during a consultation. In order to easily estimate the approximate date of birth, subtract three months from the starting date of the last period, then add one week.

A HEALTHY PREGNANCY AND A HEALTHY CHILD

During pregnancy, it is important to follow some guidelines in order to prevent certain, sometimes serious, problems, such as miscarriage and the appearance of congenital diseases in the child.

■ DO NOT CONSUME HARMFUL PRODUCTS AND DO NOT EXPOSE YOURSELF TO DANGEROUS SUBSTANCES

Tobacco, alcohol, and drugs may harm the development of the fetus and cause certain diseases, physical malformations, or mental retardation. Consuming them also increases the risk of premature childbirth and of sudden infant death syndrome. Likewise, toxic products such as paints and certain detergents are to be avoided during the first stages of pregnancy.

Fetal alcohol syndrome... page 479

■ AVOID LONG TRIPS

During long car trips, stop every hour to walk a little. For distances greater than 180 miles (300 km), the train is preferable. During a flight, move around, walk, and hydrate yourself in order to prevent phlebitis or an embolism. Avoid long trips and lengthy flights at the end of your pregnancy.

■ REST

Pregnancy, particularly the 1st and 3rd trimesters, often causes fatigue. Take time to rest when you feel the need. Avoid stress, overwork, overly intense physical activity, and the carrying of heavy loads, especially at the end of your pregnancy.

Stress management... page 28

■ EXERCISE, BUT AVOID INTENSE OR VIOLENT SPORTS

The practice of a moderate sport, such as walking, swimming, or yoga, is recommended during pregnancy. Yoga, in particular, prepares you to withstand the pains of childbirth. Avoid sports that cause jolting (horseback riding, tennis, etc.) or hitting (combat sports, group sports, etc.), as well as extreme sports (mountain climbing, scuba diving, etc.).

■ MONITOR ABNORMAL SIGNS

If signs of a miscarriage appear (bleeding, uterine contractions, etc.), stop all activity and consult a doctor as quickly as possible.

Miscarriage... page 476

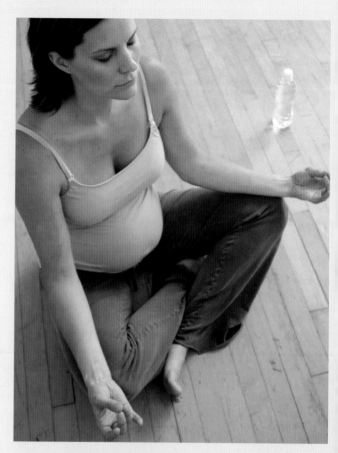

■ AVOID EXCESSIVE HEAT

Too great an increase in the mother's body temperature may cause discomfort and be dangerous for the fetus. In particular, avoid very hot baths (temperature greater than 100°F, or 38°C), whirlpool bathing, and physical activity in the heat.

■ MAINTAIN PROPER HYGIENE

Proper hygiene makes it possible to avoid infections that could harm the fetus. Wash your hands regularly. Wash the vegetables and fruits that you eat and avoid contact with cat excrement in order to minimize the risks of contracting toxoplasmosis.

Toxoplasmosis... page 478

A HEALTHY PREGNANCY AND A HEALTHY CHILD

■ ADOPT A BALANCED DIET

Nutritional deficiencies may cause fetal malformations and miscarriage. Eat three main meals, breakfast being very important, and one or two snacks per day. Eat in a varied and balanced manner, and follow your appetite without abusing products loaded with fat or sugar. In order to stay hydrated, drink at least 1½ quarts (liters) of liquid per day: water, herbal tea, fruit juice. The regular consumption of low-mercury fish is also advised.

Nutrition... page 11

■ AVOID CERTAIN FOODS

Certain foods may present a danger for the fetus, specifically in the first weeks of its development. This is the case with raw milk products, raw or poorly cooked meat and fish, undried sausages, and pâtés, which can cause diseases such as listeriosis or toxoplasmosis. Avoid these foods or cook them properly, and wash fruits and vegetables before eating them raw. Limit your consumption of sweeteners (such as aspartame), products rich in caffeine (coffee, tea, sodas, etc.), and predator fish such as tuna, swordfish, and bream, which often contain a large quantity of mercury.

Listeriosis... page 302

■ MONITOR WATER QUALITY

Consuming tap water is generally not dangerous, but it is preferable not to keep it in a pitcher for more than one day. Well water must be regularly analyzed. Do not use untreated water, whether for drinking, brushing your teeth, washing the dishes, or rinsing fruits and vegetables. Avoid drinking hot water from the tap and let the water run a bit after a long period of nonuse (in the morning, after a trip).

■ TAKE DIETARY SUPPLEMENTS

A woman's energy needs increase during pregnancy and a balanced diet may be enough to meet them. But the taking of supplements is sometimes recommended in order to increase intake of iron, iodine, calcium, Vitamin D and Vitamin B_9 (folic acid). Folic acid is found in foods such as leafy vegetables (lettuce, spinach, sorrel, cabbage), nuts, and eggs, but since the daily recommended amount of 0.4 mg is difficult to achieve, take folic acid supplements, ideally at least three months before the start of the pregnancy and until the end of the 1st trimester.

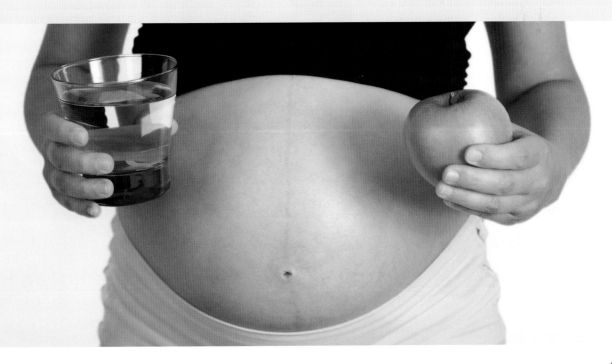

PRENATAL EXAMINATIONS

Prenatal examinations are medical examinations intended to monitor the development of the pregnancy. Most common in industrialized countries, they make it possible to monitor fetal development and to detect possible illnesses or anomalies. The pregnant woman is regularly weighed and examined. She undergoes a number of urine and blood analyses in order to detect any **infection** or disease dangerous to her health or to that of the fetus: gestational diabetes, rubella, toxoplasmosis, syphilis, etc. Blood analyses also make it possible to detect a possible Rhesus incompatibility between the mother and the child. Using **ultrasound** prenatal tests, it is possible to observe the morphology, the development, and the vitality of the fetus, as well as the position of the placenta.

Gestational diabetes... page 229
Rhesus incompatibility... page 480

PRENATAL ULTRASOUND EXAMINATION

The prenatal ultrasound examination, or obstetrical ultrasound, makes it possible to view the fetus as well as the inside of the uterus of a pregnant woman. The ultrasound probe, placed against the mother's abdomen, emits ultrasounds, which pass through the tissues. According to the density of the tissue, the ultrasounds send back a variable echo that is transformed into a rather precise image, the ultrasound. Quick and painless, the examination is generally done around the 12th, 22nd, and 32nd weeks of pregnancy. The first ultrasound examination establishes the precise fertilization and end dates of the pregnancy. It also makes it possible to detect certain malformations and to measure nuchal translucency. The second examination is done in order to detect possible morphological anomalies. It often makes it possible to determine the child's gender. During the last session, the doctor checks the position, the size, and the vitality of the fetus, as well as the amount of amniotic fluid and the position of the placenta. If an anomaly is noted (poor positioning, weak vital signs, etc.), the doctor may prescribe consultations with specialists and may determine whether specific measures will have to be taken during childbirth.

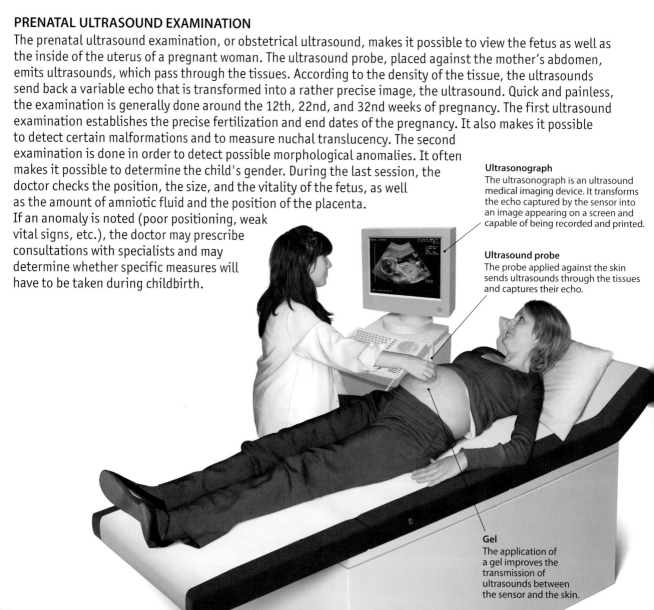

Ultrasonograph
The ultrasonograph is an ultrasound medical imaging device. It transforms the echo captured by the sensor into an image appearing on a screen and capable of being recorded and printed.

Ultrasound probe
The probe applied against the skin sends ultrasounds through the tissues and captures their echo.

Gel
The application of a gel improves the transmission of ultrasounds between the sensor and the skin.

ULTRASOUND

The ultrasound varies from black to white, passing through shades of gray according to the nature of the elements passed through by the ultrasounds. It makes it possible to monitor fetal growth and to diagnose possible malformations, specifically by measuring the size of the fetus's organs.

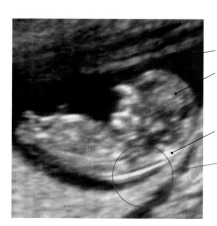

Amniotic fluid
The amniotic fluid, which lets the ultrasounds pass and produces very little echo, appears in black.

Head of the fetus

Bones
The solid structures, such as the bones, return a lot of echo and thus appear in white.

Ultrasound

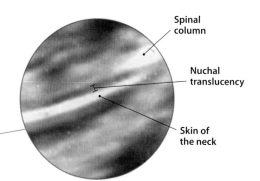

Spinal column

Nuchal translucency

Skin of the neck

Nuchal translucency
The nuchal translucency is a pocket of liquid located at the nape of the neck of the fetus. Its thickness may be evaluated during the first prenatal ultrasound examination. When it is greater than 3 mm, the probability that the fetus has a chromosomal anomaly, such as Down syndrome, is greater.

THREE-DIMENSIONAL ULTRASOUND

It is now possible to obtain a more precise image of the fetus using three-dimensional ultrasound. The examination, an addition to the standard ultrasound, is done primarily for emotional reasons. It requires a larger dose of ultrasounds, which causes heating and substantial vibrations whose effects on the fetus are still unknown. A number of health care agencies thus recommend using this technique with caution.

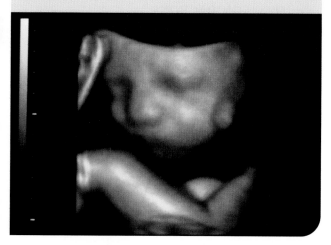

AMNIOCENTESIS

Amniocentesis is a prenatal examination that is recommended when there is a risk of chromosomal anomaly or of fetal infection, particularly when the mother is over 38 years of age, when an anomaly has been detected by ultrasound, or when a parent is a carrier of a chromosomal anomaly. The examination consists of sampling the amniotic fluid through the pregnant woman's abdominal wall in order to analyze it. Amniocentesis may be done between the 14th and the 18th week of pregnancy. The fetal cells contained in the amniotic fluid are analyzed in order to establish a chromosome map, which makes it possible to detect chromosomal anomalies and hereditary diseases. The examination also serves to verify the maturity of the fetus and to diagnose a neurological or digestive malformation, or even an infectious disease such as toxoplasmosis or cytomegalovirus. Amniocentesis involves certain risks for the fetus, specifically in the case of Rhesus incompatibility. It may also cause amniotic fluid leakage, break the amniotic sac, or transmit an infectious disease from the mother to the child (AIDS, hepatitis B). In total, it is estimated that miscarriage occurs in less than 1% of cases.

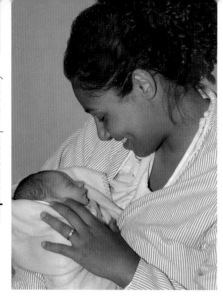

CHILDBIRTH

Childbirth is all of the phenomena occurring in the body of the pregnant woman that lead to the birth of her child. It generally occurs between the 37th and the 42nd week of pregnancy. Childbirth taking place before the 37th week is considered premature. If it occurs more than 10 days after the projected delivery date, it is referred to as a prolonged pregnancy. Childbirth normally occurs via natural means, but surgical intervention, the cesarean section, is sometimes necessary.

CHILDBIRTH IN A MEDICAL ENVIRONMENT

In industrialized countries, the majority of births take place in a medical environment in the event intervention is needed in case of complication. A nurse or a midwife follows the progress of the labor by regularly evaluating the dilation of the cervix and monitoring the uterine contractions. The fetal heartbeat is also monitored using an ultrasound sensor placed on the mother's abdomen (fetal monitoring). The midwife is authorized to deliver the baby, but a doctor intervenes in case of complication or if the birth presents certain risks, specifically in the case of premature birth or multiple pregnancy. In addition, the pain felt by the mother may be alleviated by epidural anesthesia, a technique that is also used in case of childbirth by cesarean section.

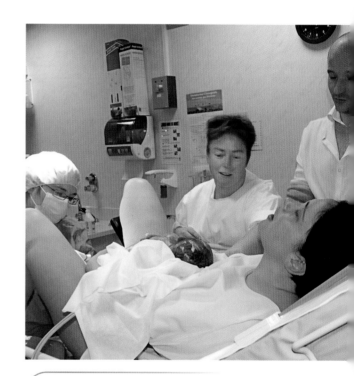

CHILDBIRTH AT HOME

Throughout the world, the majority of births take place at home, but childbirth in a medical environment is the norm in most industrialized countries. A woman may plan to give birth at home if her pregnancy does not demonstrate any risk: single fetus presenting normally, placenta in proper position, etc. However, this type of childbirth requires that certain precautions be taken. The practitioner who accompanies the labor must have the medical equipment available to handle possible complications.

THE FIRST CONTRACTIONS

During the last weeks of pregnancy, the pregnant woman may feel slightly painful and irregular contractions, but these do not necessarily indicate the start of labor. The first "real" contractions cause a wave of pain in the back and in the stomach, which hardens the uterus and which are reminiscent of menstrual cramps. The contractions are regular, then longer and longer, close together and painful, and may disturb breathing.

THE **PROGRESSION** OF **CHILDBIRTH**

During the last weeks of pregnancy, the fetus generally positions its head in the direction of the cervix. Childbirth begins when a hormone, oxytocin, triggers the dilation of the cervix and the spasmodic contractions of the uterine muscles. The amniotic sac may break, releasing the amniotic fluid, while the uterine contractions become more frequent and intensify. This is labor. The expulsion of the child occurs on average after 10 hours of labor, but this duration is often shorter in women who have already given birth. Childbirth ends with the expulsion of the placenta.

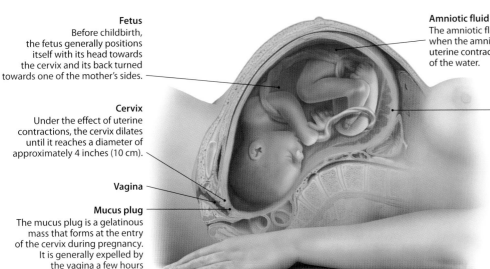

Fetus
Before childbirth, the fetus generally positions itself with its head towards the cervix and its back turned towards one of the mother's sides.

Cervix
Under the effect of uterine contractions, the cervix dilates until it reaches a diameter of approximately 4 inches (10 cm).

Vagina

Mucus plug
The mucus plug is a gelatinous mass that forms at the entry of the cervix during pregnancy. It is generally expelled by the vagina a few hours before labor starts.

Amniotic fluid
The amniotic fluid flows through the vagina when the amniotic sac is broken by the uterine contractions. This is the breaking of the water.

Uterus
At the end of labor, the uterine contractions last approximately one minute and may occur every two to three minutes.

Labor
Labor is the principal phase of childbirth, characterized by strong uterine contractions that are close together, and by the dilation of the cervix. The baby is progressively pushed towards the pelvis by the uterine contractions and its head descends into the vagina.

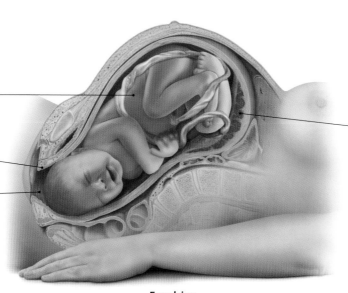

Fetus
In order to pass into the vagina, the fetus must bend its head forward and turn its back towards its mother's stomach.

Cervix

Vagina
At the moment of expulsion, the vagina and the cervix form a single pathway.

Placenta
The expulsion of the placenta generally occurs in the half-hour following the birth and may be accompanied by temporary bleeding. There must be no placental residue in the uterus in order to avoid an infection or hemorrhage.

Expulsion
The baby is expelled when labor has sufficiently dilated the cervix in order to allow it to pass. The expulsion, facilitated by the uterine contractions and the voluntary abdominal contractions of the mother, lasts one half hour on average.

TECHNIQUES FOR ASSISTING CHILDBIRTH

A number of medical techniques are used during childbirth to induce labor or to encourage the expulsion of the fetus. An artificial rupturing of the amniotic sac or an injection of oxytocin (a hormone that stimulates uterine contractions) may be used in order to induce labor. In the case of a difficult birth, forceps, a medical instrument in the form of large tongs, or a vacuum device, can be used in order to pull the fetus out of the vagina. The doctor uses them in case of insufficient uterine contractions, fatigue on the part of the mother, or slowing down of the fetal heartbeat (fetal distress). This manipulation is done under epidural anesthesia and is generally accompanied by a preventive incision of the perineum (episiotomy).

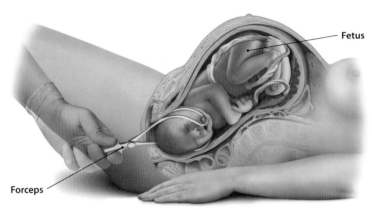

Fetus

Forceps

Forceps
In order to use the forceps, the cervix must be completely dilated,
the amniotic sac ruptured, and the head of the fetus in the mother's pelvis.
The arms of the forceps are placed on either side of the baby's head.
The doctor pulls delicately at the moment of the uterine contractions.

EPISIOTOMY

An episiotomy is a surgical incision in the wall of the vulva and of the perineum. It is performed during childbirth in order to facilitate the passage of the fetus, particularly when the child is weak, large, or in breech position. An episiotomy is also used when forceps are used or to prevent tears in the perineum, which is significantly distended during the expulsion of the baby. The incision, from 1 to 2 inches (2.5-5 cm), is done under local anesthesia, during a contraction, and during pushing. It may be done on the bias or in the direction of the anus and later requires suturing. An episiotomy takes longer to heal than a harmless tear and is normally used only in case of necessity.

EPIDURAL ANESTHESIA

Epidural anesthesia is given during childbirth in order to locally suppress the painful sensations of contractions without altering mother's consciousness. The anesthetic drug is injected into the lower back, generally between the third and forth lumbar vertebrae, in the epidural space surrounding the spinal cord. Epidural anesthesia may have some side effects for the mother: dizziness, headaches, lumbar pains, difficulties in urinating, sensation problems in the legs, etc. However, it does not present any risk for the fetus. If the labor is too advanced, it may not take effect.

CHILDBIRTH BY CESAREAN SECTION

Childbirth by cesarean section is a surgical procedure carried out to extract the fetus through an opening made in the wall of the abdomen and of the uterus. The procedure takes place in an operating room, under general or epidural anesthesia, and lasts approximately one hour. Childbirth by cesarean section is done if natural childbirth represents a danger for the mother or the child, specifically in the case of insufficient dilation of the cervix, too narrow a pelvis, a poorly positioned placenta, breech position, a particularly large or fragile fetus, or fetal distress. This type of childbirth presents few complications and leaves an unobtrusive scar, approximately 4 inches (10 cm) in length, above the pubis. However, the period that follows (postpartum) is more difficult than after a natural birth: later nursing, fatigue, abdominal pain and longer healing time. Several days of hospitalization are therefore necessary. The cesarean under epidural anesthesia enables the mother to remain conscious during childbirth and to see her child at its birth.

BREECH BIRTH

Before childbirth, it sometimes happens that the fetus is in a position with its buttocks towards the cervix. This is the breech position (3% of births). Certain maneuvers make it possible to turn the fetus around so that its head descends into in the mother's pelvis. If the maneuvers fail, natural childbirth is still possible if the size of the mother's pelvis allows it, if the baby is not too big, if the quantity of amniotic fluid is sufficient, and if the umbilical cord and the baby's head are properly positioned. If this is not the case, a cesarean section is performed. Occasionally, a baby may present itself shoulder first, which excludes any possibility of natural childbirth.

Head
The head of the fetus is at the upper end of the uterus.

Leg
Most often, the legs of the fetus are lifted up and extended in front of its chest.

Umbilical cord

Buttocks
The buttocks of the fetus are directed towards the cervix.

Cervix

THE CESAREAN IN NUMBERS

Throughout the world, approximately one of every seven births is by cesarean section, with the highest rate in Latin America and the Caribbean, and the lowest in Africa. In developing countries, this type of birth occurs approximately one out of every five births.

POSTPARTUM

The period that follows childbirth up to the return of menstruation is called postpartum or postconfinement. It lasts until the end of nursing or, in women who do not nurse, from four to nine weeks following the birth of the child. After childbirth, the woman experiences a number of physical transformations: her body progressively resumes its morphology and its normal functioning.

POSTPARTUM PHYSICAL CHANGES

With the birth of the child, the mother loses approximately 11 pounds (5 kg), then another 4-6 pounds (2-3 kg) in the days that follow. The abdomen, the uterus, and the vagina progressively return to their original size. The breasts become very sensitive and the uterus contracts painfully. Digestion is disturbed and only becomes normal after several days. Bloody vaginal discharge, lochia, occurs for several weeks.

Stretch marks
During pregnancy, the intense stretching of the skin often causes the appearance of striations, stretch marks, on the breasts, the buttocks, and the abdomen. It is possible to mitigate them by regularly applying creams softening the skin fibers, but their effectiveness is uncertain.

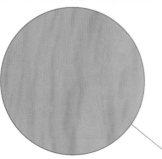

Breast
After childbirth, milk production makes the breasts sensitive and painful.

Abdomen
At childbirth, the abdomen loses a great deal of volume, but it remains soft because the abdominal muscles are distended.

Uterus
During the days following childbirth, the uterine muscles contract strongly in order to evacuate the lochia, bloody vaginal discharge consisting of uterine membrane debris.

Vagina
The lochia seeps out through the vagina. Bright red at the start of postpartum, the discharge becomes pink, then brownish, before stopping at the end of several weeks.

Perineum
The perineum is the area located between the anus and the genital organs. Severely distended by childbirth, it progressively recovers its muscle tone, possibly with the aid of perineal physiotherapy. The latter is intended to strengthen the musculature of the perineum using voluntary contraction exercises or low-intensity electrical stimulation. Perineal physiotherapy makes it possible to avoid urine leakage and may help in preventing genital prolapse.
Urinary incontinence… page 404
Genital prolapse… page 433

THE "BABY BLUES"
The significant hormonal fluctuations that follow childbirth may cause a benign and temporary emotional problem, the "baby blues." It affects most mothers and generally lasts only a few days. The "baby blues" is expressed through marked mood changes (euphoria, crying), anxiety, sadness, insomnia, and loss of appetite. More rarely, it is prolonged and evolves into postpartum depression, which requires medical monitoring. In all cases, it is important for the mother to have the support of her family.

Anus

In women who have just given birth, the blood vessels surrounding the anus are often dilated (hemorrhoids), which can cause defecation problems.

PUERPERAL FEVER

Puerperal fever is an **infectious** disease that may occur in a woman who has just given birth. It is most often the result of a bacterial infection of the uterus, the urinary tract, the vagina, the breasts, or a secondary wound following surgery (cesarean section, episiotomy). Contamination by a streptococcus, a staphylococcus, *Clostridium,* or *Escherichia coli* may occur when there is placental residue in the uterus or as the result of certain hospital manipulations during childbirth (nosocomial infection).

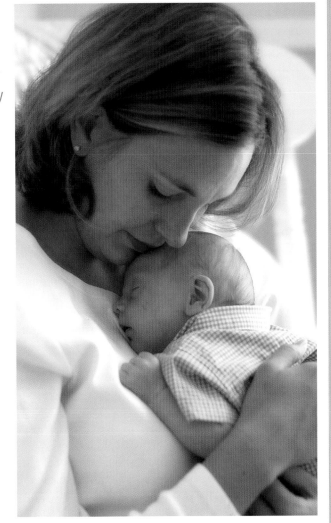

THE **RISKS** OF **PUERPERAL FEVER**

Varying in seriousness, puerperal fever is manifested by fever, pain, and foul-smelling, purulent vaginal discharges. In the absence of antibiotic treatments, the infection can spread and cause serious complications: adhesions (abnormal joining of two tissues or organs) in the pelvic cavity, generalized infection, peritonitis, embolism, sterility.

NOSOCOMIAL INFECTIONS

An infectious disease contracted in the hospital is called a nosocomial infection, or hospital infection. Primarily affecting fragile patients, such as newborns, the elderly and immunodeficient individuals, it is caused by the concentration of infectious agents and by invasive medical techniques: intravenous drip, prosthesis, probes, etc. The bacteria most often involved (staphylococcus aureus, *Clostridium difficile,* and *Escherichia coli*) come from the patient herself, from other patients, or from outside persons. They may also spread due to a lack of hygiene and as a result of a growing resistance to antibiotics.

PUERPERAL FEVER

SYMPTOMS:
Fever, pelvic pain, purulent and foul-smelling vaginal discharge.

TREATMENTS:
Antibiotics. Endouterine aspiration in case of placental residues.

PREVENTION:
Proper hygiene during and after childbirth.

MISCARRIAGE

Spontaneous abortion, or miscarriage, is an involuntary interruption of pregnancy that occurs before the fetus is viable, that is, before the 20th week of pregnancy. Often of unknown cause, it may be linked to diverse factors: chromosomal anomaly of the fetus, **infectious** disease, excess or insufficient amniotic fluid, multiple pregnancy, high fever, uterine malformation or fibroid, **anemia**, nutritional deficiency, hormonal insufficiency, gestational diabetes, **physical trauma**. The earlier the miscarriage occurs, the fewer the serious risks (serious hemorrhaging, infection) for the mother. After a miscarriage, it is recommended to have a gynecological examination and possibly to undergo a uterine curettage.

WARNING SYMPTOMS

Relatively common, particularly in the embryonic stage, a miscarriage may pass unnoticed. However, it is often preceded by warning symptoms: generally heavy bleeding and slight uterine contractions that resemble menstrual pains. Slight bleeding at the start of pregnancy does not necessarily constitute a danger. A gynecological examination helps to determine the cause of such bleeding and to diagnose a possible danger of miscarriage. It may be supplemented by an ultrasound, to verify the presence of the fetus and its placement, because an extrauterine pregnancy sometimes exhibits similar symptoms.

THE **PREVENTION** OF **MISCARRIAGES**

In order to prevent a miscarriage, the pregnant woman must abstain from smoking or consuming alcohol or drugs. She must not expose herself to dangerous substances and must avoid long trips and violent sports. Her diet must be balanced and must exclude certain foods capable of transmitting pathogenic agents (raw milk products and raw meats, etc.). In case of risk of miscarriage, complete rest as well as an antispasmodic and antalgic treatment sometimes makes it possible to bring the pregnancy to term. If the cervix appears prematurely open, a cerclage of the cervix may be done.

A healthy pregnancy and a healthy child… page 466

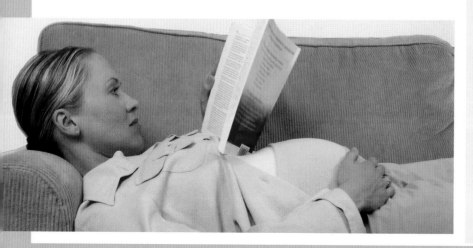

MISCARRIAGE

SYMPTOMS:
May pass unnoticed. Bleeding and more or less significant uterine contractions. Disappearance of signs of pregnancy.

TREATMENTS:
Danger of miscarriage: complete rest, antispasmodic, and antalgic treatments. After a miscarriage: uterine curettage in the case of incomplete expulsion.

PREVENTION:
Avoid tobacco, alcohol, exposure to dangerous products, long trips, violent sports, raw milk products and raw meats. Proper hygiene.

EXTRAUTERINE PREGNANCY

In approximately 1 pregnant woman out of 60, the embryo develops outside of the uterus. This is an extrauterine or ectopic pregnancy. In the majority of these cases, the fertilized egg does not manage to migrate to the uterus and remains blocked in the fallopian tube (tubular pregnancy). More rarely, it lodges in the ovary, in the cervix, or in the abdominal cavity. An extrauterine pregnancy may manifest itself by abdominal pain and uterine bleeding occurring after three to six months of **amenorrhea**. It requires increased monitoring in order to avoid a rupture of the tube, which can have serious consequences. Generally, the extrauterine pregnancy does not regress spontaneously and requires a medical or surgical treatment.

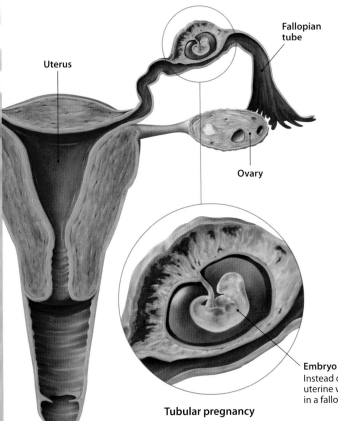

Fallopian tube

Uterus

Ovary

Tubular pregnancy

Embryo
Instead of implanting itself into the uterine wall, the embryo develops in a fallopian tube.

THE **TUBULAR PREGNANCY**

The tubular pregnancy is an extrauterine pregnancy in which the embryo develops in a fallopian tube. It occurs most often because of a malformation or a lesion disturbing the progress of the fertilized egg. An infection (salpingitis), endometriosis, surgery, or an earlier tubular pregnancy are the main causes of the tubal lesion. Smoking, the advanced age of the mother and medically assisted procreation also contribute to this type of pregnancy. After having implanted itself in the fallopian tube, the embryo generally grows for six to seven weeks, then it may become detached and die due to lack of space and nutritional resources, or cause a rupture of the tube and an internal hemorrhage.

THE RISKS OF TUBULAR PREGNANCY

When a tubular pregnancy is not diagnosed and treated in time, it may cause a rupture of the fallopian tube. The internal hemorrhage that results often causes irreversible damage or even death. Extrauterine pregnancies represent 10% of the causes of mortality in pregnant women. In addition, the lesion or the ablation of the tubes following a tubular pregnancy are significant causes of sterility.

EXTRAUTERINE PREGNANCY

SYMPTOMS:
Pain in the lower abdomen, bleeding of brownish color .

TREATMENTS:
Medical injection intended to destroy the embryo, surgery.

TOXOPLASMOSIS

Toxoplasmosis is an **infectious** disease caused by a protozoon parasite, the toxoplasma. The infection is harmless and often passes unnoticed. It may, however, have serious consequences on the development of the fetus if it is contracted by a pregnant woman. During the 1st trimester of pregnancy, the infection may result in the death of the fetus. Later on, it may cause lesions in the eyes, brain, and liver of the fetus that may only be manifested after the birth. A blood analysis makes it possible to determine whether a woman is immunized against toxoplasmosis.

CONTAMINATION BY TOXOPLASMOSIS

Residing primarily in the intestines of cats, toxoplasma is dispersed in the form of eggs contained in feline excrement, which may contaminate water, soil, vegetables, and animals eating these vegetables. A human being may contract toxoplasmosis by consuming insufficiently cooked meat or by ingesting toxoplasma eggs through a soiled carrier (hands, objects, garden vegetables, water, dirt, etc).

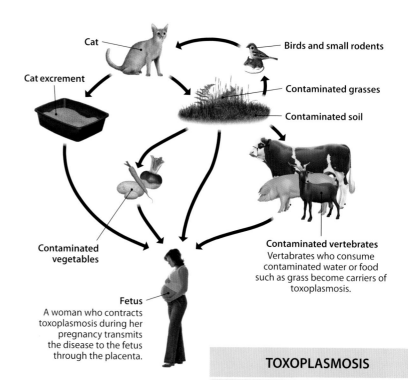

Cat

Birds and small rodents

Cat excrement

Contaminated grasses

Contaminated soil

Contaminated vegetables

Contaminated vertebrates
Vertebrates who consume contaminated water or food such as grass become carriers of toxoplasmosis.

Fetus
A woman who contracts toxoplasmosis during her pregnancy transmits the disease to the fetus through the placenta.

THE PREVENTION OF TOXOPLASMOSIS

When a pregnant woman is not immunized against toxoplasmosis, precautions must be taken throughout the pregnancy:

• Avoid contact with cats (particularly those who habitually go outside) and with their excrement.

• Eat meat or fish that is well-cooked and avoid raw eggs as well as raw or unpasteurized milk products.

• Wear gloves to garden, change cat litter, or clean shoes.

• Carefully wash fruits and vegetables.

• Wash hands regularly, especially after handling raw meat, fruits, or vegetables, as well as soil.

TOXOPLASMOSIS

SYMPTOMS:
Generally asymptomatic. Sometimes fever, inflammation of the lymph nodes, significant weakness.

TREATMENTS:
Spontaneous healing or treatment by antibiotics and corticosteroids.

PREVENTION:
Natural immunization before pregnancy. For a nonimmunized pregnant woman: do not eat raw meat, avoid contact with cat excrement, wash hands after handling soil, vegetables, etc.

FETAL
ALCOHOL SYNDROME

Fetal alcohol syndrome is a combination of problems caused by the intoxication of the embryo or of the fetus by the alcohol consumed by its mother during the pregnancy. It affects approximately 1% of births. The alcohol ingested passes through the maternal blood to the child through the placenta and interferes with the development of its organs. The consumption of alcohol, even moderate, presents a danger to the child. It is therefore recommended that pregnant women abstain from consuming alcohol during their pregnancy.

THE **CONSEQUENCES** OF **FETAL ALCOHOLISM**

Fetal alcoholism has variable consequences depending on the quantity of alcohol absorbed and the stage of the pregnancy. If intoxication takes place during the first months of pregnancy, the child may experience a slowdown in growth. It may suffer from cardiac, genital, joint, or urinary or digestive malformations, and often presents characteristic traits: small head, thin upper lip, fissure absent between the nose and the mouth, etc. When fetal alcoholism occurs after the 1st trimester of pregnancy, the toxic effect of the alcohol on the neurons of the fetus may result in malformations of the nervous system as well as motor and behavioral problems (hyperactivity, learning disabilities). Fetal alcoholism is also the primary cause of nongenetic mental retardation. In all cases, the excessive consumption of alcohol may cause a miscarriage or a premature delivery.

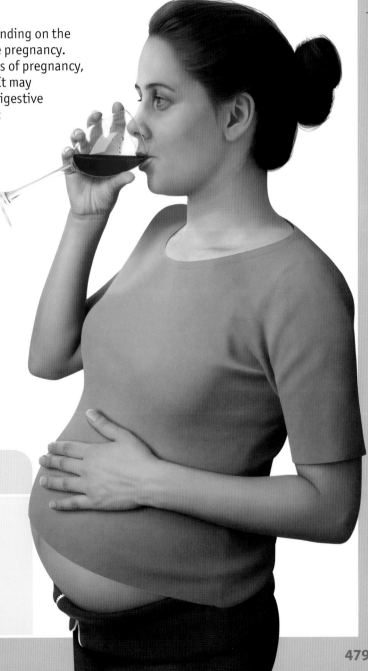

FETAL ALCOHOL SYNDROME

SYMPTOMS:
Characteristic facial features, malformations, neurological problems.

PREVENTION:
Do not consume alcohol during pregnancy.

RHESUS INCOMPATIBILITY

When two people have opposite Rhesus blood groups, their bloods are antagonists: if they come into contact, such as during a blood transfusion or a pregnancy, the Rhesus negative (Rh-) person develops an immune reaction by creating antibodies against the Rhesus positive (Rh+) blood. This is known as Rhesus incompatibility. In an Rh- pregnant woman, the Rhesus incompatibility develops following successive pregnancies where the fetuses are Rh+. It causes severe **anemia** in the child, called newborn hemolytic disease. This situation can be prevented by injecting the mother with anti-Rhesus antibodies.

The blood groups... page 237

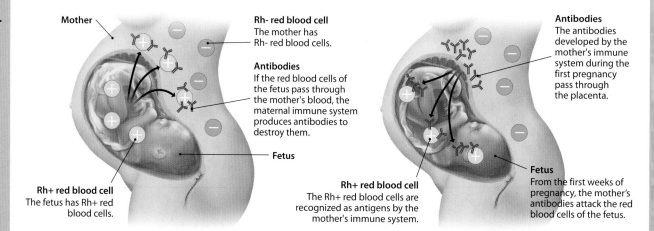

Mother

Rh- red blood cell
The mother has Rh- red blood cells.

Antibodies
If the red blood cells of the fetus pass through the mother's blood, the maternal immune system produces antibodies to destroy them.

Fetus

Rh+ red blood cell
The fetus has Rh+ red blood cells.

Antibodies
The antibodies developed by the mother's immune system during the first pregnancy pass through the placenta.

Fetus
From the first weeks of pregnancy, the mother's antibodies attack the red blood cells of the fetus.

Rh+ red blood cell
The Rh+ red blood cells are recognized as antigens by the mother's immune system.

First pregnancy
When an Rh- woman and an Rh+ man conceive an infant, it is possible that the child is Rh+. If the red blood cells of the fetus pass into the mother's blood—for example, during a hemorrhage occurring at childbirth—the mother's immune system produces antibodies to destroy them.

Subsequent pregnancy
During a subsequent pregnancy, the mother's antibodies attack the red blood cells of the fetus if the latter is also Rh+. Their bursting provokes a serious anemia that may result in heart failure, **edema**, and death of the fetus. In the newborn, the anemia is accompanied by significant icterus (jaundice), which may cause irreversible brain damage.

The immune system... page 278

RHESUS INCOMPATIBILITY

SYMPTOMS:
Anemia and icterus (jaundice) in the newborn.

TREATMENTS:
Injecting the mother with anti-Rhesus antibodies during and after the pregnancy, if there is a risk of passage of the fetal blood into the mother's blood. Fetus and newborn: blood transfusion in the case of severe attack.

PREVENTION:
Blood analyses of future parents. If they are of different blood groups, regular dosage of maternal antibodies during the pregnancy.

TWIN-TO-TWIN TRANSFUSION SYNDROME

Twin-to-twin transfusion syndrome, or feto-fetal transfusion syndrome, is a serious complication in a multiple pregnancy in which the fetuses share the same placenta. The communication of the blood vessels of the fetuses involves the transfer of blood from one of the twins (transfuser) to the other (transfusee). The twin-to-twin transfusion syndrome can cause serious damage to the fetuses (cardiovascular and neurological problems), often ending in their death. Treatment by laser occlusion of the communicating vessels makes it possible to save at least one of the fetuses, but such treatment is still not widespread.

Multiple pregnancies... page 461

MONOPLACENTAL PREGNANCY

During a monoplacental pregnancy (multiple pregnancy in which the fetuses share the same placenta), the blood vessels of the fetuses are generally connected to each other through the placenta. Depending on the number and the type of communicating vessels, a blood transfer may occur between the fetuses. The transfuser twin receives less blood, which slows its development and reduces the production of urine and of amniotic fluid. The transfused twin receives the extra blood and produces too much urine and amniotic fluid.

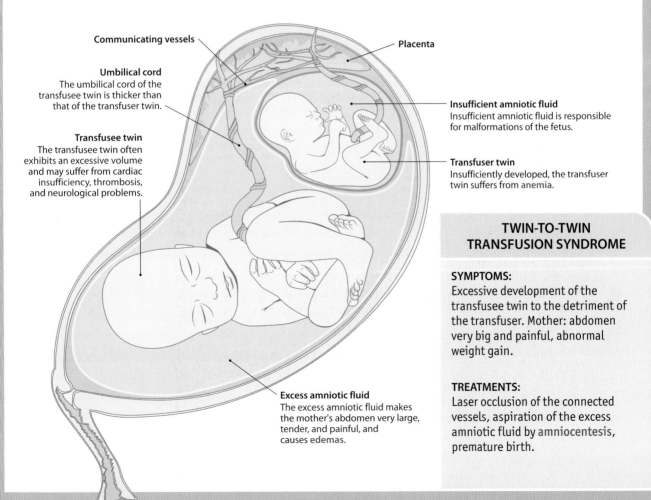

Communicating vessels

Placenta

Umbilical cord
The umbilical cord of the transfusee twin is thicker than that of the transfuser twin.

Insufficient amniotic fluid
Insufficient amniotic fluid is responsible for malformations of the fetus.

Transfusee twin
The transfusee twin often exhibits an excessive volume and may suffer from cardiac insufficiency, thrombosis, and neurological problems.

Transfuser twin
Insufficiently developed, the transfuser twin suffers from anemia.

Excess amniotic fluid
The excess amniotic fluid makes the mother's abdomen very large, tender, and painful, and causes edemas.

TWIN-TO-TWIN TRANSFUSION SYNDROME

SYMPTOMS:
Excessive development of the transfusee twin to the detriment of the transfuser. Mother: abdomen very big and painful, abnormal weight gain.

TREATMENTS:
Laser occlusion of the connected vessels, aspiration of the excess amniotic fluid by amniocentesis, premature birth.

PLACENTA PREVIA

Placenta previa is a pregnancy complication characterized by an abnormal placement of the placenta. Placed too low in the uterus, it partially or totally covers the cervix. Placenta previa is often due to the presence of uterine anomalies (malformations, scars, uterine fibroids), which disturb the implantation of the fertilized egg. This is a relatively rare problem, but one that is more frequent in women of advanced age who have had numerous pregnancies. Often asymptomatic, placenta previa may sometimes cause bleeding and early uterine contractions during the 3rd trimester of pregnancy. In the most serious cases, it causes a hemorrhage and premature birth, which may be fatal to the mother and the child.

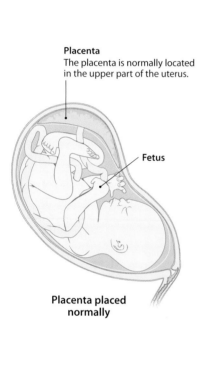

Placenta
The placenta is normally located in the upper part of the uterus.

Fetus

Placenta placed normally

TYPES OF PLACENTA PREVIA

The degree of obstruction of the cervix by the placenta is described as lateral placenta previa (without covering), marginal placenta previa (partial covering), or complete placenta previa (total obstruction). In this last case, hemorrhages are more frequent, creating a high risk of death for the fetus and the mother. Placenta previa requires greater monitoring of the pregnancy and rest for the mother. Most often, the placenta moves progressively towards the upper part of the uterus during the final trimester, which makes natural childbirth possible. However, childbirth is frequently medicalized and done by cesarean section.

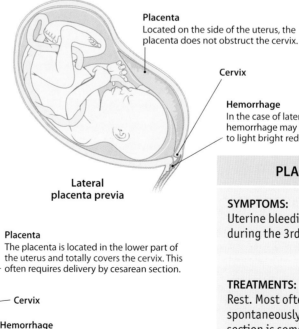

Placenta
Located on the side of the uterus, the placenta does not obstruct the cervix.

Cervix

Hemorrhage
In the case of lateral placenta previa, the hemorrhage may be heavy or limited to light bright red discharges.

Lateral placenta previa

Placenta
The placenta is located in the lower part of the uterus and totally covers the cervix. This often requires delivery by cesarean section.

Cervix

Hemorrhage
Complete placenta previa often results in significant hemorrhaging.

Complete placenta previa

PLACENTA PREVIA

SYMPTOMS:
Uterine bleeding and early contractions during the 3rd trimester of pregnancy.

TREATMENTS:
Rest. Most often, placenta moves back spontaneously. Delivery by cesarean section is sometimes necessary. In case of hemorrhage, blood transfusion.

FETAL DISTRESS

Fetal distress is the lack of oxygenation of the fetus, occurring in a **chronic** manner during the pregnancy or in an **acute** form at childbirth. This is a serious problem that can cause a slowdown in growth, brain damage or death of the fetus. Fetal distress is diagnosed by fetal monitoring (measuring of the heartbeat) or by prenatal **ultrasound** (size of the fetus).

ACUTE OR CHRONIC FETAL DISTRESS

Acute fetal distress primarily occurs during childbirth. It is most often caused by the compression of the umbilical cord or by uterine contractions that are too close, more rarely by a retroplacental hematoma. In serious cases, it may be necessary to perform a cesarean section. Chronic fetal distress occurs during pregnancy. It may be caused by a disease of the mother (cardiovascular disease, pregnancy-related hypertension, anemia, gestational diabetes), by anomalies of the umbilical cord or the placenta (placenta previa, retroplacental hematoma), or by a fetal problem (infection, malformation, physical trauma). It often results in a slowdown in fetal growth and may require a premature delivery.

Preeclampsia… page 484

Fetus
The fetus suffering from a lack of oxygenation takes on a bluish color (cyanosis).

Umbilical cord
The winding of the umbilical cord around the neck of the fetus sometimes results in a compression of the cord, a slowing down of blood circulation, and fetal distress.

Placenta

Compression of the umbilical cord

CEREBRAL MOTOR INFIRMITY

Before, during, or shortly after childbirth, the child may experience brain damage that results in a cerebral motor infirmity, commonly called cerebral palsy. This causes motor problems of variable intensity (slow and awkward movements, lack of coordination, paralysis) that may be associated with hearing and vision problems and sometimes with mental retardation. Cerebral motor infirmity may be due to several factors affecting the cerebral tissues of the fetus or newborn: fetal distress (lack of oxygenation), inflammation, infection, intoxication (medications, drugs, alcohol), cranial trauma, etc. Cerebral motor infirmity is incurable, but certain measures, such as physical therapy for movement and speech, may alleviate its symptoms.

FETAL DISTRESS

SYMPTOMS:
Chronic fetal distress: small size of the uterus. Acute fetal distress: heartbeat problems.

TREATMENTS:
Treatment of causes if possible, acceleration or premature inducement of childbirth (natural or by cesarean section).

PREECLAMPSIA

Around 5% of pregnant women suffer from preeclampsia during their pregnancy. This complication, characterized by high blood pressure and by the presence of proteins in the urine, usually develops at the start of the 3rd trimester. Preeclampsia is more common in first pregnancies and in multiple pregnancies, and is also triggered by kidney failure, blood coagulation disorders, lupus, obesity, and diabetes. It can appear as a variety of symptoms: **edema** (swelling), major weight gain, headache and stomachache, seeing spots (floating spots), buzzing in the ear, nausea, and vomiting. Preeclampsia can have serious consequences, such as eclampsia or retroplacental hematoma, which can cause fetal distress or even the death of the mother and child. Its treatment involves complete rest and monitoring arterial blood pressure. In the most severe cases, it may be necessary to induce labor before term.

PREGNANCY-INDUCED HYPERTENSION

The main cause of death of pregnant women in industrialized countries is an increase in blood pressure over the course of the pregnancy. This disorder, called pregnancy-induced hypertension, is often the consequence of poor vascularization of the placenta, which decreases blood supply and causes the arteries to contract excessively. Women under the age of 15 or over 35, with kidney disease, hypertension (high blood pressure), diabetes, or lupus or who are obese run a greater risk. Pregnancy-induced hypertension typically disappears after childbirth, but its complications can be serious: preeclampsia, eclampsia, retroplacental hematoma, cerebral vascular accident (stroke), etc.

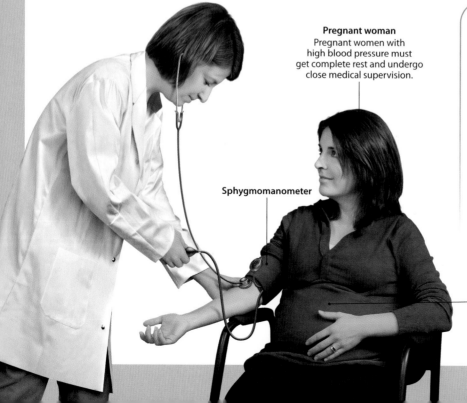

Pregnant woman
Pregnant women with high blood pressure must get complete rest and undergo close medical supervision.

Sphygmomanometer

PROTEINURIA
Proteinuria is the presence of proteins (especially albumin) in the urine. It is characteristic of several ailments (such as preeclampsia, nephrotic syndrome, glomerulonephritis, and diabetes) and often appears in the form of edemas (swelling). Proteinuria can be detected by urine testing.

Fetus
A fetus without enough nutrients and oxygen (in fetal distress) suffers a growth retardation and may be born prematurely.

Measurement of a pregnant woman's blood pressure

RETROPLACENTAL HEMATOMA

Retroplacental hematoma is a serious complication of pregnancy, characterized by an accumulation of blood (hematoma) between the uterus and the placenta. It can lead to the death of the fetus and the mother. Often caused by pregnancy-induced hypertension, retroplacental hematoma can also appear after a blow to the abdomen or abuse of toxic substances (tobacco, alcohol, cocaine, etc.). It may be triggered by several factors: advanced age, multiple pregnancy, excess amniotic fluid, and diabetes. Retroplacental hematoma appears as uterine hemorrhaging and severe abdominal pain. It decreases the supply of oxygen to the fetus, causing acute fetal distress. Furthermore, the hemorrhaging may cause hypovolemic shock in the mother. This means that an emergency blood transfusion and cesarean section will be necessary.

Hypovolemic shock... page 239

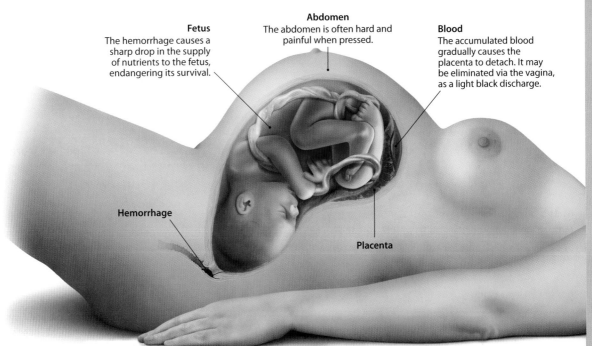

Fetus
The hemorrhage causes a sharp drop in the supply of nutrients to the fetus, endangering its survival.

Abdomen
The abdomen is often hard and painful when pressed.

Blood
The accumulated blood gradually causes the placenta to detach. It may be eliminated via the vagina, as a light black discharge.

Hemorrhage

Placenta

Retroplacental hematoma

ECLAMPSIA

Eclampsia is a serious disorder of pregnant women, characterized by convulsions and temporary loss of consciousness. These fits can occur before, during, or after childbirth, usually following preeclampsia. They are accompanied by major swelling (edema) and a sudden rise in arterial blood pressure. Eclampsia endangers the lives of the mother and child. It requires immediate hospitalization and premature delivery. Because eclampsia is typically the consequence of preeclampsia, treatment of preeclampsia can prevent it.

PREECLAMPSIA

SYMPTOMS:
Very high blood pressure, edema (swelling) in the limbs, high weight gain, headache, floating spots, buzzing in the ear, abdominal pain, nausea, vomiting, overactive reflexes.

TREATMENTS:
Hospitalization and complete rest. Treatment of hypertension and monitoring of the mother and child. Induced premature delivery, if their lives are in danger.

PREVENTION:
Close monitoring of at-risk women.

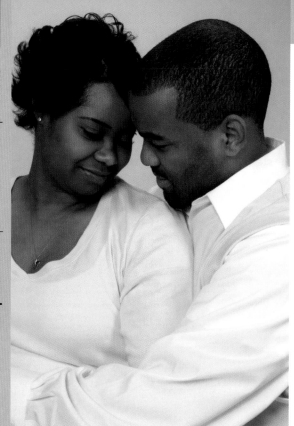

STERILITY

A couple is considered to be sterile when there has been no pregnancy after two years of regular sexual relations without contraception. Sterility, or infertility, can affect the man or the woman. It may be linked to an anomaly of the genital organs, a psychological disorder, certain medications, or the consumption of tobacco, alcohol, or drugs. However, in 10% of cases, no cause is identified. Infertility can be treated with medication or by surgery. If the treatments fail, medically assisted reproductive techniques (artificial insemination, in vitro fertilization) may be used.

MALE STERILITY

Male sterility may be linked to anomalies in the sperm, although problems with erections or ejaculation may also prevent procreation and require medical intervention.

SPERM ANOMALIES

Sperm anomalies are a common cause of male sterility. There may be too few or no sperm cells, they may lack in mobility, or they may have anomalies preventing them from fertilizing an ovum (egg). These disorders can stem from a variety of causes: infections; endocrine diseases; excess heat; stress; use of drugs, alcohol, tobacco, or certain medications; anatomical factors (overweight or malformation or obstruction of the genital tract); or immunological factors (production of antibodies acting against the sperm cells). A laboratory semen analysis (spermogram) can detect any sperm anomalies, particularly by determining the number, mobility, vitality, and shape of the sperm cells.

RETROGRADE EJACULATION

Retrograde ejaculation is an anomaly in ejaculation, characterized by the expulsion of sperm into the bladder. It is caused by a poorly functioning internal vesical sphincter, often occurring after a surgical operation on the prostate. Retrograde ejaculation can also stem from certain diseases (diabetes, neuropathy, etc.) or from the use of certain medications.

Ejaculation... page 453

ERECTILE DYSFUNCTION

Erectile dysfunction, or impotence, is the persistent inability to achieve or maintain sufficient erection of the penis for normal, satisfactory sexual relations (vaginal penetration and ejaculation). It affects men over the age of 40 in particular. Often caused by a psychological source (anxiety), erectile dysfunction can also be the result of vascular, neurological, or endocrine disorders associated with age, certain diseases (like diabetes and high blood pressure), or tobacco, alcohol, or drug use. A lesion on the spinal cord, as well as surgical ablation (removal) of the prostate, the bladder, or the rectum, can also be a cause of impotence.

FEMALE STERILITY

Female sterility is often due to problems with ovulation, an anomaly of the cervical mucus, or an obstruction of the fallopian tubes.

OVULATION DISORDERS

The main cause of female sterility is an anomaly in, or absence of, ovulation, which can be revealed by irregular or absent periods. These ovulation disorders can be caused by anomalies in the endocrine centers that send the order to ovulate (hypothalamus and pituitary gland): congenital disease, tumors, psychological shock, anorexia, etc. They may also be linked to an anatomical dysfunction of the ovaries (lesions, congenital anomaly, ovarian cysts, etc.) or be associated with a disease, such as hypothyroidism or diabetes. In some cases, medicinal or hormonal stimulation can reestablish ovulation.

ANOMALIES OF THE CERVICAL MUCUS

Female sterility may be caused by anomalies of the cervical mucus, a gelatinous substance secreted by the cervix, which encourages the movement of the spermatozoa towards the uterus at the time of ovulation. A microscopic analysis of the cervical mucus after sexual relations (postcoital test) can reveal anomalies in its consistency, quantity, or acidity, caused by an ovulation disorder, an infection, or a dysfunction of the glands that produce it. This test can also show incompatibility with the partner's sperm, which would prevent fertilization: inability of the spermatozoa to move through the mucus or presence of antibodies against the spermatozoa.

OBSTRUCTION OF THE FALLOPIAN TUBES

Obstruction of the fallopian tubes is the second leading cause of female sterility. It may be caused by a disease, such as endometriosis. It can also be a consequence of an infection (salpingitis), associated with a sexually transmitted disease, use of an intrauterine device, childbirth, or abortion. The obstruction can take the form of an accumulation of either serous fluid or scar tissue (adhesions). The diagnosis is established through an X-ray examination or through coelioscopy.

VAGINISMUS

Vaginismus is characterized by the painful, involuntary contraction of the muscles of the wall of the vagina, at the time of penetration by the penis. This disorder prevents sexual relations and can be a cause of sterility. Although usually psychological, vaginismus can sometimes be physiological, caused by malformation, irritation, or infection. Its treatment depends on the cause (psychotherapy, surgery, antibiotic therapy, etc.).

PSYCHOLOGICAL DISORDERS

A number of psychological disorders can disrupt sexual relations and be the cause behind sterility: lack of desire, traumatic memory, anxiety, stress, anger, etc. These disorders often result in erectile dysfunction in men and vaginismus in women. Their treatment is based on psychological monitoring by a psychotherapist or a sexologist.

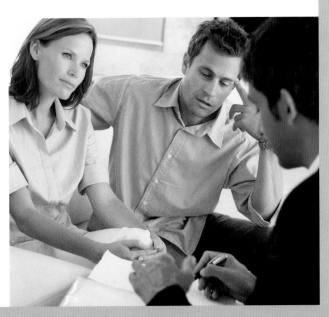

TREATMENT OF ERECTILE DYSFUNCTION

Psychological erectile dysfunction can be treated by psychotherapy. Medical treatments (impotence drugs) or mechanical treatments (penile implant or vacuum pump) may be suggested in other cases. Impotence drugs are medications that encourage the flow of blood to the penis. They come in injectable and tablet form. Penile implants are devices composed of two cylinders, implanted in the cavernous body of the penis to make it stiff. A vacuum pump is a device that sucks air into a tube placed around the penis, to stimulate an erection. Erectile dysfunction treatments can cause side effects and involve contraindications that should be taken into consideration.

ARTIFICIAL INSEMINATION

Artificial insemination is a medically assisted reproductive technique that consists in inserting sperm cells into the woman's reproductive system by means of an instrument. It is used in many industrialized countries to treat certain cases of sterility, particularly anomalies of the sperm and cervical mucus. For this technique to be effective, the woman's genital organs must not have been altered, and the period of ovulation must be known. This insemination may use the partner's sperm or, in the case of an irreversible sperm anomaly, with that of a donor from a sperm bank. The chances of success of artificial insemination are around 10% per cycle.

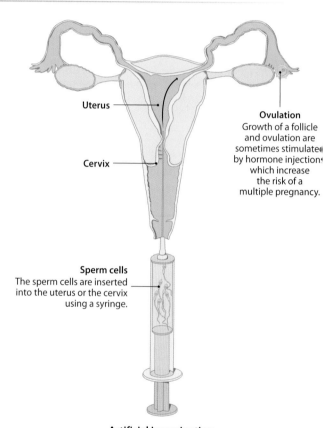

Uterus

Ovulation
Growth of a follicle and ovulation are sometimes stimulated by hormone injections which increase the risk of a multiple pregnancy.

Cervix

Sperm cells
The sperm cells are inserted into the uterus or the cervix using a syringe.

Artificial insemination

STERILITY

SYMPTOMS:
Inability to achieve pregnancy after regular attempts over at least two years.

TREATMENTS:
Hormone treatment: stimulation of ovulation or of the production of oocytes or sperm cells. Surgery of the male and female genital tracts. Medically assisted reproduction: artificial insemination, in vitro fertilization.

PREVENTION:
Prevention of sexually transmitted infections, regular gynecological examinations, healthy lifestyle.

SPERM BANKS

A sperm bank is a place that collects and stores sperm. The donors, who may or may not be anonymous, undergo examinations to verify that they are healthy. Their sperm is frozen and stored in liquid nitrogen tanks, sometimes for several years. It is later used by a sterile couple, for artificial insemination or in vitro fertilization.

IN VITRO FERTILIZATION

In vitro fertilization is a medically assisted reproductive technique in which sperm cells and ova (eggs) are collected, artificial fertilization is performed in a laboratory, and the embryo is transferred to the mother's uterus. This complex method, which requires regular follow-up, is recommended in certain cases of female (obstruction or absence of the fallopian tubes) and male sterility. Its success rate is approximately 25%. The simultaneous implantation of several embryos increases the chances of success, but also the risk of a multiple pregnancy.

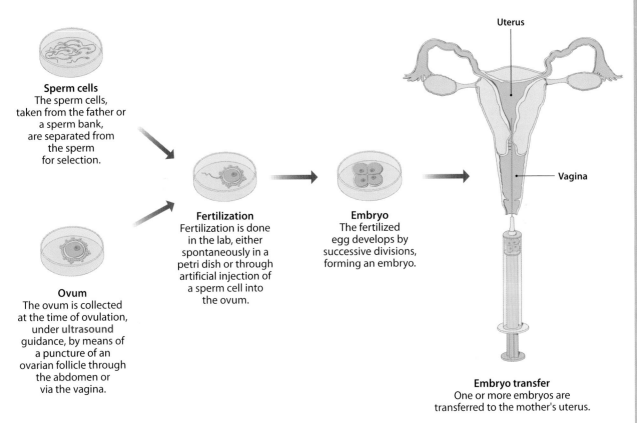

Sperm cells
The sperm cells, taken from the father or a sperm bank, are separated from the sperm for selection.

Ovum
The ovum is collected at the time of ovulation, under ultrasound guidance, by means of a puncture of an ovarian follicle through the abdomen or via the vagina.

Fertilization
Fertilization is done in the lab, either spontaneously in a petri dish or through artificial injection of a sperm cell into the ovum.

Embryo
The fertilized egg develops by successive divisions, forming an embryo.

Uterus

Vagina

Embryo transfer
One or more embryos are transferred to the mother's uterus.

A HEALTHY LIFESTYLE FOR INCREASED FERTILITY

One couple out of eight has problems conceiving a child. It is not uncommon for lifestyle to have an impact on this phenomenon, by causing certain hormonal imbalances or by damaging the genital organs.

• Maintain a healthy weight and eat a diverse, balanced diet. Avoid drastic weight-loss diets, sweets, and bad fats.

• Restrict your alcohol and caffeine intake, and avoid tobacco and drugs.

• Manage your stress, and exercise regularly and moderately.

• Protect yourself against sexually transmitted infections and make sure you have regular medical checkups.

• Avoid using douches and lubricants. Men should avoid temperatures that are too high for the testicles (hot baths, tight underwear, heated blankets and seats, etc.).

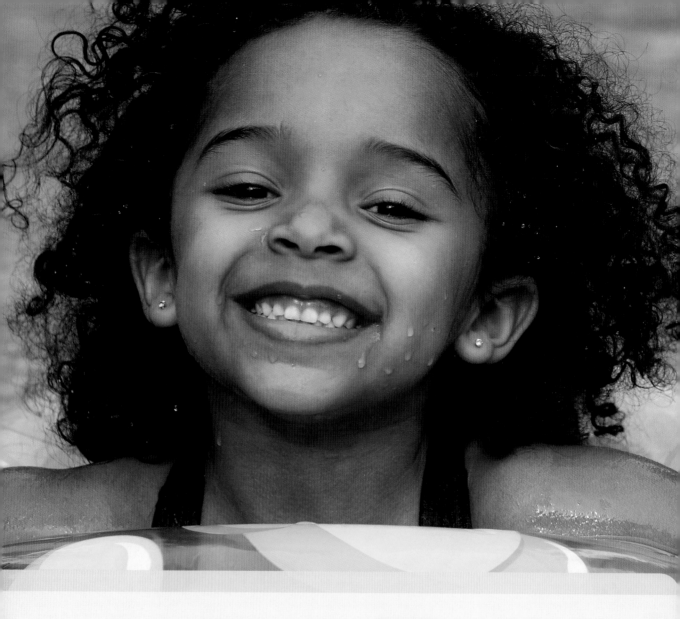

THE BODY

CHILDHOOD AND ADOLESCENCE

Childhood and adolescence are periods of major physical and psychological change. From birth to puberty, children grow and they develop their movement coordination, as well as their intellectual capacities and social skills. They learn to walk, speak, think, read, write, and create emotional ties with those around them. The maturation of the human body is completed during adolescence, with the appearance of secondary sex characteristics and the ability to reproduce.

For these stages to be successfully completed, the child's diet, sleep, and social and affective experiences are key. Complications during pregnancy or delivery, or **genetic** disease, may, however, hinder the child's development. Special medical monitoring of the child is necessary from birth, particularly in order to detect any **congenital** problems or to treat any diseases that could be harmful to the child's development.

DISEASES

DEVELOPMENT OF A HUMAN BEING

From birth to adulthood, the development of human beings occurs in successive stages, with the length of each stage varying, based on **genetic** and environmental factors. The indicators provided below represent the average.

NEWBORNS

During the first month, newborns sleep 14–20 hours per day. Their senses are functional and their attention is drawn to movement and sound. Their own movements are mainly reflexes: nursing, grasping reflex, stepping reflex when held in a standing position, etc.

INFANTS

Between the ages of 1 month and 2 years, infant development is marked by major growth. Weight is double the birth weight at 4 months and triple at 12 months. The body's proportions change. Infants learn to control their gestures and their movement from one place to another, as well as their physical and social environment. They start to speak.

CHILDREN AGES 2 TO 6

Between the ages of 2 and 6, children become independent. They develop their language, movement coordination, and relationships with others.

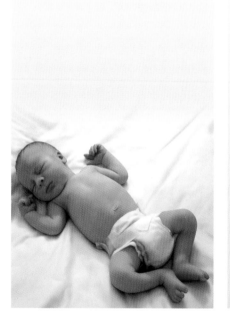

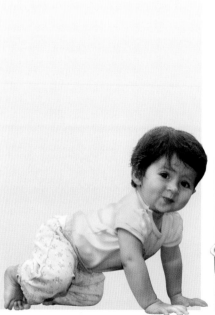

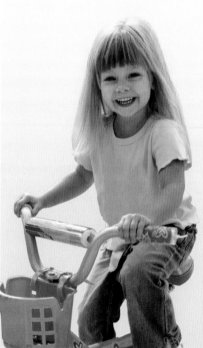

Birth	1 month	2 months	3 months	4 months	5 months	6 months	7 months	8 months	9 months
	First smile		Lengthening of periods of nighttime sleep		Grasping objects		Maintenance of a seated position		More accurate handling of objects
		Holding the head up		Head and upper body movements		First tooth		Crawling	

CHILDREN AGES 6 TO 11

The age of 6 marks the start of school for many children. This is a period in which knowledge and skills (reading, logic, etc.) are acquired, and that is also marked by learning about life in society.

ADOLESCENTS

Adolescents are in a period of physical transformation (growth, maturation of the genital organs, development of secondary sex characteristics, etc.) that ends in their sexual maturity. This transformation and the prospect of becoming an adult, with its associated responsibilities, can be difficult for adolescents to deal with.

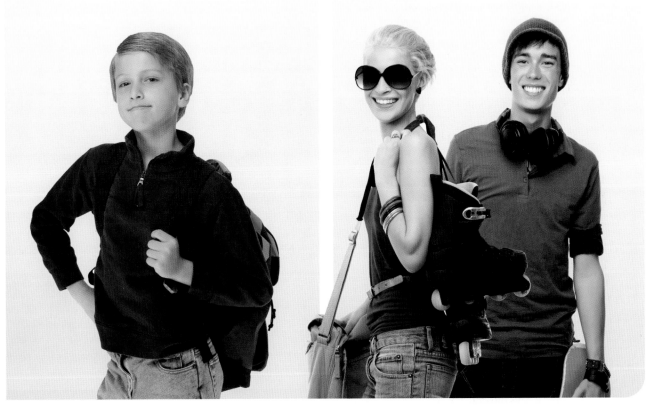

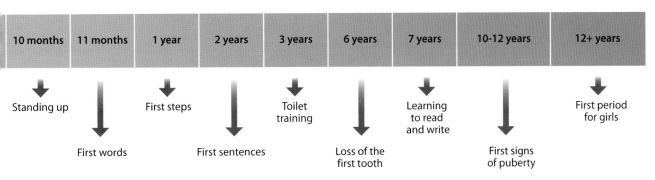

10 months	11 months	1 year	2 years	3 years	6 years	7 years	10-12 years	12+ years
Standing up		First steps		Toilet training		Learning to read and write		First period for girls
	First words		First sentences		Loss of the first tooth		First signs of puberty	

NEWBORNS

A newborn is a child under the age of 1 month. Newborns start breathing at birth and, after the umbilical cord has been cut, they are no longer dependent on the mother's placenta for food and oxygen. When delivery takes place in the presence of medical personnel, the baby undergoes multiple neonatal examinations to assess its state of health. Premature babies require special attention, due to their immaturity.

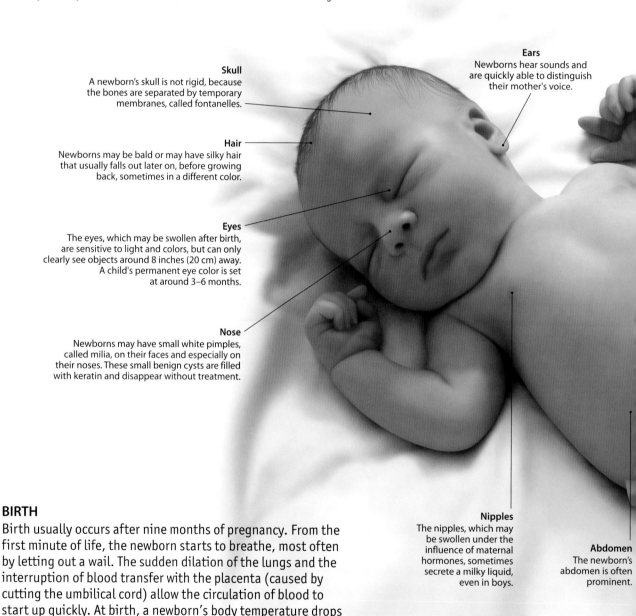

Skull
A newborn's skull is not rigid, because the bones are separated by temporary membranes, called fontanelles.

Hair
Newborns may be bald or may have silky hair that usually falls out later on, before growing back, sometimes in a different color.

Eyes
The eyes, which may be swollen after birth, are sensitive to light and colors, but can only clearly see objects around 8 inches (20 cm) away. A child's permanent eye color is set at around 3–6 months.

Nose
Newborns may have small white pimples, called milia, on their faces and especially on their noses. These small benign cysts are filled with keratin and disappear without treatment.

Ears
Newborns hear sounds and are quickly able to distinguish their mother's voice.

Nipples
The nipples, which may be swollen under the influence of maternal hormones, sometimes secrete a milky liquid, even in boys.

Abdomen
The newborn's abdomen is often prominent.

BIRTH

Birth usually occurs after nine months of pregnancy. From the first minute of life, the newborn starts to breathe, most often by letting out a wail. The sudden dilation of the lungs and the interruption of blood transfer with the placenta (caused by cutting the umbilical cord) allow the circulation of blood to start up quickly. At birth, a newborn's body temperature drops drastically, before gradually rising back up to 98.6°F (37°C). The newborn must be kept warm during this time. After being cleaned and examined, the baby is given to its mother, who feeds it for the first time (breast or bottle).

Child nutrition... page 503

THE **BODY** OF A **NEWBORN**

Newborns usually weigh between 5.7 and 8.8 pounds (2.6 and 4 kg), and measure 17.7 to 21.3 inches (45 to 54 cm) long. Their senses are already developed, although they will continue to sharpen progressively. Stimulated by the ingestion of milk, the newborn's digestive system also continues to mature over the first few weeks of life. The newborn's genital organs appear swollen. The scrotum may be dark in color, and a milky liquid, sometimes with a hint of blood, may leak from the vagina.

Skin
Newborn skin, which is soft and often covered by a protective substance, sometimes has downy hair on the back and shoulders. At birth, the skin may appear yellowish, caused by icterus (jaundice), or bluish, due to cyanosis.

Navel
The navel is the scar left after the stump of the umbilical cord has fallen off.

Limbs
Newborns' arms, fingers, and legs remain bent during the first few weeks, because their central nervous system is not fully mature.

CUTTING THE **UMBILICAL CORD**

A few minutes after birth, two clamps are placed on the newborn's umbilical cord, about an inch from the abdomen, cutting off the flow of blood between the child and the mother's placenta. Scissors are then used to cut the cord between the clamps. After around 2 weeks, the stump will have completely dried out and will fall off, leaving a scar, the navel.

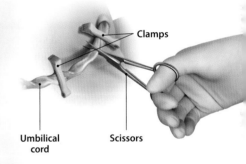

Clamps

Umbilical cord

Scissors

MECONIUM

Within a day of birth, newborns will eliminate a thick, viscous substance via the anus: meconium. This brownish-green substance is composed of bile, digestive secretions, and cells detached from the inside of the digestive tract. An absence of meconium 24 hours after birth may indicate an intestinal obstruction in the newborn. Its presence in the amniotic fluid is a sign of fetal distress.

PREMATURE BIRTH

In industrialized countries, some 7% of births are premature, meaning that they occur before 37 weeks of pregnancy. Premature birth can be spontaneous or medically induced, and may be the consequence of a complication with the pregnancy, like preeclampsia, placenta previa, or fetal distress. It is most common in cases of multiple pregnancy, and in women under 18 or over 35. Extreme cases of trauma, overexertion, or psychological stress can also lead to premature childbirth.

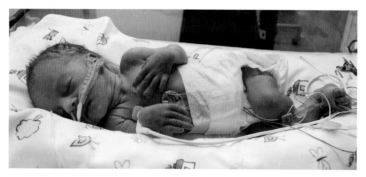

PREMATURE BABIES

A premature baby's body is well-proportioned, but is smaller and weighs less than a child born at term. Some of the organs are immature (nervous, respiratory, cardiovascular, digestive, and immune systems). The thin red skin is still covered by a fine layer of down, called lanugo. The thoracic cage is narrow and the limbs are spindly. Because they have little in the way of energy reserves, premature babies are highly sensitive to changes in temperature. Their pulse and breathing are rapid.

RISKS ASSOCIATED WITH PREMATURE BIRTH

The immaturity of a premature baby's organs can lead to complications and can be life-threatening. The child may be subject to apnea or develop a lung disease hampering its breathing. The fragility of the blood vessels increases the risk of intracranial hemorrhage, and an immature heart can be expressed as a heart murmur. A weak immune system also makes the baby more vulnerable to infection. Despite all this, premature babies born at 32-37 weeks have an excellent chance of leading a healthy life. Children born before 32 weeks (extremely premature) may retain neurological and psychomotor after-effects. In all cases, premature babies are placed in an incubator.

INCUBATOR

Fragile newborns (lightweight or premature) are placed in an incubator. This closed compartment keeps the child in conditions similar to those in the uterus. In this way, the baby can continue to develop, safe from infection in an environment where the temperature, oxygen level, and humidity are controlled. Under constant monitoring, the newborn receives care via the hand holes. The baby may be fed by a stomach tube or intravenously, may undergo phototherapy in the case of icterus (jaundice), and may receive respiratory aid.

Child
The child is usually removed from the incubator once it reaches a weight of 4.5 pounds (2 kg).

Hand hole
Hand holes with gloves are used to handle the child, so as to avoid introducing any pathological germs into the incubator.

Monitoring
A monitoring system checks the newborn's breathing, heart rhythm, level of oxygen in the blood and blood pressure.

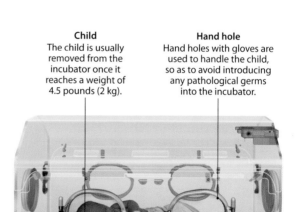

Incubator

NEONATAL EXAMINATIONS

In the case of birth in a medical setting, the newborn is quickly given a number of examinations. Its adaptation to life outside the uterus is assessed by observation of its vital functions (Apgar score). Its maturity is estimated based on its measurements (length, weight, and perimeter of the skull), the appearance of the skin (elasticity, thickness, etc.), and its spontaneous motricity (primary reflexes). The newborn's body is observed, in order to detect any lesions, malformations, or congenital anomalies: congenital dislocation of the hip, cleft lip, spina bifida, etc. Finally, a blood test is used to screen for rare diseases, so as to treat them before the onset of any symptoms.

PRIMARY REFLEXES

A primary, or automatic, reflex is a newborn's response to stimulation. For example, right from birth, newborns react by turning their heads towards any object touching their cheek or mouth (rooting reflex) and will try to suck on it if placed in the mouth (sucking reflex). When held in a standing position, the newborn's reflex is to start to take a few steps (automatic walking). When a finger is placed in a newborn's hand, it will squeeze it tightly (grasp reflex). Finally, newborns have a defensive reflex called the Moro reflex: when they are suddenly stimulated by a noise, light, or jolt, they open out their arms and hands, then bring them in towards the chest and let out a wail.

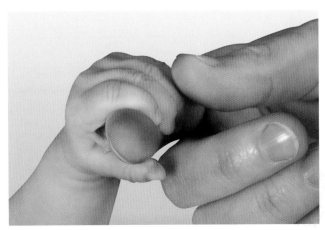

Grasp reflex

APGAR SCORE

The Apgar score is derived from a series of five examinations to assess the vitality of a newborn from its first minute alive: heart rate, respiratory activity, muscle tone, responsiveness to stimulation, and skin color. Each examination is rated from 0 to 2. If the sum of the scores is above 7, the baby is considered to be healthy. If the Apgar score is between 4 and 7, the child will have its respiratory tract unblocked and be placed under artificial respiration. If the score is below 4, the child's condition requires greater medical care (cardiopulmonary resuscitation). The tests are then repeated, five minutes later.

APGAR SCORE			
Examination Score	0	1	2
Pulse	< 80	80-100	> 100
Breathing	Absent	Slow and irregular	Good cry and normal rate
Muscle tone	Low	Medium	Normal
Responsiveness	Absent	Grimace	Active
Skin coloration	Pale or blue	Uneven	Pink

THE **SLEEP** OF **NEWBORNS**

Newborns do not differentiate between day and night. They sleep 14–20 hours a day, in blocks of around 3-4 hours. They only start to sleep more than 5 hours straight at the age of 4 months. A newborn's sleep starts out agitated, and then becomes deep and calm. It may be disrupted by various problems: gastroesophageal (acid) reflux, apnea, etc. Sleep is a vital time for the development of the brain, the assimilation of learning, and the secretion of the growth hormone. It must take place under good conditions.

GOOD SLEEP CONDITIONS

■ **USE A SUITABLE BED**

Put the baby in a cradle or crib, to avoid falls. The bed must have bars about 2 inches (5-6 cm) apart, a flat, firm surface, and a bumper guard, but no pillow or comforter. To safely keep your baby warm, you can swaddle it or put it in a baby nest. The temperature of the room should be around 66°F (19°C).

■ **PLACE YOUR CHILD IN AN APPROPRIATE POSITION**

When putting your baby to bed, place it on its back, with its face clear of any objects, so as to minimize the risk of suffocation or crib death. Your child will be able to roll over at around 6 months.

■ **ESTABLISH A ROUTINE**

Try to put your child to bed at regular times and at the first signs of fatigue (drooping eyelids, yawning, or starting to cry or whine for no apparent reason). By establishing a pre-bedtime routine (last feeding, calm environment, a story or song, cuddling, etc.), your baby will feel reassured. Leave the room before the child falls asleep and let it wake up on its own.

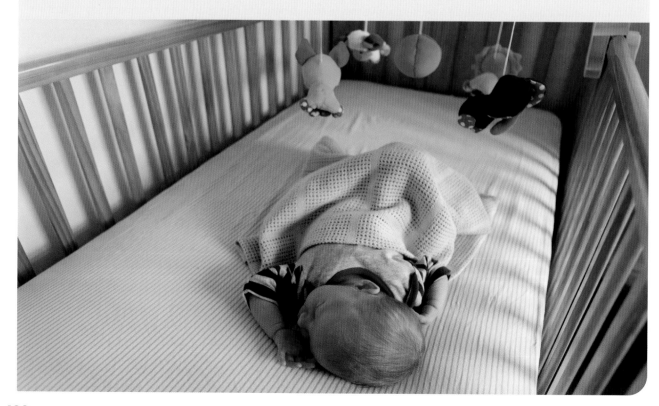

CHILDHOOD

Childhood is marked by growth: gradual overall development that occurs from birth through the end of adolescence. In particular, this period is expressed in the development of the bones, teething, and the maturation of certain organs, including the brain and the genital organs. It is accompanied by **psychomotor** development, which combines the acquisition of motor coordination with the child's sensory, intellectual, emotional, and social development.

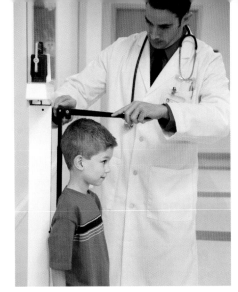

GROWTH CURVES

Children grow constantly, especially during their first years and at puberty. A child's growth will depend on diet, and on **genetic** (ethnic group, family, etc.) and hormonal (growth hormone) factors. To track a child's growth over the years, their height and weight can be recorded on a graph, forming a growth curve. This exercise makes it possible to compare a child's growth with the average values (which can differ by country and by gender), displayed as benchmark curves. A substantial deviation from these averages or an irregular curve may indicate a nutritional deficiency or a disease, such as celiac disease or cystic fibrosis. Growth comes to an end around the ages of 18–20.

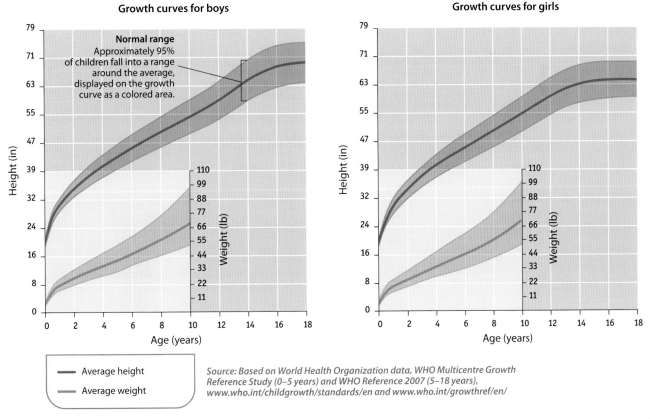

Source: Based on World Health Organization data, WHO Multicentre Growth Reference Study (0–5 years) and WHO Reference 2007 (5–18 years), www.who.int/childgrowth/standards/en and www.who.int/growthref/en/

CRANIAL PERIMETER

The cranial perimeter is the distance around the skull. The doctor will measure it regularly using a measuring tape, until the ages of 4–5 years. The brain grows considerably during the first two years, reaching almost its maximum size at around 5 years. Monitoring the growth of the cranial perimeter can help with the early detection of hydrocephalus or of a defect in the brain's development.

FONTANELLES

The bones of the skull of a young child are separated by spaces, called fontanelles. There are six fontanelles, of variable sizes. The main one is the anterior fontanelle, located at the top of the head. The presence of fontanelles allows the cranium to remain malleable and to adapt to the substantial growth of the brain during the first two years of life. When the skull's bones finally join up, they bind together via fibrous junctions, called sutures. An indented anterior fontanelle can be a sign of dehydration, and a protruding fontanelle may indicate meningitis.

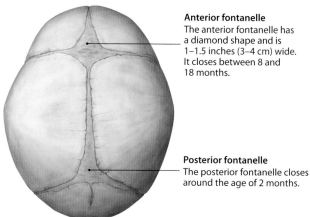

Anterior fontanelle
The anterior fontanelle has a diamond shape and is 1–1.5 inches (3–4 cm) wide. It closes between 8 and 18 months.

Posterior fontanelle
The posterior fontanelle closes around the age of 2 months.

View from above of the skull of a newborn

BONE FORMATION

Bone formation (ossification) starts in the 6th week of the embryo's development, with the beginnings of a bone composed of cartilage tissue. The cartilage is gradually replaced by bone tissue, thanks to specialized cells called osteoblasts. At birth, the epiphyses (extremities) of the long bones, still formed of cartilage tissue, start to ossify in turn, once an artery has penetrated them. The cartilage that remains between the epiphysis and the shaft, or diaphysis, is called the epiphyseal plate. It allows ossification and lengthening of the bone to continue throughout childhood.

The bones... page 94

Artery
Once an artery has penetrated the epiphysis, the cartilage tissue can be replaced by bone tissue.

Cartilage tissue
The epiphyses are made of cartilage tissue.

Epiphyseal plate
The epiphyseal plate is the cartilage tissue that remains between the diaphysis and the epiphysis of long bones during childhood, allowing them to grow in length.

Epiphysis

Diaphysis

Epiphysis

Diaphysis

Cross section of a long bone at birth

Cross section of a long bone at age 7

TOOTH FORMATION

Creation of dentition starts in the first weeks of the life of the fetus and continues until adulthood. Already present in newborns, tooth buds pierce the gums starting at the age of 6 months, yielding the mouth's 20 temporary teeth over the course of the first three years: 8 incisors, 4 canines and 8 premolars. Whiter than permanent teeth, these temporary (baby) teeth are also more vulnerable to cavities. Between the ages of 6 and 12 years, the temporary teeth are slowly replaced by 32 permanent teeth: 8 incisors, 4 canines, 8 premolars, and 12 molars.

The teeth... page 344

RELIEF OF PAIN FROM TEETHING

It is often painful when the temporary teeth break through, and a variety of problems may arise at that time: diarrhea, redness on the cheeks and buttocks, swollen gums and excessive salivation. A refrigerated teething ring to chew on will anesthetize the gums and relieve your child's pain. You can also use an age-appropriate analgesic (painkiller).

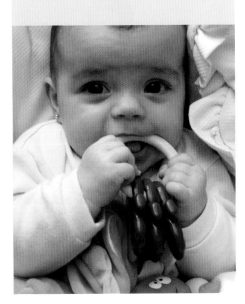

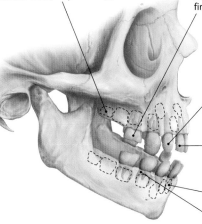

Molar
The first molars appear at around 6 years and the second set, at around 12. The third set (wisdom teeth) rarely appear before the age of 18 and, in some cases, may never appear.

Premolar
The 8 temporary premolars pierce the gums at 12–30 months. Around the age of 9, they are replaced by the first permanent premolars.

Canine
The 4 temporary canines break through at 16–20 months. The permanent canines appear around the ages of 11 or 12.

Incisor
The 8 temporary incisors appear at 6–12 months. They are replaced by permanent incisors at 6–7 years.

Permanent tooth

Root
The roots of the temporary teeth are reabsorbed as the permanent teeth develop in the jawbone.

Side view of the jaw at age 5

THUMB AND PACIFIER

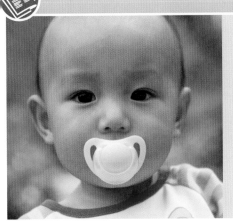

In infants, sucking is a natural need, with a calming, reassuring effect that feeding may not always fulfill. Because of this, many infants will suck their fingers or a pacifier when given to them. Multiple specialists have pointed out the drawbacks of thumb-sucking and pacifier use, especially in excess. In particular, this can disrupt the growth of the jaw and the teeth. Furthermore, excessive pacifier use could slow the development of language. What is most important is to restrict the use of the thumb or pacifier and to gradually stop it around the age of 3 years.

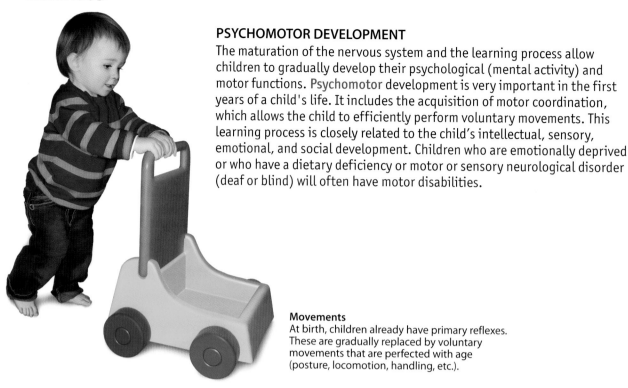

PSYCHOMOTOR DEVELOPMENT

The maturation of the nervous system and the learning process allow children to gradually develop their psychological (mental activity) and motor functions. Psychomotor development is very important in the first years of a child's life. It includes the acquisition of motor coordination, which allows the child to efficiently perform voluntary movements. This learning process is closely related to the child's intellectual, sensory, emotional, and social development. Children who are emotionally deprived or who have a dietary deficiency or motor or sensory neurological disorder (deaf or blind) will often have motor disabilities.

Movements
At birth, children already have primary reflexes. These are gradually replaced by voluntary movements that are perfected with age (posture, locomotion, handling, etc.).

TOILET TRAINING

Toilet training is often spontaneous and can take place at 2–4 years, once the child is mentally prepared and physically able to control the bladder and intestines. This training often lasts several months and must begin at a stable time in the life of the child, by the establishment of a routine: place the child on the potty when they get up, before going to bed, and after meals, while providing encouragement. The child will usually be trained during the day to start out, then at night, and will not always acquire control of urination and defecation at the same time. Children who are not toilet trained after the age of 4 may suffer from bed-wetting (enuresis).

Bed-wetting... *page 178*

SPEECH DEVELOPMENT

Speech development (the understanding and expression of language) is the result of the innate capacities of every human being and our social interactions. It starts at birth and continues through adulthood. Infants first communicate by crying. Between 4 and 18 months, they learn to make sounds (prattle), then words. At 2 years, children can express themselves using simple phrases. Their vocabulary and grammar will expand and improve greatly, up to the age of 4. At 5 years, they can start learning the written language. Children who have developmental disorders (autism, mental deficiency, etc.) or neurological disorders (e.g. brain injury, epilepsy, or myopathy) may have difficulties with understanding and speaking. Language acquisition may also be disrupted by emotional deprivation, psychological trauma, or other problems: deafness, dysphasia, dyslexia, etc.

Learning disabilities... *page 532*

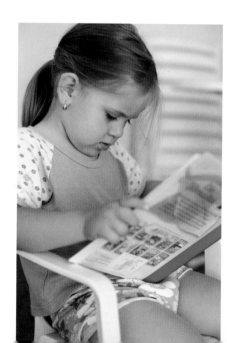

CHILD NUTRITION

During their first months, children are exclusively fed milk. This may be breast milk or baby formula (a milk preparation for infants). Starting in the sixth month, other food may be introduced into their diet. Children will gradually, depending on their age, be able to eat the same food as adults, with the exception of food that could cause suffocation, like peanuts and walnuts. Their nutritional needs will change over time, and their diet should be diverse and balanced, to ensure their growth and development.

BREAST-FEEDING

There are several advantages to feeding small children with breast milk, particularly the fact that it provides the baby with the nutrients it needs, and with immune protection, and it encourages the affective relationship between mother and child. Breast-feeding can start at the child's birth. Colostrum, a thick, yellow-orange milk secreted in the first days after birth, is of particular benefit to newborns, because it is rich in nutritive substances and antibodies. By the third day, the colostrum is gradually replaced by milk. Breast-feeding can continue for many months.

LACTATION

Lactation is the secretion and excretion of milk by the mammary glands. Controlled by hormonal factors, it starts after childbirth and continues until the baby has been weaned. Throughout pregnancy, the hormones secreted by the placenta (estrogen and progesterone) prepare the mammary glands for nursing. Childbirth causes a drop in the progesterone level, which activates the secretion (inflow) of milk, by means of another hormone, prolactin. Finally, by sucking on the areola of the mother's breast, the baby stimulates the production of oxytocin, a hormone that causes milk to be ejected in repeated spurts.

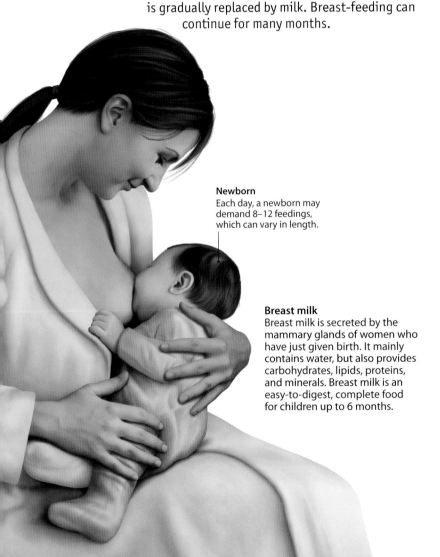

Newborn
Each day, a newborn may demand 8–12 feedings, which can vary in length.

Breast milk
Breast milk is secreted by the mammary glands of women who have just given birth. It mainly contains water, but also provides carbohydrates, lipids, proteins, and minerals. Breast milk is an easy-to-digest, complete food for children up to 6 months.

WEANING

Weaning is the end of breast-feeding. Depending on the child's age, breast milk is either replaced by baby formula (a milk preparation) or by solid foods. Weaning should be done gradually (in 15–30 days), to accustom the child to the taste of formula or other foods, and to prevent engorgement of the mother's breasts, which can be painful.

503

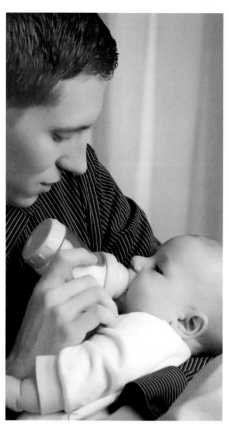

BABY FORMULA

Baby formula, a milk preparation for infants, is modified cow's milk whose composition is similar to that of breast milk. Adapted to each age, it is used to feed infants when their mother cannot or does not want to breast-feed. Baby formula is less complete and more difficult to digest than breast milk. It may give rise to certain problems: allergy, lactose intolerance, colic, etc. However, there are many different types, which allows parents to choose the one best suited to their infant.

REGURGITATION

In infants, burping up undigested milk is a common, harmless phenomenon, mainly due to the immaturity of the lower esophageal sphincter. Regurgitation usually occurs when a child drinks too much or too quickly, has swallowed too much air while feeding, or has been laid down immediately after eating. A calm meal, given in an appropriate position, as well as gently patting the child's back mid-meal and after feeding (helping the infant to burp) can usually prevent regurgitation. Regurgitation often stops once the sphincter has matured or when the child has switched to solid foods.

ADVICE ON FEEDING

Whether your child is breast-fed or bottle-fed, here is some advice to follow to ensure optimal feeding.

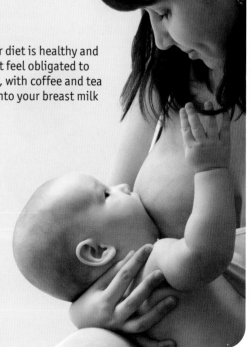

■ THE NURSING MOTHER'S DIET

When you breast-feed, you can eat as freely as you like, provided that your diet is healthy and balanced. Breast milk provides the baby with everything it needs, so don't feel obligated to eat more if you don't feel hungry. However, be sure to drink a lot of fluids, with coffee and tea in moderation. Tobacco, alcohol, and certain medications will also filter into your breast milk and could hurt your baby.

Nutrition... page 11

■ APPROPRIATE POSITION

Your child's position during feeding will ensure its success and prevent breast pain. For example, you can be seated and either hold your baby in one arm or place your child on a cushion, supporting it with one or both arms, or you can lie down on your side. Most importantly, the baby's body should be straight and facing you for easy access to the nipple.

CHILD NUTRITION

Childhood and adolescence | The body

ADVICE ON FEEDING

BREAST PAIN

Breast-feeding can cause breast pain. This pain is common —and temporary—during the first feedings, but can continue, causing serious discomfort. Breast pain may be due to the inflow of milk, poor positioning, or poor sucking by the baby and, in some cases, infection. It can often be relieved and the breast-feeding may be continued with no further problems.

- **Relieving pain caused by milk inflow and breast engorgement**
  During the inflow of milk, the breasts are warm, swollen, and very tender. To limit breast pain, feed your child frequently, starting very shortly after delivery. If your breasts are too taut, pump out some of your milk. To relieve the swelling, apply ice wrapped in a towel.

- **Treating lesions on the breast**
  After nursing, lesions (small cracks, blisters, etc.) may appear on the skin of the nipple. To treat these, adjust your child's position while nursing or try to retrain it to suck (e.g. by pressing the chin gently to help the tongue to stick out of the mouth). Then, after each feeding, apply a medicated ointment or moisturizing lotion (that is not harmful to the baby) to your nipple.

- **Detecting a breast infection**
  Lesions on the nipple or a clogged milk duct can allow pathogens to enter or spread in the breast. The resulting infection (candidosis, mastitis, etc.) may appear as fever, pain, red patches, or swelling. If it does not go away on its own, a doctor will prescribe the appropriate treatment for you.

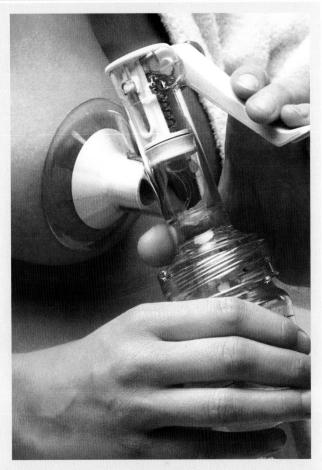
Breast pump

PUMPING MILK

You can bottle-feed your baby with your own milk, pumped manually or using a milk pump. This method is especially useful when your child has problems nursing, when you will have to be apart for several hours, or to relieve your engorged breasts. The best time to pump your milk is right after a feeding. After pumping, pour it into a glass or plastic bottle, or into a bag designed for pumped milk.

STORING AND REHEATING BREAST MILK OR FORMULA

Breast milk can be preserved for several hours at room temperature, eight days in the refrigerator, or two weeks in the freezer (or more, depending on the type of freezer). Thawed breast milk can be stored for 24 hours in the refrigerator or 1 hour at room temperature, as can bottles of formula. The milk must be given warm (pour a few drops onto your inner forearm to check the temperature). To reheat it, place the bottle in hot water. Do not use a microwave. If the milk is frozen, run it under cold water first, then hot water.

FOOD DIVERSIFICATION

Around the age of 6 months, babies can gradually start to eat new food, in addition to the milk they drink. First in pureed form, it can later be cut into small pieces, once the teeth have appeared. From 1 to 3 years of age, children develop their tastes by learning to eat a variety of foods. Starting at the age of 4, they can usually eat the same meals as adults, adapting quantities and textures as needed. A diverse, balanced diet is a source of the nutrients (vitamins, calcium, fiber, etc.) that promote the healthy growth of children by avoiding nutritional deficiencies. Each meal should contain starches (potatoes, pasta, rice, bread, cereals, etc.), dairy products, and fruit. Children should eat fresh vegetables at lunch and dinner, and meat, fish, tofu, legumes, or an egg at least once a day. Salt and sugar should be consumed in moderation. Adolescents eat more, because they have a greater need for energy. Their diet should, however, remain balanced.

Nutrition... page 11

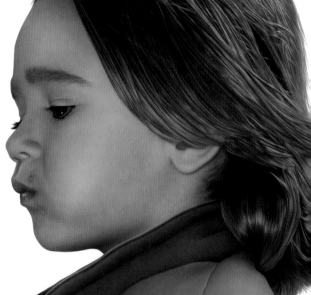

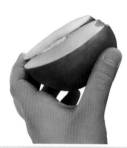

FOOD ALLERGIES

Food allergies are on the rise in industrialized countries. This increase may be linked to changes in eating habits, diversifying the diet too early, the presence of additives in food, or an overly sanitized lifestyle. Children in particular are affected, especially with regard to sensitivity to milk, soy, eggs, wheat, walnuts, sesame, peanuts, exotic fruits, and fish and shellfish. Although most allergies disappear before the age of 5, it is important to take certain precautions when you start to diversify your child's diet, particularly if your child is at risk, that is, has had a previous allergic reaction (hives, eczema, asthma, etc.) or has parents with allergies.

For at-risk children:

• Do not introduce solid foods before the age of 6 months.

• Introduce cow's milk at around 9 months to 1 year.

• Introduce one new food at a time, then wait 3–7 days before introducing the next one. Watch for the appearance of any symptoms of an allergy.

Delaying the introduction of food allergens will not necessarily protect your child from allergies. However, it is preferable that certain food allergens (soy, eggs, legumes, peanut-, walnut-, and sesame-based products, kiwi, fish, shellfish, etc.) be introduced only once your child is old enough to tell you about any problematic reactions (stinging in the mouth or other).

Allergies... page 288

INTRODUCING FOOD INTO YOUR CHILD'S DIET

Food \ Age	6 months	7 months	8 months	9 months	10 months	11 months	12+ months
Milk	From birth, breast milk or formula (milk preparation for babies).			Breast milk or baby formula, supplemented and gradually replaced by whole (3.25%) cow's milk.			
Drinks	From birth, plain water in the case of fever.	Water. Pasteurized, 100% pure, or diluted fruit juices.					
Cereal products	Simple cereals, pureed.	Mixed cereals, soy, wheat.		Pasta, bread, etc.			Whole grain cereal products, etc.
Fruits	Cooked. Pureed or very soft.			Cooked or raw (soft). In small pieces.			Whole, biting into (peeled).
Vegetables	Cooked. In a smooth puree.	Cooked. In a rough puree.		Cooked. In small pieces.			Raw or cooked. In pieces.
Legumes Tofu				Pureed or in small pieces.			
Nuts and grains							In a creamy paste.
Meats	*Well done; avoid spicy meats, deli meats, and game offal.*						
Meats	Pureed.			Ground.		In small pieces.	
Eggs		Well-cooked egg yolk.					Whole egg.
Fish		*Restrict consumption of predatory fish: lake trout, yellow pike, pike, swordfish, shark, fresh tuna, etc. Make sure to remove all bones.*					
Fish		Cooked. Pureed.			Cooked. In small pieces.		
Shellfish							In pieces.
Dairy products				Whole (3.25%) cow's milk, whole milk cheese, and yogurt, plain or with pieces or pureed fresh fruit.			
Dairy products							Ice cream, etc.
Salt							A little in cooking (limit use).
Sweets	Limit use.						

ADOLESCENCE

Adolescence is a period of physical, social, and psychological transition between childhood and adulthood. Its length varies, in different cultures and different individuals, on average lasting from 10 to 19 years of age. Adolescence is characterized by major growth and by many physiological changes associated with the increased production of sex hormones (puberty). It can involve a number of physical ailments (acne, scoliosis) and behavioral problems: mood swings, depression, drug addiction, eating disorders. Adolescence is also a period during which sexuality is a major preoccupation: first romance, first sexual relations, identification of sexual orientation, etc. Sex education can help to prevent sexually transmitted diseases and unwanted pregnancies.

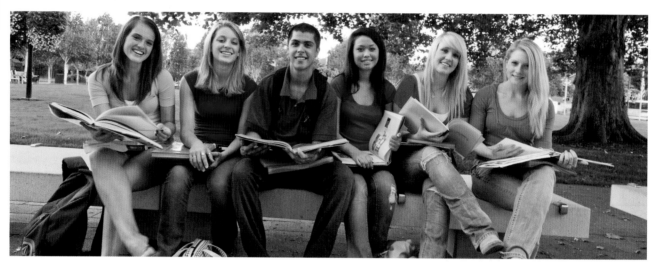

PUBERTY

Puberty is the time of life when children reach sexual maturity. They then become capable of reproduction. The age at which puberty occurs varies, depending on several different factors, particularly **genetic** factors, although it usually comes earlier in girls than in boys. It begins when the pituitary gland starts to produce gonadotropins, hormones that stimulate the growth of the gonads (ovaries or testicles) and the secretion of the sex hormones (testosterone or estrogen). The sex hormones trigger the development of the genital organs and the gradual appearance of the secondary sex characteristics, which are morphological and behavioral characteristics that differentiate the two sexes but that are not a part of the reproductive system. The secondary sex characteristics will be more or less pronounced in different people. In particular, they include height, voice, skin thickness, and the quantity and distribution of body hair, muscles, and adipose tissue (fat).

Endocrine glands and hormones... page 220

PRECOCIOUS PUBERTY

It is becoming more and more common for puberty to begin early: before the age of 8 in girls and before 10 in boys. It is difficult to determine the causes of this phenomenon. When precocious puberty is not pathological (triggered by brain injury, tumors, etc.), a genetic or environmental cause is suspected, including a diet rich in fat, a sedentary lifestyle, the presence of hormones (estrogen) in cosmetics, plastics, and chemicals, etc.

FEMALE PUBERTY

Female puberty generally starts between 10 and 13 years of age. It is characterized by an increase in breast size, the development of the genital organs, an increase in body hair (pubis and armpits), and the beginning of menstruation. Growth accelerates (just under 3 inches [7 cm] each year), then slows substantially, on average two years after the first menstrual period. Fat mass is distributed over the hips, breasts, and thighs. The skin becomes oilier.

The menstrual cycle... page 423

MALE PUBERTY

Male puberty most often occurs between 12 and 15 years of age. The genital organs (testicles and penis) develop and body hair increases over the whole body, particularly the pubis, face, armpits, torso, abdomen, and legs. Growth in adolescent boys is very fast (around 3 inches [7.5 cm] a year), especially during the first 12–18 months of puberty. Muscle mass increases, and the bones thicken, while the skin becomes oilier. The voice changes, becoming deeper. The first ejaculation usually takes place around the age of 14, although in many cases the sperm is not yet fertile.

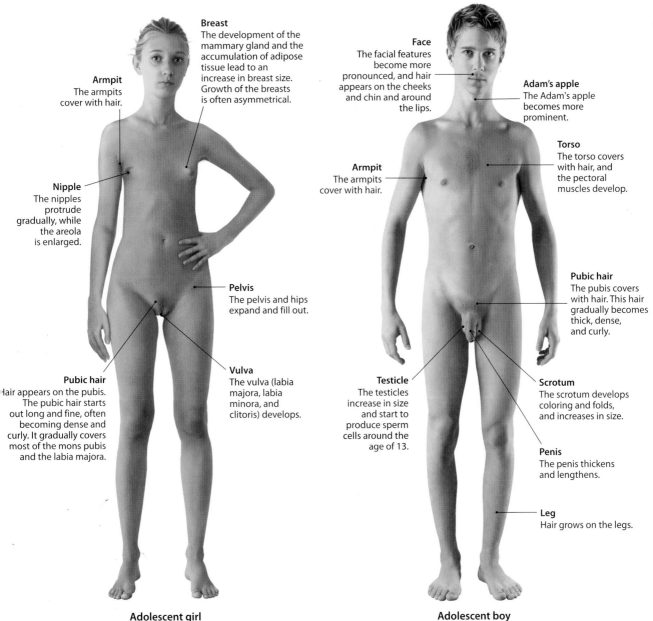

Armpit
The armpits cover with hair.

Breast
The development of the mammary gland and the accumulation of adipose tissue lead to an increase in breast size. Growth of the breasts is often asymmetrical.

Nipple
The nipples protrude gradually, while the areola is enlarged.

Pubic hair
Hair appears on the pubis. The pubic hair starts out long and fine, often becoming dense and curly. It gradually covers most of the mons pubis and the labia majora.

Pelvis
The pelvis and hips expand and fill out.

Vulva
The vulva (labia majora, labia minora, and clitoris) develops.

Face
The facial features become more pronounced, and hair appears on the cheeks and chin and around the lips.

Adam's apple
The Adam's apple becomes more prominent.

Armpit
The armpits cover with hair.

Torso
The torso covers with hair, and the pectoral muscles develop.

Pubic hair
The pubis covers with hair. This hair gradually becomes thick, dense, and curly.

Testicle
The testicles increase in size and start to produce sperm cells around the age of 13.

Scrotum
The scrotum develops coloring and folds, and increases in size.

Penis
The penis thickens and lengthens.

Leg
Hair grows on the legs.

Adolescent girl

Adolescent boy

CONGENITAL MALFORMATIONS

A **congenital** malformation is an anomaly that is present at birth, affecting one or more organs. There is a wide variety of such malformations, and the most severe types, like spina bifida and hydrocephalus, can be life-threatening. In many cases, they are relatively minor anomalies, such as clubfoot, port-wine stain, cryptorchidism, congenital dislocation of the hip, and labiopalatine clefts. There are different causes of congenital malformations: defect in the formation of an organ, immaturity of development, **genetic** disease, **infection** (toxoplasmosis, rubella), gestational diabetes, and consumption of alcohol or certain medications (anticonvulsants, cancer drugs, or **anticoagulants**) during pregnancy, etc. Depending on their severity, they must be treated more or less shortly after birth, to prevent them from becoming irreversible and from leading to potentially serious complications.

CLUBFOOT

Approximately 1 newborn in 1,000 is born with one or two clubfeet. This congenital malformation, characterized by a more or less pronounced deformation of the organs in the foot (bones, joints, tendons, muscles, skin, etc.), appears during the development of the fetus and can be detected by ultrasound. It affects boys more often than girls. Clubfoot may be associated with a serious disease, such as spina bifida or muscular dystrophy, although its causes are often unknown. The malformation can be corrected from birth by physical therapy exercises, wearing a splint, or cast or, potentially, by surgery. There are usually no long-term effects for these children, although they must be monitored through the end of their growth. When untreated, clubfoot can seriously restrict locomotion.

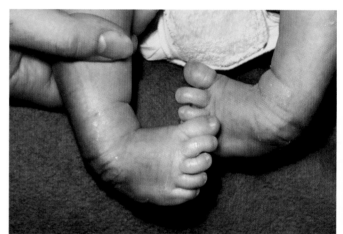

Clubfeet

CONGENITAL DISLOCATION OF THE HIP

In approximately 1% of newborns, the hip joint is badly formed: the head of the femur is not properly fitted into the socket of the iliac bone, where it normally sits. This congenital malformation, called congenital dislocation of the hip, affects girls more than boys. When detected early on, most congenital dislocations of the hip can be corrected without surgery, by means of orthopedic treatment. Otherwise, they lead to limping, in other words, difficulty walking.

Dislocation... page 111

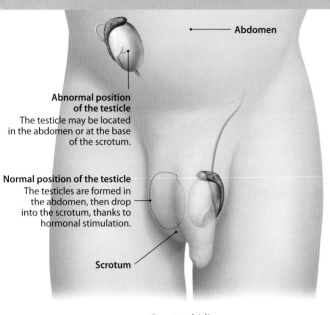

Abdomen

Abnormal position of the testicle
The testicle may be located in the abdomen or at the base of the scrotum.

Normal position of the testicle
The testicles are formed in the abdomen, then drop into the scrotum, thanks to hormonal stimulation.

Scrotum

Cryptorchidism

CRYPTORCHIDISM

Cryptorchidism is a congenital anomaly characterized by the abnormal positioning of one or both testicles. During the development of the fetus, the testicles drop from the abdomen to the scrotum. For various reasons (malformation, hormone deficiency, etc.), this movement may not be complete at birth. Cryptorchidism affects 2%-3% of boys born at term and approximately 20% of premature boys. Most of the time, the testicle completes its movement spontaneously during the first year. Otherwise, surgery may be performed between the ages of 1 and 2. Without treatment, there is a risk of sterility, atrophy, or cancer of the testicle.

PORT-WINE STAIN

A port-wine stain, also called a birthmark, is a permanent congenital malformation of the capillary network in the skin. It appears as a colored splotch of varying shape and size. Some 3 children in 1,000 are born with a port-wine stain. Although this anomaly causes no functional disturbance, it may be a major aesthetic handicap, depending on its location on the body. Laser treatment under local anesthesia can effectively lighten the mark, particularly when it is on the face. This may be performed as of the age of 1.

Blood circulation and the blood vessels... page 248

Port-wine stain
The mark (pink to purplish-red in color) is smooth and flat at birth. It tends to expand, darken, and form nodules if no treatment is administered.

CONGENITAL MALFORMATIONS

SYMPTOMS:
Clubfoot: one or both feet turned inward or outward. Congenital dislocation of the hip: often asymptomatic in the first few months. Cryptorchidism: absence of one or both testicles from the scrotum. Port-wine stain: more or less dark red splotch on the skin, varying in size.

TREATMENTS:
Clubfoot: surgery, physical therapy, splint. Congenital dislocation of the hip: manual intervention at birth. Cryptorchidism: surgical treatment. Port-wine stain: laser treatment.

PREVENTION:
Avoiding use of alcohol, tobacco, and certain medications during pregnancy.

LABIOPALATINE CLEFTS

Labiopalatine clefts are **congenital** malformations of the face, characterized by the failure of the tissues in the upper lip or the palate to knit together properly. The different forms of clefts (cleft lip, cleft palate) may be complete or incomplete and may affect one or both sides of the face. Caused by **genetic** or environmental factors (consumption of harmful products during pregnancy, nutritional deficiencies, etc.), labiopalatine clefts affect around 1 child in 700. Depending on their severity, they may pose an aesthetic problem and lead to difficulties with **phonation**, chewing, swallowing, breathing, and hearing. In 30% of cases, cleft lips and palates are associated with other malformations (of the heart, brain, etc.). They are often detected by prenatal ultrasound, and their treatment, chiefly surgical, yields good results.

CLEFT LIPS

Cleft lips are usually limited to the lip, but may extend up to the nose. If they reach the maxillary bone, they may lead to problems of malocclusion, particularly in incisors.

Dental malocclusion... page 371

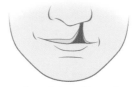
Complete unilateral cleft lip

CLEFT PALATES

Cleft palates can involve the hard palate, the soft palate, or both. They frequently lead to problems caused by the open passageway between the mouth and the nasal cavities.

The mouth... page 343

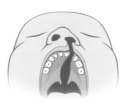
Complete unilateral cleft palate

LABIOPALATINE CLEFTS

SYMPTOMS:
Morphological malformation of the face at the lips, palate, and nose.

TREATMENTS:
Plastic surgery in the first few months of life, orthodontics, orthophony, cosmetic surgery at adolescence.

PREVENTION:
Healthy lifestyle during pregnancy (no tobacco, alcohol, drugs, pesticides, household solvents, or dietary deficiencies).

TREATMENT OF LABIOPALATINE CLEFTS

Labiopalatine clefts are treated surgically in the first few months of the child's life. Depending on the scope of the malformation, a series of surgeries may be necessary. Correction of the lip is performed first, at around 3-4 months, followed by the hard palate, at around 12-18 months. Between the two operations, a plate may be placed on the palate to block the hole between the mouth and the nasal cavity. Complementary orthodontic and orthophonic treatments may be required. The scar remaining on the lip after the operation is usually relatively discreet.

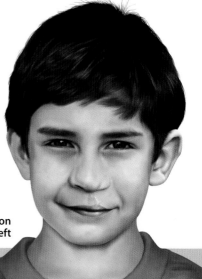
Face after operation of a labiopalatine cleft

SPINA BIFIDA

Spina bifida is a **congenital** malformation of the spinal column, linked to an anomaly in the development of the embryo's central nervous system. This malformation may lead to hernia of the meninges and of the spinal cord, protruding outside the spinal column. Spina bifida concerns approximately 1 child in 1,000, with varying degrees of severity. It can lead to a number of different neurological disorders: incontinence, erectile dysfunction, impaired locomotion, digestive disturbances, sensory impairment, and sometimes mental retardation and epilepsy. Spina bifida can be detected at 18 weeks of pregnancy, by ultrasound or by **amniocentesis**. Its treatment is based on the **reduction** of the hernia and surgically sealing the affected tissues.

The nervous system… page 132

FORMS OF SPINA BIFIDA
There are three different forms of spina bifida: two mild forms (spina bifida occulta and meningocele) and one severe form (meningomyelocele).

SPINA BIFIDA OCCULTA AND MENINGOCELE
Spina bifida occulta is the most benign and most common form of spina bifida. It is characterized by a narrow cleft at the lumbar vertebrae. It is not accompanied by a hernia, but it may cause urinary incontinence and certain minor neurological disorders. Meningocele, which is also benign, is a rare form of spina bifida, characterized by a hernia of the meninges and of the cerebrospinal fluid protruding outside the spinal column.

The meninges and the cerebrospinal fluid… page 140

MENINGOMYELOCELE
Meningomyelocele is the most serious form of spina bifida. It is characterized by a spinal cord hernia, in addition to hernias of the meninges and cerebrospinal fluid, protruding from the spinal column. It is often associated with hydrocephalus and with serious neurological disorders, like paralysis of the lower limbs and mental retardation.

HYDROCEPHALUS
Hydrocephalus, or water on the brain, is a serious neurological malformation characterized by an increase of cerebrospinal fluid in the cerebral ventricles and the meninges. It may be innate or acquired and can be caused by excessive secretion of fluid or by obstruction of the bloodstream due to tumor, congenital malformation, meningeal hemorrhage, meningomyelocele, etc. Hydrocephalus often leads to an increase in brain size and to mental and neurological disorders (impaired locomotion, incontinence, etc.).

The brain… page 140

SPINA BIFIDA

SYMPTOMS:
Spina bifida occulta: urinary incontinence, minor neurological disorders. Meningocele: mild sensory impairment. Meningomyelocele: sensory, neurological, and digestive disorders; hydrocephalus.

TREATMENTS:
Reduction of the hernia and treatment of the symptoms.

PREVENTION:
Consumption of folic acid before and during the first few weeks of pregnancy.

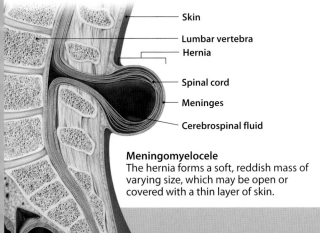

Skin

Lumbar vertebra

Hernia

Spinal cord

Meninges

Cerebrospinal fluid

Meningomyelocele
The hernia forms a soft, reddish mass of varying size, which may be open or covered with a thin layer of skin.

SUDDEN INFANT DEATH SYNDROME

Although the frequency of sudden infant death syndrome (SIDS) has clearly decreased since 1990, it is still the leading form of mortality in children between the ages of 1 month and 1 year in industrialized countries (approximately 1 death for every 2000 children). This sudden crib death, with no apparent cause, commonly occurs during sleep and more often in wintertime. Sudden infant death syndrome mainly affects babies 2–4 months old and babies with a low birth weight. Boys are affected more than girls. The causes and mechanisms of sudden infant death syndrome are still relatively unknown, although certain risk factors have been identified.

RISK FACTORS
FOR **SUDDEN INFANT DEATH SYNDROME**

Several risk factors (avoidable and unavoidable) for sudden infant death syndrome have been identified. Premature babies, lightweight infants, babies from a multiple pregnancy, and those who had a difficult birth are more susceptible to crib death than others. Some socioeconomic and environmental factors can also increase the risk: young mothers, an underprivileged social environment, exposure to tobacco smoke, sleeping position on the stomach or side, excess heat, etc.

SUDDEN INFANT DEATH SYNDROME

SYMPTOMS:
No particular symptoms.

PREVENTION:
Protection of child from tobacco smoke, sleeping position on the back, bedroom temperature at 64°F–68°F (18°C–20°C), light covers only on the child, breast-feeding, use of a pacifier during sleep (first few months).

PREVENTING SUDDEN INFANT DEATH SYNDROME

There are a number of simple measures that can be taken to reduce the risk of sudden infant death syndrome. They mainly involve establishing good sleeping conditions.

• Lay your child on its back, except in cases where this position aggravates a health problem, like gastroesophageal (acid) reflux.

• Make sure that your child can breathe freely, that the face is clear of any items, and that body temperature is kept at a normal level. Avoid overly heavy bedding (pillow, comforter, blankets) and excess clothing. Instead, dress your baby in a sleeper, which leaves the head and arms free.

• Maintain the temperature of the child's room at around 64°F–68°F (18°C–20°C).

• Do not expose your child to tobacco smoke at any point during pregnancy.

• Opt for breast-feeding when possible, especially during the first few days, because it appears to reduce the risk of SIDS.

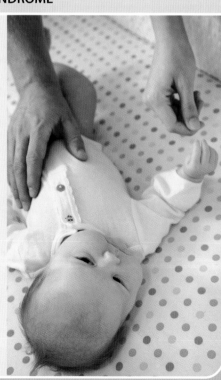

ICTERUS OF THE NEWBORN

Icterus, or jaundice, appears when a brownish-yellow pigment, bilirubin, accumulates in the blood. Bilirubin is normally eliminated by the liver, but in one-third of newborns, the immaturity of the liver causes physiological jaundice. It is benign and usually appears around the second day after birth, and disappears spontaneously around the 10th day. Breast milk jaundice, which is likewise benign, is caused by the presence of a substance in the breast milk of some women that prevents the carriage of bilirubin to the liver. It disappears when the breast milk is heated to 140°F (60°C). Pathological jaundice, which is more rare but also more serious, can have several causes: Rhesus incompatibility, infectious disease, blockage of the bile ducts, etc. Pathological jaundice can cause brain injury.

ICTERUS OF THE NEWBORN

SYMPTOMS:
Yellow coloring of the skin, the mucous membranes and the whites of the eyes. Pathological jaundice: pallor, light-colored stool, swollen liver or spleen, for more than 10 days.

TREATMENTS:
Mild icterus: exposure to daylight, phototherapy, albumin IV drip.
Severe icterus: treatment of the cause, complete blood replacement.

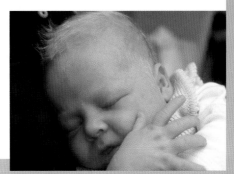

Physiological jaundice
Bilirubin accumulates in the tissues (skin, mucous membranes, etc.), which take on a yellow coloring.

ACUTE INTESTINAL INVAGINATION

Acute intestinal invagination is the slipping of one segment of the intestine into the following segment, and back again. It requires emergency treatment, because it can cause serious complications, like intestinal obstruction and peritonitis. Acute intestinal invagination mainly affects infants between the age of 2 months and 2 years and, in particular, boys 5–9 months old. It appears after an inflammation (often infectious) of the lymph nodes. It sometimes occurs in older children and adults, in which cases, it is the result of diverticulitis or a tumor.

The digestive tract... page 346

ACUTE INTESTINAL INVAGINATION

SYMPTOMS:
Sudden, intense attacks of abdominal pain (with wails and crying), vomiting, refusal to eat, pallor, lack of energy, thick, bloody mucus in the stool.

TREATMENTS:
Anal injection of pressurized air or liquid, surgery.

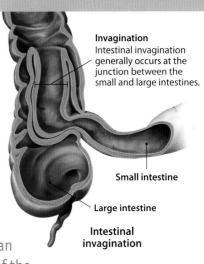

Invagination
Intestinal invagination generally occurs at the junction between the small and large intestines.

Small intestine

Large intestine

Intestinal invagination

HYPERTROPHIC PYLORIC STENOSIS

Hypertrophic pyloric stenosis is the narrowing of the pylorus, the orifice between the stomach and the duodenum, due to the thickening of the muscle around it, the pyloric sphincter. This relatively common disease, whose source is unknown, appears in infants a few weeks old, mainly boys, presenting as vomiting, followed by signs of malnutrition. Pyloric stenosis can also occur, more rarely, in adults, following a stomach lesion such as a peptic ulcer or a tumor. Hypertrophic pyloric stenosis is treated by surgery.

The digestive tract… page 346

SYMPTOMS OF HYPERTROPHIC PYLORIC STENOSIS

Hypertrophic pyloric stenosis appears around the fourth or fifth week after birth as the more or less violent vomiting of curdled milk in spurts, after each meal. Within a few days, the infant's weight levels off and may even decrease, despite an increased appetite. The infant may suffer from constipation, dehydration, and a nutritional deficiency. The condition is diagnosed by means of an ultrasound.

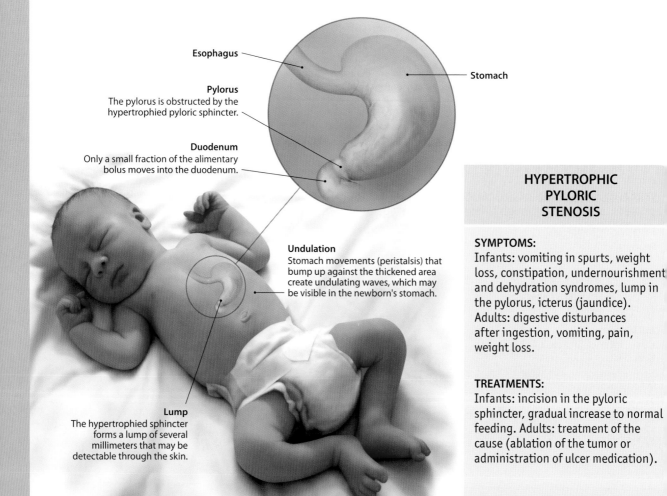

Esophagus

Stomach

Pylorus
The pylorus is obstructed by the hypertrophied pyloric sphincter.

Duodenum
Only a small fraction of the alimentary bolus moves into the duodenum.

Undulation
Stomach movements (peristalsis) that bump up against the thickened area create undulating waves, which may be visible in the newborn's stomach.

Lump
The hypertrophied sphincter forms a lump of several millimeters that may be detectable through the skin.

HYPERTROPHIC PYLORIC STENOSIS

SYMPTOMS:
Infants: vomiting in spurts, weight loss, constipation, undernourishment and dehydration syndromes, lump in the pylorus, icterus (jaundice). Adults: digestive disturbances after ingestion, vomiting, pain, weight loss.

TREATMENTS:
Infants: incision in the pyloric sphincter, gradual increase to normal feeding. Adults: treatment of the cause (ablation of the tumor or administration of ulcer medication).

INFANT SKIN DISEASES

Infants often experience skin diseases because their delicate skin is very vulnerable to attacks, whether from **infectious** agents, irritants, urine, or other. The main infant skin diseases can appear as red patches, scales, or pimples. They are usually benign, disappearing spontaneously or after following simple hygiene measures. However, some signs on the skin, such as measles, chickenpox, scarlet fever, roseola infantum, etc., may indicate an infectious disease that requires medical consultation.

Dermatitis... page 78

DIAPER RASH

Infant's bottoms, when in contact with urine and stool or with repeated rubbing of diapers, often break out in a rash (diaper rash). This very common inflammation of the skin is characterized by red patches on the buttocks, the upper thighs, and the genital organs. To prevent its onset or its aggravation, the child must be changed regularly and cleaned with a gentle soap. The buttocks must be carefully rinsed, dried, and aired. Without treatment, diaper rash can spread rapidly, becoming infected and painful. In the case of infected diaper rash, the skin is red, shiny, and presents blisters or whitish-yellowish deposits. Medical consultation is recommended in this case.

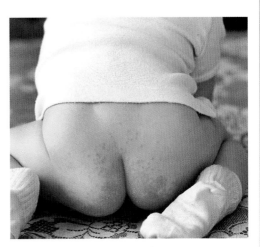

Diaper rash

CRADLE CAP

Cradle cap is a band of yellowish skin that form on the scalps of newborns. The scaly patches typically appear during the first year after birth and, most often, disappear on their own. Their cause is uncertain, although they appear to be due to excess sebum secretion.

Structure of the skin... page 64

INFANT SKIN DISEASES

SYMPTOMS:
Diaper rash: redness on the skin of the buttocks, the upper thighs, and the genital organs. Cradle cap: yellowish, dry, or oozing scales on the scalp.

TREATMENTS:
Diaper rash: good hygiene, antibiotic treatment in the case of infection.
Cradle cap: gentle shampoo, sweet almond oil, gentle scraping.

PREVENTION:
Use of nonirritating cleansing products.
Diaper rash: regular diaper changes, blot the buttocks dry, use of unscented diapers.

Cradle cap
Cradle cap forms scaly, slightly oily plaques on the scalp, forehead, eyebrows, and neck, and behind the ears. To prevent irritation, they should not be scraped when dry.

ACNE

Acne is a skin disease that affects 90% of adolescents. It is usually not serious and typically disappears by the age of 20. At puberty, the increased production of sex hormones leads to the secretion of sebum and keratin, in greater quantities, by the sebaceous glands and the cells of the epidermis. The accumulation of sebum leads to **inflammation** of the hair follicles and encourages the spread of a bacterium of the skin's flora, *Propionibacterium acnes*. The result can be a variety of lesions: papules, pustules, nodules, and cysts. Acne treatments aim to stop the blockage of the pores and the spread of the bacteria.

Structure of the skin... page 64

COMEDOS

Comedos, or blackheads, are masses of sebum and keratin that form in the orifice of a hair follicle. The upper part appears black, because it has been oxidized by its contact with the air. A blackhead prevents the evacuation of the sebum that accumulates in the follicle. If the blockage continues, the accumulation of sebum may cause more or less substantial skin lesions.

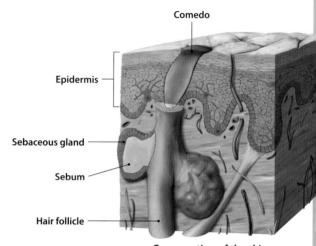

Comedo

Epidermis

Sebaceous gland

Sebum

Hair follicle

Cross section of the skin

ACNE LESIONS

Acne lesions mainly affect the face, along with the neck, chest and back. In these areas, the skin of adolescents appears shiny, due to the large amount of sebum secreted.

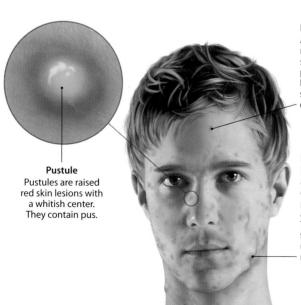

Papule
A papule is a small, red, slightly elevated skin lesion, and is potentially painful. Either it is reabsorbed spontaneously, or it develops into a pustule.

Pustule
Pustules are raised red skin lesions with a whitish center. They contain pus.

Nodule
Nodulocystic acne is a severe form of acne characterized by the presence of nodules and cysts inside the skin. These painful lesions form large bumps under the skin and may leave scars.

ACNE

SYMPTOMS:
Oily skin and lesions (blackheads, papules, pustules, nodules, cysts) on the skin of the face, back, shoulders, and torso.

TREATMENTS:
Keratolytic medications that fight blocked pores, antibiotics applied locally for mild to moderate acne or orally for resistant acne. Hormone treatments for women in some cases.

PREVENTION:
Good skin hygiene, avoid prolonged exposure to the sun.

INFECTIOUS DISEASES IN CHILDREN

Infectious diseases that specifically affect children are often highly contagious. Transmitted by the inhalation of droplets of infected saliva or by direct contact, they tend to spread chiefly in the winter and spring, especially in schools and day care centers. These diseases are usually benign, only requiring treatment of the symptoms. Some, however, such as whooping cough, measles, and epiglottitis, are more serious and can even be fatal, particularly for those who are **immunodeficient** or suffering from malnutrition. Many childhood infectious diseases can be prevented by **vaccination**.

Infectious diseases... page 284
Vaccine... page 286

CHICKENPOX

Chickenpox, which is highly contagious, mainly affects children ages 2 to 10. This infectious disease is caused by the varicella-zona virus, which remains present in the body in a latent state and may recur in adulthood, causing zona. After two weeks of incubation, chickenpox causes a rash on the chest, which gradually extends to the rest of the body. The rash may be preceded by a mild fever and slight fatigue, and is often accompanied by itching. It disappears about ten days later. A person with chickenpox is contagious two days before and five days after the appearance of the rash. Usually benign in children, recovery from chickenpox is spontaneous. Good hygiene and the administration of antihistamines to relieve the itching can help to limit the risks of secondary infection of the lesions due to scratching. The disease is more rare, but also more serious, in adults, particularly in immunodeficient people and pregnant women.

Zona... page 162

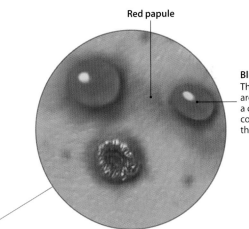

Red papule

Blister
The blisters are filled with a clear liquid containing the virus.

Skin lesion
Skin lesions caused by chickenpox appear in the form of a red papule several millimeters wide, with a blister in the middle. The blister dries out and forms a scab, which falls off after about a week without leaving any marks, except in the case of secondary infection.

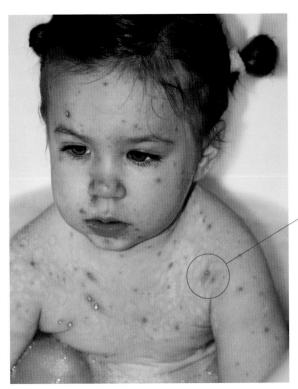

Rash (chickenpox)
The more or less intense outbreak of rashes affects the chest, scalp, limbs, back, face, and, in some cases, inside of the mouth.

Childhood and adolescence | Diseases

MEASLES

Measles is a highly contagious infectious disease caused by a virus of the Morbillivirus genus and characterized by a generalized rash. It mainly affects unvaccinated children. After 8–12 days of incubation, measles appears as a high fever (102°F–104°F [39°C–40°C]), rhinitis (common cold), conjunctivitis, and a characteristic outbreak in the mouth, called Koplik's spots. Red spots then appear on the face and gradually cover the entire body. The patient will remain contagious for four days after the outbreak of the first spots. Measles complications are fairly common and can be serious: diarrhea, acute otitis media, pneumonia, encephalitis, febrile seizures (convulsions), etc. The disease can be dangerous to young children, pregnant women, the immunodeficient, and people suffering from malnutrition. Treatment of the disease involves relieving the symptoms and treating any complications. Systematic vaccination, performed in many countries, has reduced the occurrence of the disease, although close to 350,000 people worldwide—mainly children—die from it each year.

KOPLIK'S SPOTS

Koplik's spots are small red marks with a raised whitish-bluish area in the center, which mainly appear on the inside of the cheeks, by the premolars. The spots occur two to three days before the generalized rash and only last for a few hours.

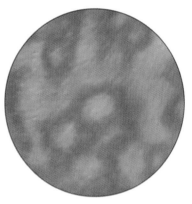

Rash (measles)
Measles causes an outbreak of more or less raised red spots that first appear behind the ears, then spread to the face and the rest of the body, forming large patches.

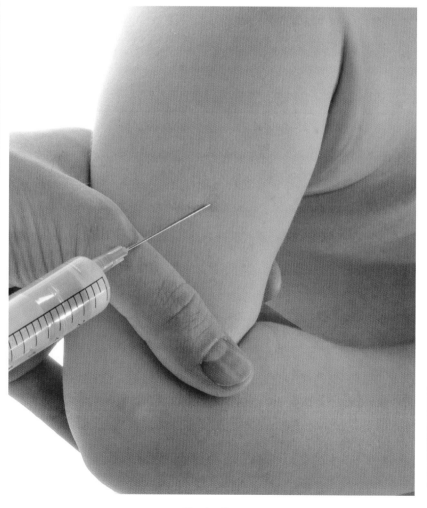

Vaccination

ROSEOLA INFANTUM

Roseola infantum is a relatively widespread, benign viral infection with a low level of contagion, affecting young children. The disease appears with the sudden onset of a high fever (102°F–104°F [39°C–40°C]) over three days. Once the fever has dropped, small pink spots appear on the skin of the torso, then the limbs and the face. The rash then disappears spontaneously after two days. Roseola requires no treatment, other than to reduce the fever.

RUBELLA

Rubella is an infectious disease caused by a virus from the Rubivirus genus, and mainly affects children and adolescents. After 15 to 20 days of incubation, the disease can appear as a moderate fever, swollen lymph nodes in the neck, headache, sore throat, and conjunctivitis. An outbreak of slight raised, small rosy spots will appear two days later. Rubella is benign, except in pregnant women who were not immunized at the start of their pregnancies, because it may cause severe malformations in the fetus. Systematic vaccination against rubella has caused it to decline considerably, and it may be completely eradicated in coming years.

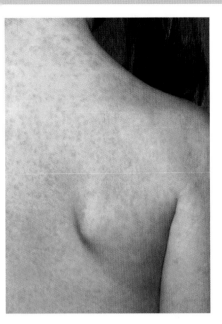

Rash (rubella)
The outbreak starts on the face, then spreads to the rest of the body, forming even patches on the skin.

MUMPS

A highly contagious infectious disease caused by a virus from the Rubulavirus genus, mumps leads to inflammation of the parotid salivary glands, located in front of the ears. The disease most often affects children ages 4 to 5, although it can also appear in older children and adults. After about three weeks of incubation, mumps can cause moderate fever, headache, and painful, sometimes spectacular, swelling of the neck. The patient, who is contagious during the week before and after onset of the symptoms, will recover spontaneously after 10 days. In some cases, the virus also affects the meninges and the testicles, which can lead to sterility in pubescent boys and adult men.

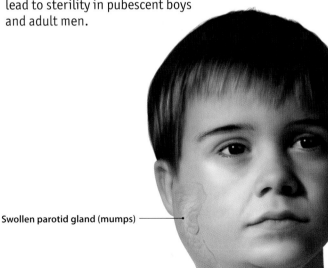

Swollen parotid gland (mumps)

THE PROS AND CONS OF VACCINATION

Children can be vaccinated at a very young age against a number of infectious diseases: measles, mumps, rubella, chickenpox, whooping cough, hepatitis B, and more. Vaccination allows the body to produce antibodies, which help to fight the development of diseases whose complications can, in some cases, be serious. This preventive technique not only reduces contagion, it can even eradicate diseases. However, some groups criticize mass vaccinations without an evaluation of the risks that these pose for each individual. According to them, the foreign agents contained in a vaccine (virus, bacteria, metals, etc.) may lead to early exhaustion of the immune system and can even provoke autoimmune diseases like multiple sclerosis and leukemia. Nevertheless, in the vast majority of cases, the side effects of vaccination are minor (fever, fatigue, swelling, etc.), and most specialists agree that the individual risks of vaccination are low, in comparison with the tremendous collective benefit they provide.

Vaccine... page 286

SCARLET FEVER

Scarlet fever is an infectious disease caused by the toxins of the group A streptococcus bacterium. It primarily affects children 5 to 10 years of age. After two to five days of incubation, it causes a sudden, high fever (102°F [39°C]) and sore throat. The lymph nodes in the neck become swollen and painful. Two days later, numerous red spots appear on the skin. The mucous membrane of the tongue is coated in a white layer, which comes off after five days, leaving a bright red color underneath. Scarlet fever is treated with antibiotics. Without treatment, it can lead to serious complications, such as glomerulonephritis and acute rheumatic fever.

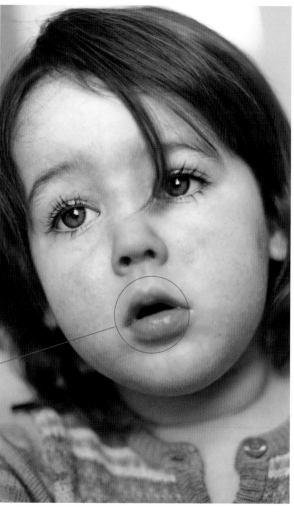

Red patches (scarlet fever)
The entire body is covered with red spots, with the exception of the palms of the hands and the soles of the feet, predominantly at folds in the skin (knees, elbows, and groin).

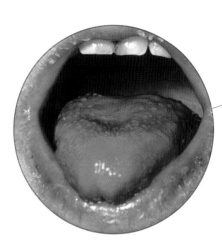

Scarlet tongue
The tongue is scarlet red, with a characteristic graininess.

WHOOPING COUGH

Whooping cough is a highly contagious infectious disease caused by the *Bordetella pertussis* bacterium and affecting the respiratory system. Although it has become relatively rare in industrialized countries, thanks to the widespread vaccination of children, it is still common in developing countries, causing 300,000 deaths each year. The first symptoms appear after about one week of incubation: runny nose, moderate fever, and dry cough, sometimes followed by vomiting. The cough then turns into violent coughing fits that end with a characteristic, noisy inhalation like a "whoop." The symptoms persist for several weeks, and an isolated cough may even last several months. Whooping cough is treated with antibiotics. Patients who are not treated will remain contagious for three weeks. The disease can affect all age ranges, but it is particularly dangerous to children under the age of 1, because of the risks of suffocation, pneumonia, and neurological ailments.

FIFTH DISEASE

Fifth disease, also known as erythema infectiosum, or slapped cheek syndrome, is an infectious disease caused by parvovirus B19. It affects mainly children 4 to 12 years of age. During incubation, which lasts for about 10 days, the patient is contagious and may display a number of ailments: mild fever, runny nose, headache, sore throat, joint pain, etc. An erythema (rash) then appears on the cheeks before spreading to the limbs, the torso, and the buttocks. These symptoms fade spontaneously after 10 days. Fifth disease is usually benign, although it can be more dangerous for the immunodeficient, those suffering from sickle-cell anemia, and pregnant women, due to the risk of miscarriage.

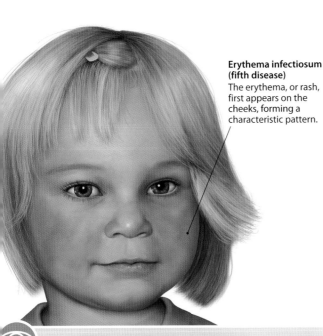

Erythema infectiosum (fifth disease)
The erythema, or rash, first appears on the cheeks, forming a characteristic pattern.

ORIGIN OF THE EXPRESSION "FIFTH DISEASE"

Fifth disease got its name from the fact that it was the fifth infectious disease characterized by rashes to have been discovered in a group of six similar pathologies. Other than fifth disease, this group also includes measles, rubella, scarlet fever, Dukes' disease (whose symptoms resemble those of rubella and scarlet fever), and roseola (sometimes referred to as sixth disease).

EPIGLOTTITIS

Epiglottitis is the acute inflammation of the epiglottis, a flap of elastic cartilage that plays an important role in deglutition (swallowing). This infectious disease is most often caused by the *Haemophilus influenzae* bacterium and chiefly affects unvaccinated children 1 to 6 years of age. It appears suddenly, as a high fever, sore throat, inability to swallow, and difficult, loud breathing. The red, swollen, purulent epiglottis blocks the movement of air to the lungs. Children with epiglottitis adopt a characteristic position (leaning forward with the mouth open) that allows them to breathe better and in which they need to be maintained. The patient's condition worsens quickly (blue coloration of the skin and suffocation), requiring emergency transportation to the hospital, where the flow of air into the respiratory tract can be reestablished and antibiotic treatment administered. Epiglottitis, which has become rare thanks to vaccination, can be very dangerous, even fatal, if not treated in time.

INFECTIOUS DISEASES IN CHILDREN

SYMPTOMS:
Depending on the case: rash, fever, headache, sore throat, cough, runny nose, etc.

TREATMENTS:
Viral infections: treatment of the symptoms (analgesics, antipyretics, rest, fluids, etc.).
Bacterial infections: antibiotics.

PREVENTION:
Vaccination of young children against: measles, mumps, rubella, whooping cough, chickenpox, *Haemophilus influenzae* infection (epiglottitis, meningitis, pneumonia). Removal of the child from school during the period of contagion to avoid spreading the disease.

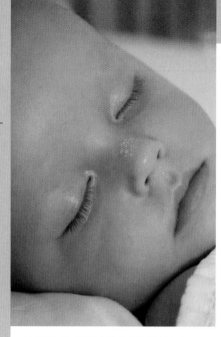

FEBRILE SEIZURES

In response to a fever higher than 102°F (39°C), the immature brain in some young children produces intense and sudden electrical activity that causes the convulsive and uncontrollable contraction of muscles in the body. These are febrile seizures. This is a common and generally benign disorder, with no connection to **infection** of the central nervous system, which often arises during the second year of life. Febrile seizures normally last only five minutes and are followed by a period of relaxation. Most of the time, they have no lasting consequence on the health of the child.

RISKS OF FEBRILE SEIZURES

During the episode, the child may be hurt by getting knocked out or choking if they are eating. Even if febrile seizures are repeated occasionally up to 5 years of age, the risk of developing neurological problems, like epilepsy or mental retardation, is low. Premature febrile seizures (occurring before the age of 1) or those that last more than five minutes are more dangerous and require a medical examination. In rare cases, they are a symptom of a more serious disorder, like meningitis.

WHAT TO DO IN THE EVENT OF FEBRILE SEIZURES

A febrile seizure in a child is manifested by rigidity of the body, loss of consciousness, upward rolling/staring of eyes, and convulsive movements of the face and limbs. Several measures can be taken to avoid injury and to lower the body temperature.

- Turn the child on his or her side in the recovery position.

- Keep away objects that may cause harm.

- Undress the child.

- Apply cool compresses on the child's body.

- Get assistance if the seizures are repeated or last more than five minutes, or if they are followed by respiratory or neurological problems.

Warning! To eliminate serious causes, a medical exam must be completed after the first episode.

First aid: Recovery position... page 543
First aid: Convulsions and fever... page 558

FEBRILE SEIZURES

SYMPTOMS:
Stiffening, unconsciousness, fixed and rolling eyes, convulsive movements of the entire body. The seizure is generally of a short duration (less than 5 minutes) and recovery is fast (less than 15 minutes).

TREATMENT:
Lowering the fever (antipyretics, cool compresses, undressing). Administering a sedative rectally.

PREVENTION:
In the event of fever, the preventative effect of antipyretics has not been proven. A preventative anticonvulsant treatment may be prescribed in some cases.

SKELETAL DEFORMITIES

Skeletal development, which occurs until the end of adolescence, may be disrupted by several factors: dietary deficiency, **trauma**, congenital malformation, etc. The resulting deformities are reversible if they are treated without delay. Certain skeletal deformities may also affect adults: osteomalacia (adult equivalent of rachitis), osteoporosis, Paget's disease, ankylosing spondylitis.

RACHITIS
Rachitis is a disease caused by a vitamin D deficiency. This vitamin is present in certain foods (dairy products, cod liver oil, salmon, egg yolk, etc.) and is created by the body when the skin is exposed to sunlight. A vitamin D deficiency leads to bone growth problems in young children: the bones, less dense, are subject to deformities. Other problems can also arise (weak muscle tone, **psychomotor** development handicap, incomplete dentition). Rachitis particularly affects children between the ages of 4 and 18 months, with dark skin, suffering from a dietary deficiency, or living in a region that has little sun. Through screening and vitamin D supplements, this disease has become rare in industrialized countries.

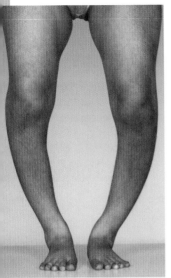

Rachitis
The lower limbs are curved.

SKELETAL DEFORMITIES

SYMPTOMS:
Rachitis: skeletal deformity, bloating, weak muscle tone, development handicap.
Scoliosis: deformity of the spinal column, dorsal pain.

TREATMENT:
Rachitis: calcium and vitamin D supplements. Scoliosis: regular monitoring, **physical therapy**, **orthopedic** corset, surgery in severe cases.

PREVENTION:
Rachitis: calcium and vitamin D supplements.
Scoliosis: premature screening.

SCOLIOSIS
Scoliosis is a deviation in the spinal column. Most often of unknown cause, it can also be the result of a birth defect, tumor, poor posture, trauma, or a neuromuscular problem. Scoliosis particularly affects girls and generally appears from infancy. The deformity of the spinal column is accentuated during puberty, then normally stabilizes at the end of development. Scoliosis is treated by wearing an orthopedic corset, physical therapy, and, more rarely, by surgery.

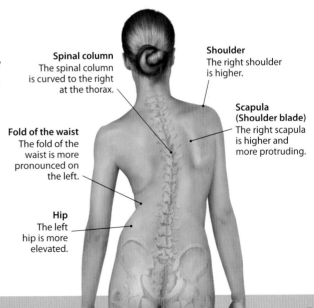

Spinal column
The spinal column is curved to the right at the thorax.

Shoulder
The right shoulder is higher.

Scapula (Shoulder blade)
The right scapula is higher and more protruding.

Fold of the waist
The fold of the waist is more pronounced on the left.

Hip
The left hip is more elevated.

Right thoracic scoliosis
Scoliosis results in a change in posture. Adolescents often adopt a "scoliotic attitude" when their legs are different lengths or when they adopt poor posture, but generally this isn't real scoliosis.

DWARFISM

Dwarfism is a **chronic** condition characterized by a much smaller than average size. Dwarfism can be proportionate or disproportionate, meaning that it may or may not respect body proportions. Depending on its origin, it can manifest itself during fetal development or appear after birth. The main causes of dwarfism (e.g. in the cases of achondroplasia and Turner syndrome) are **genetic** or chromosomal. The growth deficiency can also be the result of a growth hormone deficiency (hypophyseal or thyroid failure), a prolonged dietary deficiency, or an affective deficiency.

ACHONDROPLASIA

Achondroplasia is an incurable genetic bone development disease that affects approximately 1 in 20,000 people in the world. This common form of dwarfism particularly halts the growth of long bones, which results in a disproportion between the small size limbs and the rest of the body. It has no effect on the intellectual development of affected individuals, but it can lead to certain complications, particularly the compression of the cerebral trunk or spinal cord.

Bones... page 94

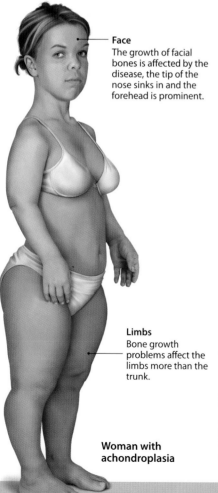

Face
The growth of facial bones is affected by the disease, the tip of the nose sinks in and the forehead is prominent.

Limbs
Bone growth problems affect the limbs more than the trunk.

Woman with achondroplasia

TURNER SYNDROME

Turner syndrome is a chromosomal disease characterized by the partial or total absence of an X chromosome. This disease affects 1 in 2,500 women in the world and results in proportionate dwarfism and the absence of genital organ development during puberty, which generally causes sterility. Other problems may also arise: cardiac malformations, deafness, lymphedema, thyroid anomaly, etc. Hormone treatments reduce the growth deficiency and stimulate the development of secondary sex characters: injection of growth hormone during infancy, administration of estrogen and progesterone during puberty.

DNA and genes... page 48

DWARFISM

SYMPTOMS:
Much smaller than average size of individuals of the same gender and age, taking into account ethnic and familial factors. There are several other symptoms that vary depending on the causes.

TREATMENT:
Some forms may be treated by hormone supplements (growth hormone, thyroid hormone).

EATING DISORDERS

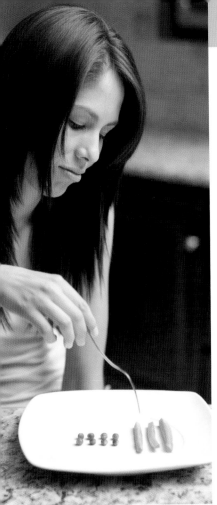

Eating disorders are psychological disorders characterized by a pathological relationship with food. It may be the refusal to eat, the sudden and irrepressible desire to consume a large quantity of food, the ingestion of inedible materials, or the voluntary regurgitation of food. There are multiple causes for these disorders: affective deficiency, conflict in the person's family and social circles, low self-esteem, stress, depression, mental retardation, schizophrenia, sociocultural causes, etc. Eating disorders most often affect children, adolescents, and young women. In the absence of treatment, they can have serious health repercussions: dietary deficiencies, intoxication, **metabolism** problems.

Nutritional deficiencies... page 360

ANOREXIA NERVOSA

Anorexia nervosa is an eating disorder characterized by the pathological fear of gaining weight and results in significant food restriction. It must be distinguished from anorexia, which is the loss of appetite caused by disease. Anorexia nervosa mainly affects young women in industrialized countries, particularly during adolescence, and may be accompanied by bulimia. Its causes can be psychological (low self-esteem, perfectionism, introversion, conflict in the person's family and social circles), sociocultural (female stereotype) or genetic (familial predisposition). The disease, which may be undetected at first, results in significant weight loss that leads to a halting of periods and several other potentially serious issues: dehydration, cardiac problems, growth delay, dietary deficiency, etc. Treatment often requires hospitalization and the intervention of several specialists, particularly nutritionists and psychologists.

Weight loss
A person with anorexia nervosa may lose up to 30% of their initial weight.

527

BULIMIA

Bulimia is an eating disorder that is characterized by hyperphagia, meaning the uncontrollable and excessive ingestion of food, followed by compensation behavior: voluntary vomiting, using laxatives and diuretics, excessive exercising, food restriction. It mainly affects adolescents and young women in industrialized countries and results from sociocultural and psychological causes: low self-esteem, stress, depression, sexual abuse, etc. Bulimia does not cause significant weight fluctuations, but it can have serious health consequences leading to cardiac problems and serious digestive system problems. Vomiting and laxative use may in fact cause inflammation of the gums, esophagus, stomach, and intestines as well as digestive bleeding, cavities, etc.

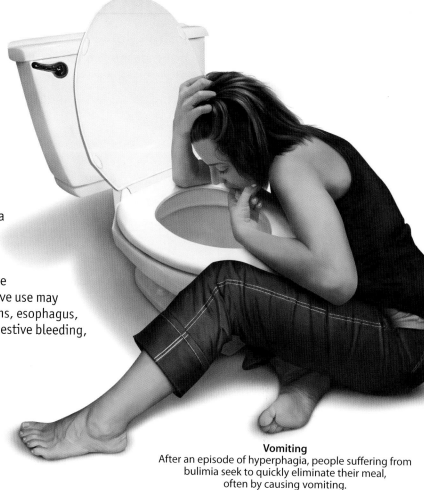

Vomiting
After an episode of hyperphagia, people suffering from bulimia seek to quickly eliminate their meal, often by causing vomiting.

HYPERPHAGIA

Hyperphagia, or compulsive eating, is characterized by the uncontrollable ingestion of large quantities of food during a short period of time. Often linked to psychological problems (low self-esteem, depression, etc.), this eating disorder affects men almost as much as women. Hyperphagia is often accompanied by weight gain and may entail, in the long term, complications like obesity, type 2 diabetes, hypercholesterolemia.

MERYCISMUS

Merycismus is an eating disorder that consists in voluntarily regurgitating food and chewing it before swallowing or spitting it out. It appears in young children, both male and female, from the age of 6 months. Merycismus is generally linked to a relational problem between a child and their parents (lack of attention, affective deficiency, etc.). In older children, it may be the sign of mental retardation. Merycismus appears a few minutes after eating. The child, seeming absent or occupied, begins chewing, sometimes for one to two hours, and stops when receiving attention. Merycismus resolves sometimes spontaneously, but it may require psychotherapy involving the parents. Hospitalization is sometimes necessary if the disorder is accompanied by dehydration or dietary deficiencies.

PICA

Pica is characterized by the ingestion of inedible materials. Normal in children under the age of 2, this behavior is considered pathological beyond that age group. Pica mainly affects young children, but it can occasionally affect pregnant women. When it is not associated with psychiatric problems like pervasive developmental disorder, mental retardation, or schizophrenia, it is often linked to familial problems (affective deficiency, dysfunctional family, parental negligence, etc.), and sometimes an iron deficiency. Pica can have serious health consequences that vary depending on the substances ingested: food poisoning, heavy metal (lead or mercury) poisoning, intestinal parasitic infections, intestinal occlusion, perforation of the digestive tract, etc.

PICA IN PREGNANT WOMEN

Certain compulsions like the desire to eat dirt, clay, or even burned matches are surprising, but not that rare in pregnant women. This behavior is linked to an iron deficiency and not psychiatric problems.

Grit ingestion
The ingestion of certain materials can endanger the life of a child: paint containing lead, dirt containing infectious agents, etc.

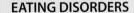

EATING DISORDERS

SYMPTOMS:
Anorexia nervosa: food restriction, weight loss, absence of menstruation. Bulimia: hyperphagia followed by compensation. Merycismus: regurgitation and chewing of food. Pica: ingestion of inedible materials.

TREATMENT:
Psychotherapy that sometimes includes parents, antidepressants, nutrition therapy.

PREVENTION:
Paying attention to young children and showing them affection.

PERVASIVE DEVELOPMENTAL DISORDERS

Pervasive developmental disorder (PDD) is a disorder characterized by social interaction and communication difficulties in addition to repetitive behavior, which hinders the normal development of the child. There are five forms of this disorder, of which autism is the most common. PDD appears during the first years of life for reasons that are not yet clearly known (**genetic** anomaly, complication during pregnancy, **metabolism** or cerebral activity problems, environmental factors, etc.). PDD may be associated with neurological problems like epilepsy, blindness, or deafness, as well as psychiatric problems: mental retardation, self-mutilation, depression, and obsessive compulsive disorders. There is no cure, but there are pedagogical methods that allow children suffering from PDD to develop independence.

FORMS OF PDD

The five forms of PDD are autism, nonspecified pervasive developmental disorder, Asperger's syndrome, Rett syndrome and childhood disintegrative disorder. Childhood disintegrative disorder and Rett syndrome, more severe and more rare, manifest themselves particularly through a serious intellectual deficiency, as well as a significant language and psychomotor handicap. Nonspecified pervasive developmental disorder and Asperger's syndrome, not as severe, are characterized by social interaction difficulties, without language or intellectual development handicaps, and by restricted activities and interests that are sometimes associated with exceptional performance (music, math, etc.). Autism has a large number of symptoms that present themselves in varying degrees from one person to another.

AUTISM

Autism affects 10 to 15 people out of 10,000 in the world and 3 to 4 times more boys than girls. It is characterized by an alteration in verbal and nonverbal communication, reduced or atypical social interaction, stereotypical behavior, and restricted interests. Autism appears before the age of 3 and manifests itself in aversion of the eyes, through unadapted contextual reactions, social isolation, language handicap, tireless repetition of heard words, repetitive use of objects, swaying of the body and hands, etc. Some autistic people possess higher than average abilities in particular domains while lacking in others. Autism is sometimes accompanied by insomnia, anxiety, eating disorders, and motor skill problems. The development of an autistic child depends on the prematurity of the diagnosis, the degree of the affliction, and the psychopedagogical methods implemented.

PERVASIVE DEVELOPMENTAL DISORDER

SYMPTOMS:
Alteration of social interaction, verbal and nonverbal communication deficiency, limited interests and repetitive behavior.

TREATMENT:
Special education programs.

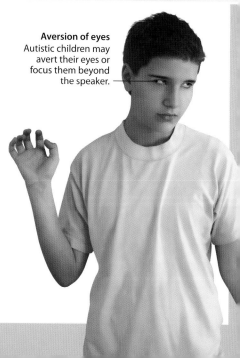

Aversion of eyes
Autistic children may avert their eyes or focus them beyond the speaker.

MENTAL RETARDATION

Mental retardation, or mental delay, is a developmental disorder that manifests itself through an intellectual ability deficiency: reasoning, communication, learning, etc. It has multiple causes and presents varying degrees of severity, measured through tests to assess cognitive and **psychomotor** functions. Mental retardation affects 1% to 3% of the population of industrialized countries and generally constitutes a handicap for life in society. However, special education programs, an adapted environment, and supervision improve the condition of affected individuals in many cases.

CAUSES OF MENTAL RETARDATION

The causes of mental retardation are known in only about 50% of cases. Often it is a case of incidents arising during pregnancy: genetic or chromosomal anomalies (trisomy, fetal malformation), infections in the mother (rubella, toxoplasmosis), exposure to toxic substances (fetal alcohol syndrome), preeclampsia, prematurity. Mental retardation may also be caused by events surrounding the birth such as encephalitis, meningitis, asphyxia, or a trauma. More rarely, mental retardation is caused by events that occur after birth: infection, heavy metal poisoning, trauma, brain tumor, etc.

DNA and genes... page 48

INTELLIGENCE QUOTIENT

The intelligence quotient, or IQ, is the score from tests to quantify intellectual abilities. It is obtained by dividing the mental age determined by the tests by the actual age of the individual, multiplied by 100. The normal score of an IQ test is 100. Scores lower than 70 indicate a more or less significant mental retardation: slight retardation (50–69), medium retardation (35–49), serious retardation (25–34), profound retardation (20–24). Scores above 140 signify gifted individuals. The validity of this test and the exact nature of what it measures are subject to numerous controversies.

MENTAL RETARDATION

SYMPTOMS:
Deficiency in intellectual capacities (reasoning, learning, communication), psychomotor disorders.

TREATMENT:
Special education allows a certain degree of independence to be acquired.

PREVENTION:
Avoiding infections and intoxications (particularly by alcohol) during pregnancy.

- IQ below 85
- IQ between 85 and 115
- IQ above 115

Distribution of the intelligence quotient among the population

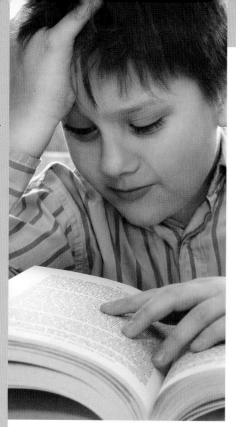

LEARNING DISABILITIES

A learning disability is a deficiency in the acquisition of specific abilities, not associated with mental retardation nor with a sensory deficiency or pervasive developmental disorders like autism. Learning disabilities can affect oral (stuttering, dysphasia) and written (dyslexia, dysgraphia) language, math (dyscalculus), and motricity (dyspraxia). They can be caused by various factors, particularly of **genetic** and neurological origin, and can lead to social insertion problems. Learning disabilities can be reduced or overcome when they are handled by specialists: neuropsychologists, orthophonists, special educators.

DYSLEXIA

Dyslexia is a reading learning disability that leads to writing difficulties in children of a normal intelligence. At varying degrees, it affects approximately 10% of children and more specifically boys. Its causes are not clear, but they can be neurological, genetic, psychological or pedagogical. Dyslexia, generally screened at 6 to 8 years of age, leads to academic difficulties. In most cases, monitoring by an orthophonist allows the child to overcome the deficiency and attend normal schooling.

DYSPHASIA

Dysphasia is an oral language learning disability, characterized by a difficulty of expression, comprehension or both, without a hearing deficiency. Communication problems with people in the child's surroundings can lead to aggressive behavior. The diagnosis of dysphasia is generally established between the ages of 3 and 5 when the parents notice a language handicap in their child: lack of vocabulary, absence of phrases, poor pronunciation, use of miming. Treatment of a child by an orthophonist and neuropsychologist reduces the deficiencies and, in some cases, allows the child to go to school.

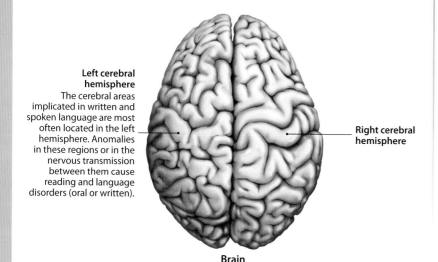

Left cerebral hemisphere
The cerebral areas implicated in written and spoken language are most often located in the left hemisphere. Anomalies in these regions or in the nervous transmission between them cause reading and language disorders (oral or written).

Right cerebral hemisphere

Brain

STUTTERING

Stuttering is a word disorder characterized by hesitations, convulsive speech, repetition of sounds, syllables, or words, sometimes accompanied by unusual mimics (grimaces, gestures). It can be the result of intense emotional shock, disturbed family life, a language disorder and genetic factors. Stuttering manifests itself in episodes, particularly in the event of stress or excitation, and disappears when the person who suffers from it sings, yells, or whispers. Common, especially in young boys, it often disappears at adolescence. Orthophonic retraining or behavioral psychotherapy can counter it.

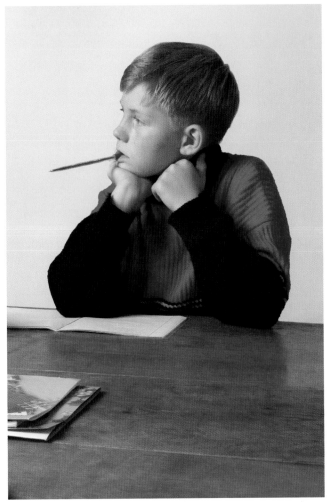

ATTENTION DEFICIT DISORDER
WITH OR WITHOUT **HYPERACTIVITY**

Attention deficit disorder, with or without hyperactivity (ADD or ADHD) is a neurological disorder that appears during childhood and often persists to adult age. It affects approximately 5% of children and 4% of adults. Its causes are still poorly defined, but an excess of dopamine linked to a genetic predisposition is suspected. ADD or ADHD is characterized by difficulties paying attention and concentrating, sometimes associated with hyperactivity: the constant need to move, impulsiveness, mood swings, etc. This disorder may disturb learning and social relations. To overcome these deficiencies, the child may be supported by various professionals: psychologist, special educator, etc. Medication treatment for ADD or ADHD is still controversial.

Dopamine... page 184

PREJUDICES SURROUNDING ADD AND ADHD
People suffering from ADD or ADHD are often the subject of unfounded prejudices. In no case is ADD or ADHD linked to mental retardation, sensory disorders, social or affective problems, lack of motivation, immaturity, or even poor education.

LEARNING DISABILITIES

SYMPTOMS:
Developmental handicap or nonverbal and verbal communication deficiency in a child, academic difficulties. ADD or ADHD: agitation, difficulty paying attention and concentrating, impatience, impulsiveness, etc.

TREATMENT:
Retraining by an orthophonist, monitoring by a neuropsychologist. Special education depending on the severity of the disorder. ADD or ADHD: adaptation of social environment (school, hobbies, etc.), multidisciplinary approach: psychotherapist, social worker, special educator, medication, etc.

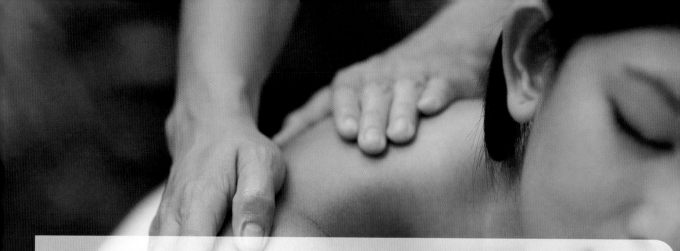

ALTERNATIVE MEDICINE

Alternative medicine, or unconventional medicine, treats health problems naturally. It does not use synthetic medications. This type of medecine is also characterized by a holistic approach to health problems: it considers the spirit and body to be closely linked and that both must be taken into account to determine the cause of disease and to stimulate healing.

NATURAL PRODUCT THERAPY

Natural vegetable, animal, or mineral products are the basic curing elements in alternative medicine such as **phytotherapy**, aromatherapy, or nutritional therapy. Their use can also be integrated with other therapeutic practices, such as naturopathy or Chinese medicine.

NATUROPATHY

Naturopathy was developed at the end of the 19th century, but its principles were proclaimed by Hippocrates approximately 2,500 years ago: the body is provided with natural self-healing mechanisms and diseases result from an imbalance in the body caused by an unhealthy lifestyle. Naturopathy aims to reestablish this balance and stimulate the self-healing ability through a multidisciplinary approach integrating different natural methods (nutrition, phytotherapy, osteopathy, massage, yoga, etc.). During the first consultation, the practitioner tries to determine the cause of the health problem by asking questions and completing different exams: blood pressure reading, reflex test, auscultation, etc. Once the diagnosis is established, the naturopathologists propose a treatment borrowed from various forms of alternative medicine that may range from a change in diet to the use of plant-based remedies. They may also direct their client towards conventional medicine when necessary. Several principles of naturopathy—such as the influence on health of diet, emotional balance, and the environment—are now emphasized by conventional medicine.

AROMATHERAPY

Aromatherapy is a practice dating back to antiquity and uses essential oils. These oils are strong-smelling chemical substances extracted from certain plants and are most often applied during a massage or by compresses. They can also be added to bath water or inhaled. Essential oils must be used carefully because they can irritate the skin and mucous membranes and cause allergies.

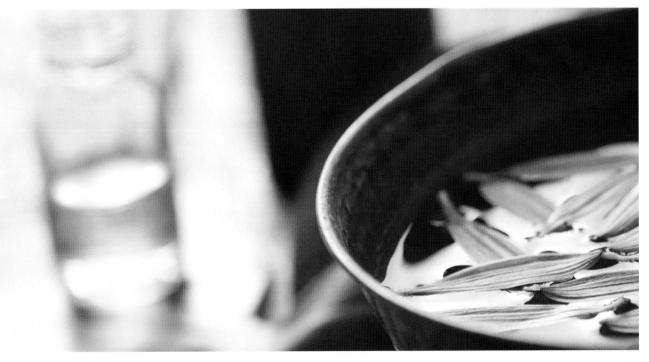

Alternative medicine

HOMEOPATHY

Homeopathy consists of treatment through the ingestion of extremely diluted natural vegetable, animal, or mineral substances. Its foundation, established at the beginning of the 19th century, rests on the following principle: a substance causing symptoms similar to those of the disease in a person of good health can stimulate the body's ability to heal itself, when it is given to a sick person in small quantities. During the first consultation, the homeopath creates a physical and psychological profile of the patient as well as a list of symptoms. Then one or several homeopathic medications are prescribed. Remedies come in various forms: pills, seeds, or powder to dissolve under the tongue. In some countries, particularly in Europe, homeopathy is taught in medical schools and some doctors include it in their conventional practice. While homeopathy claims to treat most diseases, no study concludes a true effectiveness of this method. However, it does not induce any side effects or present any danger, and the treatments can be followed at the same time as conventional medical treatments.

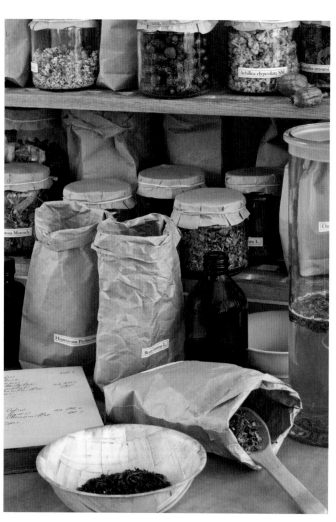

PHYTOTHERAPY

Phytotherapy uses chemical substances contained in certain plants for treatment. The use of plants for therapeutic purposes is a traditional and universal practice that is a part of medicine in many cultures. Phytotherapy is notably included in traditional Chinese and Indian medicine and it is at the origin of numerous modern medications. During a consultation, the phytotherapists question the sick person on their symptoms, their life habit and the circumstances surrounding the appearance of their disease. They then prescribe plants or parts of plants (root, flowers, leaves) that may be used in different forms (infusion, brew, gel, pill, salve, etc.), depending on the dose established by the practitioner. Some plants contain substances that can act on the body's chemistry and several synthetic medications are derived from natural vegetable substances (e.g. aspirin). Plants must be used with caution because some may be toxic or interfere with other treatments.

TOUCH THERAPY

Several alternative treatment methods use the manipulation of the body (massotherapy, reflex therapy, chiropractic, osteopathy, acupuncture, etc.) or its movement (Qigong, tai chi, yoga, etc.).

CHIROPRACTIC

Founded in Canada in 1895, chiropractic consists of manipulating the spinal column and joints to rectify vertebrae alignment. According to the principles of chiropractic, all of the functions of the body are controlled by the central nervous system. Consequently, any pressure exerted on a nerve of the spinal column would interfere with the functioning of a body part and result in a health problem. During the first consultation, chiropractors establish their diagnosis by observing the posture and movements of the patient. They examine the spinal column and the mobility of its joints and may request radiological or other exams. The treatment only begins during the second session and consists of different manipulations of the limbs and back. Chiropractic has achieved a certain success in treating dorsal pain and migraines, but its effectiveness remains to be seen for other health problems.

ACUPUNCTURE

Practiced for thousands of years in China, acupuncture developed in the West mainly during the 1970s. In the Chinese medical tradition, the body is composed of material and energy that circulates in the body following well-defined paths, called meridians. Disease is the imbalance in the circulation of energy that may be reestablished by the application of needles in precise points, sometimes completed by applying heat or suction cups. During a the consultation, acupuncturists assess their patients' state of health by asking questions, observing them, auscultating them, and conducting a series of palpations, including taking the pulse. They ask them then to lie down and apply, without causing any pain, a series of needles of which the position varies depending on the diagnosis. Acupuncture claims to be able to treat most health problems. Even though the principles on which it rests are difficult to quantify, studies show a certain effectiveness in treating pain (back pain, headaches) and nausea.

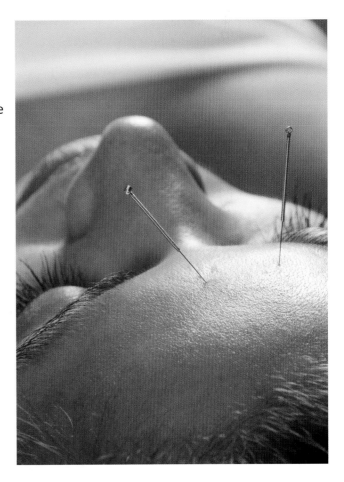

Alternative medicine

OSTEOPATHY

Osteopathy, which appeared at the end of the 19th century in the United States, uses the manipulation of the body in the form of pressure or movements to prevent and heal numerous health problems. The foundation of this therapeutic method is based on the intimate relationship that connects the musculoskeletal system and the other systems and organs of the body. All muscle, joint or skeletal problems result in local tension, discernible by touch, and cause functional problems. Osteopaths examine their patients by asking them questions about their symptoms and in particular looking for muscle tension, asymmetry in different postures, or changes in skin temperature. The treatment then consists of pressure and movements of varying speed, conducted on the joints. The effectiveness of osteopathy is mainly recognized in the treatment of dorsal pain and exogenous joint problems (sprain, tendinitis). For other health problems, the studies, which are few in number, do not allow any definitive conclusion.

MASSOTHERAPY

Massotherapy, the origins of which are difficult to establish because it is ancient, uses numerous different techniques depending on the school of thought and the countries where they were developed. Their principle, however, is identical and rests on the manipulation of the body, essentially with the hands. Different forms of pressure are exerted on the skin and underlying muscles, with the goal to relax muscle and nerve tension and stimulate blood and lymphatic circulation. Massotherapy can be effective in alleviating muscular pain and problems associated with stress: anxiety, insomnia, headaches, digestive problems. It is safe, but the massages are contraindicated in some cases—among others, for people suffering from cardiovascular problems, in the event of fever, or on the site of a recent wound. In case of doubt, seeking a medical opinion is advisable.

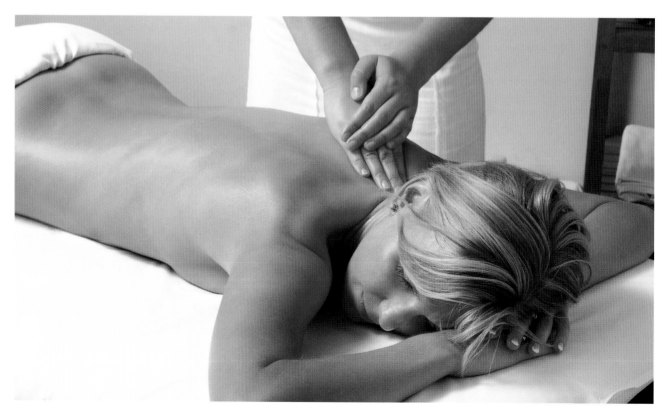

MENTAL THERAPY

In alternative medicine, the mind is a component of global health just as much as the physical and environmental components. Maintaining good mental health, therefore, contributes to disease prevention, and the mind participates in the healing process when a disease arises. It is this psychic aspect that several therapies (sophrology, music therapy, art therapy, etc.) have developed in their approach to health.

PSYCHOTHERAPY

Psychotherapy gathers all of the methods and approaches that aim to treat ailments with a psychological origin. Its principles were largely established at the end of the 19th century by Sigmund Freud, who studied the mechanisms of the human psyche (mental activity) and founded psychoanalysis. Psychotherapy generally occurs over several sessions. The treatment consists of making the patient conscious of events that are at the source of their problem. These can go back to childhood and are lost in the subconscious. Methods to bring these out differ depending on varying schools of thought. Psychotherapy is effective in treating numerous psychological problems like depression, anxiety, phobias, relationship problems, mourning, eating disorders, and psychosomatic diseases. The choice of psychotherapist and the method is a fundamental element in the success of the treatment. Therapists' areas of expertise can be obtained through their professional order or association. It is advisable to change therapists if a relationship of trust is not established after a few sessions.

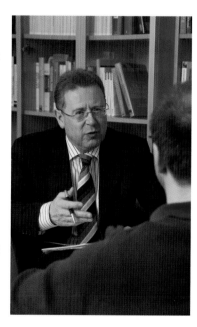

MEDITATION

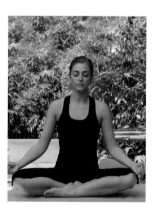

While it finds its origin in numerous religions, meditation is an exercise that can be practiced outside of any belief system. It aims to achieve a state of deep mental relaxation, which has a positive effect on the body. There are several meditation techniques, but they all emphasize the importance of a calm environment, a position promoting relaxation, and, above all, slow and deep breathing. Meditation is an excellent relaxation exercise and helps prevent stress-related diseases. Meditation is more effective, however, if practiced, at least in the beginning, under the guidance of someone who has several years of experience.

SOPHROLOGY

Appeared in the 20th century in Spain, sophrology is a form of psychotherapy that uses a collection of techniques inspired by meditation, hypnotherapy, visualization, and other practices. These techniques concentrate the patient's attention on a particular problem, which may be physical or psychological, in the effort to resolve it and allow better personal development. Depending on the problems that led to the consultation, sophrologists suggest different dynamic relaxation exercises (e.g. borrowed from yoga). With the patient's consent, they can also guide the resolution of the problem through suggestion and visualization techniques used in hypnosis. Sophrology may be used to treat anxiety, stress, and pain, as well as in preparation for birth. Some health professionals have received accredited sophrology training and include it in their practice.

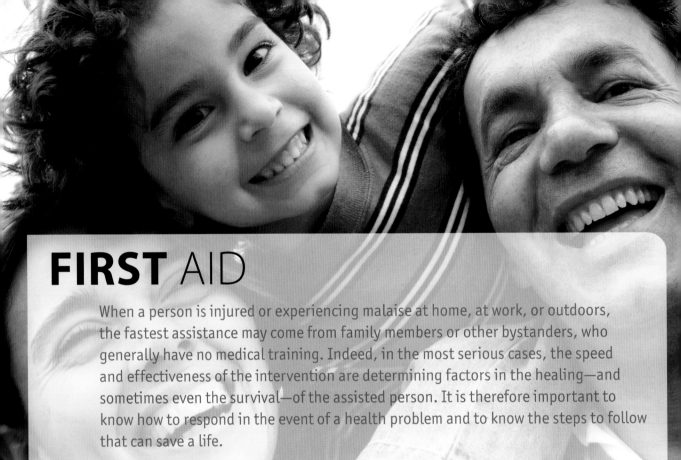

FIRST AID

When a person is injured or experiencing malaise at home, at work, or outdoors, the fastest assistance may come from family members or other bystanders, who generally have no medical training. Indeed, in the most serious cases, the speed and effectiveness of the intervention are determining factors in the healing—and sometimes even the survival—of the assisted person. It is therefore important to know how to respond in the event of a health problem and to know the steps to follow that can save a life.

FIRST AID MATERIALS AND SERVICES

EMERGENCY NUMBERS

Most countries have easy to remember and dial phone numbers to contact emergency medical assistance. Knowing them, programming them in your phone, or posting them near phones will make it possible to obtain help quickly if a situation arises. In North America, for example, the emergency telephone number for medical assistance is 911.

Links and resources... page 606

FIRST AID KIT

It is crucial to have a proper first aid kit at home, in your car, and in your backpack while hiking, and to know where to find one at work. Care should be taken to ensure that it is complete and kept in good condition. This first aid kit contains the materials required to treat most benign problems. It also helps to stabilize a more serious situation while waiting for professional medical assistance. The basic kit, of which the elements are numbered below, may be completed at home with a thermometer and acetaminophen or ibuprofen based analgesics and, for hiking, with sunscreen, insect repellent, and calming lotion for sunburn and insect bites (calamine). Metallic instruments must be disinfected with alcohol before and after use. Materials that are outdated or partially used, or whose packaging has been damaged by humidity, must be thrown out and replaced.

A basic first aid kit includes:

- Metal scissors with rounded ends

- Splinter tweezers

- Disposable gloves and masks to protect against infection

- Different sized safety pins to fasten a bandage

- Different sized adhesive bandages, sterile and individually wrapped, to protect a wound

- Gauze compresses, sterile and individually wrapped, to cover an extended wound or stop bleeding

- Different sized gauze bandages in rolls, sterile and individually wrapped

- Thick compress dressings, sterile and individually wrapped, to stop bleeding

- Elastic cloth bands

- Triangular bandages, to make a sling or to keep a splint or compress dressing in place

- Roll of adhesive tape, to secure dressings

- Swabs soaked in antiseptic, individually wrapped, to clean an injury

- Antiseptic cleanser

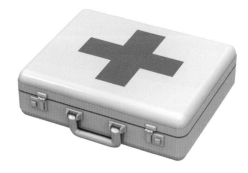

RISK OF INFECTION

All wounds are a means of entry for pathogenic agents and present a risk of infection. Superficial wounds must therefore be cleaned gently with soap and water and treated with gloved or clean hands, an antiseptic product and sterile dressing. Signs of wound infection are increase in pain, swelling and redness around the wound, increase in skin heat, and appearance of pus.

FIRST STEPS

Knowing the first steps to follow in an emergency often helps to prevent the worst outcome and can provide the time required to obtain professional medical assistance.

WHAT TO **DO**

1. Remain calm and quickly analyze the situation. Reduce the risk of aggravation by securing the premises (cut electrical power, stop cars, etc.). Avoid placing yourself in danger or hurting yourself.

2. Call for emergency assistance, indicate your location, the state of the victim, and the cause of the accident.

3. **If the victim is conscious:**

   A. Reassure the victim. If they suffered a trauma, ask them not to move. Control all excessive bleeding *(page 550)*.

   B. Disengage or clear the airways, if needed *(page 547)*.

   C. While waiting for assistance, monitor the victim's state of consciousness, breathing, and pulse, and establish their assessment (**SAMDLE**):

      • **S**igns and symptoms: How does the victim feel? In the event of malaise, what were the signs before the current situation?

      • **A**llergies: Does the victim have allergies?

      • **M**edications: Does the victim take any medication? If so, which one(s)? If they take medication for the problem that is affecting them at that moment, help them take it according to the dose.

      • **D**iseases: Does the victim have known medical issues? Do they have a medical bracelet?

      • **L**ast meal: What was the last meal consumed by the victim and when?

      • **E**vent: How did the accident occur?

4. **If the victim is semiconscious or unconscious,** assess their state of breathing.

   A. **If they are breathing**, place them in the recovery position *(page 543)*.

   B. **If they are not breathing**, conduct cardiopulmonary resuscitation *(page 546)*.

   C. Assess the state of the victim's blood circulation while controlling serious bleeding *(page 550)*.

5. Examine the victim from head to toe to detect injuries and give necessary first aid (wound dressing, immobilization of fractures, etc.).

6. Regularly monitor vital signs (breathing, pulse) until assistance arrives.

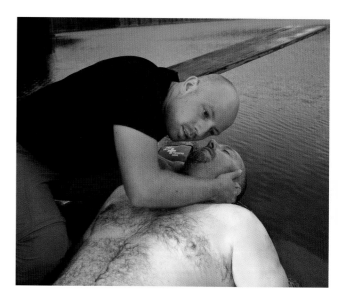

HOW TO ASSESS A VICTIM'S STATE OF CONSCIOUSNESS

A person is unconscious if they do not open their eyes when asked to or when their skin is pinched, or if they do not respond to any questions. A person who gives incoherent or incomprehensible responses may be partially conscious. In an emergency situation, the state of consciousness may change and must be verified regularly.

HOW TO ASSESS BREATHING

To verify if someone is breathing, first be sure that their airways are clear. Lay your cheek close to the nose and mouth of the victim, turning your face towards their chest. Try to make out breathing, listen for noises caused by breathing, and observe their chest to see if it rises by placing your hand on it. Count the number of rises for 15 seconds and multiply the number by 4 to know the number of breaths per minute. In adults, a rate below 10 breaths per minute or more than 24 breaths per minute requires examination by specialized medical personnel. A respiratory problem can manifest itself by breathing that is loud, too slow, too fast, superficial (panting), deep, or irregular. Blue coloring of the skin is a sign of respiratory deficiency.

Warning! If the victim is unconscious, is not breathing, and does not have any thoracic wounds, cardiopulmonary resuscitation must be performed quickly *(page 546)* **and emergency responders must be notified that a defibrillator may be needed.**

HOW TO TAKE A PULSE

The radial pulse is taken by placing your index and middle fingers on the inside of the wrist, on the side of the thumb. The carotid pulse is taken on the neck with two or three fingers. The fingers are placed on the Adam's apple, then progressively slid to the side to a dip located between the Adam's apple and neck muscles, where slight pressure is exerted. Then, the number of pulsations are counted for 30 seconds and the result is multiplied by 2. In the event of cardiopulmonary arrest, circulation must be reestablished immediately. Since taking a pulse delays medical intervention, it is recommended to conduct cardiopulmonary resuscitation as soon as unconsciousness and absence of breathing are established.

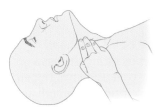 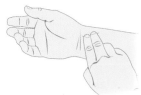

Carotid pulse   Radial pulse

NORMAL BREATHING FREQUENCY	
Age	Frequency (breaths per minute)
Under than 1 year old	30 to 50
1 to 8 years old	20 to 30
Over 8 years old	12 to 20

NORMAL PULSE FREQUENCY	
Age	Frequency (beats per minute)
Under 1 year old	100 to 140
1 to 8 years old	80 to 100
Over 8 years old	50 to 100

RECOVERY POSITION

If the injuries allow it, a semiconscious or unconscious victim must be placed in the recovery position to keep airways open and to prevent choking.

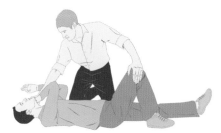

2. Roll
Roll the victim towards you by pulling on the folded knee; protect the head while proceeding with the rotation. Adjust the head back and block it in extension, resting it on the hand you placed against the cheek. Position the arms and legs in a way to stabilize the body. Cover the victim.

1. Placement
Get into position next to the victim who is lying down. Place the arm closest to you perpendicular to the body. Fold the other arm to place the back of the hand on the cheek. Lift the knee that is further away.

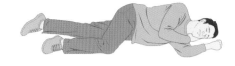

CARDIOPULMONARY ARREST

Pulmonary arrest is the interruption of breathing: the lungs no longer receive the oxygen essential to the life of each cell and, ultimately, of the body. Pulmonary arrest is often accompanied by cardiac arrest: the heart stops beating, blood circulation stops, and the pulse disappears. This serious situation requires emergency cardiopulmonary resuscitation.

SIGNS OF CARDIOPULMONARY ARREST

Cardiopulmonary arrest: Unconsciousness, skin pallor, grayish or bluish complexion, blue lips, lack of breathing and rising of the chest, absence of pulse.

CARDIOPULMONARY ARREST
WHAT **TO DO**

1. Call for emergency assistance.

2. Lay the victim on their back on a flat, hard surface. Open the airways by tilting the head back and lifting up on the chin using two fingers placed under the jaw. Look inside the mouth and remove any visible foreign bodies blocking the way. Move the head carefully if you suspect neck or head injuries.

    - **For a child under 1 year old**, slide a folded cloth, not too thick, under the shoulders to lift them. The head is then stretched back and the airways are cleared.

3. Verify that the victim is breathing by placing your ear close to the mouth and nose and attempting to hear any breathing noise or breath. Observe if the chest is rising.

    A. **If the victim is breathing** at a rate of less than 12 breaths per minute and does not present any trauma, put them in the recovery position *(page 543)* and wait for emergency assistance.

    B. **If the victim is not breathing**, give two rescue breaths of approximately one second each *(page 545)*.

C. **If the victim is still not breathing**, conduct cardiopulmonary resuscitation *(page 546)*.

    - If the victim vomits, turn them on their side until the vomiting stops. Verify that the mouth is empty and continue cardiopulmonary resuscitation while laying them on their back.

D. **If the victim displays signs of consciousness and their breathing returns**, in the absence of trauma, place them in the recovery position *(page 543)* while waiting for emergency assistance.

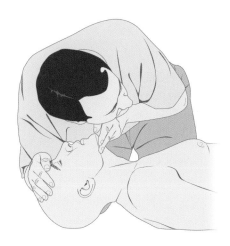

**Clearing the airways
and verifying breathing**

RESCUE BREATHS

1. Pinch the victim's nose to close the nostrils. Take a deep breath, cover the victim's mouth completely with yours, and blow into it.

   • **For an adult**, complete two rescue breaths each lasting approximately one second.

   • **For a child 1 to 8 years old**, also complete two rescue breaths of approximately one second each. The rescue breath must stop when the chest rises (do not blow all of your air).

   • **For a child under 1 year old**, two rescue breaths are given covering the nose and mouth of the child with your mouth. Each breath must last one second and stop as soon as the chest rises.

2. Move your mouth away and release the nostrils while observing whether the victim's chest lowers. If the chest of the victim does not move on the first try, move the head back into position and blow into the mouth again. If the air still does not pass, the airways are obstructed and you must clear them *(page 547)*.

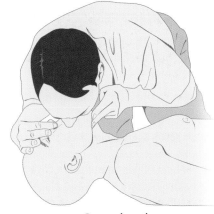

Rescue breath

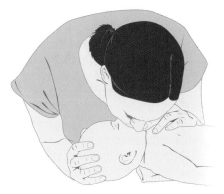

Rescue breath for a child under 1 year old

DROWNING

Drowning is a suffocation or near suffocation caused by flooding of the airways. It can occur in a very small amount of water, such as in a bath or wading pool. Always remove the victim from the water before performing cardiopulmonary resuscitation.

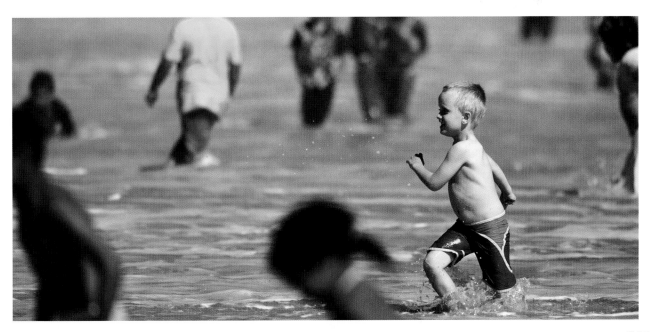

CARDIOPULMONARY RESUSCITATION (CPR)

1. After calling for emergency assistance, lay the victim on their back on a hard, flat surface and open their airways *(page 544)*.

2. Kneel next to the victim, facing their chest.

3. Slide two fingers along the last rib of the victim until you reach the base of their sternum, the point where the ribs join, at the center of the rib cage. Place the heel of your hand there (the one that is closer to the victim's head) and place the other hand on top of the first.

4. With your hands in place, align your shoulders directly above the sternum so that your arms form a vertical axis.

5. Keeping your elbows locked and arms straight, compress the victim's chest approximately 2 inches (5 cm), then reduce the pressure, at the rate of 15 compressions every 10 seconds. You can, to help you, count each compression out loud, as follows: "1 and 2 and 3 and 4 and 5 and 1 and 2 and 3 and 4 and 10 and 1 and 2 and 3 and 4 and 15." After 30 compressions, give 2 rescue breaths *(page 545)*, all of which is equivalent to one CPR cycle. Continue this cycle until emergency assistance arrives. Discontinue the maneuver and reassess breathing if the victim displays signs of consciousness (movement, making sounds, opening eyes, etc.).

- For a child 1 to 8 years old, the chest compressions, which must not exceed 1 inch (3 cm), are done with the palm of only one hand (or both, if the use of one hand is ineffective due to the size of the child) at the rate of 15 compressions every 10 seconds. Each CPR cycle has 30 compressions, followed by 2 rescue breaths.

- For a child younger than 1 year old, the compressions are done with two fingers at the rate of 15 compressions every 10 seconds. The pressure exerted is not very strong, limited to about ½ inch (1–2 cm) in depth. Each CPR cycle has 30 compressions, followed by 2 rescue breaths.

6. Maintain this rhythm of compressions and rescue breaths until signs of consciousness appear (then place the victim in the recovery position *(page 543)*), or until emergency assistance arrives. CPR can be performed by two people, one doing the compressions and the other giving the rescue breaths.

Warning! If the victim has suffered a trauma, try to keep their head in alignment with the spine and perform the maneuver carefully *(page 554)*.

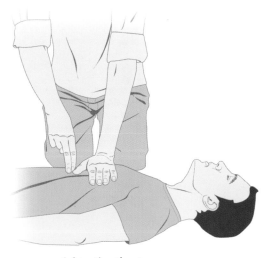

1. Locating the sternum

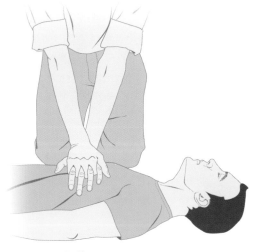

2. Chest compression

AIRWAY OBSTRUCTION

Choking is generally caused by the presence of a foreign body in the airways. This can partially or totally block the passage of air.

SIGNS OF AIRWAY OBSTRUCTION

Partial obstruction: Panic, hands on the throat, red face, cough, abnormal loud breathing, difficulty making sound or talking.

Complete obstruction: Panic, hands on the throat, absence of cough, inability to make sound, grayish or bluish face.

WHAT **TO DO**

1. Call for emergency assistance.

2. **If the victim can cough**, encourage them to do so and reassure them.

3. **If the victim cannot cough or if their breathing seems labored**, practice abdominal thrusts until the foreign body is dislodged.

4. **If the victim loses consciousness,** lay them on their back and proceed to 30 thoracic compressions, like for CPR. Lift the chin and examine the inside of the mouth all the way back to the base of the tongue. Using a finger, remove any visible foreign object then perform two rescue breaths of one second each *(page 545)*. If the air does not penetrate, repeat the compressions until the foreign body is dislodged and air passes through, or until assistance arrives.

5. **If the victim's breathing returns,** place them in the recovery position *(page 543)*.

Warning! Even if the maneuver to clear the airways is successful, a medical examination must be carried out to ensure that its application did not cause any internal injuries.

ABDOMINAL THRUSTS (HEIMLICH MANEUVER)
The principle of abdominal thrusts consists in expelling the air remaining in the lungs through a sudden pressure on the diaphragm. The maneuver can dislodge a foreign body that is obstructing the airways.

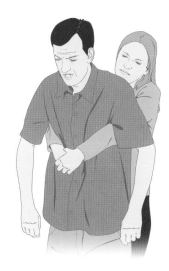

Conscious child and adult
Encircle the victim with your arms, without leaning on the ribs. Place a fist (thumb inside) just above their navel, under the sternum. Grab the fist with your other hand and exert a quick and strong pressure in and up. If you are alone and you are choking, use a piece of furniture (like the back of a chair) or your own hands to exert pressure.

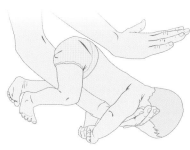

Child under 1 year old
Lay the child out on your forearm, with your arm in a downward inclination (if needed, support your arm on your thigh). Your hand should support the head, holding it firmly at the jaw. Tap the child five times on the back with the palm of your hand, between the shoulder blades. Then turn the child, keeping the head lower than the trunk, and use two fingers to apply slight pressure (about ½ inch, or 1–2 cm) five times on the sternum. This is where the ribs meet, at the center of the rib cage. Repeat the steps until the foreign body is dislodged.

RESPIRATORY DIFFICULTIES

Diseases like asthma, serious allergic reaction, or hyperventilation can cause respiratory failure and endanger a person's life.

SIGNS OF RESPIRATORY DIFFICULTY

Asthma: Shortness of breath, difficulty speaking, wheezing, quick and superficial breathing, cough, pallor, bluish coloring of lips and nails, panic, chest pains, rapid and irregular pulse, fatigue caused by breathing effort.

Allergic reaction: Swelling of the throat, tongue, lips, or eyelids; cough; wheezing; difficulty speaking; panic; face reddening.

Hyperventilation: Quick and deep breathing, sensation of suffocation, difficulty swallowing, rapid pulse but good skin color, headache, thoracic pain, dizziness.

WHAT TO DO

1. Place the victim in the most comfortable position, generally sitting or partially lying down.

   - **If the person is asthmatic**, ask them to use their inhaler (pump) or help them if they are unable to do so. Shake it. Remove the mouth end cover. Ask the person to breathe out deeply. Place the end at a distance of approximately four fingers width away from their mouth and press on the top of the pump at the same time as the person breathes in. If their condition does not improve within 10 minutes of using the inhaler, call for medical assistance.

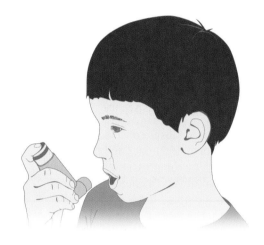

Use of an inhaler

   - **If the person suffers from a serious allergy** (swelling, difficulty breathing), ask them to use their EpiPen® adrenaline self-injector. Check the expiration date and do not proceed if it has expired or if the liquid is not transparent and uncolored. Immediately call medical emergency services.

   - **In the event of hyperventilation**, instruct the person to breathe calmly and try to calm them down. Ask them if they are taking any medication for the problem that they are experiencing. If necessary, help them find and take their medication. If their condition does not improve within 10 minutes of taking the medication, call for medical assistance.

2. If the state of consciousness of the victim changes and their breathing is no longer discernible, perform cardiopulmonary resuscitation *(page 546)*.

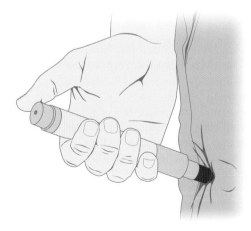

Adrenaline self-injector

CAUTION

- Do not make the person breathe in a paper bag in the event of hyperventilation.

POISONING

Poisons are most often absorbed by ingestion or inhalation, sometimes through injection or contact with the skin.

SIGNS OF POISONING

Through ingestion: Nausea, vomiting, abdominal cramps, diarrhea, burns inside and around the mouth, lip discoloration, particular breath odor.

Through inhalation: Coughing, sneezing, thoracic pains, difficulty breathing, headaches, dizziness, loss of consciousness, bluish skin color, pulmonary arrest, cardiac arrest.

Through the skin: Rash, blisters, swelling, burns.

Through injection: Rash and irritation at injection site.

WHAT TO DO

Before intervening, be sure that there is no risk of toxic gas release or contact with a toxic or corrosive substance. Protect yourself by airing out the room or wearing a mask or protective clothing, if needed.

1. Call emergency assistance or the poison control center and verify the vital signs of the victim *(page 543)*.

2. Identify the toxic substance, save a sample of vomit for poison identification, estimate the quantity of substance absorbed, and the time elapsed since its absorption.

3. If it is poisoning:

   • **Through ingestion:** rinse the inside and perimeter of the mouth with water.

   • **Through inhalation:** keep the victim away from the source of gas and place them in a ventilated place.

   • **Through skin contact:** thoroughly rinse the skin with cold water.

4. **If the victim is breathing:** lay them down in the recovery position *(page 543)* and wait for assistance.

5. **If the victim is not breathing:** perform cardiopulmonary resuscitation *(page 546)* being careful not to enter in contact with the poison. If the poison was ingested, clean the perimeter and the inside of the victim's mouth or insufflate air through the nose. In the event that the poison was inhaled, complete CPR thoracic compressions *(page 546)*, but only proceed with insufflations if you are using a pocket mask with a one-way valve and stop if you feel the slightest discomfort.

6. If the victim vomits, clean and rinse their mouth.

TO AVOID POISONING

• Keep products in their original packaging.

• Read the label of a product before use and follow the instructions for use.

• Air out the premises when using toxic substances.

• Do not run a motor in a closed space.

• Follow medication doses.

• Keep dangerous products and medications separately and in places that are inaccessible to children.

• Be informed on the toxicity of indoor plants.

CAUTION

• Do not make the victim vomit, as this may aggravate digestive tract burns caused by a corrosive substance or trigger choking if they are semiconscious.

BLEEDING

Bleeding is the flow of blood from a blood vessel. It is external when the blood flows from a wound and internal when the bleeding happens inside the body. If the organs do not receive enough blood, they progressively stop working. In this case, the person is said to be in shock (or **hypovolemic shock**), which can lead to death if not treated quickly.

Bleeding... page 239

SIGNS OF BLEEDING

External bleeding: Wound and visible blood flow.

Internal bleeding: Hematoma, swelling, difficulty breathing, vomiting blood, pain. Intracranial bleeding: bleeding in the ear or nose, blood present in the eye. Pulmonary bleeding: foamy spit with bright red blood. Digestive bleeding: granular vomiting, bright red or brownish, presence of blood in stools.

Shock: Pallor and coolness of skin; bluish coloring of lips and extremities; rapid and weak pulse; rapid, irregular, and sometimes loud breathing; confusion, disorientation, and sometimes agitation; extreme thirst; nausea; loss of consciousness.

EXTERNAL BLEEDING
WHAT **TO DO**

1. **For a chest wound,** which may cause damage to the lungs and serious breathing difficulties, call for emergency medical assistance, then:

   - Cover the entire wound with a clean plastic film. Fasten it on three sides, leaving the lower side open.

   - Cover the victim. If they did not suffer a trauma to the spine, place them in the sitting or recovery position *(page 543)* until assistance arrives.

2. **For a serious wound to a limb,** call for emergency medical assistance, then:

   - Bring the ends of the wound close together and compress it with one or several sterile dressings or even with a cloth (the cleanest possible). Place a compression bandage around the dressing, then a second, if needed.

   - If the bleeding continues after the application of the second compression bandage, exert indirect pressure *(page 551)*.

   - If a foreign body protrudes from the wound, do not try to remove it. You could aggravate the bleeding. Instead, place the dressing around in such a way as to compress the wound and immobilize the object without exerting any pressure on it.

- Verify blood circulation around the dressing by comparing the temperature and color of the skin to that of the intact member. If you notice a difference, slightly loosen the bandage.

- Make the victim lie down or sit. If the limb does not appear to be fractured, raise it above heart level.

3. **For a superficial wound** (scratch, shallow cut, etc.), rinse it with soap and water to eliminate potential foreign bodies. Dry it, apply antiseptic, and cover it with a sterile dressing.

Warning! Consult a physician for any severe or particularly dirty wounds.

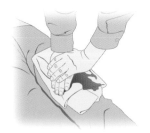
Direct compression on the wound

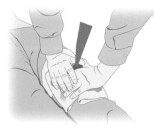
Wound dressing containing a foreign body

INDIRECT COMPRESSION

When direct compression is ineffective, the blood flow may be interrupted by compressing the main artery upstream from the injury, meaning between the wound and the heart (as close as possible to the wound). This technique is applicable only to external bleeding affecting a limb artery or neck artery.

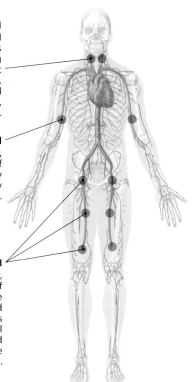

Neck wound
The carotid, located next to the trachea, is compressed by squashing it with the thumb against the neck vertebrae. The other fingers, placed on the nape of the neck, serve as support.

Arm or hand wound
The brachial artery, located on the inside of the arm, is compressed by pressing the thumb firmly against the bone.

Leg wound
The femoral artery, located in the crease of the groin, on the inside of the thigh and behind the knee (where it is called the popliteal artery), is compressed by leaning on it with the fist, arm extended.

Main compression points

APPLYING A COMPRESSION BANDAGE

A simple bandage consists of placing the end of the band on the wound (two turns) and progressively wrapping the wound up, covering a third of the band already placed in each turn. The bandage is then fastened with a safety pin. The bandage must be tight enough without cutting off blood circulation.To be sure of this, compare the temperature and color of the skin with another limb and adjust the bandage if necessary.

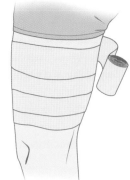

Simple bandage

NOSEBLEEDS

Nosebleeds are controlled by slightly tilting the head forward and pinching the nose under its bony section for 10 minutes. Once the bleeding stops, you must avoid blowing your nose for several hours. If the cause of the bleeding is a violent shock to the head, a cranial or face trauma may have occured (page 554). Therefore, let the blood run and call emergency medical assistance.

SHOCK AND INTERNAL BLEEDING

WHAT **TO DO**

1. Call for emergency assistance.

2. Reassure and calm the victim. Moisten their lips with a damp cloth if they are thirsty.

3. Keep the victim in the position that they are found in. If needed, support the head, without pulling it.

4. Loosen the victim's clothing and cover them.

5. Monitor the victim's breathing and their pulse (page 543) and if needed perform cardiopulmonary resuscitation while waiting for medical assistance (page 546).

CAUTION

• Do not give an internal bleeding victim something to eat or drink.

• Do not remove a blood-soaked dressing. (Instead add supplementary dressings on top.)

• Do not give aspirin or derived medications to a bleeding victim.

• Do not massage a hematoma or apply heat on it.

FALLS AND TRAUMAS

Falls and false movements can cause muscle, joint, or bone **traumas** of varying severity: elongation, laceration, sprain, dislocation, fracture.

SIGNS OF TRAUMA

Elongation, tear: Intense muscle pain, appearance of a bruise and swelling, reduction of mobility.

Muscle injuries... page 125

Sprain: Pain that is accentuated by movement, reduction of mobility, joint swelling.

Sprain... page 110

Dislocation: Intense pain, deformity and swelling of the joint, loss of mobility of dislocated joint.

Dislocation... page 111

Fracture: Sensitivity or pain in the fractured region (made worse when touched), reduction or loss of mobility and sensitivity, deformation or abnormal position of a limb, change in color and temperature, swelling, hematoma, bone fragment that may exit the wound.

Bone fractures... page 102

ELONGATION OR BENIGN SPRAIN (SPRAIN)
WHAT **TO DO**

1. Avoid applying weight to or moving the injured region.

2. Apply ice on the painful region, as soon as possible, in alternating periods of 15 minutes (never more than 20) with and without ice.

3. Immobilize the painful region while ensuring not to obstruct blood circulation.

4. If possible, raise the injured region.

5. Consult a physician if you do not notice improvement.

SERIOUS SPRAIN, DISLOCATION, OR FRACTURE
WHAT **TO DO**

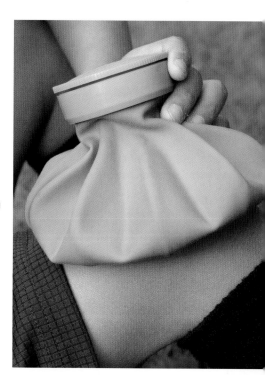

1. In the event of head or spinal injuries, do not move the victim. In other cases, place the victim in a comfortable position, while keeping the injured limb immobilized.

2. If there is a wound, clean it delicately and cover it with a sterile dressing, without exerting pressure.

3. Immobilize, without trying to readjust, the injured region.

4. Verify blood circulation (temperature, skin color, pulse) in the hand or foot of the injured limb. A sign of absence of circulation requires emergency medical treatment.

5. Depending on the situation and the severity of the injury, call emergency medical assistance or quickly obtain a medical consultation. In the meantime, apply ice on the painful region, in alternating periods of 15 minutes (never more than 20 so as not to cause hypothermia) with and without ice.

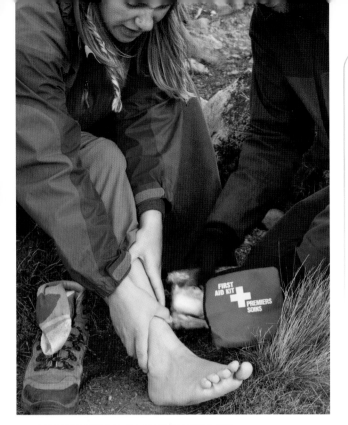

CAUTION

- Do not move a victim of a spinal injury.
- Do not attempt to readjust a displaced joint or bone.
- Do not manipulate or move a painful joint or limb.
- Do not apply ice directly on the skin or on a wound.
- Do not apply a compress bandage on a fracture.
- Do not make a fracture victim drink or eat, which is especially not recommended before surgical operation under anesthesia.

IMMOBILIZATION OF AN INJURED LIMB

Before moving a person suffering from a trauma (elongation, sprain, dislocation, fracture), be sure to immobilize the injured limb, from the joint above the injury to the one below it. Immobilization limits the pain and avoids damage caused by a bone to a nerve or blood vessel while moving. This is done by attaching the injured limb to a stiff support like a board, umbrella, ski pole, cane, etc. It is preferable to insert padding (piece of thick cloth, foam, etc.) between the object and the limb. The straps (band, scarf, tie, belt) must be quite tight to keep the limb in place, but must never cut off the circulation, nor be fixed directly on the injury or joint. In the absence of a stiff object, a pillow may be used to wrap the injured limb. The legs can be kept immobile by attaching them together. An arm can be rested against the body and immobilized with a scarf.

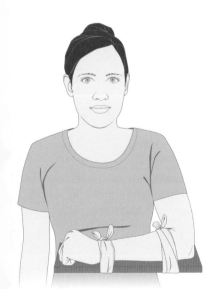

Immobilization of a forearm

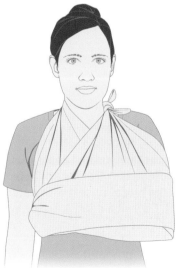

Scarf

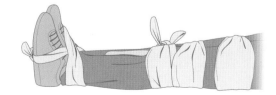

Immobilization of a leg

HEAD AND SPINAL INJURIES

Even if head and back injuries are not serious, vigilance is required to monitor for signs of a more serious injury. The skull and spinal column house nervous centers (brain, spinal cord) and their damage may be irreversible.

Cranial traumas... page 150

SIGNS OF BRAIN AND SPINAL CORD INJURIES

Brain injury: Swelling or deformation of the skull; bruising on the skull or around the eyes; blood or clear liquid emanating from the scalp, nose, or ears; pain and difficulty turning the head or swallowing; difference in size between the two pupils or absence of reaction to light; weakness or paralysis of limbs; nausea; vomiting; alteration in state of consciousness (confusion, memory loss, speech problems, vision, or hearing problems); convulsions; shock; temporary unconsciousness.

Spinal cord injury: Swelling or bruising on the back, abnormal sensation in one or several limbs (tingling, numbness), difficulty moving, paralysis of limbs, shock.

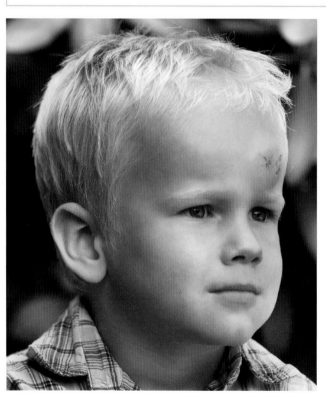

CONTUSION
WHAT **TO DO**

Contusion, which manifests itself through a purple-blue bump on the skin, is a common injury in children. Most often benign, it can also be accompanied by a concussion or cerebral compression caused by a hematoma developing under the bones of the skull.

1. Be sure that the child does not have other more serious injuries.

2. Quickly apply a cold compress or ice for 15-minute periods.

3. Monitor the child. If they present signs of a brain injury, even a few days after the incident, quickly obtain medical assistance.

MOUTH INJURIES
In the event of bleeding, ask the victim to spit out the blood and apply a small sterile compress on the wound until bleeding stops. If a tooth is accidentally uprooted, roll a piece of a compress the size of the tooth and apply it on the gums to replace the tooth. If you find the tooth, rinse it with water and save it in a damp compress, only touching it by the crown, never by the root. Consult a dentist. In the event of jaw fracture, support the jaw without closing it and obtain medical assistance.

HEAD OR SPINAL INJURIES
WHAT **TO DO**

A shock to the head can cause a hematoma between the brain and skull bones, without leaving a visible trace on the skin surface. At first, the victim may be conscious and feel good, but their condition may change in a few minutes or several hours. Therefore, it is important to not neglect a head injury and to monitor the victim. If you suspect a spinal injury, do not move the victim.

1. **If the person is conscious and up**, make them sit down. Apply a dressing on the wounds, without compressing them. Then remain with the victim until medical assistance is obtained.

2. **If the person is conscious and lying down**, ask them not to move, stabilize the head without pulling it, and call for emergency assistance.

    • Keep the head in the same position or stabilize it with clothing, pillows, or thick linens.

    • Treat bleeding *(page 550)*.

    • Investigate a potential injury to the spine by questioning the victim on the circumstances of the accident and asking them if they feel pain or other sensations in the limbs. Ask them to move a finger and toe on each limb.

3. **If the victim is partially conscious or unconscious**, clear the airways, and verify breathing *(page 543)*.

    • If they are breathing normally, keep them in position until assistance arrives and regularly verify breathing.

    • If they are not breathing, perform cardiopulmonary resuscitation *(page 546)* while keeping the head and neck in the spinal column axis.

4. If the victim vomits, turn them on their side until the vomiting stops, while moving the body and head in one block (it is preferable to seek assistance). Clean the mouth and place the victim back on their back. Resume CPR, if needed.

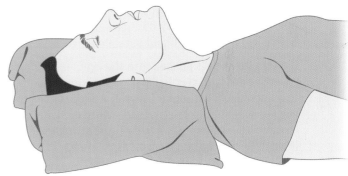

**Immobilization
of the head with objects**

EAR BLEEDING
In the event of ear bleeding, carefully examine the blood.

• If it is mixed with clear liquid, call for assistance, as this may be a sign of a skull fracture. Stabilize the head and cover the ear with a bandage without tightening it, to absorb the blood without preventing flow.

• If the blood is pure, the head must be inclined to the side of the bleeding. Place a dressing without tightening it and immediately consult a physician.

First aid | At home and in daily life

EYE INJURIES
WHAT **TO DO**

The eye is a fragile and very sensitive organ. Any contact with the surface causes significant disturbance, irritation, tearing, reddening of the white part of the eye, and sometimes pain.

1. **If a foreign body is in contact with the surface of the eye** (eyelash, dust), you can try to remove it without injuring the eye by rinsing the eye or using the corner of a clean, damp cloth (handkerchief or gauze compress). Wash your hands before any contact and turn toward a light source to better spot the foreign body.

    •   If the foreign body is located under the upper eyelid, pull the eyelid downward, over the lower eyelid, holding it by the eyelashes. In relaxing it, friction between the two eyelids may be enough to remove the foreign body. If this maneuver does not work, ask the affected person to look down. Then, by delicately turning the upper eyelid over, remove the foreign body with the point of a clean and damp linen while pushing it towards the exterior of the eye.

    •   If it is located under the lower eyelid, ask the affected person to look up. While pulling the lower eyelid down and to the outside, remove the foreign body with the corner of a clean, damp cloth.

2. If you cannot remove the foreign body or **if you have injured the eye or surrounding tissues**, cover the injured eye with a dry and sterile dressing while taking care to not exert pressure on the eyeball. Ask the victim to avoid all eye movement (cover both eyes, if necessary) and obtain medical assistance.

3. **If a foreign body is pushed into the eye**, leave it in place and cover the eye with sterile damp gauze, surrounding the object to immobilize it without moving it. Ask the victim to avoid all eye movement (you can cover the other eye with a dry dressing to avoid any involuntary movement that would aggravate the injury). Quickly obtain medical assistance.

4. **If the eye was in contact with a chemical product**, obtain medical assistance. Thoroughly rinse the surface of the eye while avoiding the contamination of the other eye (tilt the head to the side of the affected eye).

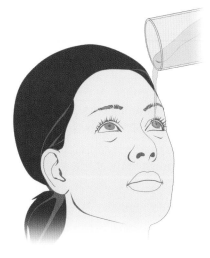

Rinsing the eye

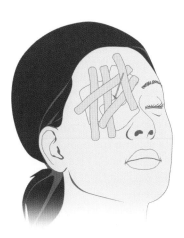

Dressing around the foreign body that entered the eye

> ### CAUTION
>
> •   Do not immediately lift a child who has fallen. It is better to wait and see if they get up on their own and then examine them.
>
> •   Do not move a victim of a head or spinal injury.
>
> •   Do not rub an injured eye or apply pressure or a compress dressing on top.

BURNS AND ELECTROCUTION

The severity of a thermal, chemical, electrical, or radiation burn is assessed based on the extent of the burn, its depth, and the region of the body that is affected.

Burns... page 72

SIGNS OF BURNS

First-degree burn: Red and dry skin, swelling, pain.

Second-degree burn: Red skin, liquid filled blisters, intense pain.

Third-degree burn: Shiny white or black skin, visible subcutaneous tissues, absence of sensitivity to the burn or extreme pain.

Burn through inhalation: Burned facial hair or hair, cough, wheezing, pallor, cyanosis, difficulty breathing.

WHAT **TO DO**

1. If the burn is deep, is extensive, affects the airways (burn located on the face or neck or following gas inhalation), or is of electrical or chemical origin, complications may arise. Immediately call for emergency assistance.

2. Before intervening, be sure to secure the intervention premises or move the victim to a secure location (well-ventilated, far from cut wires or live electrical appliances).

3. Find the cause of the burn.

    • **If caused by a flame, hot water, or hot object**, submerge the burn in cold water, place it under running water, or cover it with damp compresses. Then remove clothing or jewelry (unless they are stuck to the skin) and cover the wound with a dry, sterile dressing. If the burned area is extensive, use a napkin or clean cloth.

    • **If of electrical origin**, monitor the vital signs of the victim while waiting for assistance, as heart rate problems may occur. It may then be necessary to perform CPR *(page 546)*. Find the entry and exit points of the electrical current (which are very localized burns) and cover the wounds with a dry dressing.

    • **If caused by a chemical product**, be careful to avoid contaminating yourself or recontaminating the victim. Consult the product label for information. If it is a powder product, first brush away residue with an object (brush, dry sponge, paper, etc.). Rinse the contaminated zone with plenty of water for 30 minutes, unless contraindicated. Have the victim remove all clothing and jewelry that has been in contact with the toxic product. Apply dry dressings and cover the victim. Monitor their state while waiting for assistance.

    • **If it arises following the inhalation of a vapor or chemical product**, move the victim to a well-ventilated area and attentively monitor their vital signs while waiting for assistance. In the event of cardiopulmonary arrest following poisoning, avoid inhaling air exhaled by the victim *(page 549)*.

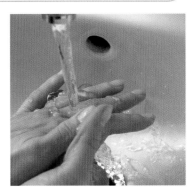

Immersion or rinsing of the burn in cold water

CAUTION

• Do not touch an electrocution victim if the electrical source is not disconnected.

• Do not touch a burn with a bare hand.

• Do not pierce blisters.

• Do not remove clothing that is stuck to the burn.

• Do not apply fatty products like a cream or ointment.

• Do not place a dressing that leaves fibers on the skin.

CONVULSIONS AND FEVER

Convulsions are uncontrolled passing muscular contractions, generally benign, most often caused by epilepsy or by a spike in fever (especially in children younger than 3 years old). Fever is an elevation in temperature above the normal temperature, which is approximately 99.5°F (37.5°C), and is the body's way of fighting **infection**.

SIGNS OF CONVULSIONS OR FEVER

Convulsions: Muscle stiffening, convulsive contractions and movements of one body part or the entire body, temporary loss of consciousness, loud breathing, grinding teeth, foaming at the mouth, bluish lips.

Fever: Temperature higher than 100°F (37.8°C), shivers and sensation of cold when the fever increases, sweat and sensation of heat when it lowers, fatigue, muscle soreness, headaches. In young children: agitation or apathy, uninterrupted crying, rapid breathing, reddening, accelerated heart rate, bright eyes.

CONVULSIONS
WHAT **TO DO**

1. Support and lay down the victim. Loosen the clothing. Slide a thin cushion under the head or support it with your hands without exerting resistance. Keep away any objects that may harm the victim.

2. If the convulsions are due to fever, try to lower the victim's temperature.

3. At the end of the attack, if the victim is unconscious, search for potential injuries and verify their breathing and pulse. Place them in the recovery position *(page 543)* and cover them.

4. Call for assistance if the attack lasts more than five minutes, if it repeats, or if it is followed by breathing or neurological difficulties.

Epilepsy... page 166
Febrile seizures... page 524

FEVER
WHAT **TO DO**

1. Immediately consult a physician:

   - In the event of fever, even a slight one, in a child under 6 months old

   - In the event of elevated fever (104°F [40°C] and higher)

   - If a child presenting a moderate fever becomes very irritable, no longer responds when spoken to, refuses to drink, no longer urinates, or presents other symptoms, such as flushing, coughing, or wheezing

   - If the fever persists more than 72 hours

2. Have the person drink a lot of liquids.

3. Cool the person down by dressing them in light clothing (under garments, camisole) and moistening their skin with a sponge with tepid water (which is more effective than a bath). If they are shivering, cover them.

4. You can give the person an acetaminophen or ibuprofen-based medication (following the dosage according to their weight in the case of a child), which will temporarily lower the fever by 2°F–4°F (1°C–2°C).

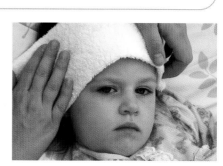

Sponging with tepid water

CAUTION

- Do not give aspirin to children.

- Do not use very cold water to lower temperature.

- Do not try to restrain the movements of the seizing person.

- Do not try to introduce something in the mouth of the seizing person.

MALAISE AND LOSS OF CONSCIOUSNESS

Malaise is a sensation of weakness, discomfort, and decline of the physical condition, resulting in a health problem that can be benign or more serious. This condition can disappear spontaneously, but it can also develop into loss of consciousness (fainting).

SIGNS OF MALAISE OR LOSS OF CONSCIOUSNESS

Malaise: Discomfort, anguish, weakness, dizziness, glare, chest pain, difficult, loud or irregular breathing, sleepiness or agitation, pallor, perspiration, confusion, difficulty talking, loss of movement coordination.

Loss of consciousness: Closed eyes, no reaction to voice, insensitivity to pain (pinching skin).

MALAISE AND LOSS OF CONSCIOUSNESS
WHAT TO DO

1. **If a person is conscious:**

   • Lay them down on their back, raising the legs. If this is not possible, make them sit, tilted forward, placing the head lower than the shoulders.

   • Loosen clothing around the neck, chest, and waist.

   • Ventilate the premises, if possible.

   • Reassure the person and remain at their side until they feel better.

2. **If a person has lost consciousness:**

   • Call for emergency assistance.

   • **If the victim is breathing**, place them in the recovery position *(page 543)* and loosen their clothing.

   • **If the victim is not breathing**, perform CPR *(page 546)*.

CEREBRAL VASCULAR ACCIDENT AND HEART ATTACK

Cerebral vascular accident (stroke) can be preceded by malaise associated with various symptoms: violent headache, paralysis of facial muscles, difficulty speaking, loss of saliva, numbness or weakening of limbs (often unilateral), loss of vision, mental confusion, dizziness, and loss of consciousness. A heart attack is associated with the following symptoms: sensation of oppression in the chest, tightening or burning, pain in the arm or jaw, pallor, nausea, perspiration, fatigue, shortness of breath . If you suspect a stroke or heart attack:

1. Immediately call for emergency medical assistance.

2. Place the victim in the most comfortable position. Cover them and reassure them.

3. If they lose consciousness, place them in the recovery position *(page 543)*. Monitor their vital signs and prepare to perfom CPR *(page 546)*.

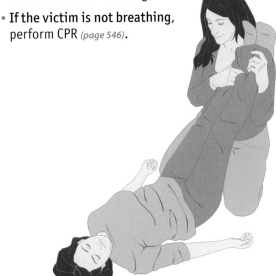

Raising the legs

DIABETIC MALAISE

If the victim of malaise tells you that they are diabetic or wears a pendant or bracelet indicating this, help them take their medication or give them sugar in solid or liquid form (the victim must be alert and give their consent). If they lose consciousness, call for emergency assistance and place them in the recovery position *(page 543)*. Do not put anything in their mouth.

SUNBURN

Sunburn is a burn caused by prolonged exposure to sun rays, without protection. It may be accompanied by heatstroke.

Burns... page 72

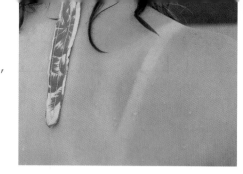

SIGNS OF SUNBURN

Sunburn: Reddening or significant sensitivity of the skin (sometimes to the point of being unable to endure the friction of clothing), blister forming on the skin when the burn is more severe.

WHAT **TO DO**

1. Apply cold compresses to alleviate pain.
2. Obtain a cream or specific lotion for sunburn from a pharmacist or physician. You can also apply an aloe-based gel (composed of at least 70% pure aloe) on the burn.
3. Drink plenty of water.
4. If you must go out and are exposed to the sun, cover the burned area with opaque clothing.
5. Consult a physician if the pain does not decrease in 48 hours or if the symptoms of heatstroke appear.

PREVENTING SUNBURN

Prolonged exposure to the sun can cause sunburn and, in the long term, accelerate aging of the skin and increase the risk of developing skin cancer. It is therefore necessary to protect the skin against the harmful effects of the sun. Here is some useful information:

- The sun is most intense between 10 a.m. and 3 p.m., particularly in the summer.
- The strength of sun rays increases with altitude.
- Opaque and thick clothing as well as hats offer good protection against ultraviolet rays.
- Sunglasses offer relative protection against sun rays (anti-UV treatments strengthen this protection).
- Sunscreens in cream form applied to the skin have limited effectiveness, even when they are adequately used. They are complementary measures of protection. The cream must be applied half an hour before exposure, in a thick and even layer. It must be reapplied regularly (following instructions), particularly after swimming.
- Car windows, even tinted, do not protect against ultraviolet rays.
- Reflected solar light (water, sand, snow, etc.) has similar harmful effects on the skin.

HEATSTROKE

Physical activity that is not adapted to the context, or prolonged exposure to heat can cause health problems that are due to dehydration or the inability of the body to regulate its temperature (sunstroke or heatstroke).

SIGNS OF HEATSTROKE

Dehydration: Muscle cramps; fatigue; skin that is abnormally pale, cold, and clammy; dilated pupils; rapid and weak pulse; rapid and superficial breathing; nausea; vomiting; dizziness; thirst; dry mouth; dark urine; mental confusion; progressive loss of consciousness.

Insolation (heatstroke): Dry skin that is red and warm, rapid pulse, loud breathing, headache, confusion, agitation, dizziness, convulsions, progressive loss of consciousness.

Eye burning: Inability to tolerate light, swelling of eyelids, eye irritation, pain, sensation of burning or having grains of sand under the eyelid, vision problems, temporary blindness, tearing.

DEHYDRATION AND HEATSTROKE
WHAT **TO DO**

1. Place the victim in the shade, if possible in a cool location.

   - **In the event of dehydration**, the priority is to rehydrate the victim by making them drink a lot, but in small quantities. Do not give them anything if they vomit.

   - **In the event of sunstroke**, the priority is to cool down the victim by any available means: electric or handheld fan, cold damp cloth, bath, etc. Stop when the skin temperature seems normal to touch.

2. **If the person is conscious:**

   - Lay them down on their back, raising the legs.

   - Remove as much clothing as possible or loosen it.

   - Obtain medical treatment.

3. **If the person is unconscious:**

   - Place them in the recovery position (page 543).

   - Call for emergency assistance.

   - Monitor their breathing and pulse (page 543) while waiting for assistance.

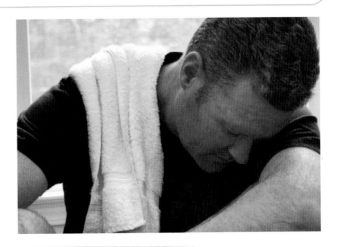

EYE BURNING BY THE SUN

Sun rays, direct or reflected, as well as certain particularly intense light sources, can cause damage to the cornea and retina. Symptoms may appear quickly or a few hours after exposure.

WHAT **TO DO**

1. Apply cold damp opaque compresses on both closed eyes. Prevent the victim from rubbing their eyes.

2. Keep the compresses in place using an opaque bandage around the head (it should cover the eyes, but not exert pressure on them).

3. Reassure the victim and obtain medical assistance.

561

HYPOTHERMIA AND FROSTBITE

A person suffers from **hypothermia** when their internal temperature drops below 95°F (35°C). Hypothermia leads to a slowing of the functions of the body (breathing, heart rate, etc.), then their complete arrest, if hypothermia continues. Frostbite is an injury of the skin and subcutaneous tissues caused by the cold.

SIGNS OF HYPOTHERMIA OR FROSTBITE

Hypothermia: Shivering that intensifies then disappears, slow and weak pulse, superficial breathing slowing with the degree of hypothermia, alternating state of consciousness until loss of consciousness.

Frostbite: Signs develop depending on the aggravation of the frostbite: cold skin turns from white and waxy to tough, bluish, and grayish; redness around the frostbitten area; pain; sometimes formation of blisters; numbness then progressive loss of sensitivity.

HYPOTHERMIA
WHAT **TO DO**

1. Depending on the situation and severity of hypothermia, call for medical assistance.

2. Limit the sources of cold:

   • Protect the victim from the ground and the wind with a cover or clothing. Cover exposed body parts and keep the head, neck, and trunk warm. If you can, slowly move them inside a heated room.

   • Replace wet clothing with dry clothing, or dry wet clothing before putting it back on.

3. **If the person is unconscious:**

   • Check their breathing *(page 543)*. If needed, perform CPR *(page 546)*.

   • If they are breathing and you do not suspect fracture, put the victim in the recovery position *(page 543)*.

FROSTBITE
WHAT **TO DO**

1. Delicately remove clothing covering the frostbitten area.

2. Heat the frostbitten area with body heat (placing under the arm, against the abdomen, etc.) or by submerging it in room temperature water.

3. Once the normal temperature of the frostbitten area is restored, apply a dry dressing.

4. Cover the victim and, if they are conscious, make them drink a warm beverage.

5. Obtain medical treatment.

CAUTION

• Do not make a victim of hypothermia drink alcohol or caffeinated beverages.

• Do not let a hypothermia victim smoke.

• Do not rub or massage frostbite.

• Do not directly apply a source of heat on frostbite.

• Do not rub a frostbitten area with snow.

• Do not walk with frostbite of lower limbs.

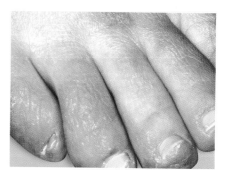

Frostbite

INSECT BITES, BITE WOUNDS, AND STINGING PLANTS

Outdoor activities can lead to insect bites and animal bites as well as contact with stinging or venomous plants. While the majority of these incidents are not severe, some complications (poisoning, **infection**, allergic reaction) can occur.

SIGNS OF A BITE, INSECT BITE, OR CONTACT WITH A STINGING PLANT

Bite: Wound, wound infection. Venomous serpent: localized burn, swelling, skin discoloration, intense pain, weakness, perspiration, vomiting, shivers, possibility of respiratory problems.

Insect bite: Intense itching or pain, swelling, reddening of skin. Possibility of serious allergic reaction *(page 548)*.

Stinging (or venomous) plant: Itching, pain, reddening, swelling, presence of small oozing vesicles on the skin, poisoning *(page 549)*.

WHAT **TO DO**

1. Regardless of whether the injury is caused by an animal or a plant, clean the wound with antiseptic soap. Then dress the wound and check for signs of infection. Seek medical assistance when a bite leads to a wound. Some animals can transmit rabies *(page 160)*.

2. **In the event of a venomous snake bite**, place the victim in a semireclined position and ask them not to move. Clean and dress the wound, and immobilize the affected limb. Seek medical assistance.

3. **In the case of an insect bite**, apply ice or an ointment specifically formulated to ease the itching and slow the reaction.

   - **Bee or wasp:** Remove the stinger by scratching the skin with a flat and blunt object or with the fingernails. Do not grab it with tweezers, as this may increase the quantity of venom injected. If the person suffers from allergies, ask them if they have adrenaline in their possession so that they can inject it in the event of respiratory difficulties *(page 548)*.

   - **Tick:** Remove the tick by grabbing it by the head with tweezers and pulling, without crushing it. Save it for analysis, because ticks are carriers of various diseases, particularly Lyme disease *(page 303)*.

4. **In the event of contact with a stinging plant**, the victim must not touch the affected area even if it is itchy. Clean it with soap and water. Remove and wash clothing that has been in contact with the plant.

CAUTION

- Do not apply ice on a bite wound.

- Do not allow a person to walk if they have been bitten by a venomous snake, as this can accelerate diffusion of the venom.

- Do not try to remove the venom by sucking on the wound (risk of poisoning).

- Do not apply dirt or mud on an insect bite.

EXTRACTING A **SPLINTER**

To remove a splinter, cleanse the skin with soapy water or antiseptic. With fine tweezers, remove the splinter in the direction of penetration, without splitting it. Clean the wound and protect it, if needed, with sterile dressing. For deep splinters or those with a curved point, obtain medical assistance.

Tick

563

DIRECTORY OF SYMPTOMS

The Directory of Symptoms assembles the main symptoms associated with the pathologies presented in this medical encyclopedia. It is a navigational tool for quick identification of the pages where the different pathologies are described. **In no instance should this directory be used for diagnosis. It cannot replace a doctor's opinion.**

The Directory of Symptoms is divided into nine sections. Eight of them list the symptoms associated with a group of organs. The "General Symptoms" section presents signs that cannot be associated with a specific part of the body. Each section includes several subsections, corresponding to a symptom or group of symptoms. Here, the diseases cited in the book are associated with the different symptoms that may characterize them.

References ("See also...") are provided to guide the reader towards other sections in the Directory of Symptoms or in the encyclopedia itself. In addition, pictograms are used to relate a pathology to a specific group of people or to signal an emergency situation.

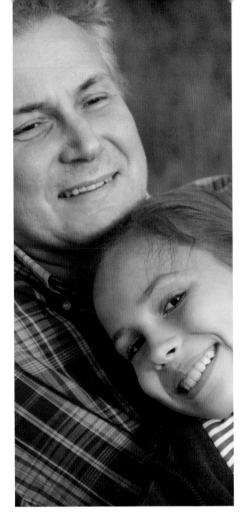

Pictogram key

Ailments that only or mainly affect:

Women ....

Men ....

Children ....

Pregnant women ....

Ailments associated with aging ....

Ailments requiring a call or visit to the emergency room, as quickly as possible .... *Emergency*

GENERAL SYMPTOMS

FEVER, FATIGUE, WEAKNESS AND WEIGHT LOSS

Fatigue and weakness

- Thirst, dry mouth, dark urine, muscle cramps, fatigue, pallor, rapid and weak pulse, rapid and shallow breathing, nausea and vomiting, confusion and dizziness.
  Dehydration... page 561

- Pain in the lower abdomen, mood swings, headache, fatigue and insomnia, vertigo, acne, digestive disturbances (bloating, abdominal pain), weight gain, swollen limbs and breasts, tender breasts.
  Premenstrual syndrome... page 424

- Absence of menstruation, nausea and vomiting, swollen breasts, mood swings, intense fatigue, etc.
  Pregnancy... page 462

- Snoring, disturbed sleep, fatigue, drowsiness, decreased alertness, irritability and depression.
  Sleep apnea... page 316

- Constant fatigue, insomnia, negative feelings about oneself and others, discouragement, cognitive impairment and physical ailments associated with stress (pains, skin problems, high blood pressure), etc.
  Burnout... page 182

- Weakness (pallor, fatigue, dizziness, shortness of breath), palpitations, cold sensation and headache.
  Anemia... page 242

- Pressure pain (neck, chest, shoulders, buttocks, elbows, knees), headache, fatigue and sleep disturbances.
  Fibromyalgia... page 122

- Digestive disturbances (diarrhea, abdominal pain, bloating, etc.) and weakness (weight loss and fatigue).
  Dietary intolerances... page 362
  Intestinal parasites... page 380
  Colitis... page 382

- Yellow coloring of the skin, whites of the eyes and mucus; spider-shaped red patches (arterial spiders) and reddening of the palms of the hands; significant weakness; weight loss; swollen legs and stomach; etc.
  Cirrhosis of the liver... page 392
  Hepatic failure... page 393 ....Emergency

- Nausea and vomiting, major fatigue, back pain, rare or frequent urination, shortness of breath and swollen legs.
  Kidney failure... page 412

- Goiter (swollen neck), significant weakness, weight fluctuations, cold or hot sensation, disruption of the heart rhythm, intestinal disturbances, shaking, change in the appearance of the skin or hair, etc.
  Diseases of the thyroid gland... page 225

- Sudden pain, generalized faintness (weakness, pallor, sweating) and, in some cases, a lump in a superficial artery.
  Aneurysm rupture... page 270 ....Emergency

- Fatigue, difficulty breathing (at night, feeling of a lack of air), disruption of the heart rhythm, etc.
  Cardiac arrhythmia... page 264
  Cardiac insufficiency... page 262

Fever, fatigue and weakness

- Fever, fatigue, headache, congestion and runny nose, dry cough, etc.
  Infectious diseases... page 284
  Respiratory infections... page 318
  Flu... page 320
  Bronchitis... page 322
  Sinusitis... page 318

- Moderate fever, headache and painful swelling of the neck.
  Infectious diseases... page 284
  Infectious diseases in children... page 519 ....

- Fever over 102°F (39°C), stiffness, loss of consciousness and convulsive movements of the whole body.
  Febrile seizures... page 524 ....Emergency

- Moderate fever, runny nose, dry cough and violent coughing fits.
  Whooping cough... page 522 ....Emergency

- Sudden high fever, sore throat, inability to swallow, and difficult, noisy breathing.
  Epiglottitis... page 523 ....Emergency

- High fever and change in overall condition (significant weakness, pallor).
  Septicemia... page 285 ....Emergency

- Fever, pelvic pain and purulent, foul-smelling vaginal discharge.
  Puerperal fever... page 475 ....Emergency

- Back and abdominal pain, high fever with shivering and urinary disturbances (burning, frequent urge, abnormal urine, etc.).
  Pyelonephritis... page 407

- Fever, fatigue, muscle and joint pain, cough, runny nose, headache, memory impairment, behavioral disturbances, drowsiness, etc.
  Encephalitis... page 159

Fever, fatigue and weakness (cont'd)

- High fever and headache, sensitivity to light, vomiting, stiff neck and convulsions.
  Meningitis... page 161 ....*Emergency*

- Fever, swollen lymph nodes, significant weakness, etc.
  Infectious diseases... page 284
  Infectious mononucleosis... page 295
  Toxoplasmosis... page 478
  Adenitis... page 305
  Lymphoma... page 307
  Leukemia... page 245
  Primary HIV infection... page 292

- Fever, respiratory discomfort, disruption of the heart rhythm or chest pains.
  Pneumonia... page 323
  Myocarditis... page 269 ....*Emergency*
  Pericarditis... page 269 ....*Emergency*

Fever, fatigue, weakness and weight loss

- Fever and intense fatigue, perspiration, red patches, pallor, and joint and muscle pain.
  Infectious endocarditis... page 269

- Rapid weight loss, swollen lymph nodes, fever, persistent diarrhea, and skin and respiratory infections.
  AIDS... page 292

Weight loss

- Very limited food intake and major weight loss, absence of menstruation, and numerous other ailments (dehydration, heart problems, etc.).
  Anorexia nervosa... page 527

- Digestive disturbances (diarrhea, abdominal pain, bloating, etc.) and weakness (weight loss and fatigue).
  Dietary intolerances... page 362
  Intestinal parasites... page 380
  Colitis... page 382

- Weight loss, abdominal and back pain, and soft, foul-smelling, oily stool.
  Chronic pancreatitis... page 396

- Digestive disturbances after meals, vomiting, abdominal pain and weight loss.
  Hypertrophic pyloric stenosis... page 516 ....*Emergency*

- Intense thirst, heavy urination and loss of consciousness or weight loss.
  Diabetes... page 228

- Difficulty swallowing, weight loss, chest pain and, in some cases, bloody vomit.
  Esophagitis... page 373
  Esophageal cancer... page 375 ....

See also:

First aid: Convulsions and fever... page 558
Red patches, rash, and fever... page 569
Muscular weakness... page 572

BALANCE DISTURBANCES

Balance disturbances or vertigo

- Transitory dizzy spells caused by changes in position.
  Benign paroxysmal positional vertigo... page 216

- Vertigo, loss of hearing, tinnitus.
  Labyrinthitis... page 217
  Cholesteatoma... page 215
  Ménière's disease ... page 216

- Very high blood pressure, headache, loss of balance, memory loss and vision problems.
  High blood pressure - stage 2... page 254

- Loss of consciousness or bleeding from the nose or ears; head pain or head wound; impaired balance, speech and vision; sensory impairment (paralysis); nausea and vomiting; abnormal behavior or convulsions.
  Severe cranial trauma... page 150 ....*Emergency*

- Sudden paralysis, sensory impairment, impaired vision, speech or coordination, vertigo, loss of consciousness, headache or convulsions, etc.
  Cerebrovascular accidents... page 156 ....*Emergency*

- Motor impairment (muscular weakness, balance disturbances, paralysis, etc.), visual, sensory, sexual and psychological problems (depression, difficulty concentrating, etc.), acute, chronic pain and major fatigue; recurring symptoms.
  Multiple sclerosis... page 164

- Headache, nausea and vomiting, vertigo, and visual, behavioral, cognitive, motor and sensory impairment.
  Tumors of the nervous system... page 158

Dizziness

- Thirst, dry mouth, dark urine, muscle cramps, fatigue, pallor, rapid and weak pulse, rapid and shallow breathing, nausea and vomiting, confusion and dizziness.
  Dehydration... page 561

- Weakness (pallor, fatigue, dizziness, shortness of breath), palpitations, cold sensation and headache.
  Anemia... page 242

- Cough, chest pain, difficulty breathing, headache, dizziness or respiratory or cardiac arrest.
  Inhalation poisoning... page 549 ....*Emergency*

- Substantial loss of blood (external hemorrhaging), cold, pale extremities, dizziness, vomiting, rapid, weak pulse, rapid breathing and intense thirst.
  Shock... page 239 ....*Emergency*

See also:
Sensory and motor impairment... page 576
Impaired consciousness (drowsiness, loss of consciousness and sleep disturbances)... page 577
Psychological and behavioral disorders... page 579

SWELLING

Swelling

- Extensive or localized swelling.
  Edema... page 53

- Swelling or redness of the skin localized around a wound, sharp pain, weakness, perspiration, shivering, etc.
  Infected wound... pages 70 and 541

- Red patches, blisters, swelling, hives, burning, etc.
  Allergies... page 288
  Contact poisoning... page 549 ....*Emergency*

Swollen face or mouth

- Red eye, swollen eyelids, stinging and watery eyes.
  Conjunctivitis ... page 204

- Red, swollen gums, painful or shifting teeth, etc.
  Gingivitis ... page 364
  Periodontitis... page 364
  Dental abscess... page 367

Swollen face or mouth and neck

- Swollen lips, tongue, larynx, pharynx and eyelids.
  Infectious diseases... page 284
  Allergies (Quincke's edema)... page 290 .....*Emergency*

Swollen neck or goiter

- Fever, swollen neck, headache, sore throat, rash, etc.
  Infectious diseases... page 284
  Infectious diseases in children... page 519 ....

- Moderate fever, headache and painful swelling of the neck.
  Infectious diseases... page 284
  Infectious diseases in children... page 519 ....

- Goiter (swollen neck), significant weakness, weight fluctuations, cold or hot sensation, disruption of the heart rhythm, intestinal disturbances, shaking, change in the appearance of the skin or hair, etc.
  Diseases of the thyroid gland... page 225

Swollen lymph nodes (neck, groin, armpits, etc.)

- Fever, swollen lymph nodes, significant weakness, etc.
  Infectious diseases... page 284
  Infectious mononucleosis... page 295
  Toxoplasmosis... page 478
  Adenitis... page 305
  Lymphoma... page 307
  Leukemia... page 245
  Primary HIV infection... page 292

- Rapid weight loss, swollen lymph nodes, fever, persistent diarrhea and skin and respiratory infections.
  AIDS... page 292

Swollen abdomen

- Intense abdominal pain, vomiting, swollen abdomen, and absence of emissions of gas and stool.
  Intestinal obstruction... page 385 ....*Emergency*

- Painless swelling of the abdomen (navel, groin or scrotum) that can be reduced by pressure from the fingers.
  Hernia... page 386

Swollen abdomen and limbs

- Yellow coloring of the skin, whites of the eyes and mucus; spider-shaped red patches (arterial spiders) and reddening of the palms of the hands; significant weakness; weight loss; swollen legs and stomach; etc.
  Cirrhosis of the liver... page 392
  Hepatic failure... page 393 ....*Emergency*

Swollen limbs

- Swelling of one or more limbs, sensation of pressure, heaviness, tingling, stretched skin and pain.
  Edema... page 53
  Lymphedema... page 306

- Pain in the lower abdomen, mood swings, headache, fatigue and insomnia, vertigo, acne, digestive disturbances (bloating, abdominal pain), weight gain, swollen limbs and breasts, tender breasts.
  Premenstrual syndrome... page 424 ....

- Sensation of heavy legs, swelling and dilation of the veins (blue cords).
  Venous insufficiency... page 272
  Varicose veins... page 272

Swollen limbs (cont'd)

- Intense muscle pain, infirmity, swelling and bruising after exercise or movement.
  Torn or pulled muscle... pages 125 and 552

- Very high blood pressure, swollen limbs and substantial weight gain, headache and stomachache, spotty vision, buzzing in the ears, nausea and vomiting, convulsions, loss of consciousness.
  Preeclampsia... page 484 ....*Emergency*
  Eclampsia... page 485 ....*Emergency*

- Fatigue, major respiratory discomfort at night, disruption of the heart rhythm, and swelling (veins of the neck, legs, liver, etc.).
  Cardiac insufficiency... page 262

- Swelling of a vein and the tissues around it, fever and sharp pain (calf, ankle).
  Venous thrombosis... page 274 ....*Emergency*

Swollen joints

- Pain and swelling in the joints.
  Sprain... pages 110 and 552
  Rheumatoid arthritis... page 119
  Gout... page 121
  Bursitis... page 121
  Tenosynovitis... page 126

Swollen genital organs

- Fever, pain, swelling, red patches or itching at the genital organs, disturbances when urinating or during sexual relations, and bloody, purulent or foul-smelling discharge.
  Genital infections... page 441

- Sudden pain in the testicle, spreading to the groin, and swelling of the testicle.
  Testicular torsion... page 429 ....

- Hard mass on one testicle and swelling of the testicle or sterility. No pain.
  Testicular cancer... page 428 ....

Swollen breasts

- Pain in the lower abdomen, mood swings, headache, fatigue and insomnia, vertigo, acne, digestive disturbances (bloating, abdominal pain), weight gain, swollen limbs and breasts, tender breasts.
  Premenstrual syndrome... page 424 ....

- Absence of menstruation, nausea and vomiting, swollen breasts, mood swings, major fatigue, etc.
  Pregnancy... page 462 ....

- Swelling, thickening of the skin, orange-peel skin on one breast.
  Benign breast tumors... page 437 ....
  Breast cancer... page 438 ....

See also:

First aid: Hemorrhage... page 550
First aid: Insect bites, bite wounds, and stinging plants... page 563
Red patches and rash with itching... page 569

SKIN PROBLEMS (SKIN, NAILS, BODY HAIR, HAIR)

SKIN PROBLEMS

Wounds

- Swelling or redness of the skin localized around a wound, sharp pain, weakness, perspiration, shivering, etc.
  Infected wound... pages 70 and 541

- Chronic wound.
  Skin ulcers... page 76
  Skin cancer... page 88

- Pain at the site of a bite, fever followed by difficulty swallowing, mood disturbances (despondency, excitation, etc.), pathological fear of water, hallucinations, contractures and paralysis.
  Rabies... page 160 ....*Emergency*

Head wounds

- Brief loss of consciousness or bleeding from the nose or ears; head pain or head wound; impaired balance, speech and vision; sensory impairment (paralysis); nausea and vomiting; abnormal behavior or convulsions.
  Severe cranial trauma... page 150 ....*Emergency*

Red patches

- Swelling or redness of the skin localized around a wound, sharp pain, weakness, perspiration, shivering, etc.
  Infected wound... pages 70 and 541

- Red skin, flaking, in some cases blisters.
  Burns... page 72
  Discoid lupus... page 304

- Red, hot, dry or moist skin, rapid pulse, loud breathing, headache, confusion, agitation, dizziness, convulsions and gradual loss of consciousness.
  Heatstroke... page 561

- Hot, painful redness in irregular streaks on the skin.
  Lymphangitis... page 305

Red patches under the breast

- Constant redness under a breast.
  Benign breast tumors... page 437 ....
  Breast cancer... page 438 ....

Red patches on the buttocks

- Red patches on the buttocks, upper thighs and genital organs.
  Diaper rash... page 517 ....

Red patches and rash

- Red patches, blisters, swelling, hives, burning, etc.
  Allergies... page 288
  Dermatitis... page 78
  Herpes zoster... page 162
  Contact poisoning... page 549 ....Emergency

- Oily skin and various lesions (blackheads, papules, pustules, nodules, cysts) on the skin of the face, back, shoulders and torso.
  Acne... page 518
  Premenstrual syndrome... page 424........................

- Pustules or swelling around hairs, especially on the face, the arms and the legs.
  Folliculitis... page 82
  Styes... page 204

- Circular red patch in the shape of a ring (tick bite), followed several weeks later by neurological, inflammatory or cardiac disturbances.
  Lyme disease... page 303

- Red patches and small blisters that form scabs when they burst.
  Ringworm... page 84
  Impetigo... page 83

- Yellow coloring of the skin, whites of the eyes and mucus, spider-shaped red patches (arterial spiders) and reddening of the palms of the hands, significant weakness, etc.
  Hepatic failure... page 393 ....Emergency

Red patches, rash, and fever

- Fever, outbreak of red spots and conjunctivitis (red, watery eyes), headache, sore throat or runny nose, etc.
  Infectious diseases in children... page 519..................

- Very swollen, very painful red patches covered with scabs, often on the face or legs, and high fever.
  Erysipelas... page 83 ....Emergency

Red patches and rash with itching

- Red patches and itching.
  Hives... page 79
  Psoriasis... page 80
  Intertrigo... page 85

- Red patches, small blisters, stinging, itching, burning sensation, etc.
  Infectious diseases in children... page 519 ....
  Cold sores... page 86
  Genital herpes... page 447
  Eczema... page 78

- Itching and typically painful lesions (redness, scabs, scales, cracking) between the toes.
  Athlete's foot... page 84

- Intense itching and dark lines on the skin, especially on the hands and forearms.
  Scabies... page 87

See also:
First aid: Head and spinal injuries... page 554
First aid: Insect bites, bite wounds, and stinging plants... page 563
Rash on the genital organs... page 588

Tumefaction (small lump)

- Small, usually painless, smooth or rough lump that is more or less prominent and pigmented, appearing especially on the feet and hands.
  Warts... page 75

- Rounded lump.
  Mole... page 89
  Cysts... page 52
  Benign tumors... page 54
  Skin cancer... page 88

Spots

- Brown, more or less prominent spot, with an even coloring and well-defined contours.
  Mole... page 89

- Smooth, white, clearly-defined spots.
  Vitiligo... page 91

- More or less prominent spot with blurred contours and uneven coloring, or beauty mark that changes in appearance, itches or bleeds.
  Skin cancer... page 88

Bluish skin, bruising

- Intense muscle pain, infirmity, swelling and bruising after exercise or movement.
  Torn or pulled muscle... page 125

- White or blue fingers and toes and loss of sensitivity.
  Raynaud's disease... page 67 ....

- Sensation of heavy legs, swelling and dilation of the veins (blue cords).
  Varicose veins... page 272

569

Directory of Symptoms | Skin Problems

Bluish skin, bruising (cont'd)

- Chest pain (at the base of a lung), feeling of suffocation, rapid breathing and bluish skin.
Pulmonary embolism... page 275 ....*Emergency*

- Prolonged bleeding that may begin with no apparent cause.
Hemophilia... page 244
Side effects of anticoagulant and antiplatelet medications... pages 261 and 274

Blue or pale lips

- Dry cough, difficulty breathing (shortness of breath, wheezing, rapid, shallow breathing), feeling of oppression in the chest, rapid, irregular pulse, pale face, bluish lips and nails, and clear sputum.
Asthma... page 326
Allergies... page 288

Yellowish skin (icterus)

- Yellow coloring of the skin, whites of the eyes and mucus; spider-shaped red patches (arterial spiders) and reddening of the palms of the hands; significant weakness; etc.
Cirrhosis of the liver... page 392
Hepatic failure... page 393 ....*Emergency*

- Yellow coloring of the skin, whites of the eyes and mucus, pain in the upper abdomen and deterioration of general state of health (loss of appetite, weight loss and significant weakness).
Hepatitis... page 390
Pancreatic cancer... page 397 ....

See also:

First aid: Obstruction of the respiratory tract... page 547
First aid: Hemorrhage... page 550
First aid: Falls and trauma... page 552
First aid: Burns and electrocution... page 557
First aid: Hypothermia and frostbite... page 562
First aid: Insect bites, bite wounds, and stinging plants... page 563
Fatigue and weakness... page 565
Swelling... page 567
Mouth and tongue lesions... page 574

NAIL DISEASES

Yellowish or whitish nails

- Deformation, thickening and yellowish coloring of the nail, superficial white spots, detachment of the nail, pressure pain and inflammation around the nail.
Onychomycosis... page 85

Bluish nails

- White or blue fingers and toes and loss of sensitivity.
Raynaud's disease... page 67 ....

- Dry cough, difficulty breathing (shortness of breath, wheezing, rapid, shallow breathing), feeling of oppression in the chest, rapid, irregular pulse, pale face, bluish lips and nails, and clear sputum.
Asthma... page 326
Pulmonary embolism... page 275 ....*Emergency*
Emphysema... page 329

Redness next to a nail

- Redness and painful swelling, often at the edge of a nail, potentially with the appearance of pus.
Whitlow... page 82
Ingrown nails... page 71

SCALP DISORDERS AND PILOSITY

Scales

- Fine, dry or oily scales, sometimes with itching.
Dandruff... page 85

- Yellowish, dry or oozing scales on the scalp.
Cradle cap... page 517 ....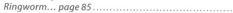

Itching on the head

- Intense itching and red dots on the skin.
Lice... page 87

Hair loss

- Gradual, permanent hair loss.
Baldness... page 66

- Plaques on the scalp covered with pus or scales, and hair breakage.
Ringworm... page 85 ....

Abnormal pilosity (hairiness)

- Change in physical appearance (skin, pilosity, goiter, etc.), impaired growth and lactation, sexual impairment, diabetes, headache, impaired vision, etc.
Diseases of the pituitary gland... page 226

BONE, JOINT, AND MUSCULAR DISORDERS (LIMBS, BACK, JOINTS, ETC.)

BONE AND JOINT DISORDERS

Upper and lower back pain

- Back pain.
  Backache... page 114

- Intense pain in the back, possibly extending along the nerves, pins and needles, and stiffness.
  Herniated disk... page 112

- Presence of blood in urine, painful urination, nausea, vomiting and intense lower back pain.
  Urolithiasis... page 408

- Swelling, especially of the face, dark, foamy urine in small quantities, lower back pain, headache and vomiting.
  Glomerulonephritis... page 410 ....

- Back and abdominal pain, high fever with shivering and urinary disturbances (burning, frequent urge, abnormal urine, etc.).
  Pyelonephritis... page 407

Upper back pain and deformation of the spinal column

- Upper and lower back pain, decreased height and fractures caused by mild trauma.
  Osteoporosis... page 106 ....
  Lumbar arthrosis... page 117 ....

- Deformation of the spinal column and back pain.
  Scoliosis... page 525 ....

- Pelvic and back pain, gradual ankylosis followed by deformation of the spinal column.
  Ankylosing spondylitis... page 120 ....

Painful and deformed limbs

- Painful, deformed or crippled limb, sometimes with a protruding bone and external hemorrhaging.
  Bone fracture... pages 102 and 552

Painful and swollen limbs

- Intense pain and inflammation of the affected bone, crippled limb, fever, shivering, fatigue, nausea, faintness, and refusal to walk or limping in young children.
  Osteitis... page 108

Joint and muscle pain

- Fever, muscle and joint pain, fatigue, headache, runny nose and dry cough.
  Flu... page 320

- Fever and muscle and joint pain or diarrhea.
  Listeriosis... page 302

- Fever and intense fatigue, perspiration, red patches, pallor, and joint and muscle pain.
  Infectious endocarditis... page 269

Joint pain

- Joint pain related to effort, morning stiffness developing in bursts and deformation of certain joints (fingers).
  Arthrosis... page 117
  Rheumatoid arthritis... page 119

- Low fever, runny nose, headache, sore throat, joint pain followed by red patches on the cheeks, limbs, torso and buttocks.
  Fifth disease... page 523 ....

Painful, deformed joints

- Intense pain and deformed, crippled joint after a trauma.
  Dislocation... page 111

- Joint pain related to effort, morning stiffness developing in bursts and deformation of certain joints (fingers).
  Arthrosis... page 117
  Rheumatoid arthritis... page 119

Painful, swollen joints

- Pain and swelling in the joints.
  Sprain... pages 110 and 552
  Rheumatoid arthritis... page 119
  Gout... page 121
  Bursitis... page 121
  Tenosynovitis... page 126

Back, limb, joint pain, etc. and limb deformation

- Bone pain, swelling, sometimes with fever, fractures.
  Bone cancer... page 109

- Bone, joint and nerve pain, stiffness, headache, bone deformations (arched legs and arms, enlarged skull), spontaneous fractures and increased skin temperature around lesions.
  Paget's disease... page 108 ....

See also:

First aid: Falls and trauma... page 552
Swollen limbs... page 567
Swollen joints... page 568

MUSCULAR DISORDERS

Muscle contractions

- Muscle stiffness, pain, and limited movement or inability to move.
  Contracture... page 123

- Contracture of certain muscles in the neck, leading to abnormal positioning of the head.
  Torticollis... page 123
  Spasmodic torticollis ... page 128

- Thirst, dry mouth, dark urine, muscle cramps, fatigue, pallor, rapid and weak pulse, rapid and shallow breathing, nausea and vomiting, confusion and dizziness.
  Dehydration... page 561

- Pain at the site of a bite, fever followed by difficulty swallowing, mood disturbances (despondency, excitation, etc.), pathological fear of water, hallucinations, contractures and paralysis.
  Rabies... page 160 ....Emergency

Finger spasms

- Spasms and locking of the fingers when flexed or extended, during certain precise, repetitive movements.
  Writer's cramp... page 128

Anal spasms

- Bright red bleeding from the anus in small quantities during or shortly after defecation, sometimes with itching, sharp pain and spasms around the anus.
  Hemorrhoids... page 388
  Anal fissures... page 389

Muscle pain

- Temporary muscle pain related to effort.
  Temporary muscle pains and aches... page 122

- Intense muscle pain, infirmity, swelling and bruising after exercise or movement.
  Torn or pulled muscle... page 125

- Tendon pain.
  Tendinitis... page 126
  Tenosynovitis... page 126

- Pain in the heel.
  Plantar fasciitis... page 127

- Sudden cracking, intense pain and infirmity after an effort or a trauma.
  Ruptured tendon... page 127

- Pressure pain (neck, chest, shoulders, buttocks, elbows, knees), headache, fatigue and sleep disturbances.
  Fibromyalgia... page 122

- Fever, headache, muscle pain and general weakness, sore throat, and swollen ganglions in the neck, armpits and groin, etc.
  Infectious diseases... page 284
  Infectious mononucleosis... page 295

See also:
Convulsions... page 577

Muscular weakness or lack of muscle tone

- Motor impairments (muscular weakness, balance disturbances, paralysis, etc.), visual or sensory impairment, etc.
  Cerebrovascular accidents... page 156
  Lou Gehrig's disease... page 163
  Multiple sclerosis... page 164

- Abrupt sleeping fits and drop in muscle tone over the course of the day.
  Narcolepsy... page 178

- Gradual weakening of the muscles, posture anomalies, inexpressive face and functional disabilities.
  Muscular dystrophy... page 130

- Vision problems, joint impairment, difficulty chewing and swallowing, inexpressive face, weak limbs and general fatigue.
  Myasthenia... page 129

See also:
First aid: Falls and trauma... page 552
Pain along the nerves... page 574
Difficulty moving or inability to move... page 576

EYE, EAR, AND MOUTH PROBLEMS

EYE DISORDERS

Poor visual acuity

- Imperfect vision at a distance.
  Myopia... page 202

- Imperfect vision close up, causing headache.
  Hyperopia... page 202

- Imperfect vision at all distances.
  Astigmatism... page 202

- Imperfect vision at short distances, headache and visual fatigue.
  Presbyopia... page 202 ....

- Decreased visual acuity.
  Cataracts... page 206
  Chronic glaucoma... page 207 ....

- Decreased visual acuity, red eye and pain.
  Acute glaucoma... page 207 ....*Emergency*
  Keratitis... page 204

Various visual impairments (decreased acuity, deformed vision, floating spots, etc.)

- Impaired central vision and deformed vision.
  Macular degeneration... page 210 ....

- Deviation of one eye from the other, poor visual acuity and two-dimensional vision.
  Strabismus... page 211 ....

- Difficulty adapting to darkness, appearance of floating spots, shrinking of the visual field followed by a decline in visual acuity.
  Retinopathy... page 208

- Sudden appearance of floating spots and flashes, followed by a dark veil over the visual field.
  Retinal detachment... page 208 ....*Emergency*

- Redness around the cornea, deformed pupil, decreased visual acuity, sensitivity to light or impaired vision.
  Uveitis... page 204

- Vision problems, joint impairment, difficulty chewing and swallowing, inexpressive face, weak limbs and general fatigue.
  Myasthenia... page 129

- Brief loss of consciousness or bleeding from the nose or ears; head pain or head wound; impaired balance, speech and vision; sensory impairment (paralysis); nausea and vomiting; abnormal behavior or convulsions.
  Severe cranial trauma... page 150 ....*Emergency*

- Sudden paralysis, sensory impairment, impaired vision, speech or coordination, vertigo, loss of consciousness, headache or convulsions, etc.
  Cerebrovascular accidents... page 156 ....*Emergency*

- Motor impairment (muscular weakness, balance disturbances, paralysis, etc.), visual, sensory, sexual and psychological problems (depression, difficulty concentrating, etc.), acute, chronic pain and major fatigue, recurring symptoms.
  Multiple sclerosis... page 164

- Very high blood pressure, headache, loss of balance, memory loss and vision problems.
  High blood pressure - stage 2... page 253

- Headache, nausea and vomiting, vertigo, visual impairment (double vision), and behavioral, cognitive, motor and sensory impairment.
  Tumors of the nervous system... page 158

Light sensitivity

- Headache, nausea, vomiting, and sensitivity to light and noise.
  Migraines... page 148
  Glaucoma... page 207 ....

- High fever and headache, sensitivity to light, vomiting, stiff neck and convulsions.
  Meningitis... page 161 ....*Emergency*

- Convulsions, fever, confusion, memory impairment, sensory impairment (photophobia) and motor impairment (impaired coordination, paralysis).
  Severe encephalitis... page 159 ....*Emergency*

- Decreased visual acuity, red, watery eye, pain and increased sensitivity to light.
  Keratitis... page 204

- Redness around the cornea, deformed pupil, decreased visual acuity, sensitivity to light or impaired vision.
  Uveitis... page 204

Pain or inflammation of the eye

- Painful boil on the eyelid.
  Styes... page 204

- Redness along the edge of the eyelid, watering of the eye and discomfort.
  Blepharitis... page 204

- Small lump under the skin of the eyelid.
  Chalazion... page 204

- Discomfort, burning or stinging in the eye, and sometimes red eye.
  Dry eye... page 205
  Allergies... page 288

- Red eye, swollen eyelids, stinging and watery eyes.
  Conjunctivitis... page 204
  Infectious diseases in children... page 519 ....

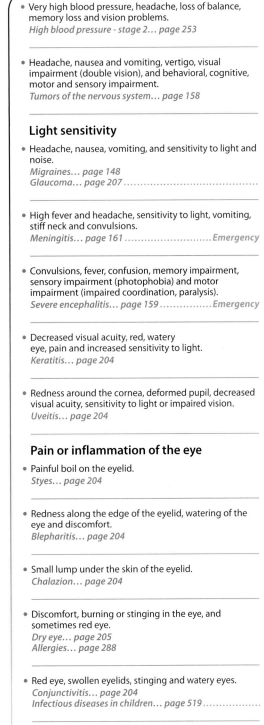

Eye pain or inflammation and impaired vision

- Decreased visual acuity, red eye and pain.
  Acute glaucoma... page 207 ....*Emergency*
  Keratitis... page 204

- Redness around the cornea, deformed pupil, decreased visual acuity, sensitivity to light or impaired vision.
  Uveitis... page 204

EAR DISORDERS

Hearing loss and tinnitus

- Hearing loss and, in some cases, tinnitus.
  Deafness... page 212

- Dizzy spells, hearing loss and tinnitus.
  Labyrinthitis... page 217
  Ménière's disease ... page 216

Hearing loss, tinnitus and ear pain

- Ear pain, itching, hearing loss, tinnitus, sometimes fever and discharge from the ear, etc.
  Otitis... page 214

- Ear pain, tinnitus, vertigo and irreversible hearing loss.
  Cholesteatoma... page 215

MOUTH DISORDERS

Gum and tooth disease

- Red, swollen gums with frequent bleeding.
  Gingivitis... page 364

- Red, swollen gums, loosening and shifting of the teeth.
  Periodontitis... page 364

- Tooth pain, sometimes sharp, triggered by cold, heat or pressure on the tooth, or by certain foods.
  Cavities... page 367

- Constant pain in one tooth, swelling and redness in the gums, possibly extending to the cheek.
  Dental abscess... page 367

Mouth and tongue lesions

- Small, round or oval yellowish spot, surrounded by a red, painful halo, on the mucous membrane of the mouth.
  Aphta... page 366

- Outbreak of blisters.
  Cold sores... page 86

- Change in the appearance of the tongue (swelling, smoothed surface, intense red color), pain and discomfort when chewing, swallowing or speaking.
  Glossitis... page 365

- Whitish coating over the mucous membrane in the mouth.
  Thrush... page 365
  Lichen planus... page 79
  Scarlet fever... page 522

- Worsening lesion (small cut, red patch, ulceration, nodule) on or around the mouth, bleeding, persistent pain and numbness in the mouth and throat, and difficulty chewing, swallowing or moving the tongue.
  Mouth cancer... page 366

See also:
Swollen face or mouth... 567

DISORDERS OF THE BRAIN AND NERVOUS SYSTEM (HEAD, NERVES, COGNITIVE, OR PSYCHOLOGICAL DISTURBANCES, ETC.)

PAIN ALONG THE NERVES

Pain in the limbs

- Pain on the back side of a lower limb, possibly extending from the buttocks to the foot, and intensified by a standing position.
  Sciatica... page 146

- Sensory and motor impairment, pins and needles, numbness and nerve pain in a limb.
  Canal syndrome... page 147
  Herniated disk... page 112

Facial pain

- Very short, violent fits of pain, comparable to electric shock.
  Migraines... page 148
  Facial neuralgia... page 146

Pain in the back, face or limbs

- Burning sensation, outbreak of red patches and blisters on the skin along a nerve path, and intense pain, especially in the back, face or limbs.
  Herpes zoster... page 162

See also:
Bone, joint, and muscular disorders... page 571

HEAD PAIN

Headache

- Cranial pain.
  Headache... page 148

- Headache, nausea, vomiting and sensitivity to light and noise.
  Migraines... page 148

- Imperfect vision at short distances, headache and visual fatigue.
  Presbyopia... page 202 ....

- Imperfect vision close up, causing headache.
  Hyperopia... page 202

- Pain in the lower abdomen, mood swings, headache, fatigue and insomnia, vertigo, acne, digestive disturbances (bloating, abdominal pain), weight gain, swollen limbs and breasts, tender breasts.
  Premenstrual syndrome... page 424 ....

- Brief loss of consciousness or bleeding from the nose or ears; head pain or head wound; impaired balance, speech and vision; sensory impairment (paralysis); nausea and vomiting; abnormal behavior or convulsions.
  Severe cranial trauma... page 150 ....Emergency

- Very high blood pressure, headache, loss of balance, memory loss and vision problems.
  High blood pressure - stage 2... page 253

- Very high blood pressure, swollen limbs and substantial weight gain, headache and stomachache, spotty vision, buzzing in the ears, nausea and vomiting.
  Preeclampsia... page 484 ....Emergency

- Snoring or wheezing, sleep apnea, headache, nasal congestion and nose bleeds.
  Lesions of the nasal septum... page 317

- Nausea accompanied by headache and sleep disturbances.
  Altitude sickness... page 335

- Cough, chest pain, difficulty breathing, headache, dizziness or respiratory or cardiac arrest.
  Inhalation poisoning... page 549 ....Emergency

- Pressure pain (neck, chest, shoulders, buttocks, elbows, knees), headache, fatigue and sleep disturbances.
  Fibromyalgia... page 122

- Sudden paralysis, sensory impairment, impaired vision, speech or coordination, vertigo, loss of consciousness, headache or convulsions, etc.
  Cerebrovascular accidents... page 156 ....Emergency

- Headache, nausea and vomiting, vertigo, visual, behavioral, cognitive, motor and sensory impairment.
  Tumors of the nervous system... page 158

Headache and fever

- Fever, fatigue, headache, congestion and runny nose, dry cough, etc.
  Infectious diseases... page 284
  Respiratory infections... page 318
  Flu... page 320
  Sinusitis... page 318

- Fever, headache, sore throat, outbreak of red spots, etc.
  Infectious diseases in children... page 519..................

- Moderate fever, headache and painful swelling of the neck.
  Infectious diseases... page 284
  Infectious diseases in children... page 519 ....

- High fever and headache, sensitivity to light, vomiting, stiff neck and convulsions.
  Meningitis... page 161 ....Emergency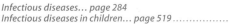

- Fever, headache, muscle pain and general weakness, sore throat and swollen ganglions in the neck, armpits and groin, etc.
  Infectious mononucleosis... page 295

- Fever, fatigue, muscle and joint pain, cough, runny nose, headache, memory impairment, behavioral disturbances, drowsiness, etc.
  Encephalitis... page 159

See also:
First aid: Head and spinal injuries... page 554
First aid: Convulsions and fever... page 558
Fever, fatigue and weakness... page 565

SENSORY AND MOTOR IMPAIRMENT (ABNORMAL MOVEMENTS, DIFFICULTY MOVING OR INABILITY TO MOVE, LOSS OF SENSITIVITY, ETC.)

Difficulty moving or inability to move

- Muscle stiffness, pain, and difficulty moving or inability to move.
Contractures... page 123

- Contracture of certain muscles in the neck, leading to abnormal positioning of the head.
Torticollis... page 123
Spasmodic torticollis ... page 128

- Spasms and locking of the fingers when flexed or extended, during certain precise, repetitive movements.
Writer's cramp... page 128

- Painful, deformed or crippled limb, sometimes with a protruding bone and external hemorrhaging after a trauma.
Bone fracture... pages 102 and 552

- Intense pain and deformed, crippled joint after a trauma.
Dislocation... page 111

- Pain and swelling in a joint.
Sprain... page 110

- Intense muscle pain, infirmity, swelling and bruising after exercise or movement.
Torn or pulled muscle... page 125

- Sudden cracking, intense pain and infirmity after an effort or a trauma.
Ruptured tendon... page 127

- Intense pain in the back, possibly extending along the nerves, pins and needles, and stiffness.
Herniated disk... page 112

- Joint pain related to effort, morning stiffness and deformation of certain joints (fingers).
Arthrosis... page 117

- Pain, hot sensation, swelling and morning stiffness in the joints, fatigue and weight loss.
Rheumatoid arthritis... page 119

- Convulsions, fever, confusion, memory impairment, sensory impairment (photophobia) and motor impairment (impaired coordination, paralysis).
Severe encephalitis... page 159 ....*Emergency*

- Muscular dysfunctions (paralysis, atrophy, excessive stiffness, cramps, spontaneous, irregular contractions) and impaired breathing, speech or swallowing. Slow evolution.
Amyotrophic lateral sclerosis... page 163

- Vision problems, joint impairment, difficulty chewing and swallowing, inexpressive face, weak limbs and general fatigue.
Myasthenia... page 129

- Bone, joint and nerve pain, stiffness, headache, bone deformations (arched legs and arms, enlarged skull), spontaneous fractures and increased skin temperature around lesions.
Paget's disease... page 108 ....

- Pelvic and back pain, gradual ankylosis followed by deformation of the spinal column.
Ankylosing spondylitis... page 120 ....

- Intense pain and inflammation of the affected bone, crippled limb, fever, shivering, fatigue, nausea, faintness, and refusal to walk or limping in young children.
Osteitis... page 108

- Appearance of hard, painless nodules under the skin of the palm of the hand and at the base of the fingers, and gradual, irreducible bending of the fingers.
Dupuytren's contracture... page 129 ....

- Pain at the site of a bite, fever followed by difficulty swallowing, mood disturbances (despondency, excitation, etc.), pathological fear of water, hallucinations, contractures and paralysis.
Rabies... page 160 ....*Emergency*

Abnormal movements (shaking, tics, etc.), difficulty moving or inability to move

- Motor impairment (epilepsy, shaking, paralysis) and mental impairment (confusion, hallucinations, delirium).
Chronic alcohol intoxication... page 358

- Shaking while at rest, slow movements or inability to move, change in posture, difficulty walking, impaired memory and concentration, fatigue, depression and an inexpressive face.
Parkinson's disease... page 167 ....

- Gradual weakening of the muscles, posture anomalies, inexpressive face and functional disabilities.
Muscular dystrophy... page 130

- Goiter (swollen neck), significant weakness, weight fluctuations, cold or hot sensation, disruption of the heart rhythm, intestinal disturbances, shaking, change in the appearance of the skin or hair, etc.
Diseases of the thyroid gland... page 225

- Twitching, use of obscene words, or repetition of words or phrases.
  Tourette's syndrome... page 168 ....

- Sudden, uncoordinated involuntary movements, impaired motor coordination, psychological disturbances (depression, psychosis) and cognitive disturbances (language, attention, memory).
  Huntington's disease... page 168

Difficulty moving or inability to move and sensory impairment

- White or blue fingers and toes and loss of sensitivity.
  Raynaud's disease... page 67 ....

- Sensory and motor impairment, pins and needles, numbness and nerve pain in a limb.
  Canal syndrome... page 147

- Intense pain in the back, possibly extending along the nerves, pins and needles, and stiffness.
  Herniated disk... page 112

- Brief loss of consciousness or bleeding from the nose or ears; head pain or head wound; impaired balance, speech and vision; sensory impairment (paralysis); nausea and vomiting; abnormal behavior or convulsions.
  Severe cranial trauma... page 150 ....*Emergency*

- Localized motor and sensory impairment, psychological disturbances (hallucinations, behavioral change); short in duration and recurring.
  Partial epilepsy... page 166

- Sudden paralysis, sensory impairment, impaired vision, speech or coordination, vertigo, loss of consciousness, headache or convulsions.
  Cerebrovascular accidents... page 156 ....*Emergency*

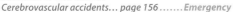

- Motor impairment (muscular weakness, balance disturbances, paralysis, etc.), visual, sensory, sexual and psychological problems (depression, difficulty concentrating, etc.), acute, chronic pain and major fatigue; recurring symptoms.
  Multiple sclerosis... page 164

- Inability to perform a voluntary movement and, in some cases, loss of sensitivity.
  Paralysis... page 151

- Headache, nausea and vomiting, vertigo, visual, behavioral, cognitive, motor and sensory impairment.
  Tumors of the nervous system... page 158

See also:
First aid: Falls and trauma... page 552
First aid: Head and spinal injuries... page 554
Balance disturbances... page 566

Convulsions

- Fever over 102°F (39°C), stiffness, loss of consciousness and convulsive movements of the whole body.
  Febrile seizures... page 524 ....*Emergency*

- Convulsive attacks and absence.
  Generalized epilepsy... page 166

- Convulsions, temporary loss of consciousness, significant swelling of the limbs, and sudden, sharp rise in blood pressure.
  Eclampsia... page 485 ....*Emergency*

- Brief loss of consciousness or bleeding from the nose or ears; head pain or head wound; impaired balance, speech and vision; sensory impairment (paralysis); nausea and vomiting; abnormal behavior or convulsions.
  Severe cranial trauma... page 150 ....*Emergency*

- Convulsions, fever, confusion, memory impairment, sensory impairment (photophobia) and motor impairment (impaired coordination, paralysis).
  Severe encephalitis... page 159 ....*Emergency*

- Sudden paralysis, sensory impairment, impaired vision, speech or coordination, vertigo, loss of consciousness, headache or convulsions.
  Cerebrovascular accidents... page 156 ....*Emergency*

- Major deterioration of the overall condition (stopping eating, crying, grayish tint, lack of muscle tone, drowsiness, bulging fontanelle, convulsions, appearance of red spots on the skin, etc.).
  Meningitis (in infants)... page 161 ....*Emergency*

- High fever and headache, sensitivity to light, vomiting, stiff neck and convulsions.
  Meningitis... page 161 ....*Emergency*

See also:
First aid: Convulsions and fever... page 558
Muscular disorders... page 572

IMPAIRED CONSCIOUSNESS

Loss of consciousness

- Abrupt sleeping fits and drop in muscle tone over the course of the day.
  Narcolepsy... page 178

Loss of consciousness (cont'd)

- Brief loss of consciousness or bleeding from the nose or ears; head pain or head wound; impaired balance, speech and vision; sensory impairment (paralysis); nausea and vomiting; abnormal behavior or convulsions.
  Severe cranial trauma... page 150 ....Emergency

- Thirst, dry mouth, dark urine, muscle cramps, fatigue, pallor, rapid and weak pulse, rapid and shallow breathing, nausea and vomiting, confusion and dizziness.
  Dehydration... page 561

- Sudden paralysis, sensory impairment, impaired vision, speech or coordination, vertigo, loss of consciousness, headache or convulsions.
  Cerebrovascular accidents... page 156 ....Emergency

- Fever over 102°F (39°C), stiffness, loss of consciousness and convulsive movements of the whole body.
  Febrile seizures... page 524 ....Emergency

- Intense thirst, heavy urination and loss of consciousness or weight loss.
  Diabetes (hypoglycemia)... page 228

- Convulsions, temporary loss of consciousness, significant swelling of the limbs and sudden, sharp rise in blood pressure.
  Eclampsia... page 485 ....Emergency

- Loss of consciousness, pale, grayish or blue coloration of the skin and lips, and absence of breath, chest movement and pulse.
  Cardiorespiratory arrest... page 544 ....Emergency

See also:

First aid: Airway obstruction... page 547
First aid: Poisoning... page 549
First aid: Hemorrhage... page 550
First aid: Malaise and loss of consciousness... page 559
First aid: Hypothermia and frostbite... page 562

Sleep disturbances

- Difficulty falling asleep and obtaining sufficient or satisfactory sleep.
  Insomnia... page 177

- Absence of menstruation, changing body (skin, nails, hair, mucus, breasts), hot flashes and night sweats, mood and sleep disturbances, high vulnerability to urinary infections, etc.
  Menopause... page 426 ....

- Constant fatigue, insomnia, negative feelings about oneself and others, discouragement, cognitive impairment and physical ailments associated with stress (pains, skin problems, high blood pressure), etc.
  Burnout... page 182

- Pressure pain (neck, chest, shoulders, buttocks, elbows, knees), headache, fatigue and sleep disturbances.
  Fibromyalgia... page 122

- Unconscious walking at night.
  Sleepwalking... page 176 ....

- Sudden waking and panic attacks (screaming, crying, accelerated heart and respiratory rates, etc.) during the night.
  Night terrors... page 176 ....

See also:

Loud breathing (snoring)... page 581

COGNITIVE DISTURBANCES (MEMORY, CONCENTRATION, ETC.)

Impaired memory

- Temporary or permanent, total or partial loss of memory or of the ability to acquire new memories.
  Amnesia... page 169
  Partial epilepsy... page 166

- Very high blood pressure, headache, loss of balance, memory loss and vision problems.
  High blood pressure - stage 2... page 253

- Fever, fatigue, muscle and joint pain, cough, runny nose, headache, memory impairment, behavioral disturbances, drowsiness, etc.
  Encephalitis... page 159

- Convulsions, fever, confusion, memory impairment, sensory impairment (photophobia) and motor impairment (impaired coordination, paralysis).
  Severe encephalitis... page 159 ....Emergency

- Cognitive disturbances (memory, speech, logic, attention) and behavioral disturbances (aggressiveness, delirium, anorexia, etc.), sleep disturbances and depression.
  Alzheimer's disease and other dementias... page 170 ....

Impaired memory and concentration

- Difficulty focusing attention and concentrating, agitation, impatience, impulsiveness, etc.
  Attention deficit disorder with or without hyperactivity... page 533

- Shaking while at rest, slow movements or inability to move, change in posture, difficulty walking, impaired memory and concentration, fatigue, depression and an inexpressive face.
  Parkinson's disease... page 167 ....

- Motor impairment (muscular weakness, balance disturbances, paralysis, etc.), visual, sensory, sexual and psychological problems (depression, difficulty concentrating, etc.), acute, chronic pain and major fatigue; recurring symptoms.
  Multiple sclerosis... page 164

Speech impairment

- Difficulty learning to read and difficulty writing.
  Dyslexia... page 532

- Difficulty expressing oneself or understanding others, or both (lack of vocabulary, poor pronunciation, etc.).
  Dysphasia... page 532

- Impaired speech (hesitation, halting speech, repetition of sounds or words) and, sometimes, unusual facial expressions.
  Stuttering... page 533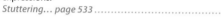

- Slowed reflexes, difficulty speaking and moving, loss of inhibitions, mood swings, nausea and vomiting, dehydration and hypothermia.
  Acute alcohol intoxication... page 358

- Brief loss of consciousness or bleeding from the nose or ears; head pain or head wound; impaired balance, speech and vision; sensory impairment (paralysis); nausea and vomiting; abnormal behavior or convulsions.
  Severe cranial trauma... page 150 ....Emergency

- Sudden paralysis, sensory impairment, impaired vision, speech or coordination, vertigo, loss of consciousness, headache or convulsions.
  Cerebrovascular accidents... page 156 ....Emergency

- Twitching, use of obscene words, or repetition of words or phrases.
  Tourette's syndrome... page 168 ....

Various cognitive disturbances (memory, speech, logic, attention, etc.)

- Constant fatigue, insomnia, negative feelings about oneself and others, discouragement, cognitive impairment and physical ailments associated with stress (pains, skin problems, high blood pressure), etc.
  Burnout... page 182

- Cognitive disturbances (memory, speech, logic, attention) and behavioral disturbances (aggressiveness, delirium, anorexia, etc.), sleep disturbances and depression.
  Alzheimer's disease and other forms of dementia... page 170 ....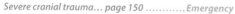

- Intellectual deficiency.
  Mental retardation... page 531

- Change in social interaction, communication deficiency, limited interests and repetitive behaviors.
  Pervasive developmental disorder... page 530

- Sudden, uncoordinated involuntary movements, impaired motor coordination, psychological disturbances (depression, psychosis) and cognitive disturbances (language, attention, memory).
  Huntington's disease... page 168

- Headache, nausea and vomiting, vertigo, visual, behavioral, cognitive, motor and sensory impairment.
  Tumors of the nervous system... page 158

PSYCHOLOGICAL AND BEHAVIORAL DISORDERS

Confusion

- Thirst, dry mouth, dark urine, muscle cramps, fatigue, pallor, rapid and weak pulse, rapid and shallow breathing, nausea and vomiting, confusion and dizziness.
  Dehydration... page 561

- Motor impairment (epilepsy, shaking, paralysis) and mental impairment (confusion, hallucinations, delirium).
  Chronic alcohol intoxication... page 358

Confusion and behavioral disturbances

- Obsessions, compulsions, phobias, anxiety, sexual disorders, difficulty interacting with others, etc.
  Neurosis... page 173

- Impaired perception, judgment, logic and behavior.
  Psychosis... page 172

- Localized motor and sensory impairment, and psychological disturbances (hallucinations, behavioral change); short in duration and recurring.
  Partial epilepsy... page 166

Mood disturbances

- Pain in the lower abdomen, mood swings, headache, fatigue and insomnia, vertigo, acne, digestive disturbances (bloating, abdominal pain), weight gain, swollen limbs and breasts, tender breasts.
  Premenstrual syndrome... page 424 ....

- Absence of menstruation, nausea and vomiting, swollen breasts, mood swings, major fatigue, etc.
  Pregnancy... page 462 ....

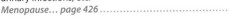

Mood disturbances (cont'd)

- Absence of menstruation, changing body (skin, nails, hair, mucus, breasts), hot flashes and night sweats, mood and sleep disturbances, high vulnerability to urinary infections, etc.
  Menopause... page 426 ....

- Despondency and negative thoughts, combined with a strong tendency to sleep and overeat.
  Seasonal affective disorder... page 180

- Constant fatigue, insomnia, negative feelings about oneself and others, discouragement, cognitive impairment and physical ailments associated with stress (pains, skin problems, high blood pressure), etc.
  Burnout... page 182

- Despondency and negative thoughts (profound sorrow and despair), mental suffering and inability to function normally in everyday life.
  Depression... page 180

- Alternating episodes of depression (despondency and negative thoughts) and mania (euphoria, elation).
  Bipolar affective disorder... page 179

- Motor impairment (muscular weakness, balance disturbances, paralysis, etc.), vision, sensory, sexual and psychological problems (depression, difficulty concentrating, etc.), acute, chronic pain and major fatigue; recurring symptoms.
  Multiple sclerosis... page 164

Mood and behavioral disturbances

- Slowed reflexes, difficulty speaking and moving, loss of inhibitions, mood swings, nausea and vomiting, dehydration and hypothermia.
  Acute alcohol intoxication... page 358
  Drug addiction... page 184

- Cognitive disturbances (memory, speech, logic, attention) and behavioral disturbances (aggressiveness, delirium, anorexia, etc.), sleep disturbances and depression.
  Alzheimer's disease and other forms of dementia... page 170 ....

- Sudden, uncoordinated involuntary movements, impaired motor coordination, psychological disturbances (depression, psychosis) and cognitive disturbances (language, attention, memory).
  Huntington's disease... page 168

- Pain at the site of a bite, fever followed by difficulty swallowing, mood disturbances (despondency, excitation, etc.), pathological fear of water, hallucinations, contractures and paralysis.
  Rabies... page 160 ....*Emergency*

Behavioral disturbances

- Agitation, difficulty focusing attention and concentrating, impatience, impulsiveness, etc.
  Attention deficit disorder with or without hyperactivity... page 533

- Brief loss of consciousness or bleeding from the nose or ears; head pain or head wound; impaired balance, speech and vision; sensory impairment (paralysis); nausea and vomiting; abnormal behavior or convulsions.
  Severe cranial trauma... page 150 ....*Emergency*

- Fever, fatigue, muscle and joint pain, cough, runny nose, headache, memory impairment, behavioral disturbances, drowsiness, etc.
  Encephalitis... page 159

- Change in social interaction, communication deficiency, limited interests and repetitive behaviors.
  Pervasive developmental disorders... page 530

- Headache, nausea and vomiting, vertigo, visual, behavioral, cognitive, motor and sensory impairment.
  Tumors of the nervous system... page 158

Eating disorders

- Very limited food intake and major weight loss, absence of menstruation, and numerous other ailments (dehydration, heart problems, etc.).
  Anorexia nervosa... page 527

- Uncontrolled, excessive food consumption followed by compensation behaviors: voluntary vomiting, use of laxatives and diuretics, excessive exercise, etc.
  Bulimia... page 528

- Voluntary regurgitation of food and rechewing before swallowing or spitting out.
  Merycism... page 528 ....

- Ingestion of inedible substances.
  Pica... page 529 ....

See also:

First aid: Head and spinal injuries... page 554
Weight loss... page 566

PULMONARY AND RESPIRATORY DISORDERS (NOSE, THROAT, LUNGS)

NASAL DISORDERS

Congestion and runny nose

- Congestion, runny, irritated nose, sneezing, fatigue and, sometimes, fever.
  Common cold... page 318

- Fever, fatigue, headache, congestion and runny nose, dry cough, etc.
  Infectious diseases... page 284
  Respiratory infections... page 318
  Flu... page 320
  Bronchitis... page 322
  Sinusitis... page 318

- Snoring or wheezing, sleep apnea, headache, nasal congestion and nose bleeds.
  Lesions of the nasal septum... page 317
  Nasal polyps... page 336

- Fever, runny nose, outbreak of red spots and headache, sore throat, etc.
  Infectious diseases in children... page 519...................

- Moderate fever, runny nose, dry cough and violent coughing fits.
  Whooping cough... page 522 ....Emergency

THROAT DISORDERS

Sore throat

- Intense sore throat and swollen neck.
  Pharyngitis... page 319

- Inflammation of the nose and throat, itching, sneezing, etc.
  Allergies... page 288

- Fever, muscle and joint pain, fatigue, headache, runny nose, dry cough and pain in the respiratory tract (throat, thorax, etc.).
  Flu... page 320

- Dry, throaty cough, sore throat and hoarse voice.
  Laryngitis... page 319

- Fever, headache, swollen neck, outbreak of red spots, etc.
  Infectious diseases in children... page 519...................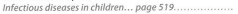

- Sudden high fever, sore throat, inability to swallow, and difficult, loud breathing.
  Epiglottitis... page 523 ....Emergency

- Worsening lesion (small cut, red patch, ulceration, nodule) on or around the mouth, bleeding, persistent pain and numbness in the mouth and throat, and difficulty chewing, swallowing or moving the tongue.
  Mouth cancer... page 366

LUNG AND RESPIRATORY DISORDERS

Loud breathing (snoring)

- Snoring, disturbed sleep and fatigue, drowsiness, loss of alertness, irritability and depression.
  Sleep apnea... page 316

- Snoring or wheezing, sleep apnea, headache, nasal congestion and nose bleeds.
  Lesions of the nasal septum... page 317

Rapid breathing

- Thirst, dry mouth, dark urine, muscle cramps, fatigue, pallor, rapid and weak pulse, rapid and shallow breathing, nausea and vomiting, confusion and dizziness.
  Dehydration... page 561

- Substantial loss of blood (external hemorrhaging), cold, pale extremities, dizziness, vomiting, fast, weak pulse, rapid breathing and intense thirst.
  Shock... page 239 ....Emergency

Rapid, difficult breathing

- Rapid, difficult breathing and feeling of a lack of air, skin and mucus turning blue, cardiac arrhythmia, substantial sweating and, sometimes, loss of consciousness.
  Respiratory insufficiency... page 332 ....Emergency

Rapid, difficult, noisy breathing

- Difficult, wheezing, rapid breathing.
  Bronchiolitis... page 322 ....

Difficult, noisy breathing

- Sudden high fever, sore throat, inability to swallow, and difficult, loud breathing.
  Epiglottitis... page 523 ....Emergency

Difficulty breathing

- Sharp drop in blood pressure, difficulty breathing and various other symptoms: shivering, perspiration, vomiting, bloody diarrhea, hives, Quincke's edema, etc.
  Anaphylactic shock... page 290 ....Emergency

- Fatigue, significant respiratory discomfort, disruption of the heart rhythm, etc.
  Cardiac insufficiency... page 262

Difficulty breathing and chest pain

- Chest pain (at the base of a lung), feeling of suffocation, rapid breathing and bluish skin.
  Pulmonary embolism... page 275 ....*Emergency*

- Fever, difficulty breathing, disruption of the heart rhythm or chest pain.
  Pericarditis... page 269 ....*Emergency*
  Myocarditis... page 269 ....*Emergency*

Difficulty breathing and cough

- Difficulty breathing, cough, sputum, fatigue and weight loss.
  Emphysema... page 329

- Difficulty breathing, cough, pinkish, foamy sputum and, sometimes, impaired consciousness, sweating, cold fingers and toes, and marbled skin.
  Pulmonary edema... page 335

Difficulty breathing, cough and chest pain

- Dry cough, difficulty breathing (shortness of breath, wheezing, rapid, shallow breathing), feeling of oppression in the chest, rapid, irregular pulse, pale face, bluish lips and nails, and clear sputum.
  Asthma... page 326

- Cough, chest pain, difficulty breathing, headache, dizziness or respiratory or cardiac arrest.
  Inhalation poisoning... page 549 ....*Emergency*

- High fever, dry cough, chest pain, difficulty and discomfort in breathing, etc.
  Pneumonia... page 323
  Tuberculosis... page 324

- Chest pain accentuated by a dry cough and difficulty breathing.
  Pneumothorax... page 330
  Pleurisy... page 330

- Impaired speech, breathing and swallowing, cough, coughing up blood, chest pain.
  Malignant tumors of the respiratory system... page 336

Shortness of breath

- Weakness (pallor, fatigue, dizziness, shortness of breath), palpitations, cold sensation and headache.
  Anemia... page 242

- Palpitations, fatigue, shortness of breath and, sometimes, feeling of oppression or sudden, complete loss of consciousness.
  Cardiac arrhythmia... page 264

- Shortness of breath and, sometimes, loss of consciousness, chest pain, palpitations.
  Cardiac valve disease... page 268

Shortness of breath and cough

- Shortness of breath related to effort, dry cough and high vulnerability to infections.
  Nicotine addiction... page 338
  Pneumonia... page 323
  Pneumoconiosis... page 331

Absence of breathing

- Loss of consciousness, pale, grayish or blue coloration of the skin and lips, and absence of breath, chest movement and pulse.
  Cardiorespiratory arrest... page 544 ....*Emergency*

Sleep apnea

- Snoring, disturbed sleep and fatigue, drowsiness, loss of alertness, irritability and depression.
  Sleep apnea... page 316

- Snoring or wheezing, sleep apnea, headache, nasal congestion and nose bleeds.
  Lesions of the nasal septum... page 317

Cough, sneezing

- Congestion, runny, irritated nose, sneezing, fatigue and, sometimes, fever.
  Infectious diseases... page 284
  Common cold... page 318

- Dry, throaty cough, sore throat and hoarse voice.
  Laryngitis... page 319

- Dry then loose cough, sputum, runny nose and mild fever.
  Bronchitis... page 322

- Chronic cough and thick, liquid sputum.
  Chronic bronchitis... page 322

- Moderate fever, runny nose, dry cough and violent coughing fits.
  Whooping cough... page 522 ....*Emergency*

Cough and chest pain

- Fever, muscle and joint pain, fatigue, headache, runny nose, dry cough and pain in the respiratory tract (throat, thorax, etc.).
  Flu... page 320

- Violent fits of dry coughing, sometimes becoming loose, and feeling of discomfort in the chest.
  Tracheitis... page 319

See also:

First aid: Cardiorespiratory arrest... page 544
First aid: Airway obstruction... page 547
First aid: Hemorrhage... page 550
First aid: Hypothermia and frostbite... page 562
Chest pain... pages 582 and 584

BLOOD, VASCULAR, AND CARDIAC DISORDERS
(BLOOD, BLOODSTREAM, HEART)

BLEEDING

Bleeding from a wound

- Painful, deformed or crippled limb, sometimes with a protruding bone and external hemorrhaging.
  Bone fracture... pages 102 and 552

- Substantial loss of blood (external hemorrhaging), cold, pale extremities, dizziness, vomiting, fast, weak pulse, rapid breathing and intense thirst.
  Shock... page 239 ....*Emergency*

Bleeding from the nose and ears

- Breef loss of consciousness or bleeding from the nose or ears; head pain or head wound; impaired balance, speech and vision; sensory impairment (paralysis); nausea and vomiting; abnormal behavior or convulsions.
  Severe cranial trauma... page 150 ....*Emergency*

Bleeding in the mouth

- Red, swollen gums with frequent bleeding.
  Gingivitis... page 364

- Worsening lesion (small cut, red patch, ulceration, nodule) on or around the mouth, bleeding, persistent pain and numbness in the mouth and throat, and difficulty chewing, swallowing or moving the tongue.
  Mouth cancer... page 366

Bleeding from the anus

- Bright red bleeding from the anus in small quantities during or shortly after defecation, sometimes with itching, sharp pain and spasms around the anus.
  Hemorrhoids... page 388
  Chronic colitis... page 382
  Colorectal cancer... page 376

Presence of blood in sputum

- Coughing up blood, chest pain, difficulty breathing, fever, night sweats, fatigue, loss of appetite and weight loss.
  Tuberculosis... page 324
  Pulmonary embolism... page 275 ....*Emergency*

- Impaired speech, breathing and swallowing, cough, coughing up blood, chest pain.
  Malignant tumors of the respiratory system... page 336

Presence of blood in the urine

- Presence of blood in the urine.
  Urinary infections... page 406
  Urolithiasis... page 408

- Presence of blood in the urine and upper back or abdominal pain.
  Polycystic kidney disease... page 410 ....
  Urolithiasis... page 408
  Tumors of the urinary system... page 411
  Prostate adenoma... page 429 ....
  Prostate cancer... page 430 ....

Bleeding (nose, urine, anus, etc.)

- Prolonged bleeding that may begin with no apparent cause.
  Hemophilia... page 244
  Side effects of anticoagulant and antiplatelet medications... pages 261 and 274

See also:

First aid: Hemorrhage... page 550
Bloody stool... page 586
Bleeding between periods... page 587
Abnormal discharge... page 588

VEIN DISORDERS

Protruding vein

- Sensation of heavy legs, swelling and dilation of the veins (blue cords).
  Venous insufficiency... page 272
  Varicose veins... page 272

Inflamed vein

- Swelling of a vein and the tissues around it, pain.
  Venous thrombosis... page 274 ....*Emergency*

See also:

Swelling... page 567

Directory of Symptoms | Blood, Vascular, and Cardiac Disorders

CHEST PAIN IN THE STERNUM

Chest pain in the sternum

- Chest pain (crushing, burning sensation in the middle of the thorax), possibly extending to the neck and left arm, sometimes preceded by generalized weakness, respiratory discomfort, nausea, vertigo, digestive disturbances and heavy perspiration.
Angina pectoris... page 257
Myocardial infarction... page 257 .... Emergency

- Fever, chest pain and respiratory discomfort.
Pericarditis... page 269 .... Emergency

See also:

Chest pain... page 582

DISRUPTION OF THE HEART RHYTHM

Heart rhythm anomalies

- Palpitations, fatigue, shortness of breath and, sometimes, feeling of oppression or sudden, complete loss of consciousness.
Cardiac arrhythmia... page 264

- Fatigue, significant respiratory discomfort, disturbance of the heart rhythm, etc.
Cardiac insufficiency... page 262

- Rapid, difficult breathing and sensation of a lack of air, skin and mucus turning blue, cardiac arrhythmia, substantial sweating and, sometimes, loss of consciousness.
Respiratory insufficiency... page 332 .... Emergency

- Fever, difficulty breathing and disruption of the heart rhythm.
Myocarditis... page 269 .... Emergency

- Heart murmur, blue skin, impaired growth and shortness of breath.
Cardiac malformations... page 267

- Shortness of breath and, sometimes, loss of consciousness, chest pain, palpitations.
Cardiac valve disease... page 268

- Goiter (swollen neck), significant weakness, weight fluctuations, cold or hot sensation, disruption of the heart rhythm, intestinal disturbances, shaking, change in the appearance of the skin or hair, etc.
Diseases of the thyroid gland... page 225

Rapid pulse, palpitations

- Palpitations, fatigue, shortness of breath and, sometimes, feeling of oppression or sudden, complete loss of consciousness.
Cardiac arrhythmia... page 264

- Weakness (pallor, fatigue, dizziness, shortness of breath), palpitations, cold sensation and headache.
Anemia... page 242

Rapid, weak pulse

- Thirst, dry mouth, dark urine, muscle cramps, fatigue, pallor, rapid and weak pulse, rapid and shallow breathing, nausea and vomiting, confusion and dizziness.
Dehydration... page 561

- Substantial loss of blood (external hemorrhaging), cold, pale extremities, dizziness, vomiting, fast, weak pulse, rapid breathing and intense thirst.
Shock... page 239 .... Emergency

Absence of pulse

- Loss of consciousness, pale, grayish or blue coloration of the skin and lips, and absence of breath, chest movement and pulse.
Cardiorespiratory arrest... page 544 .... Emergency

- Cough, chest pain, difficulty breathing, headache, dizziness or respiratory or cardiac arrest.
Inhalation poisoning or poisoning by ingestion... page 549 .... Emergency

- Blood vessel pain, pallor, coldness and absence of pulse.
Arterial thrombosis... page 274 .... Emergency

See also:

First aid: Hemorrhage... page 550
First aid: Hypothermia and frostbite... page 562

DIGESTIVE DISTURBANCES (ESOPHAGUS, STOMACH, LIVER, PANCREAS, INTESTINES, ANUS)

IMPAIRED INGESTION AND DIGESTION

Difficulty swallowing

- Acidic regurgitation, burning at the top of the stomach, moving up along the esophagus, difficulty swallowing and nighttime cough.
  Gastroesophageal reflux... page 372

- Change in the appearance of the tongue (swelling, smooth surface, more or less intense red color), pain and discomfort when chewing, swallowing or speaking.
  Glossitis... page 365

- White coating of the mucus in the mouth, throat and esophagus, stinging, burning, difficulty swallowing and loss of appetite.
  Thrush... page 365

- Sudden high fever, sore throat, inability to swallow, and difficult, loud breathing.
  Epiglottitis... page 523 ....Emergency

- Difficulty swallowing and regurgitation.
  Esophageal stenosis... page 373

- Impaired speech, breathing and swallowing, cough, coughing up blood, chest pain.
  Malignant tumors of the respiratory system... page 336

- Difficulty swallowing, weight loss, chest pain and, in some cases, bloody vomit.
  Esophagitis... page 373
  Esophageal cancer... page 375 ....

See also:
Sore throat... page 581

Nausea, vomiting and abdominal pain

- Diarrhea, vomiting, abdominal cramps and pains, sometimes fever.
  Gastroenteritis... page 378

- Nausea and vomiting, abdominal pain, bloating and headache.
  Indigestion... page 363

- Absence of menstruation, nausea and vomiting, swollen breasts, mood swings, major fatigue, etc.
  Pregnancy... page 462 ....

- Slowed reflexes, difficulty speaking and moving, loss of inhibitions, mood swings, nausea and vomiting, dehydration and hypothermia.
  Acute alcohol intoxication... page 358

- Nausea and vomiting, abdominal pain, burning inside and around the mouth, discoloration of the lips and odd-smelling breath.
  Poisoning by ingestion... page 549 ....Emergency

- Continuous pain in the lower right or left of the abdomen, nausea and vomiting, loss of appetite, constipation and fever.
  Appendicitis... page 387
  Diverticulitis... page 385

- Digestive disturbances (diarrhea, abdominal pain, bloating, etc.) and weakness (weight loss and fatigue).
  Dietary intolerances... page 362
  Intestinal parasites... page 380
  Colitis... page 382

- Fits of intense, violent abdominal pain (screaming and crying), nausea and vomiting, refusal to eat, pallor, lack of muscle tone, and thick, bloody mucus in the stool.
  Acute intestinal invagination... page 515 ....Emergency
  Intestinal obstruction... page 385

- Very high blood pressure, swollen limbs and substantial weight gain, headache and stomachache, spotty vision, buzzing in the ears, nausea and vomiting.
  Preeclampsia... page 484 ....Emergency

- Intense, continuous abdominal pain and hardening of the abdomen, vomiting, constipation, high fever, weakness, pallor, and disrupted breathing, heart rhythm and blood pressure.
  Peritonitis... page 387 ....Emergency
  Diverticulosis... page 385

- Bloody stool, diarrhea or constipation, abdominal pain and vomiting.
  Chronic colitis... page 382

- Digestive disturbances after meals, vomiting, abdominal pain and weight loss.
  Stomach cancer... page 376
  Colorectal cancer... page 376
  Hypertrophic pyloric stenosis... page 516 ....Emergency

Abdominal pain

- Alternating diarrhea and constipation, abdominal pain and cramps, bloating, mucus in stool.
  Irritable bowel syndrome... page 384

Directory of Symptoms | Digestive Disturbances

Abdominal pain (cont'd)

- Acidic regurgitation, burning at the top of the stomach, moving up along the esophagus, difficulty swallowing and nighttime cough.
  Gastroesophageal reflux... page 372

- Abdominal pain and cramps in the stomach, possibly extending to the middle of the back and, in severe cases, bloody vomit and dark-colored stool.
  Gastroduodenal ulcer... page 374 ....

- Intense pain on the right, below the sternum and below the ribs.
  Cholelithiasis... page 395

- Intense pain in the mid- and upper abdomen, radiating out on the sides and in the back, especially after meals, bloating and vomiting.
  Acute pancreatitis... page 396

- Loss of appetite and weight loss, fever, weakness and liver (upper abdomen) pain.
  Liver cancer... page 394

- Yellow coloring of the skin, whites of the eyes and mucus, pain in the upper abdomen and deterioration of general state of health (loss of appetite, weight loss and significant weakness).
  Hepatitis... page 390
  Pancreatic cancer... page 397 ....

See also:

Swollen abdomen... page 567
Pain or discomfort in the lower abdomen... page 587

DEFECATION DISORDERS (PAIN, ABNORMAL STOOL)

Diarrhea

- Diarrhea, vomiting, abdominal cramps and pains, etc., and sometimes fever.
  Gastroenteritis... page 378

- Digestive disturbances (diarrhea, abdominal pain, bloating, etc.) and weakness (weight loss and fatigue).
  Dietary intolerances... page 362
  Intestinal parasites... page 380
  Colitis... page 382

- Fever and muscle and joint pain or diarrhea.
  Listeriosis... page 302

- Rapid weight loss, swollen lymph nodes, fever, persistent diarrhea and skin and respiratory infections.
  AIDS... page 292

Diarrhea or constipation

- Alternating diarrhea and constipation, abdominal pain and cramps, bloating, and mucus in the stool.
  Irritable bowel syndrome... page 384

- Bloody stool, diarrhea or constipation, abdominal pain and vomiting.
  Chronic colitis... page 382
  Colorectal cancer... page 376

- Diarrhea and constipation, in some cases bloody stool.
  Colon polyps... page 383

Pain at defecation

- Very painful burning and tearing sensation during defecation.
  Anal fissures... page 389

- Bright red bleeding from the anus in small quantities during or shortly after defecation, sometimes with itching, sharp pain and spasms around the anus.
  Hemorrhoids... page 388
  Colorectal cancer... page 376

Light-colored stool

- Yellow coloring of the skin, whites of the eyes and mucus, pallor, light-colored stool and swelling of the liver and spleen, lasting more than 10 days.
  Pathological icterus of the newborn... page 515 ....Emergency

- Yellow coloring of the skin, whites of the eyes and mucus, light-colored stool, dark urine, loss of appetite, weakness, weight loss, fever and painful discomfort around the liver.
  Hepatitis... page 390

Oily stool or containing mucus

- Alternating diarrhea and constipation, abdominal pain and cramps, bloating, mucus in the stool.
  Irritable bowel syndrome... page 384

- Weight loss, abdominal and back pain, and soft, foul-smelling, oily stool.
  Chronic pancreatitis... page 396

Bloody stool

- Diarrhea, vomiting, abdominal cramps and pains, sometimes fever.
  Gastroenteritis... page 378

- Digestive disturbances (diarrhea, abdominal pain, bloating, etc.) and weakness (weight loss and fatigue).
  Intestinal parasites... page 380

- Fits of intense, violent abdominal pain (screaming and crying), nausea and vomiting, refusal to eat, pallor, lack of muscle tone, and thick, bloody mucus in the stool.
  Acute intestinal invagination... page 515 ....Emergency

- Bloody stool, diarrhea or constipation, abdominal pain and vomiting.
  Chronic colitis... page 382
  Colorectal cancer... page 376

- Diarrhea and constipation, in some cases bloody stool.
  Colon polyps... page 383

- Intense weakness, yellow coloring of the skin, whites of the eyes and mucus, spider-shaped red patches (arterial spiders) and reddening of the palms of the hands, bloody stool, repeat infections and neurological disturbances (confusion, drowsiness, coma, etc.).
  Hepatic failure... page 393 ....Emergency

See also:
Weight loss... page 566

DISORDERS OF THE GENITAL ORGANS (SEX, BREASTS, OVARIES, TESTICLES, UTERUS, VAGINA, PROSTATE, ETC.) AND THE URINARY SYSTEM (KIDNEYS, BLADDER, URETHRA, ETC.)

DISORDERS OF THE GENITAL ORGANS

Pain or discomfort in the lower abdomen

- Pain in the lower abdomen, mood swings, headache, fatigue and insomnia, vertigo, acne, digestive disturbances (bloating, abdominal pain), weight gain, swollen limbs and breasts, tender breasts.
  Premenstrual syndrome... page 424 ....

- Feeling of weightiness in the lower abdomen, lower back pain, impaired urination and constipation.
  Genital prolapse... page 433 ....

- Back and abdominal pain, high fever with shivering and urinary disturbances (burning, frequent urge, abnormal urine, etc.).
  Cystitis... page 406 ....
  Pyelonephritis... page 407

- Violent pain in the lower abdomen, and sometimes fever.
  Twisting, rupture or infection of an ovarian cyst... page 436 ....

- Very high blood pressure, swollen limbs and substantial weight gain, headache and stomachache, spotty vision, buzzing in the ears, nausea and vomiting.
  Preeclampsia... page 484 ....Emergency

- Abdominal pain and swelling, change in frequency and appearance of stool, and weakness (fatigue, weight loss).
  Ovarian cancer... page 436

Pain or discomfort in the lower abdomen and heavy periods

- Heavy periods, debilitating abdominal pain and, sometimes, fatigue and shortness of breath.
  Heavy periods... page 423 ....

- Abdominal pain, especially during periods and sexual relations, and long, heavy, irregular periods.
  Endometriosis... page 432...................................

Pain or discomfort in the lower abdomen and bleeding between periods

- Feeling of weightiness in the lower abdomen and pain during sexual relations, bleeding between periods, absence of menstruation, and difficulty urinating.
  Ovarian cysts... page 436 ....

- Yellowish, foul-smelling vaginal discharge, pain in the lower abdomen, vaginal bleeding, inflammation and discharge from the urethra, fever and burning during urination.
  Sexually transmitted infections... page 444
  Chlamydias... page 446

Pain or discomfort in the lower abdomen, heavy periods and bleeding between periods

- Heavy periods and spotting between periods or after menopause, urinary disorders (frequent or uncontrollable urge), constipation pain and feeling of weightiness in the lower abdomen, and white discharge.
  Uterine fibroids... page 434 ....
  Uterine cancer... page 434 ....

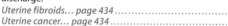

Pain or discomfort in the lower abdomen and spotting during pregnancy

- Uterine bleeding and uterine contractions or abdominal pain.
  Ectopic pregnancy... page 477 ....Emergency
  Miscarriage... page 476 ....Emergency
  Placenta previa... page 482 ....Emergency
  Abruptio placentae... page 485 ....Emergency

Pain or discomfort in the testicles

- Feeling of heaviness in the testicles.
  Varicocele... page 429 ....

Pain or discomfort in the testicles (cont'd)

- Sudden pain in the testicle, spreading to the groin, and swelling of the testicle.
  Testicular torsion... page 429 ....

Pain or discomfort in the genital organs and abnormal discharge

- Fever, pain, swelling, red patches or itching at the genital organs, disturbances when urinating or during sexual relations, and bloody, purulent or foul-smelling discharge.
  Genital infections... page 441
  Sexually transmitted infections... page 444

- Yellowish, foul-smelling vaginal discharge, pain in the lower abdomen, vaginal bleeding, inflammation of and discharge from the urethra, fever, and burning during urination.
  Chlamydias... page 446

- Inflammation of the vagina (itching, heavy, foul-smelling greenish discharge) or the urethra, and disturbed urination.
  Trichomoniasis... page 449

Pelvic pain and abnormal discharge

- Abnormal discharge from the vagina or urethra, accompanied by burning during urination and pelvic pain.
  Gonorrhea... page 449

- Fever, pelvic pain and purulent, foul-smelling vaginal discharge.
  Puerperal fever... page 475 ....Emergency

Abnormal discharge

- Bleeding during sexual relations and white discharge streaked with blood.
  Cervical cancer... page 434 ....

Absence of menstruation

- Absence of menstruation, changing body (skin, nails, hair, mucus, breasts), hot flashes and night sweats, mood and sleep disturbances, high vulnerability to urinary infections, etc.
  Menopause... page 426 ....

- Absence of menstruation, nausea and vomiting, swollen breasts, mood swings, major fatigue, etc.
  Pregnancy... page 462 ....
  Diseases of the thyroid gland... page 225
  Diseases of the pituitary gland... page 226

- Very limited food intake and major weight loss, absence of menstruation, and numerous other ailments (dehydration, heart problems, etc.).
  Anorexia nervosa... page 527

Lump on a testicle

- Hard mass on one testicle and swelling of the testicle or sterility. No pain.
  Testicular cancer... page 428 ....

Lump on a breast

- Palpable mass in a breast.
  Benign breast tumors... page 437 ....
  Breast cancer... page 438 ....

Rash on the genital organs

- Fever, pain, swelling, red patches or itching at the genital organs, disturbances when urinating or during sexual relations, and bloody, purulent or foul-smelling discharge.
  Genital infections... page 441
  Sexually transmitted infections... page 444

- Herpes blisters on the genital organs, open wound, scabs and burning, stinging and itching.
  Genital herpes... page 447

- Cauliflower-like growths on the skin or mucous membrane.
  Genital warts... page 448

- Cankers on the skin or mucous membrane followed by swelling of the lymph nodes in the groin, rash, etc.
  Syphilis... page 445
  Venereal lymphogranuloma... page 446

See also:

Swollen genital organs... page 568

DISORDERS OF THE URINARY SYSTEM

Uncontrollable or involuntary urination

- Slight emission of urine during contraction of the abdominal muscles.
  Effort incontinence... page 404 ....
  Genital prolapse... page 433 ....

- Sudden, uncontrollable need to urinate.
  Hyperactive bladder... page 404

- Involuntary urination during sleep.
  Bed-wetting... page 178 ....

Frequent, uncontrollable urination

- Heavy periods, spotting between periods or after menopause, urinary disorders (frequent or uncontrollable urge), constipation, pain and feeling of weightiness in the lower abdomen, and white discharge.
  Uterine fibroids... page 434 ....
  Uterine cancer... page 434 ....

Frequent, painful urination

- Frequent, painful, urgent urination producing cloudy, foul-smelling urine containing blood.
  Urinary tract infection... page 406

- Urinary disturbances (frequent urge, discomfort, blood, etc.).
  Adenoma of the prostate... page 429 ....
  Prostate cancer... page 430 ....

- Back and abdominal pain, high fever with shivering and urinary disturbances (burning, frequent urge, abnormal urine, etc.).
  Pyelonephritis... page 407

Frequent, heavy urination

- Intense thirst, heavy urination and loss of consciousness, weight loss.
  Diabetes... page 228

- Nausea and vomiting, major fatigue, lower back pain, infrequent or absent urination or thirst and frequent urination, shortness of breath and swollen legs.
  Kidney failure... page 412

Painful urination

- Painful urination.
  Urinary tract infection... page 406
  Urolithiasis... page 408

- Abnormal discharge from the vagina or the urethra, burning during urination, etc.
  Sexually transmitted infections... page 444
  Genital infections... page 441
  Chlamydias... page 446
  Gonorrhea... page 449
  Trichomoniasis... page 449

Infrequent urination or in small quantities

- Nausea and vomiting, major fatigue, lower back pain, infrequent or absent urination or thirst and frequent, heavy urination, shortness of breath and swollen legs.
  Kidney failure... page 412

- Swelling, especially of the face, dark, foamy urine in small quantities, lower back pain, headache and vomiting.
  Glomerulonephritis... page 410 ....

- Feeling of weightiness in the lower abdomen and pain during sexual relations, bleeding between periods, absence of menstruation and difficulty urinating.
  Ovarian cysts... page 436 ....

Presence of blood in the urine

- Presence of blood in the urine.
  Urinary tract infection... page 406
  Urolithiasis... page 408

- Presence of blood in the urine, and upper back or abdominal pain.
  Polycystic kidney disease... page 410 ....
  Urolithiasis... page 408
  Tumors of the urinary system... page 411
  Prostate adenoma... page 429 ....
  Prostate cancer... page 430 ....

Abnormal urine

- Mid-back and abdominal pain, high fever with shivering and urinary disturbances (burning, frequent urge, cloudy or reddish urine, etc.).
  Pyelonephritis... page 407

- Swelling, especially of the face, dark, foamy urine in small quantities, lower back pain, headache and vomiting.
  Glomerulonephritis... page 410 ....

- Yellow coloring of the skin, whites of the eyes and mucus, light-colored stool, dark urine, loss of appetite, weakness, weight loss, fever and painful discomfort around the liver.
  Hepatitis... page 390

See also:

Bleeding... page 583

Directory of Symptoms | Disorders of the Genital Organs and the Urinary System

INDEX

The main subjects are indicated in **bold**.

GLOSSARY

Acute
Describes a disease that appears suddenly and develops rapidly, or a pain that is intense and penetrating.

Amenorrhea
Absence of menstruation in a woman of an age to have her period.

Amniocentesis
Prenatal examination in which amniotic fluid is drawn through the pregnant woman's abdominal wall, then analyzed to verify the health of the fetus (maturity, malformation, chromosomal defect, hereditary or infectious disease, etc.).

Analgesic
Medication or substance that reduces or eliminates pain. Syn. antalgic.

Anemia
Drop in the quantity of hemoglobin in the blood, notably causing fatigue and pallor.

Anesthesia or anesthetics
Partial or total loss of sensitivity in all or a part of the body. Anesthesia may be caused by disease or by an anesthetic agent.

Anorexia
Reduction or stoppage of food intake due to loss of appetite or refusal to eat.

Antalgic
See analgesic.

Antibiotic
Natural or synthetic substance capable of destroying or preventing the development of certain bacteria, allowing the body to fight the infections that they cause.

Anticoagulant
Substance that prevents or delays coagulation of the blood.

Anticonvulsant or antispasmodic
Medication or substance that fights cramps, contractions, and convulsions.

Antiemetic
Medication that prevents or stops nausea and vomiting.

Antifungal
Medication or substance that destroys fungus and fights the infections that it causes by preventing its development.

Antihistamine
Medication that counters the actions of histamine, a substance produced by the body that triggers, in particular, the effects of allergic reactions.

Antipyretic
Medication that prevents, reduces, or eliminates fever.

Antiseptic
Product that destroys germs.

Antitussive
Medication that calms or eliminates coughing.

Anxiolytic
Medication designed to fight anxiety.

Apathy
Decreased activities and interests due to a state of pronounced emotional indifference.

Autoimmune
Describes a disease caused by a breakdown in the immune system, which produces defenses (lymphocytes and antibodies) against certain components of the body itself.

Beta-blocker
Medication or substance that counters the actions of some of the body's neurotransmitters (adrenalin, norepinephrine, and dopamine), mainly used in treating cardiovascular disorders.

Biopsy
Taking a tissue or organ sample to examine it under a microscope.

Biotherapy
Type of treatment that uses living organisms or substances produced by living organisms.

Brachytherapy
Radiotherapy technique that consists of introducing a radioactive substance directly into a cancerous tumor or a hollow cancerous organ, in this way limiting the side effects of radiotherapy on the surrounding tissues.

Celioscopy
Endoscopy of the abdominal cavity via an incision close to the navel.

Celiosurgery
Surgical operation using an endoscope inserted through the abdominal wall.

Chemotherapy
Treatment with chemical substances, used to fight infection and cancer.

Chronic
Describes a disease or ailment that evolves slowly and that continues over a long period of time.

Colectomy
Removal of all or part of the colon.

Colonoscopy
Endoscopic examination of the colon, performed with or without general anesthesia for the purpose of taking samples for analysis and/or removing polyps.

Congenital
Describes a hereditary or nonhereditary characteristic (disease, lesion, malformation, etc.) that is present from birth.

Contusion
Lesion caused by a blow without tearing of the skin or fracture of the bones, often appearing as a bruise.

Convulsion
Sudden, spasmodic, and involuntary contraction of the muscles, localized or generalized throughout the body.

Corticoid or corticosteroid (steroid anti-inflammatory drug)
Medication used to alleviate certain symptoms of an inflammation or an inflammatory disease, derived from natural corticosteroids (hormones secreted by the adrenal glands).

Cryotherapy
Treatment using intense cold.

Degeneration or degenerative
Aggravation of a disease or deterioration of a cell, tissue, or organ, resulting in a change in its functions.

Deglutition or swallowing
Action of moving food or liquid from the mouth to the esophagus (swallowing).

Diuretic
Medication or substance that increases the production and evacuation of urine.

Ecchymosis
Or bruise. Hematoma under the skin, often caused by an impact, resulting in a blackish or bluish coloration of the skin, reabsorbed after a few days.

Edema
Accumulation of fluid in a tissue, appearing as swelling.

Electrocoagulation
Technique that uses the heat released by an electric current to stimulate coagulation of a tissue.

Endoscopy
Exploration of the inside of an organ or body cavity (bronchial tubes, colon, abdominal cavity, etc.) using an optical tube equipped with a lighting system, which allows for diagnosis and treatment of certain disorders.

Enzyme
Protein that stimulates the body's biochemical reactions.

Ergonomics
Scientific discipline that studies working conditions (resources, methods, and environments) with the aim of improving them to optimize worker comfort, safety, and efficiency.

Expectorant
Describes a medication that helps with the expulsion of secretions from the respiratory tract via the mouth.

Genetics
Science that studies the transmission of characteristics from one generation to the next (heredity).

Glycemia
Glucose level in the blood.

Heart tonic
Medication that increases the strength of the heart's contractions.

Hematoma
Accumulation of blood in a tissue or organ, appearing after a blood vessel has burst.

Hemodialysis
Blood purification technique, consisting of pumping the blood, filtering it through an artificial membrane outside the body, then reintroducing it into the bloodstream.

Hormone therapy
Treatment using hormones.

Hypoglycemia
Insufficient quantity of glucose in the blood.

Hypothermia
Abnormal drop in body temperature.

Hypovolemic shock
Sudden weakening of the body's operations (state of shock), caused by a significant decrease in blood volume.

Immunosuppressant or immunodepressant
Medications that inhibit the immune system's activities.

Immunosuppression or immunodeficiency
Decrease in the immune defenses; person whose immune defenses have been diminished.

Immunotherapy
Treatment designed to modify the activity of the immune system by stimulating or inhibiting it.

Infection or infectious
Invasion of the body by pathogenic microorganisms (viruses, bacteria, fungus, or parasites).

Infirmity
Condition of a person who cannot move or who can only move with great difficulty.

Inflammation or inflammatory
The body's reaction to an attack, resulting in redness, swelling, a hot sensation, and pain, localized around a tissue or an organ.

Laxative
Substance that stimulates the evacuation of fecal matter.

Metabolism or metabolic
Set of biological and chemical reactions that take place in the cells and provide the energy needed for the body to function.

Necrosis
Death of a body cell or tissue.

Non-steroidal anti-inflammatory drug (NSAID)
Medication used to alleviate certain symptoms of an inflammation or an inflammatory disease, not derived from natural corticosteroids (hormones secreted by the adrenal glands).

Orthopedic
Relating to the treatment of disorders of the musculoskeletal system (skeleton, joints, muscles, and tendons).

Orthopedic corset
More or less rigid apparatus fitted around the torso to maintain the spinal column in a proper position.

Orthophony
Therapeutic technique whose purpose is to diagnose and treat oral and written language disorders (speech therapy).

Orthosis
Orthopedic apparatus designed to stabilize part of the body and to compensate for or correct a deficient locomotor function.

Oxygen therapy
Treatment consisting of inhaling oxygen-rich air.

Palliative
That alleviates the symptoms of a disease without curing it.

Phlebotonic
Medication that increases the resistance of the walls of the veins.

Phonation
Set of phenomena that contribute to the production of the voice and language, articulated by the vocal organs.

Photocoagulation
Therapeutic technique involving the application of a powerful beam of light (laser) to the retina in order to reduce certain lesions that could cause it to become detached.

Phototherapy
Treatment involving exposure of the skin to light or to a portion of its rays (ultraviolet or infrared).

Physical therapy
Therapeutic technique that uses active movements (gymnastics) and passive movements (massage, mobilization, etc.) or physical agents (electric currents, waves, etc.), particularly to treat motor and respiratory disorders.

Phytotherapy
Use of the chemical substances contained in certain plants to treat diseases (herbal medicine).

Prosthesis
Apparatus implanted in the body, designed to replace part or all of an organ or a limb in order to restore an altered function.

Psychomotor
Relating to both motor and psychological functions.

Psychotropic
Substance whose chemical actions change mental activity.

Radiation therapy or radiotherapy
Treatment based on the administration of ionizing rays, used in particular to treat cancer.

Reduction
Medical or surgical intervention aiming to reposition a displaced organ, dislocated bone, or the fragments of a fractured bone.

Repetitive strain
Trauma that is mild but, if repeated, can cause injury.

Sclerotherapy
Treatment consisting of the injection of an atrophying product into varicose veins to make them disappear.

Septicemia
Generalized infection caused by the regular release of large quantities of pathogenic microorganisms into the blood from an initial focus of infection.

Steroid anti-inflammatory drug
See corticoid.

Syncope
Complete loss of consciousness for a short time after a sudden decrease in the supply of oxygen or blood to the brain.

System
Set of organs and structures whose complementary functions combine towards a collective function (reproduction, digestion, breathing, etc.).

Tinnitus
Abnormal auditory sensation (whistling, ringing, buzzing in the ears) perceived by the brain without any external sound stimulus.

Tissue
Set of cells with a relatively similar structure and function.

Trauma
Set of physical disorders following after a lesion or injury accidentally caused by an external agent. In psychology: set of psychological disorders following after an event caused by an external agent.

Ultrasound
Medical imaging technique used to view the body's internal organs thanks to the echoes produced by ultrasound waves passing through the body. The image produced by this examination.

Vaccine
Substance prepared from a transformed infectious agent (virus, parasite, microbe, or toxin) that, after inoculation of a human being or an animal, forces the body to produce antibodies that immunize it against the disease caused by the infectious agent.

Vasoconstrictor
Describes something (nerve, substance, etc.) that reduces blood vessel diameter through contraction of the muscle fibers.

Vasodilator
Describes something (nerve, substance, etc.) that increases blood vessel diameter through relaxation of the muscle fibers.

LINKS AND RESOURCES

EMERGENCY AND SUPPORT RESOURCES

Emergency assistance (police, fire and ambulance) 911

American Association of Poison Control Centers .... www.aapcc.org
1 800 222-1222

Child Welfare Information Gateway .... www.childwelfare.gov

National Center on Elder Abuse .... www.ncea.aoa.gov

The National Domestic Violence Hotline .... www.ndvh.org
1 800 799 SAFE (7233)

National Clearinghouse on Family Violence .... www.phac-aspc.gc.ca/ncfv-cnivf/index-eng.php

National Suicide Prevention Lifeline... 1 800 273 TALK (8255)

Gay, Lesbian, Bisexual & Transgender National Help Hotline................. 1 888 THE GLNH(1 888 843 4564)

Alchoholics Anonymous .... www.aa.org

Narcotics Anonymous .... www.na.org

Gamblers Anonymous .... www.gamblersanonymous.org

GOVERNMENT ORGANIZATIONS

U.S. Department of Health & Human Services .... www.hhs.gov

Centers for Disease Control & Prevention... www.cdc.gov

The National Women's Health Information Center............................... www.womenshealth.gov

NIH Senior Health .... www.nihseniorhealth.gov

National Institute on Drug Abuse.. www.nida.nih.gov

Substance Abuse & Mental Health Services Administration .... www.samhsa.gov

National Council on Problem Gambling... www.ncpgambling.org

World Health Organization .... www.who.int

GENERAL INFORMATION

Healthfinder.. www.healthfinder.gov

MedlinePlus .... www.nlm.nih.gov/medlineplus

American Red Cross .... www.redcross.org

Mayo Clinic .... www.mayoclinic.com

USDA Food Pyramid .... www.mypyramid.gov

National Cancer Institute .... www.cancer.gov

National Diabetes Education Program .... www.ndep.nih.gov

National Mental Health Information Center .... www.mentalhealth.samhsa.gov

American Medical Association .... www.ama-assn.org

La Leche League .... www.lllusa.org

PHOTO CREDITS